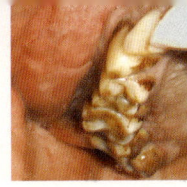
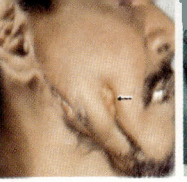
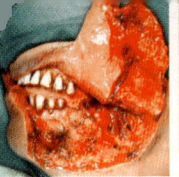
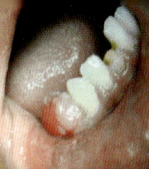

SRB's Surgery *for* DENTAL Students

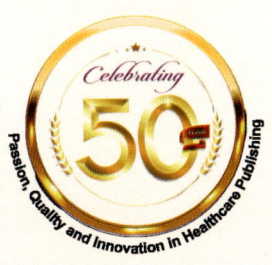

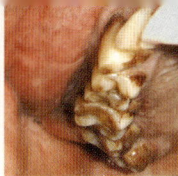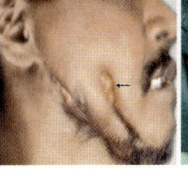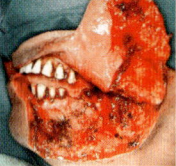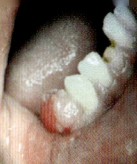

SRB's Surgery *for* DENTAL Students

3rd Edition

Sriram Bhat M MS (General Surgery)
Professor and Head
Department of Surgery
Kasturba Medical College Mangalore
Mangaluru, Karnataka, India

Honorary Surgeon
Government Wenlock District Hospital
Mangaluru, Dakshina Kannada, Karnataka, India
e-mail: *meera_sriram2003@yahoo.com*

Foreword
V Surendra Shetty

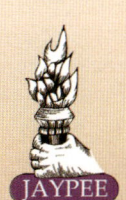

JAYPEE BROTHERS MEDICAL PUBLISHERS
The Health Sciences Publisher
New Delhi | London

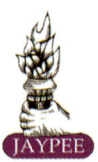 **Jaypee Brothers Medical Publishers (P) Ltd**

Headquarters
Jaypee Brothers Medical Publishers (P) Ltd
4838/24, Ansari Road, Daryaganj
New Delhi 110 002, India
Phone: +91-11-43574357
Fax: +91-11-43574314
Email: jaypee@jaypeebrothers.com

Overseas Office
J.P. Medical Ltd
83 Victoria Street, London
SW1H 0HW (UK)
Phone: +44 20 3170 8910
Fax: +44 (0)20 3008 6180
Email: info@jpmedpub.com

Website: www.jaypeebrothers.com
Website: www.jaypeedigital.com

© 2020, Jaypee Brothers Medical Publishers

The views and opinions expressed in this book are solely those of the original contributor(s)/author(s) and do not necessarily represent those of editor(s) of the book.

All rights reserved. No part of this publication may be reproduced, stored or transmitted in any form or by any means, electronic, mechanical, photocopying, recording or otherwise, without the prior permission in writing of the publishers.

All brand names and product names used in this book are trade names, service marks, trademarks or registered trademarks of their respective owners. The publisher is not associated with any product or vendor mentioned in this book.

Medical knowledge and practice change constantly. This book is designed to provide accurate, authoritative information about the subject matter in question. However, readers are advised to check the most current information available on procedures included and check information from the manufacturer of each product to be administered, to verify the recommended dose, formula, method and duration of administration, adverse effects and contraindications. It is the responsibility of the practitioner to take all appropriate safety precautions. Neither the publisher nor the author(s)/editor(s) assume any liability for any injury and/or damage to persons or property arising from or related to use of material in this book.

This book is sold on the understanding that the publisher is not engaged in providing professional medical services. If such advice or services are required, the services of a competent medical professional should be sought.

Every effort has been made where necessary to contact holders of copyright to obtain permission to reproduce copyright material. If any have been inadvertently overlooked, the publisher will be pleased to make the necessary arrangements at the first opportunity.

The **CD/DVD-ROM** (if any) provided in the sealed envelope with this book is complimentary and free of cost. **Not meant for sale**.

Inquiries for bulk sales may be solicited at: jaypee@jaypeebrothers.com

SRB's Surgery for Dental Students

First Edition	:	2004
Second Edition	:	2014
Third Edition	:	**2020**

ISBN 978-93-89587-56-2

Printed at Replika Press Pvt. Ltd.

Dedicated to

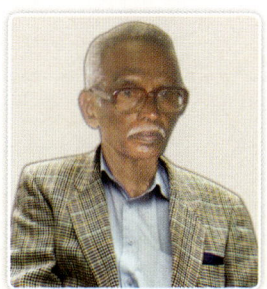

My Beloved Father—Mr Sri Krishna Bhat

and also to

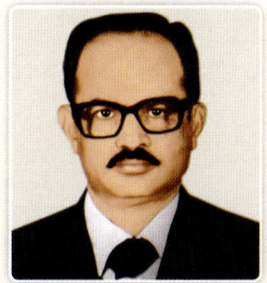

My Beloved Father-in-Law—Late Dr Krishna Karanth

Foreword

I am delightful to write a foreword for this book entitled *SRB's Surgery for Dental Students*, third edition, by Dr Sriram Bhat M.

It is a manual of surgery covering all general surgical topics for dental students with clinical methods in brief. All topics are covered in detail as needed for dental students with adequate diagrams, photographs and illustrations. This book will be very useful to all BDS students as well as MDS students in relation to basic general surgery and topics like wounds, shock, trauma, vascular diseases, burns, thyroid, basic orthopedics, basic ENT topics and instruments.

A comprehensive manual of this standard can be best compiled only by a person with depth of knowledge in the subject and teaching experience to understand the requirements of the dental students. It is very apt that Dr Sriram Bhat a person to whom the above description applies to has come out with this book.

I wish Dr Bhat the very best in this and all his other professional endeavors.

V Surendra Shetty
Pro Vice-Chancellor
Manipal Academy of Higher Education (MAHE)
Mangaluru, Karnataka, India

Preface to the Third Edition

SRB's Surgery for Dental Students is book mainly written for dental students. As the previous second edition was released in 2014, the contents of the book needed revision and editing. Topics of general surgery and chapters like Oral Cavity, Salivary Glands, Laryngeal Tumors, Thyroid, Neck, Tonsils, and Maxillofacial Injuries are been adequately edited and changed as per the new syllabus. Recent advances in treatment, staging and classification in various topics are updated. New photographs and tables are included wherever necessary. History, sterilization and fluid and electrolytes chapters are rewritten completely again with newer concepts. This will help students to update themselves about these topics. These topics are also brought highlighting importance in managing as well as patients who are critically ill.

I hope this edition will be of more use to the students. Any suggestions and criticisms are welcomed.

Sriram Bhat M

Preface to the First Edition

My first book *SRB's Manual of Surgery* is well accepted by medical students in our country. But I felt, it will be much comprehensive for dental undergraduate (BDS) students and it should be condensed and be selective. Keeping the surgery subject syllabus of BDS students in mind I wrote *SRB's Surgery for Dental Students* mainly concentrating on general surgery, head and neck, oral cavity and maxillofacial injuries. I also included Basic Orthopedics, Neurosurgery, Adjuvant Therapy, Sterilization and Instruments in the book. Miscellaneous chapter contains clinical examination of swelling/hernia/hydrocele/arterial diseases/varicose veins/thyroid/oral cavity/salivary gland to complete the fulfillment of the clinical surgical university examinations so that it will be easier for students to get required subject in a single text. I essentially eliminated gastrointestinal and urology topics. Adequate diagrams, photographs, tables and illustrations are added wherever needed. I also discussed about the topics with staff members of few dental colleges. I hope the book will be appreciated by the dental faculty and students. Any suggestions and criticisms are well accepted.

Sriram Bhat M
e-mail: meera_sriram2003@yahoo.com

Acknowledgments

I have great pleasure to bring out the third edition of the book—*SRB's Surgery for Dental Students*.

I thank our Chancellor Dr Ramdas M Pai; Pro-Chancellor Dr HS Ballal; Vice-Chancellor of Manipal Academy of Higher Education (MAHE) Dr Professor Vinod Bhat, our beloved Dean Professor Venkatraya Prabhu, Registrar Dr Narayana Sabhahit, additional Dean, Dr Alfred Augustine, our Vice-Deans Professor Nuthan Kamath and Professor Unnikrishnan, for their academic support.

I acknowledge Dr V Surendra Shetty, Pro Vice-Chancellor, MAHE, Mangaluru, Karnataka, India, for writing foreword to this book as well as for encouraging me in my all works.

I thank and remember Dr Rajendra Prasad, Ex-Dean AB Shetty, Institute of Dental Sciences, Mangaluru; Dean, Yenepoya Dental College, Mangaluru; Dean, KVG Dental College, Sullia, Karnataka, and all dental staff members and consultants at various dental colleges of the district and state, for their kind help.

I thank Dr Jagadishchandra, MDS, Associate Professor and Dr Veena Jagadischandra, MDS, for their affectionate help. Dr Jagadish has provided photographs, X-rays and syllabus for dental students.

I thank district surgeon, for providing enough clinical materials from Government District Wenlock Hospital, Mangaluru, where I am working.

I thank Dr Ganapathy, MD, Director, Mangala Hospital, Mangaluru, for his encouragement.

I thank my dear friend Dr Ashok Pandit, MCh (Urology), for his constant guidance to me in all my endeavors.

Heads of all departments in Kasturba Medical College (KMC), Mangaluru and colleagues from my department always stood with me for all my work. I remember all of them always for their kind heart.

I remember all staff members of surgery department and postgraduates of KMC, Mangaluru, for their affection and support.

I appreciate Dr Ishwarkeerthi, MBBS, who has helped me by writing diagrams needed to this book.

My beloved daughter Ananya, did many diagrams beautifully and helped me to reduce my work.

My wife Dr Meera Sriram, MD (Obstetrics and Gynecology), has done the corrections in the script and I owe her a lot.

I thank all my patients and all who have directly or indirectly helped me in bringing out this book.

I am very grateful to the whole team of M/s Jaypee Brothers Medical Publishers (P) Ltd, who helped and guided me, Shri Jitendar P Vij (Group Chairman), Mr Ankit Vij (Managing Director), Mr MS Mani (Group President), Dr Madhu Choudhary (Publishing Head–Education), Ms Pooja Bhandari (Production Head), Ms Sunita Katla (Executive Assistant to Group Chairman and Publishing Manager), Mr Venugopal V (Associate Director–South), Mr Rajesh Sharma (Production Coordinator), Ms Seema Dogra (Cover Visualizer), Mr Kapil Dev Sharma and Mr Akshay Thakur (Typesetters), Mr Laxmidhar Padhiary and Ms Geeta Rani (Proofreaders), Mr Gopal Singh Kirola (Graphic Designer) and their team members, for all their support to work in this project and make it a success.

I remember everybody working in editing the book in M/s Jaypee Brothers Medical Publishers (P) Ltd, New Delhi, to bring out book more effectively.

Contents

1A. History of Surgery   1

1B. Sterilization and Disinfection   3
- Different Methods of Disinfection   4
- Gaseous Sterilization   9

2. Fluid, Electrolytes, Acid-Base Balance and Nutrition   11
- Water Loss   11
- Water Excess   11
- Hyponatremia   12
- Hypernatremia   15
- Hypokalemia   16
- Hyperkalemia   18
- Anion Gap   19
- Acid-Base Balance   20
- Metabolic Alkalosis   21
- Respiratory Alkalosis   21
- Metabolic Acidosis   22
- Respiratory Acidosis   22
- Fluid Therapy   22
- Nutrition   23
- Gastrostomy   25
- Jejunostomy   25
- Total Parenteral Nutrition   26
- Obesity   27

3. Wounds, Inflammation, Sinus, Fistula and Ulcer   28
- Wound   28
- Problems with Wound Healing   36
- Compartment Syndrome   36
- Crush Syndrome   36
- Keloid (Like a 'Claw')   37
- Hypertrophic Scar   38
- Sinus   39
- Fistula   39
- Median Mental Sinus   41
- Ulcer   42
- Trophic Ulcer   48
- Diabetic Ulcer (Diabetic Foot)   49
- Meleney's Ulcer   51
- Traumatic Ulcer   51
- Arterial/Ischemic Ulcer   51
- Rodent Ulcer   53
- Melanotic Ulcer   53
- Tropical Ulcer   53
- Venous Ulcer (Gravitational Ulcer)   54
- Tuberculous Ulcer   55
- Lupus Vulgaris   55
- Ulcer due to Chilblains   55
- Ulcer due to Frostbite   55

4. Infectious Diseases   56
- Cellulitis   56
- Lymphangitis   58
- Erysipelas   59
- Dangerous Area of Face   59
- Pyogenic Abscess   59
- Cold Abscess (Tuberculous Abscess)   62
- Boil (Furuncle)   64
- Carbuncle   65
- Pott's Puffy Tumor   66
- Pyogenic Granuloma (Granuloma Pyogenicum)   66
- Pyemia   68
- Tetanus   68
- Gas Gangrene   71
- Tuberculosis   72
- Leprosy (Hansen's Disease)   73
- Syphilis (Great Pox, French Disease)   74
- Actinomycosis   75
- Madura Foot (Mycetoma Pedis)   76
- Rabies (Hydrophobia)   77
- Anthrax   79
- Nosocomial Infection (Hospital-acquired Infection)   80
- Opportunistic Infections   81
- Necrotizing Fasciitis   81
- Acute Pyomyositis   82

Hepatitis   83
HIV Infection and AIDS   87
Needle Stick Injury in Surgical
   Practice   90
Gonorrhea   91
Surgical Site Infection   92

5. Swellings   97
Lipoma   97
Papilloma   99
Cysts   100
Dermoids   101
Sebaceous Cyst   103
Glomus Tumor   104
Lymph Cyst (Lymphatic Cyst)   104
Neuroma   105
Neurofibroma   105
Neurilemmoma (Schwannoma)   107
Fibroma   107
Ganglion   107
Bursae   108
Morrant Baker Cyst   110
Calcinosis Cutis   110
Epignathus   110
Chordoma   111

6. Shock, Hemorrhage and Blood Transfusion   112
Shock   112
Cardiogenic Shock   117
Central Venous Pressure   117
Pulmonary Capillary Wedge
   Pressure   118
Systemic Inflammatory Response
   Syndrome   119
Oxygen Therapy   119
Hyperbaric Oxygen   120
Cardiac Arrest   120
Mechanism of Blood Coagulation   122
Hemorrhage   123
Blood Transfusion   127
Blood Fractions   128
Massive Blood Transfusion   129
Blood Substitutes   129
Autologous Blood Transfusion   130
Recycled Blood   130

Artificial Blood   130
Tourniquets   130

7. Burns   132
Burns   132
Management of Burns   135
Eschar   137
Burns Contracture   138
Electrical Burns   138
Inhalation Burns   140
Chemical Burns   140

8. Reconstruction and Transplantation   142
Skin Grafting   142
Flaps   145
Transplantation   151
Renal Transplantation   151
Liver Transplantation   152
Bone Marrow Transplantation   152
Graft Rejection   152
Cimino Fistula   152
Immunosuppressive agents   153

9. Hand and Foot   154
Surgical Anatomy of the
   Hand   154
Hand Infections   155
Acute Paronychia   156
Chronic Paronychia   157
Terminal Pulp Space Infection
   (Felon)   157
Infection of Webspaces   158
Deep Palmar Space Infection   159
Acute Suppurative Tenosynovitis   159
Hand Injuries   160
Compound Palmar Ganglion   161
Dupuytren's Contracture   162
Syndactyly   162
Mallet Finger (Base Ball Finger)   163
Heberden's Nodes   163
Spina Ventosa   163
Callosity   163
Corn   163
Plantar Fasciitis (Policeman's
   Heel)   164
Ingrowing Toe Nail
   (Onychocryptosis)   164

10. Trauma 165

Triage 165
Spinal Injury 168
Neck Injuries 169
Bullet Injuries 169
Blast Injuries 170
Penetrating Injury 170
Abdominal Trauma 170
Duodenal Injury 171
Pancreatic Injury 172
Small Bowel Injury 172
Colonic Injury 172
Liver Injury 172
Splenic Injury 173
Renal Injury 173
Urinary Bladder Injury 173
Abdominal Compartment
  Syndrome 173

11. Arterial Diseases 174

Surgical Anatomy of Thoracic
  Outlet 174
Arteries of Upper Limb 175
Raynaud's Phenomenon 180
Acrocyanosis 182
Polyarteritis Nodosa 182
Scleroderma/Systemic Sclerosis 183
Thakayasu's Pulseless Arteritis 183
Temporal Arteritis 184
Erythromelalgia/Erythralgia 184
Livedo Reticularis 184
Subclavian Steal Syndrome 184
Arteries of Lower Limb 184
Arterial Diseases 185
Atherosclerosis 190
Thromboangiitis Obliterans 192
Acute Arterial Occlusion 197
Compartment Syndrome 197
Reperfusion Injury 197
Embolism 198
Aneurysms 201
Carotid Artery Aneurysm 205
Gangrene 206
Ainhum 209
Vascular Anomalies 209
Cirsoid Aneurysm 212
Arteriovenous Fistula 212

12. Venous Diseases 216

Anatomy of Veins of Lower Limb 216
Physiology of Venous Blood Flow in
  Lower Limb 217
Deep Vein Thrombosis 218
Varicose Veins 220
Venous Ulcer 228
Thrombophlebitis 230
Anticoagulants 230

13. Lymphatics 232

Lymphangiography 232
Isotope Lymphoscintigraphy 233
Lymphangitis 233
Lymphedema 233
Differential Diagnosis for (Cervical)
  Lymphadenopathy 238
Lymphomas 240
Hodgkin's Lymphoma 240
Non-Hodgkin's Lymphoma 243
Tuberculous Lymphadenitis 245

14. Nerves and Tendon 248

Peripheral Nerve Injuries 248
Brachial Plexus Injuries 250
Causalgia 251
Median Nerve Injuries 251
Carpal Tunnel Syndrome 252
Ulnar Nerve Injuries 253
Claw Hand 253
Radial Nerve Lesions 254
Common Peroneal Nerve 255
Axillary Nerve Injury 255
Long Thoracic Nerve 256
Trigeminal Neuralgia 256
Tendon 256
Tendon Repair 257
Tendon Transfer 257
Tendon Graft 257

15. Neoplasm and Soft Tissue Tumors 258

Neoplasm 258
Spread of Malignant Tumors 260
Paraneoplastic Syndromes 261
Investigations for Neoplasm 262
Soft Tissue Tumors (Sarcomas) 263
Kaposi's Sarcoma 270

16. Skin Tumors — 271

Classification of Skin Tumors 271
Skin Adnexal Tumors 271
Merkel Cell Carcinoma 272
Dermatofibroma 272
Dermatofibrosarcoma
    Protuberance 272
Keratoacanthoma (Molluscum
    Sebaceum) 273
Rhinophyma (Potato Nose) 273
Premalignant Conditions of the
    Skin 274
Squamous Cell Carcinoma
    (Epithelioma) 274
Marjolin's Ulcer 276
Basal Cell Carcinoma (Rodent
    Ulcer) 277
Nevi/Naevi 279
Melanoma 280

17. Neck — 285

Anatomy of Lymphatics of
    Head and Neck 285
Branchial Cyst 287
Branchial Fistula 287
Pharyngeal Pouch 288
Laryngocele 289
Cystic Hygroma (Cavernous
    Lymphangioma) 289
Ludwig's Angina 291
Parapharyngeal Abscess 292
Retropharyngeal Abscess 293
Carotid Body Tumor 294
Torticollis (Wry Neck) 295
Sternomastoid Tumor 296
Subhyoid Bursitis 296
Secondaries in Neck
    Lymph Nodes 297
Pancoast Tumor 303

18. Thyroid — 304

Development 304
Anatomy 304
Congenital Anomalies 306
Thyroid Function Tests 309
Classification of Goiter 310
Diffuse Hyperplastic Goiter 310
Nodular Goiter 311
Solitary Thyroid Nodule 312
Retrosternal Goiter 312
Thyrotoxicosis 313
Thyroid Neoplasm 321
Papillary Carcinoma 322
Follicular Carcinoma 323
Anaplastic Carcinoma 325
Medullary Carcinoma
    of Thyroid 325
Malignant Lymphoma 326
Hashimoto's Thyroiditis 326
De Quervain's Subacute
    Granulomatous Thyroiditis 327
Reidel's Thyroiditis 327
Thyroidectomy 327
Emil Theodor Kocher 330
Hypothyroidism 330

19. Parathyroid and Adrenal Glands — 332

Anatomy of Parathyroid 332
Hyperparathyroidism 333
Tetany 335
MEN Syndrome
    (MEA Syndrome) 335
Adrenal Glands 336

20. Salivary Glands — 340

Anatomy 341
Sialography 343
Salivary Calculus 343
Sialosis 345
Sialectasis 345
Sialadenitis 345
Parotid Abscess 345
Parotid Fistula 346
Sjögren's Syndrome 347
Mikulicz Disease 348
Salivary Neoplasms 348
Management of Malignant
    Salivary Tumors 355
Minor Salivary Gland Tumors 357
Parotidectomy 357
Frey's Syndrome (Auriculotemporal
    Syndrome, Gustatory
    Sweating) 359

21. Oral Cavity — 361

Retromolar Trigone 362
Ranula 364
Sublingual Dermoids 365

Cancrum Oris (Noma)   366
Leukoplakia   366
Erythroplakia   367
Oral Submucosal Fibrosis   367
Premalignant Conditions of the Oral Cavity   368
Oral and Upper Aerodigestive Cancers   368
Carcinoma Cheek (Buccal Mucosa)   370
Neoplasm of Lip   377
Carcinoma of Lip   377
Tongue   379
Carcinoma Tongue   384
Nasopharyngeal Carcinoma   388
Maxillary Tumors   389
Carcinoma Hard Palate   392

22. Laryngeal Tumors   394
Surgical Anatomy of Larynx   394
Benign Lesions of Larynx   397
Malignant Tumors   398
Care after Total Laryngectomy   401
Total Laryngectomy   401

23. Tonsils   402
Anatomy of the Tonsils   402
Acute Tonsillitis   403
Chronic Tonsillitis   403
Peritonsillar Abscess (Quinsy)   404
Tonsillectomy   405
Acute Pharyngitis   406

24. Cleft Lip, Cleft Palate and Jaw Tumors   407
Cleft Lip and Cleft Palate   407
Diseases of the Palate   411
Orthopantomogram   411
Preauricular Sinus   412
Jaw Tumors   412
Epulis   413
Ameloblastoma   414
Dentigerous Cyst   415
Dental Cyst   416
Osteomyelitis of Jaw   417
Alveolar Abscess   417
Cherubism   418
Fibrous Dysplasia of Bone/Jaw   418

25. Maxillofacial Injuries   421
Primary Care (Early Care) in Maxillofacial Injuries   421
Fracture Middle Third Area   423
Fracture Mandible   430
Complications of Maxillofacial Injuries   437

26. Tracheostomy   439
Tracheostomy   439
Tracheostomy Tubes   439

27. Basic Orthopedics   445
Anatomy of the Bone   445
Fracture   446
Plaster of Paris   450
Arthrodesis   451
Arthroplasty   451
Osteotomy   452
Infections of the Bone   453
Paget's Disease of Bone   454
Rickets   455
Bone Disease of Hyperparathyroidism   455
Osteoporosis   455
Scurvy   456
Osteogenesis Imperfecta   456
Achondroplasia   456
Tendinitis   456
Diaphyseal Achalasia   456
Enchondromatosis   457
Arthritis   457
Rheumatoid Arthritis   457
Osteoarthrosis   458
Ankylosing Spondylitis   459
Kyphosis   459
Scoliosis   459
Spondylolisthesis   459
Intervertebral Disc Prolapse   459
Bone Tumors   460

28. Esophagus   464
Anatomy   464
Lower Esophageal Sphincter   465
Dysphagia   466
Achalasia Cardia   467
Gastroesophageal Reflux Disease   468
Barrett's Esophagus   470

Hiatus Hernia   470
Reflux Esophagitis   471
Corrosive Stricture of Esophagus   471
Plummer-Vinson Syndrome   472
Mallory-Weiss Syndrome   472
Boerhaave's Syndrome   472
Tracheoesophageal Fistula   473
Carcinoma Esophagus   473

29. Neurosurgery   477
Head Injuries   477
Extradural Hematoma   481
Subdural Hematoma   483
Depressed Skull Fracture   484
Subarachnoid Hemorrhage   484
Intracranial Abscess   485
Intracranial Aneurysm   486
Hydrocephalus   486
Intracranial Tumors   487
Pituitary Tumors   490
Spina Bifida   490

30. Adjuvant Therapy   492
Radiotherapy   492
Chemotherapy   494
Immunosuppression   496
Hormone Therapy   496
Immunotherapy   496
Hybridoma   497
Gene Therapy   497

31. Instruments and Suture Materials   498
Instruments   498
Suture Materials   510

32. Cautery, Laser, Cryosurgery and Day Care Surgery   513
Diathermy (Electrocautery)   513
Lasers in Surgery   514
Cryosurgery   514
Day Care Surgery   515

33. Advanced Imaging Methods   516
Ultrasound   516
Doppler   517

CT Scan   518
Magnetic Resonance Imaging   519

34. Anesthesia   521
Preoperative Assessment   521
General Anesthesia   522
Muscle Relaxants   522
Reversal Agents   523
Instruments in Anesthesia   523
Steps in General Anesthesia   524
Complications in General Anesthesia   524
Postoperative Care   524
Regional Anesthesia   525
Spinal Anesthesia   526
Epidural Anesthesia   527
Caudal Anesthesia   527

35A. Clinical Methods in Surgery for Dental Students   528
Clinical Examination of Sinus or Fistula   535
Examination of an Ulcer   536
Examination of a Swelling/Lump   540
Examination in Arterial Disease   546
Examination of Varicose Veins   553
Examination of Thyroid Gland   556
Examination of Oral Cavity   564
Examination of Jaw and Temporomandibular Joint   571
Examination Salivary Gland   575
Examination of Inguinoscrotal Swellings   581
Definition of Hernia   587
Examination of Hydrocele   591

35B. Laboratory Values   593
Urine   593
Blood   594
Stool Examination   596

Index   597

CHAPTER 1A

History of Surgery

The word 'surgery' is derived from French term *CHIRURGIEN* which came from Latin which in turn derived from Greek words—*CHEIR* means HAND and *ERGON* means WORK. Surgery has got a long history to begin with.

Edwin Smith Papyrus is one of the oldest scripts about surgery written in 1600 BC.

Sushruta of ancient India described more than 100 surgical instruments and is best known for plastic surgery of nose and ear (Fig. 1A.1).

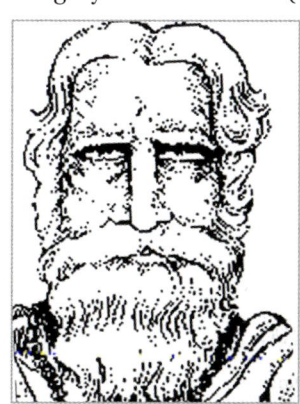

Fig. 1A.1: Sushruta.

Hippocrates has written books on fractures, dislocations and surgical disorders.

Celsus described inflammation and wrote 'De medicina'.

Ambroise Pare was popular in sixteenth century, a French surgeon.

John Hunter was superb anatomist and teacher and is called as father of experimental surgery. He described many surgeries for many surgical conditions.

Sir Astley Cooper was the most popular surgeon from London in nineteenth century.

William TG Morton a Boston dentist successfully demonstrated ether anesthesia in October 16th, 1846.

Joseph Lister was the originator of antisepsis in surgery and is called as father of modern surgery (Fig. 1A.2).

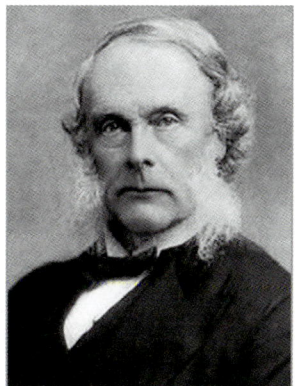

Fig. 1A.2: Jopseph Lister.

Louis Pasteur (1895) brought the germ theory of diseases and infectious diseases and operation theater infections later came into picture widely.

In the sweetness of friendship let there be laughter and sharing of pleasures

Rudolph Matas pioneered in vascular surgery.

William S Halsted (1922) an American surgeon contributed about surgeries of thyroid, breast, hernia and blood vessels. He introduced usage of rubber gloves during surgery.

Bernard von Langenbeck a German surgeon is considered as father of modern residency system in surgery (1887).

Thodor Billroth a pioneer abdominal surgeon who did different types gastrectomies and brought into practice.

Emil Thedor Kocher, Swiss surgeon from Bern, Switzerland. He did extensive work on thyroid surgery and got Nobel Prize in 1909 for the same (Fig. 1A.3).

John H Gibbon (1973) cardiothoracic surgeon developed extracorporeal circulation.

Alfred Blalock detailed pathogenesis of the shock also a pioneer innovator in the field of cardiac surgery.

Owen H Wangensteen did extensive work in surgical field and also a very good teacher at University of Minnesota.

Francis D Moore described metabolism in surgical patients.

Jonathan Rhoads introduced proper total parenteral hyperalimentation (1960).

Charles B Huggins received Nobel Prize in 1966 for his work on the effects of hormones on tumor growth.

Wilhelm K Rontgen discovered X-rays in 1895.

Alexander Fleming invented penicillins as an antibiotic.

Gaspare Tagliacozzi an Italian surgeon was doing rhinoplasty in sixteenth century.

Alexis Carrel in 1912 got Nobel Prize for his work on blood vessel anastomosis, organ transplantation.

Michael E DeBakey an American surgeon did extensive work on cardiothoracic surgery. He introduced occlusive roller pumps in extracorporeal circulation. He did first carotid endarterectomy. He reported first the successful use of a saphenous vein bypass graft for coronary artery occlusion in 1964.

Christiaan Neethling Barnard from Cape Town, South Africa, did first successful heart transplantation (Fig. 1A.4).

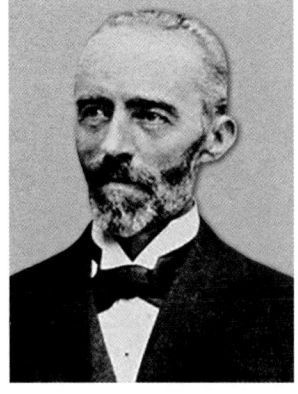

Fig. 1A.3: Emil Thedor Kocher.

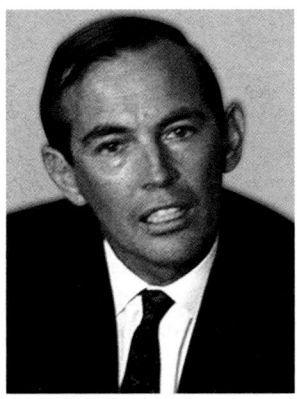

Fig. 1A.4: Christiaan Neethling Barnard.

Work is love made visible

CHAPTER 1B

Sterilization and Disinfection

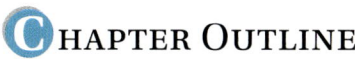

- Different Methods of Disinfection
- Gaseous Sterilization

Bearing in mind that it is from the vitality of the atmospheric particles that all the mischief arises, it appears that all that is requisite is to dress the wound with some material capable of killing these septic germs, provided that any substance can be found reliable for this purpose, yet not too potent as a caustic. —**Joseph Lister, 1867**

Joseph Lister is called as father of modern surgery and father of antisepsis. He introduced carbolic acid as an antiseptic agent. He presumed that infection can be prevented by proper asepsis and antisepsis. Concept of asepsis is started in 19th century. Ignaz Semmelweis showed reduction of the puerperal fever by washing hands prior to delivery. Lawson Tait introduced principles of asepsis.

Asepsis

Asepsis means organisms are prevented to access the patient or individual. It is a state of being free from disease causing contaminants or preventing contact with microorganisms. Term is used to those methods to promote or to induce asepsis in an operative field to prevent infection to make the surgical field "sterile"; means it is free of all biological contaminants; but it is difficult to achieve; and so elimination of infection is the goal of asepsis, not sterility. There are two types of asepsis—medical and surgical (Ayliffe et al. 2000). Medical or clean asepsis reduces the number and prevents the spread of organisms; surgical or sterile asepsis eliminates microorganisms from surgical area.

The practice of surgical asepsis begins with cleaning the object in question using the principles of medical asepsis followed by a sterilization process creating an environment in a surgical suite or special procedure room, to avoid any possible infection to the patient also with proper attire (scrubs, cap, mask, gloves, shoe covers).

Antisepsis

It means prevention of infection by inhibiting the growth and multiplication of microorganisms so that making the field free of microorganisms.

Disinfection

It is the killing of as many micoorganisms as possible from a surface by physical or chemical means. Articles or surfaces that cannot be sterilized in the operation theater or special procedure room must be disinfected. Disinfectant may be with or without tuberculocidal activity. It eliminates many or all pathogenic microorganisms, except bacterial spores (usually) *on inanimate objects.* The Center of Disease Control and Prevention (CDC) has given three levels of disinfection— High; Intermediate and Low.

Sterilization

It is freeing an article by removing or killing all bacteria, spores, fungi and viruses.

DIFFERENT METHODS OF DISINFECTION

PHYSICAL AGENTS

Burning or *incineration* is used to disinfect contaminated articles like dressings.

Hot-air oven: Here temperature used is 160°C for one hour or 180°C for 20 minutes. Glassware, scissors, scalpel, forceps and oil, powders are sterilized by this method.

Boiling: It kills bacteria but not spores and viruses. Temperature is between 90 to 99 degrees. It is used to disinfect syringes, utensils. It is not useful for gloves, rubber materials.

Autoclave: It is steam under pressure. Temperature attained is between 120 and 135 degrees. It is sterilized for 20 minutes with 15 pounds/sq. inch pressure. It kills all organisms including spores. Completeness of sterilization is confirmed by using specific gelatin protein which precipitates only in steam under pressure for 20 minutes. Green colored strip turns to black if autoclave is complete (*signaloc*). Surgical gloves, linen, cotton, dressings, surgical instruments are sterilized by this method. Sharp and plastic instruments cannot be sterilized by this method. *Bacillus thermophillus* spores are used to assess the completeness of the sterilization in mass scale. Double autoclaving is done for instruments of orthopedic or ophthalmic surgeries (Fig. 1B.1).

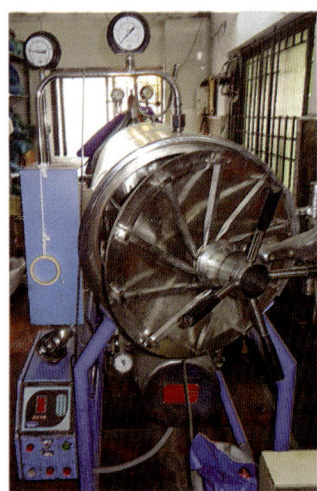

Fig. 1B.1: Autoclave machine.

Radiation: *Ionizing type of radiation:* Atomic gamma radiation is used as commercial method to sterilize suture materials, disposable materials in packets. It is viable, safe and cheaper. *Non-ionizing radiation* either infra-red radiation or ultraviolet radiation is used to reduce the bacteria in air, water. Bacteria and virus are vulnerable to ultraviolet rays below 3000A°. Exposure to eyes and skin can cause burn injury.

CHEMICAL AGENTS

Chemicals are used when heat sterilization is inappropriate for materials like electronic, fiber optics, plastics, etc. (heat sensitive instruments). Gas or liquid chemicals are used. Chemicals used should be compatible when such sterilized articles are being used.

Physical agents	Chemical agents
• Sunlight • Drying • Dry heat is most reliable and rapid without any residue. Incineration, flaming using Bunsen burner, hot-air oven are the different methods • Moist heat like pasteurization (63°C for 30 minutes Holder method or 72°C for 20 seconds—flash method), boiling, autoclaving • Filtration • Radiation ionizing or non-ionizing	• Phenol • Cresol • Lysol • Hibitane • Hexachlorophene • Dettol • Savlon • Halogens like Eusol, iodophors • Alcohols • Formaldehyde • Glutaraldehyde • Hydrogen peroxide • Gases like ethylene oxide • Dyes like acriflavine

It is performed by soaking item in the solution. It kills the organisms by coagulation/alkylation of proteins and also by enzymatic degradation and lysis of cell membranes.

The criteria to be satisfied in the chemical methods are: Must be capable of killing spores; should be non-corrosive; should be non-irritant; should be economical; should be stable; should penetrate grease and fibers; should be non-toxic.

Phenolic Compounds

They are used as standard to compare the efficacy of other agents. They are intermediate to low level disinfectants. It is derived from carbolic acid (phenol), one of the oldest germicides. It is the oldest known disinfectant used by Lister.

Phenol (5%) is prepared from coal tar. It is obtained by distillation of coal in 170°C.

They are bactericidal (at 1%), fungicidal and viricidal but not sporicidal. They are active in the presence of organic matter. They are irritant to skin and mucous membranes, have bad odor. They are absorbed by rubber and residual disinfectant may cause tissue irritation.

Cresol is more powerful and nontoxic (5% solution). It is obtained by distillation of coal in 270°C.

Lysol is emulsified cresol with soap. 2% solution is effective.

Hexachlorophene, thymol [derived from herb thyme (intermediate level disinfectant)], amylmetacresol (is present in strepsils), α phenylphenol, chloroxylenol, triclosan are other phenolic products. *Triclosan* is organic phenyl ether which acts against Gram-positive bacteria and to some extent against many Gram-negative bacteria. It also acts on fungi and viruses.

They are bactericidal, fungicidal, mycobactericidal but are inactive against spores and most viruses. They are not inactivated by organic matter. The corrosive phenolics are used for disinfection of ward floors, in discarding jars in laboratories and disinfection of bedpans. Phenol is considered as standard and measurement of effectiveness of other compounds is assessed as *"phenol coefficient"*. Disinfectant is compared with phenol using *Salmonella typhi* and *Staphylococcus aureus*. Disinfectants which are more effective than phenol has got phenol coefficient >1; and less effective one has got coefficient <1. *Disadvantages*: Phenols are often toxic and irritant.

Halogens

Iodophors

It is a combination of iodine and carrier with a resulting complex providing sustained

*Out of suffering have emerged the strongest souls; the most massive characters are seared with scars—**Kalil Gibran***

release reservoir of iodine. They are bactericidal, viricidal and tuberculocidal but not sporicidal. These are intermediate to low level disinfectants. They corrode the metallic items and non-metallic items may be stained or discolored. They are non-irritant and do not stain skin. Tincture iodine is 2% iodine in 70% alcohol. Iodine when combined with neutral carrier polymers like polyvinylpyrrolidone forms iodophors. *Povidone iodine is a good example.* Iodophores allow slow release and so minimize the irritation. For hand-washing iodophores are diluted in 50% alcohol. 10% povidone iodine is used undiluted in preoperative and postoperative skin disinfection.

Chlorine and Chlorine Compounds

They are intermediate level disinfectants. They are active against bacteria and viruses but not spores. They are available both in liquid (sodium hypochlorite) and solid (calcium hypochlorite, bleaching powder) forms. They are most widely used, inexpensive and fast acting. *EUSOL: Edinburgh University Solution* contains sodium hypochlorite, boric acid and calcium hydroxide. *Eusol bath* is dipping the ulcer bearing part in dilute eusol solution for 30 minutes 2–3 times a day. It is highly effective against HIV. Household bleach is an inexpensive and excellent source of sodium hypochlorite. A *1:100 to 1:1000* dilutions is effective against HIV. *1:5 to 1:10* dilution is effective against hepatitis.

Alcohols

Alcohol dehydrates cells, disrupts membrane and causes coagulation of proteins. Ethyl or isopropyl alcohols (ethanol or isopropanol) are used. It is intermediate level disinfectants. Ethyl alcohol is bactericidal in 60–90% concentration and isopropyl alcohol in 60% concentration. 70% ethyl alcohol (spirit) is better. They kill bacteria but not spores, action against viruses is variable. Recommendation is—exposure to 70% ethanol for *15 minutes* to inactivate the hepatitis virus but *1 minute for HIV*. Their effectiveness is limited because of rapid evaporation, lack of ability to penetrate organic matter. They are used mainly to disinfect external surfaces of equipment like thermometers, stethoscopes, ventilators, fiberoptic cables. They can damage mounting of lensed instruments and tend to swell and harden rubber. Methyl alcohol kills fungal spores.

Alcohols are basically antiseptics rather than disinfectant as it is used mainly on living tissue surfaces. They are noncorrosive, but due to limited contact time as it gets evaporated rapidly their effects get reduced unless surface is submerged into the liquid. They are more effective when combined with distilled water which facilitates the diffusion through cell membrane. 70% ethanol diluted in water is effective against many bacteria. 80% ethanol and 5% isopropanol is effective to deactivate viruses like HIV, hepatitis B and C. Alcohol efficacy is enhanced by adding wetting agent dodecanoic acid (coconut soap) which is also effective against *Clostridium difficile*.

Aldehydes

Aldehydes act through alkylation of amino, carboxy and hydroxyl groups damaging nucleic acids. They kill all microorganisms including spores.

Formaldehyde

It is useful to disinfect the rooms like operation theater. It is effective at a high temperature and humidity of 80–90%. It is commonly used to fumigate the room. 500 mL of formalin with one liter of water is boiled to get formaldehyde vapor. Adding potassium permanganate to the same solution can create formaldehyde vapor. Room is kept closed for 12 hours. It is less expensive and has got longer half life.

Paraformaldehyde is used to get the vapor formaldehyde. It is used principally in water-based solution called formalin. Vapor can be generated from paraformaldehyde tablets which contain 95% formaldehyde in a polymerized form. 40% formaldehyde (formalin) is used for surface disinfection and fumigation of rooms, chambers, operation theaters, wards, sick rooms. Fumigation is achieved by boiling formalin, heating paraformaldehyde or treating formalin with potassium permanganate. It also sterilizes bedding, furniture and books. 10% formalin with 0.5% tetraborate sterilizes clean metal instruments. It is a high level disinfectant. It is non-corrosive and is not inactivated by organic matter. It is widely used for sterilization of endoscopic equipment, catheters, etc. For better effect it needs relative humidity of 60–80% and temperature of 37°C. Residual formaldehyde may affect the skin, but it can be neutralized by ammonia. Its use is limited by its pungent odor and fumes. It should be handled as a potent sensitizer and probable carcinogen. Methanol is added to increase its half life.

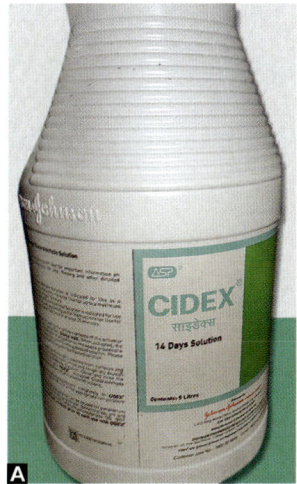

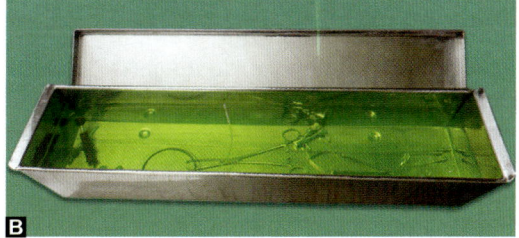

Figs. 1B.2A and B: Cidex—glutaraldehyde solution (2%).

Glutaraldehyde (Cidex 2%)

It is used to sterilize sharp instruments. Instruments should be dipped for 22 hours to achieve complete sterilization. It is potent bactericide, sporicide, fungicide and viricide. The presence of solid materials and block of tissues need still longer time as it will take more time to penetrate these tissues. It is volatile and toxic to skin and also on inhalation. Its half life is short—less than 2 weeks.

It is a saturated dialdehyde. It is used in 1.0% concentration (but highly effective in 2% concentration). It is *high level disinfectant*. It kills spores within 12 hours and viruses within 10 minutes. It is widely used because of their excellent biocidal properties, activity in the presence of organic matter, non-corrosiveness and noncoagulation of proteinaceous material. 2% glutaraldehyde is used to sterilize thermometers, cystoscopes, bronchoscopes, centrifuges, anesthetic equipments. An exposure of at least 3 hours at alkaline pH is required for action by glutaraldehyde. 2% formaldehyde at 40°C for 20 minutes is used to disinfect wool and 0.25% at 60°C for six hours to disinfect animal hair and bristles. Glutaraldehyde requires alkaline pH and only those articles that are wettable can be sterilized (Figs. 1B.2A and B).

Disadvantages: It is noxious and irritating to tissues and hence thorough rinsing of all exposed materials is mandatory. Prepackaging is not possible and equipment will be wet. Pseudomembranous laryngitis has been linked to disinfection of tracheal tubes with glutaraldehyde.

Hydrogen Peroxide (H_2O_2)

It is used as topical oxygen therapy. Because of its effervescence and release of nascent oxygen it removes the tissue debris. It is used to clean wounds, cavities, ulcers and as mouth wash, as ear drops to clear ear wax.

H_2O_2, being a strong oxidant is used to sterilize rigid scopes and heat sensitive articles. Its cycle time is less (<30 minutes). It is available as both liquid and vaporized form. It is an effective bactericidal, fungicidal, viricidal and sporicidal. It is commercially available as 3% solution but can be used up to 25% concentration. It is non-corrosive and not inactivated by organic matter but irritant to skin and eyes. Vapor can be used to sterilize/disinfect the rooms/aircrafts. It gets decomposed in light; proteinaceous organic materials reduce its activity. 3% should be used for skin, ulcers and wounds. 6% is used to decontaminate the instruments.

Detergents

They are surface active agents. They contain fat soluble long chain hydrocarbons and water soluble ions which concentrate between cell membrane and surrounding medium causing membrane disruption. Detergents can be anionic or cationic. Negatively charged long chain hydrocarbons are anionic detergents. Cationic detergents are fat soluble with positive charges and combine with quaternary nitrogen atom and are called as **quaternary ammonium compounds (quats)**. Cetrimide and bezalkonium compounds are quats. 2% detergent solutions are used. They are active against vegetative cells, mycobacteria and enveloped viruses.

Dyes

Acridine and aniline dyes are used as antiseptics and disinfectants. They interact with bacterial nucleic acids and so microicidal. Aniline dyes such as crystal violet, malachite green and brilliant green; Acridine dyes such as acriflavine and aminacrine are commonly used dyes. Acriflavine is a mixture of proflavine and euflavine; only euflavine has effective antimicrobial properties. They are more effective against Gram-positive bacteria. They may be used topically as antiseptics to treat mild burns. They are used as paint on the skin to treat bacterial skin infections. Melachite green is used in Lowenstein Jenson medium for growth of *Mycobacterium tuberculosis*.

Others

Chlorhexidine (hibitane) is useful antiseptic. It is a nondetergent chemical disinfectant usually used in the concentration of 0.5% in 70% alcohol for skin. Tubes, masks, etc. are sterilized by keeping for 20 min in 0.1% aqueous solution. Chlorhexidine can be used in an isopropanol solution for skin disinfection, or as an aqueous solution for wound irrigation. It is also used as an antiseptic handwash. 20% chlorhexidine gluconate solution is used for preoperative hand and skin preparation. Chlorhexidine gluconate is also mixed with quaternary ammonium compounds like cetrimide to get better antimicrobial effects (Savlon). Chlorhexidine is inactivated by soap water.

Cetrimide is cationic surfactant (cetavlon). 2% solution is used. *Savlon* is combination of cetrimide and hibitane (chlorhexidine). It is very commonly used antiseptic in operation theaters and wards.

Hexachlorophene (cinthol): It is not used in infants and children because it can get absorbed through intact skin in this age group causing severe neurotoxicity. Hexachlorophene is chlorinated diphenyl and is less irritant. It has marked effect over Gram-positive bacteria but not over Gram-negative bacteria, mycobacteria, fungi and viruses.

Let there be spaces in your togetherness—**Kalil Gibran**

Dettol (chloroxylenol) 5% solution is used. Chloroxylenol is less irritant and is used for topical purposes; is more effective against Gram-positive bacteria than Gram-negative bacteria. Chloroxylenol is inactivated by hard water.

Acriflavine and proflavine are orange-red colored dyes used as antiseptics. It is effective against Gram-positive and few Gram-negative organisms. It retains its activity in pus and body fluids.

The polymer of polyaminopropyl biguanide is bactericidal at very low concentrations (10 mg/L). The polymer strands are incorporated into the bacterial cell wall, which disrupts the membrane and reduces its permeability. It is also known to bind to bacterial DNA, alter its transcription, damages DNA. It shows very low toxicity to human cells.

Sodium bicarbonate and lactic acids are other disinfectants often used.

Beta-propiolactone (BPL): It is a condensation product of ketane with formaldehyde.

It is an alkylating agent which by alkylation of carboxyl and hydroxyl groups becomes microcidal. It is a colorless liquid with pungent to sweetish smell. It is an effective sporicidal agent. 0.2% is used to sterilize biological products. It is more efficient in fumigation than formaldehyde. It is used to sterilize vaccines, tissue grafts, surgical instruments and enzymes. But it is poor penetrating power and carcinogenicity limits its use.

Potassium permanganate ($KMnO_4$): It is a purplish-black crystalline powder that colors everything it touches, through a strong oxidizing action. It stains "stainless" steel, which somehow limits its use and makes it necessary to use plastic or glass containers. It is used to disinfect aquariums and is used in community swimming pools to disinfect ones feet before entering the pool. It is widely used to disinfect community water ponds and wells in tropical countries, as well as to disinfect the mouth before pulling out teeth. It can be applied to wounds in dilute solution.

GASEOUS STERILIZATION

ETHYLENE OXIDE STERILIZATION

Ethylene oxide (ETO) is used for 70% of sterilizations and 50% of medical devices. It is done with a temperature of 30–60°C with more than 30% humidity and gas concentrations of 200–800 mg/L. Ethylene oxide penetrates well through paper, plastics, clothes, etc. It kills bacteria, spores, viruses, fungi and is highly effective and compatible. But it is inflammable, toxic and can be carcinogenic and may affect the reproductive system. ETO sterilizer needs biological validation after installation, repair and failure. Gas chamber and micro-dose methods—are two methods used. Ethylene oxide is delivered into a chamber containing ethylene oxide and diluents gases like carbon dioxide and halogenated hydrocarbon. Now commonly 100% ethylene oxide is used. Micro-dose sterilization method is done using 100% ethylene oxide in specialized bags and is called as gas diffusion sterilization. Ethylene oxide $(CH_2)_2O$ is a colorless, odorless, and flammable gas. It acts through alkylations of sulphydryl, amino, hydroxyl and carboxyl groups on proteins and amino groups of nucleic acids. The concentration ranges (weight of gas per unit chamber volume) from 800–1200 mg/L for ethylene oxide with operating temperatures of 45–63°C. Gas is potentially mutagenic and crcinogenic; can produce acute toxicity; irritation of the skin, conjunctiva and nasal mucosa (Fig. 1B.3).

Phases are—initial preconditioning phase, an exposure phase, a phase of post-sterilization aeration to remove ethylene oxide residues like ethylene glycol and ethylene chlrorohydrine. Here instrument is packed in a sealed plastic cover. It is kept in the ethylene oxide sterilizer.

Your children are not your children. They are the sons and daughters of Life's longing for itself—**Kalil Gibran**

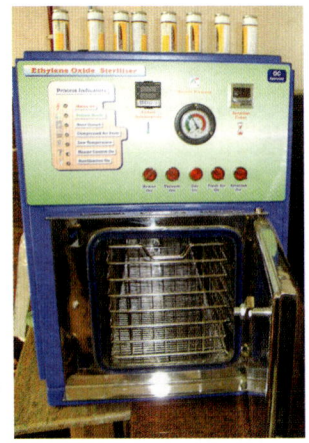

Fig. 1B.3: Ethylene oxide sterilizer.

Total 12 hours sterilization is needed; 6 hours for gas sterilization and another 6 hours for gas to come out. It is good way of sterilization. Once instrument is sterilized, it can be kept and used for 6 months. Problem is cost factor, time duration needed (minimum 12 hours) for sterilization.

Formaldehyde (HCHO): It is similar to ethylene oxide with similar action from a range of 15–100 mg/L with a temperature of 70–75°C. **Low temperature steam formaldehyde (LTSF) sterilizer:** It operates with subatmospheric pressure steam; air is removed by evacuation and steam is admitted to the chamber.

Instruments/objects	Sterilization method
All theater appliances	Autoclave
Sharp instruments (scissors, needles, blades)	Glutaraldehyde 2%, Lysol
Plastic materials; endoscopes; rubber equipments	Glutaraldehyde 2%
Syringes	Autoclave, hot air oven, gamma radiation
Heart-lung machine	Ethylene oxide
Disposable articles	Gamma radiation
Operation theater and rooms	Ideally by UV radiation or by formaldehyde
Sera and biological materials	Filtration
Laboratory glassware	Hot-air oven
Ward, sick room, furniture	Formaldehyde, iodophor spray, glutaraldehyde
Clothes, bed sheets on operation theater and for burns patients	Autoclaving
Soiled dressings, materials, animal carcasses	Incineration, lysol, iodophors
Excreta	Lysol, iodophors
Cleaning of skin before surgery	Iodophors 2%, savlon, spirit
For cleaning infected wounds	Iodophors, acriflavine, savlon, H_2O_2
To remove slough from the wounds	EUSOL, H_2O_2
Before injection	Spirit is used to clean the skin
Cleaning the ward	Phenol, cresol, lysol
Handwash	Chloroxylenol, savlon, spirit, iodophors
Bladder wash	0.1% potassium permanganate solution (Condy's lotion), solution of acetic acid and silver nitrate
Water	Chlorination, potassium permanganate
Fruits, vegetables	Potassium permanganate

Ever has it been that love knows not its own depth until the hour of separation—**Kalil Gibran**

CHAPTER 2

Fluid, Electrolytes, Acid-Base Balance and Nutrition

Chapter Outline

- Water Loss
- Water Excess
- Hyponatremia
- Hypernatremia
- Hypokalemia
- Hyperkalemia
- Anion Gap
- Acid-Base Balance
- Metabolic Alkalosis
- Respiratory Alkalosis
- Metabolic Acidosis
- Respiratory Acidosis
- Fluid Therapy
- Nutrition
- Gastrostomy
- Jejunostomy
- Total Parenteral Nutrition
- Obesity

NORMAL PHYSIOLOGY

Total body water is 60% of body weight in males, 50% of body weight in females, i.e. 30 liters.

Intracellular water (ICF)—20 liters (2/3).
Extracellular water (ECF)—10 liters (1/3).
  Plasma (1/4) (2.5 liters)
  Interstitial fluid (7.5 liters).

Three hormones—aldosterone, antidiuretic hormone (ADH), atrial natriuretic hormone, control ECF volume and osmolality regulation.

Ion	ICF	ECF and plasma
Sodium	10 mmol/L	140 mmol/L
Potassium	150 mmol/L	4.5 mmol/L
Chloride	Trace only	105 mmol/L

WATER LOSS

It is decrease in the whole body fluid volume—both ECF and ICF.

Causes: Poor intake; diabetes insipidus.

Drop in ECF is balanced by drop in ICF. So clinically patient is not dehydrated even though there is water drop. Thirst, confusion and hypothermia are the clinical features.

Investigations: Rise in plasma sodium and urea.

Treatment: Oral water or IV isotonic fluid, 5% dextrose.

WATER EXCESS (Water Intoxication; ECF Volume Excess)

Causes
- Excessive infusion of intravenous dextrose 5%.

Worry does not empty tomorrow of its sorrow. It empties today of its strength.

- If water is used instead of saline for colorectal bowel wash, at the time of preparation for surgery of large bowel, especially in children.
- In transurethral resection of prostate (TURP) when excess irrigating fluid is used (glycine is commonly used).
- In syndrome of inappropriate antidiuretic hormone (SIADH) which is commonly associated with lobar pneumonia, empyema, oat cell carcinoma and head injury.

Clinical features

- Drowsiness, weakness.
- Convulsions and coma.
- Nausea, vomiting.
- Passage of dilute urine.
- Distended neck veins.
- Pedal edema.
- *Gain in body weight*—most sensitive and consistent sign.
- Circulatory overload—tachycardia, pulmonary edema, hypertension.
- Bilateral basal crepitations, ascites.
- Raised central venous pressure (CVP), pulmonary capillary wedge pressure (PCWP).

Investigations

- Hematocrit, serum electrolytes, blood urea (shows fall in serum Na$^+$, low K$^+$ and low blood urea).

Treatment

- Water restriction and observation.
- ICU monitoring with proper management of fluid and electrolyte balance.
- Infusion of hypotonic sodium chloride.

Note: Administration of diuretics and hypertonic saline should be avoided. as it may cause rapid changes in serum sodium and water level which in turn leads to neuronal demyelination and *fatal outcome*.

ECF loss

- Here only ECF loss is present with normal ICF
- It is seen in vomiting, diarrhea, and intestinal obstruction
- Treatment is infusion of normal saline

ECF excess

- There is only ECF excess without any ICF excess.
- Due to excessive infusion of saline with impaired excretion.
- Raised JVP, cardiac failure and peripheral edema.
- Treatment is fluid restriction and diuretics like frusemide.

HYPONATREMIA

Hyponatremia is defined as a serum sodium concentration less than 135 mEq/L. The normal serum sodium concentration is 135–145 mEq/L. It is the most common electrolyte disorder; incidence is 1%; prevalence is 2.5% (in surgical ward 4.4%; in ICU patients it is 30%). It is more common in elderly patients, and one with hepatic/cardiac/renal failures.

Classification of hyponatremia

According to serum sodium level:
- *Mild:* 130–134 mmol/L.
- *Moderate*: 125–129 m mol/L.
- *Profound*: <125 mmol/L.

Often considered *Severe*: <115 mmol/L—brain edema, seizures, coma.
Occasionally hyponatremia can be asymptomatic.

According to volume status:
- *Hypovolemic*: Decrease in total body water with more decrease in total body sodium.
- *Normovolemic/euvolemic*: Increase in total body water with normal body sodium.
- *Hypervolemic*: Great increase in total body water with increase in total body sodium.

According to the onset:
- *Acute:* Onset in <48 hours.
- *Chronic:* Onset in >48 hours.

Contd...

---

*The teacher who is indeed wise does not bid you to enter the house of his wisdom but rather leads you to the threshold of your mind—**Kalil Gibran***

Contd...

> **According to the osmolality:**
> - **Hypotonic:** >280
> - **Isotonic:** 280–295—hyperlipidemia; hyperproteinemia (multiple myeloma).
> - **Hypertonic:** >295—hyperglycemia; mannitol or glycerol therapy.
>
> **Note:**
> **Hypotonic hyponatremia** has three main etiologies: *Hypovolemic*—both water and sodium decreased (water < sodium)—due to obvious losses like diarrhea, vomiting, dehydration, malnutrition. *Euvolemic*—water increased and sodium stable—SIADH, thyroid disease (hypothyroidism with TSH >50 units), primary polydipsia. *Hypervolemic*—water increased and sodium increased (water increase > sodium)—due to like obvious CHF, cirrhosis, renal failure.
>
> In euvolemic hyponatremia, **urine osmolali**ty should be checked. If *urine osmolality <100*—means excess water intake due to—primary polydipsia, tap water enemas, post-TURP. If urine osmolality >100—means impaired renal concentration—SIADH, hypothyroidism, cortisol deficiency.
>
> *Urine sodium should be checked and FeNa% (Fractional excretion of sodium) should be calculated.* Low *urine sodium (<20)* and *low FeNa (<1%)* implies the kidneys are appropriately reabsorbing sodium. High *urine sodium (>20)* and *high FeNa (>1%)* implies the kidneys are not functioning properly.

Note:
- Mechanism of hyponatremia is almost always the result of an increase in circulating arginine vasopressin and/or increase renal sensitivity to arginine vasopressin, combined with any intake of free water.
- Glucose produces a drop in the serum sodium level of 1.6 mEq/L for each 100 mg/dL of serum glucose greater than 100 mg/dL. This calculation is nonlinear as there is greater reduction in plasma sodium level with glucose level over 400 mg/dL, making 2.4 mEq/L for each 100 mg/dL increase in glucose over 100 mg/dL.

Causes of Hypotonic Hyponatremia

Hypovolemic

- *When urinary [Na^+] >20 mEq/L:* Diuretic use; salt-wasting nephropathy (renal tubular acidosis, chronic renal failure, interstitial nephritis); osmotic diuresis (glucose, urea, mannitol, hyperproteinemia); mineralocorticoid (aldosterone) deficiency (Addison's); cerebral salt syndrome.
- *When urinary [Na^+] <20 mEq:* Volume replacement with hypotonic fluids; GI loss (vomiting, diarrhea, fistula, tube suction); trauma; third-space loss (burns, hemorrhagic pancreatitis and peritonitis).

Hypervolemic

- *Urinary [Na^+] >20 mEq/L:* Renal failure (inability to excrete free water).
- *Urinary [Na^+] <20 mEq/L:* Congestive heart failure; nephrotic syndrome; cirrhosis.

Euvolemic

Here urine [Na^+] usually >20 mEq/L.

- *SIADH* (syndrome of inappropriate secretion of antidiuretic hormone).
- *Hypothyroidism* (possible increased ADH or deceased glomerular filtration rate).
- *Pain, stress, nausea, psychosis* (stimulates ADH).
- *Drugs:* ADH, nicotine, sulfonylureas, morphine, barbiturates, NSAIDs, acetaminophen, carbamazepine, phenothiazines, tricyclic antidepressants, colchicine, clofibrate, cyclophosphamide, isoproterenol, tolbutamide, vincristine, monoamine oxidase inhibitor.

If you reveal the secrets to the wind, you should not blame the wind for revealing them to the trees—**Kalil Gibran**

- *Water intoxication.*
- *Glucocorticoid deficiency.*
- *Positive pressure ventilation.*
- *Porphyria.*
- *Essential* (reset osmostat or sick cell syndrome—usually in the elderly).

Causes of Acute Hyponatremia

- Polydypsia.
- MDMA ingestion.
- Exercise induced.
- Multifactorial, e.g. thiazide and polydypsia.
- Iatrogenic: Postoperative premenopausal women; hypotonic fluids with cause of increase vasopressin; glycine irrigation during TURP; colonoscopy preparation; recent institution of thiazides.

Acute hyponatremia causes brain edema and tentorial herniation which is an emergency situation. It needs aggressive sodium correction using 3% hypertonic saline.

Clinical Features of Hyponatremia

- Nausea, vomiting, anorexia, headache, muscle cramps, confusion, disorientation, restlessness, convulsions, lethargy, tremors, hypotension.
- Seizures and coma—seizures are quite likely at [Na$^+$] of 113 mEq/L or less.
- *In acute hyponatraemia*: Brain edema, *tentorial herniation* and sudden death can occur.
- *In chronic hyponatremia*: Brain adapts to keep the edema within limits and rapid correction leads on to cell shrinkage and demyelination—*osmotic demyelination syndrome* with spastic/flaccid quadriplegia, dysarthria, dysphagia which can develop as late as 2 weeks after therapy (ODS/pontine demyelination).

Evaluation

- Serum electrolytes and urinary electrolytes estimation.
- Evaluation for specified causes.
- *Sodium deficit formula*: (Desired change in Na) × TBW (Total body water); TBW is 0.6 × body weight in kg in men and 0.5 × body weight in kg in women. For example, the amount of Na needed to raise the Na from 106 to 112 in a 70-kg man can be calculated as: 112 mEq/L –106 mEq/L) × (0.6 L/kg × 70 kg) = 252 mEq.

Treatment

- *Fluid restriction is the mainstay of treatment.*
- *In acute type however rapid correction is needed* but the rise in [Na$^+$] should be no greater than 0.5 to 1.0 mEq/L per hour. Hypertonic (3%) saline (containing 513 mEq Na/L) is used, but only with frequent (2 to 4 hourly) electrolyte determinations. Sodium correction should be 6 mmol/L per day and should not exceed 12 mmol/L per day.
- In hypovolemia 0.9% normal saline (154 mEq Na/L) may be used as slow gradual correction.
- Often associated hypokalemia needs to be corrected.
- Cause should be treated.
- *Chronic hyponatremia is treated by*: Water restriction; Demeclorcycline 300–600 mg tid (causes nephrogenic diabetes inspipidus); Lithium; Oral urea; VAPTANS. Chronic hyponatremia when presents with seizures should be treated using careful monitored infusion of hypertonic saline 3%.
- *Vaptans* are vasopressin receptor antagonists [Arginine, Vasopressin, Antagonists] (V1A and V2 receptors) used mainly in hypervolemic hypontremia and in cirrhotics and heart failure. Conivatan

Only when you drink from the river of silence shall you indeed sing—**Kalil Gibran**

(intravenous) and Tolvaptan (oral) are used commonly. They are useful in chronic hyponatremia and SIADH but should not be used in acute or euvolemic or hypovolemic hyponatremia.
- Loop diuretics (frusemide) are useful in SIADH.

HYPERNATREMIA

It is raise in serum sodium concentration more than 145 mmol/L. It is a hyperosmolar condition related to total body water (TBW) related to electrolyte content. It is common in aged, with impaired thirst, poor access to needed water, increased fluid loss. There is net water loss or sodium gain or both. Serum sodium concentration more than 160 m mol/L is severe hypernatremia.

Acute hypernatremia occurs within 24 hours and should be corrected rapidly whereas *chronic type* develops in more than 24 hours and should be corrected slowly otherwise cerebral edema develops.

Normal plasma osmolality (Posm) is 275 to 290 mOsm/kg. Calculated Posm is—2(Na) mEq/L + serum glucose (mg/dL)/18 + BUN (mg/dL/2.8). Posm and plasma sodium concentration is regulated by antidiuretic hormone [ADH/arginine vasopressin (AVP)] and thirst mechanism. When there is thirst raised Posm occurs with hypernatremia which draws water from cells dehydrating the neuronal cells which stimulates ADH release initiating the thirst mechanism causing adequate water intake and thus correction of the hypernatremia.

Causes

- It is commonly observed in ICU, patients in shock, in old aged, mental illness, uncontrolled diabetes mellitus, diabetes insipidus, polyuria, diuretic therapy, tube feeding, lactulose therapy, sedatives, and mechanical ventilation. Diabetes insipidus is due to deficiency of ADH.
- It can be central wherein pituitary gland cannot secrete adequate ADH causing diuresis. It can also be nephrogenic wherein there are systemic diseases involving kidney making kidney (nephrons) inability to response to ADH.

Features

- *Features of volume depletion*: Tachycardia, hypotension, dry skin.
- *Features of neuronal inactivity*: Irritability, seizures, lethargy, confusion.
- *General features*: Weakness, polyuria, polydispia.

Investigations

- Serum electrolytes, blood glucose estimation, blood urea and serum creatinine, urine electrolytes.
- Plasma and urine osmolality, 24 hours urine volume, plasma AVP level estimation, tests relevant to suspected cause.

Treatment

- *In acute type* (hypernatremia <24 hours): Serum sodium correction rate is 3 mEq/L/hour for 3 hours with maximum correction per day is 12 mEq/L. Serum and urine electrolytes, plasma and urine osmolality should be measured every two hours.
- *In chronic hypernatremia* correction rate are 0.5 mEq/L/hour with total correction per day of 8 mEq/L.

Trust in dreams, for in them is hidden the gate of eternity

Note:
- Rapid correction may cause cerebral edema and herniation of brain and myelinolysis.
- Proper formula should be used to calculate the need using total body water (TBW). TBW = Weight in kg × correction factor; correction factor is 0.6 for children and adult male; 0.5 for adult female and elderly male; 0.45 for elderly female.
❖ *Common infusates used are:* 5% dextrose (0 mmol/L); 0.2% NaCl in 5% dextrose in water (D5 2 NS) with 34 mmol/L; 0.45% NaCl in water (0.45 NS) with 77 mmol/L; Ringer lactate with 130 mmol/L; 0.9% NaCL in water (0.9 NS) with 154 mmol/L.
❖ *Oral fluid* (water) is also helpful.
❖ *Drugs* may be used in specific situations. Thiazide diuretics, desmopressin (DDAVP oral or nasal as vasopressin analog) in diabetes insipidus.
❖ *Hemodialysis* may be needed in pulmonary edema.
❖ *Treating the cause* and monitoring is also very important.

HYPOKALEMIA

It is defined as plasma concentration of potassium <3.5 mEq/L. Normal value is 3.5–5.0/5.5 mEq/L.

98% of body potassium is intracellular. Gradient is maintained by sodium/potassium pump. Total body potassium store is 50 mEq/kg (3500 mEq in a 70 kg adult). Normal daily intake is 60 mEq/day. 90% of potassium excretion occurs through kidney; at cortical collecting duct with presence of adequate sodium in distal convoluted tubule under the effect of aldosterone. Aldosterone, insulin, alkalosis, beta adrenergic agents decrease the plasma potassium level whereas acidosis, alpha adrenergic agents, cell damage, succinylcholine increases the plasma potassium level.

- **Mild hypokalemia**: 3.0–3.5 mEq/L—asymptomatic
- **Moderate hypokalemia**: <3.0 mEq/L—symptomatic
- **Severe hypokalemia**: <2.5 mEq/L

Causes

❖ Decreased intake.
❖ *Redistribution into cells*; metabolic alkalosis; hypothermia; hypomagnesemia (magnesium is essential for potassium absorption).
❖ *Increased loss* which may be either due to renal or extrarenal.
- *Renal causes* are—diabetes insipidus, hyperaldosteronism (primary hyperaldosteronism/Conn's syndrome), hyperreninemia, European licorice (liquorice) ingestion, Cushing's syndrome, dialysis.
- *Extrarenal causes* are—vomiting (pyloric stenosis, gastroenteritis); diarrhea (villous tumor of the rectum, ulcerative colitis); duodenal/pancreatic fistula, ileostomy; after ureterosigmoidostomy; malabsorption syndrome; laxative abuse.
❖ *Drugs* like frusemide, thiazides, steroids, amphotericin B, cisplatin, insulin excess, chloroquine, beta 2 agonist and alpha antagonist.
❖ Myocardial infarction and acute asthma are associated with hypokalemia as there is activation of sympathetic (beta 2 adrenergic) system causing transcellular potassium shift.
❖ *Rare hereditary defects like*—Bartter or Gitelman syndrome (familial hypokalemic alkalosis syndrome) wherein renal salt transportation is defective.

- *Hypokalemic periodic paralysis*: It is an autosomal dominant genetic disorder with sudden hypokalemia during awakening, after exercise, after high carbohydrate or sodium meals, after change in temperature. There will be muscle weakness of one part or entirely which gradually recovers; occasionally muscle weakness may persist for days. Thyrotoxic periodic paralysis is hypokalemia causing muscle paralysis in thyrotoxic patient.
- *Pseudohypokalemia* can occur as seasonal in summer or in acute myeloid leukemia due to increased white cell count or in stored blood with large quantity of leukocytes.
- *Other causes*—total parenteral nutrition (TPN); hypothermia; barium toxicity; trauma, post-surgery.

Features

- Muscle weakness/cramps, constipation, hypoventilation, reduced reflexes and paralysis. Cardiac arrhythmias and heart blocks are known to occur.
- Hypokalemia ccurs in 20% of hospitalized patients. It shows 10 fold increase in mortality rates by its adverse effects on cardiac rhythm, blood pressure, respiratory depression. It precipitates hepatic encephalopathy in patients with liver disease. It worsens blood pressure in hypertension patients on treatment with diuretics. Prolonged hypokalemia leads to acute kidney injury. Hypokalemic myopathy often leads into rhabdomyolysis. It increases the risk of arrhythmias in patients who are on digitalis therapy.
- *Evaluation*: Serum potassium, sodium and magnesium estimation. ECG changes (QRS prolongation, T wave inversion, presence of U wave); electromyography (EMG to assess muscle weakness); investigations for specific causes. Urine potassium excretion is best measured by a 24-hour urine collection. A spot urine potassium concentration can also be measured (less accurate, but easier to obtain) with a value of <15 mEq/L indicating extrarenal loss (poor oral intake, GI loss, intracellular shift) and a value of >15 mEq/L indicating renal potassium wasting.

> The **trans-tubular potassium gradient** (**TTKG**) is an index reflecting the conservation of potassium in renal cortical collecting ducts. It is used in identifying the causes of hypo- or hyperkalemia. It assesses the ratio of potassium in the lumen of the cortical collecting ducts to that of peritubular capillaries. *Formula for calculating the TTKG*: Urine potassium divided by plasma potassium ÷ Urine osmolality divided by plasma osmolality. *Note*: Formula is valid only when urinary osmolality (U_{osm}) >300 and urinary sodium (U_{Na}) >25
>
> *TTKG in a normal person* on a normal diet is 8–9.
> *During hyperkalemia*, TTKG should be above 10 with increased urinary excretion of potassium.
> *During hypokalemia*, the TTKG should fall to less than 3 with reduced urinary excretion of potassium.

Treatment

- **Prevention of potassium loss**: Avoiding diuretics/laxatives; treat vomiting or diarrhea; control hyperglycemia.
- **Repletion of potassium loss:**
  - *Oral potassium (potassium chloride) syrup is ideal*, safer and simpler way. But often it may not be tolerated by patients. Diet rich in potassium should be encouraged. Magnesium supplementation may be added along with oral therapy. In hypokalemic patient with acidosis, potassium bicarbonate/citrate may be used. Oral potassium phosphate in patients with associated hypophosphatemia. Usually dose of 20 mEq 3-4 times a day is given and should not exceed 200 mEq/day.

---

*Generosity is giving more than you can, and pride is taking less than you need—**Kalil Gibran***

- In *moderate and severe cases*, intravenous potassium should be used. It should be given slowly in a normal saline bottle (not in dextrose) as 20–40 mEq (potassium chloride) in *four hours* under cardiac monitoring with a daily maximum total dose of 240 mEq. Correction should be done gradually over 4 days. Rapid infusion should be avoided as it will precipitate cardiac asystole. Phlebitis, thrombosis, cardiac arrhythmias are the complications of intravenous potassium therapy. Hourly potassium estimation should be done to avoid occurrence of hyperkalemia. Angiotensin converting enzyme (ACE) inhibitors like captopril and enalapril, potassium sparing diuretics like amiloride, spironolactone and triamterene cause increased risk of hyperkalemia. Concomitant use with corticosteroids and corticotropins is not recommended.
- *Hypokalemia due to loop diuretics* is treated with potassium sparing diuretics (amiloride, spiranolactone, eplerenone), oral potassium supplements.
- In *both familial and nonfamilial periodic paralysis* (e.g. from thyrotoxicosis), hypokalemia can be life-threatening. Oral propranolol (nonselective beta blocker) at the dose of 1–2 mg/kg is an effective treatment to treat an acute attack of thyrotoxic periodic paralysis.
- Patients who are receiving *digitalis therapy* and have hypokalemia are prone to develop serious cardiac arrhythmias (especially in overdose situations) and must be treated urgently.
- Patients with significant *magnesium deficiency* have renal potassium wasting and often must have their magnesium levels corrected before therapy for hypokalemia is initiated.

HYPERKALEMIA

Hyperkalemia is defined as serum potassium level more than the normal to the age; in adult it is >5.5 mEq/L. Level more than 7 causes significant hemodynamic and neurologic changes and level more than 8.5 will cause muscle paralysis, respiratory failure and cardiac arrest.

	Hyperkalemia
Mild	5.5–6.0 mEq/L
Moderate	6.1–7.0 mEq/L
Severe	>7.0 mEq/L
Fatal	>8.5 mEq/L

Hyperkalemia can be acute which is often critical and fatal needing emergency management; *or can also be chronic* which is not critical but needs ongoing management.

Causes

- *Excessive intake:* Intravenously or orally with compromised kidney function; packed red cell transfusion. Effect may not be significant if glomerular filtration rate (GFR) is >60 mL/minute.
- *Decreased excretion*: Renal failure; renal tubular acidosis; metabolic acidosis; diabetic nephropathy; hypoaldosteronism; drugs like potassium sparing diuretics, ACE inhibitors, nonsteroidal anti-inflammatory drugs (NSAIDs), cyclosporine, heparin, septran, ketoconazole; Addison's disease; hyporeninemic hypoaldosteronism.
- *Shift from intracellular space to extra-cellular space*: Hyperosmolality due to hyperglycemia, mannitol, contrast agents, hypernatremia; rhabdomyolysis; tumor lysis syndrome; propofol infusion syndrome; digitalis or fluoride intoxication; malignant hyperthermia; *hyperkalemic periodic paralysis* with myotonia; electric/thermal burns.

Progress lies not in enhancing what is, but in advancing toward what will be—Kalil Gibran

* *Pseudohyperkalemia*: It occurs after drawing of blood due to hemolysis which is found to be more if fisting is done; thrombocytosis and leukocytosis are other causes.

Features

* Often hyperkalemia can be asymptomatic.
* Weakness, muscle pain and tenderness, paralysis, bradycardia, tachypnea, arrhythmias and sudden cardiac arrest can occur.

Evaluation

* *ECG changes*: Tall T wave, shortened QT interval, ST segment depression, prolonged PR interval.
* *Blood*: Serum electrolytes, blood sugar, blood urea, serum creatinine estimation, arterial and venous blood gas analysis; serum aldosterone and cortisol estimation; serum uric acid and phosphate level for tumor lysis; serum creatinine phosphokinase (CPK) and calcium measurement for rhabdomyolysis and crush injury.
* *Urine* analysis; urine myoglobin test, urine sodium, potassium and creatinine level estimation; TTKG measurement.

Treatment

* Avoid potassium rich diet and drugs causing hyperkalemia.
* Intravenous calcium gluconate 10 mL 10% (contains 2.26 mmol of calcium) in 3–5 minutes or calcium chloride 10 mL 10% solution (contains 6.8 mmol of calcium); it protects the heart. Calcium chloride contains three times more elemental calcium than calcium gluconate and so calcium chloride is more effective in emergency cardiac situation due to hyperkalemia. 6.8 mmol of elemental calcium is required to correct the ECG changes of hyperkalemia.
* Intravenous insulin as 10 units in 50% of 50 mL glucose.
* Frusemide diuresis intravenously.
* Sodium polystyrene sulfonate ion (cation) exchange resin orally or rectally—30 gram in 33% sorbitol; Patiromer sorbitex calcium is a nonabsorbed, cation exchange polymer is also used.
* Albuterol/salbutamol nebulization as beta adrenergic agent.
* Intravenous sodium bicarbonate in metabolic acidosis.
* In severe cases, hemodialysis is a must as a life-saving measure.

ANION GAP

The *anion gap* is the difference between primary measured cations (sodium Na^+ and potassium K^+) and the primary measured anions (chloride Cl^- and bicarbonate HCO_3^-) in serum. The normal value for the serum anion gap is 8–16 mEq/L. It is the calculated estimation of unmeasured or undetermined anions in the blood.

Serum anion gap $= (Na + K) - (Cl + HCO_3)$. Sample collection should be as plasma or serum or in heparin in serum separator tube with refrigeration. EDTA, oxalate or citrate

Decreased anion gap (<6 mEq/L)	*Normal anion gap (6–12 mEq/L)*	*Increased anion gap (>12 mEq/L)*
• Hypoalbuminemia • Plasma cell dyscrasia • Monoclonal proteins/myeloma • Bromide toxicity	• Diarrhea—HCO_3 loss • Ileostomy, GI fistulas • Carbonic anhydrase inhibitors like acetazolamide • Arginine and lysine parenteral nutrition	• Uremia (renal failure) • Diabetic ketoacidosis • Lactic acidosis • Methanol, ethanol intoxication • Propylene glycol, isoniazid, salicylates toxicity • Rhabdomyolysis

Trust in dreams, for in them is hidden the gate of eternity

> **Buffers**
>
> Buffers—resist change in pH.
> *Buffer is a solution of weak acid and corresponding salt. It is an acid-base mixture which resists sudden change in pH.*
>
> **Two types:**
> 1. Mixture of weak acids with their salt with a strong base.
> 2. Mixture of weak bases with their salt with a strong acid.
>
> *Examples*: Bicarbonate buffer (H_2CO_3/$NaHCO_3$); Acetate buffer (CH_3COOH/CH_3COONa); Phosphate buffer (Na_2HPO_4/NaH_2PO_4).
>
> **Uses of buffer:**
> 1. Standard buffer solution is used with indicator for determination of pH.
> 2. Buffers are used to check the performance of electrode used for determination of pH.
> 3. Used for many chemical reactions including those catalyzed by enzymes.
> 4. Used in the pathological laboratory to control pH of culture media for bacteria tissues.
> 5. Very important in regulating the pH of body fluids, e.g. blood, interstitial fluid, lymph.
>
> *Regulation of acid-base balance and control of pH occurs by three mechanisms:*
> 1. *Blood buffers*: First line of defense
> 2. *Respiratory regulation*: Second line of defense
> 3. *Renal regulation*: Third line of defense
>
> **Blood buffers:**
> They cannot remove H^+ ions from the body; but temporarily but very rapidly acts as a shock absorbant to reduce the free H^+ ion.
>
> **Three blood buffer systems are:**
> 1. Bicarbonate buffer.
> 2. Phosphate buffer.
> 3. *Protein buffer*: Hemoglobin buffer (RBCS); amino acid buffer; plasma protein buffer.

tubes should not be used. Report should be done within 30 minutes.

In *urine anion gap*, the most important unmeasured anion is ammonia. If urine anion gap is more than 20 mEq/L, usual cause is metabolic acidosis. If the urine anion gap is zero or negative, the cause is most likely to be gastrointestinal (diarrhea or vomiting).

ACID-BASE BALANCE

Normal blood pH: 7.36–7.44

Maintenance of blood pH is important homeostatic mechanism of the body. pH less than 7.35 leads to acidosis and pH more than 7.45 leads to alkalosis.

$pH = -\log[H^+]$, dimensionless quantity. $[H^+]$ means gram of hydrated H^+ ion present as H_3O^+ per liter of fluid.

{E.g. H_2O contains $1/1000000$ g of hydrogen ion in 1 liter, means $[H^+] = 10^{-7}$}. Decrease of one pH unit represents a tenfold increase in the H^+ activity. The pH 7.40 corresponds to a hydrogen ion concentration of 40 nmol/L. If H^+ is high solution is acidic with pH <7; if H^+ is low solution is alkali with pH >7. Small change in pH can produce major changes in the metabolic system.

pK (pk' or pKa): It represents the negative logarithm of the ionization constant of a weak acid (ka). Pk is the pH at which an acid is half dissociated. Acids have pk value less than 7 and bases have more than 7. Lower pk = stronger acid; higher pk = stronger base. Urine pH is (6.0) normally lower than that of blood; urine is acidic.

Acids are proton donors. Bases are proton acceptors.

HCL is strong acid; carbonic acid is weak acid. Carbonic acid (Oxidation of c-compounds); sulfuric acid (oxidation of sulfur containing amino acids); phosphoric acid (metabolism of dietary phosphoproteins, nucleoproteins, phosphatides); organic acid

*To understand the heart and mind of person, look not at what he has already achieved, but what at he aspires to be—**Kalil Gibran***

(oxidation of carbohydratesfats and proteins, e.g. pyruvic acid, lactic acid, acetoacetic acid); iatrogenic (certain medicine like NH_4Cl, mandelic acid).

NaOH and KOH are strong alkali; $NaHCO_3$ and NH_3 are weak alkali. Bicarbonate (HCO_3^-) and biphosphate is physiologically important base.

Note:
Diet rich in animal protein results in more acid production. Vegetarian diet has an alkalizing effect.

When H^+ increases pH decreases. An acid is a substance that dissociates water to release hydrogen ion. A base is a substance that takes hydrogen ion. A buffer is a combination of weak acid and conjugate base. These buffers maintain the H^+ concentration in blood within fine limits. Natural buffers are extracellular or intracellular. Bicarbonate/carbonic acid buffer, phosphate buffer and plasma proteins are extracellular natural buffers. Hemoglobin and other proteins are intracellular buffers. Bicarbonate/carbonic acid buffer is most important as carbonic acid levels are regulated by lungs which eliminates excess of it as CO_2. Bicarbonate part is separately controlled by kidney. Acidosis is pH of blood less than 7.35. Alkalosis is pH more than 7.45.

Henderson equation (used to assess hydrogen ion concentration)

$$H^+ (nmol/L) = K \times \frac{H_2CO_3 \text{ mmol/L}}{HCO_3^- \text{ mmol/L}} \quad \text{OR}$$

$$K \times \frac{\alpha \, PCO_2 \text{ mmol/L}}{HCO_3^- \text{ mmol/L}}$$

Here constant K is 800 (for H_2CO_3/HCO_3^- buffer).

Henderson-Hasselbalch equation (used to assess pH)
It is used to find out pH of the blood using logarithm. Negative logarithm of constant K (800 for carbonic buffer) is called as pKa. It is 6.1 for H_2CO_3/HCO_3^- buffer system.

pH = pKa + log HCO_3^-/ H_2CO_3 means 6.1 + log 24 divided by 1.2 = 6.1 + log 20 = 6.1 + 1.3 = 7.4.

METABOLIC ALKALOSIS

It is primary base excess, i.e. HCO_3^-. Standard bicarbonate is above 27 mmol/L. It causes overexcitability of central and peripheral nervous system with numbness, muscle spasm, convulsions. pH will be >7.45; body compensates completely or partially through different mechanisms like buffer/respiratory/renal systems.

Causes

- Repeated vomiting due to any cause. Commonly seen in pyloric stenosis. Here *hypokalemic alkalosis* occurs, which is important to be corrected before managing the patient.
- Excess alkali ingestion, e.g. antacids.
- Cortisol excess either due to over administration or Cushing's syndrome.
- Potassium wasting diuretics.

Feature

- Cheyne Stokes breathing with period of apnea of 5–30 seconds.
- **Tetany** due to alkalosis. More often it is *latent tetany*, which is revealed by *Trousseau's sign.*
- **Investigations**: Serum electrolytes, arterial blood gas analysis.
- **Treatment:** IV infusion of normal saline or double strength saline, with slow IV potassium chloride 40 mmol/L in saline—*under ECG monitoring.* Treating the cause.

RESPIRATORY ALKALOSIS

Arterial PCO_2 is below normal.

*Optimism is the faith that leads to achievement. Nothing can be done without hope and confidence—**Hellen Keller***

Causes

- Hyperventilation during anesthesia.
- High altitude.
- Hyperpyrexia.
- Encephalitis, hypothalamic tumors, drugs like salicylates.
- Hysteria.

It may lead to tetany.

Respiratory suppression due to alkalosis is treated by CO_2.

METABOLIC ACIDOSIS

It is an excess acid or base deficit. Standard bicarbonate is below 21 mmol/L.

Causes

Increase in fixed acid:
- Diabetic ketoacidosis.
- Starvation.
- Hypoxia.
- Renal insufficiency.
- Cardiac arrest.
- Excessive exercise.
- Intestinal strangulation. Here anion gap is increased.

Loss of base:
- Diarrhea.
- Ulcerative colitis.
- Gastrocolic fistula.
- Intestinal fistula.
- Ureterosigmoidostomy causes hyperchloremic hypokalemic acidosis. Here anion gap is normal.

Features

- Rapid, deep, noisy breathing (air-hunger).
- Cold clammy skin, tachycardia, right heart strain, altered level of consciousness.
- Capillary stasis.
- Urine is strongly acidic.
- Low standard HCO_3 level.
- Base deficit.

Treatment

- Correction of hypoxia.
- 50 mmol of 8.4% sodium bicarbonate infusion IV.

Sodium bicarbonate required in mEq/L = ***Body weight in kg × 0.3 × Base deficit.***

RESPIRATORY ACIDOSIS

It is a feature of respiratory failure with high arterial PCO_2 causing fall in pH.

Causes

- During and after anesthesia.
- Chronic bronchitis.
- Emphysema.
- Thoracic diseases.
- Upper abdominal surgeries and diseases.
- Respiratory airway obstruction.
- Myasthenia gravis.
- Poliomyelitis.

FLUID THERAPY

- Osmolality of a solution is assessed by the amount of solute dissolved in a solvent like water measured in weight (kg).

Osmolality is calculated by two methods

a. Osmolality of plasma = $\dfrac{0.54}{1.86} \times 10^3$ mOsm/kg

It is based on the fact that solution of 1 mOsmol/kg freezes at – 1.86°C; whereas normal plasma freezes at – 0.54°C.

b. Osmolality of plasma = $2 \times (Na) + \dfrac{(Glucose\ mg\ \%)}{18} + \dfrac{(Blood\ urea\ mg\ \%)}{6}$

With a new day comes a new strength and a new thought—**Eleanor Roosevelt**

- Osmolarity of a solution is assessed by the amount of solute dissolved in a solvent like water measured in volume (liter).
- Normal plasma osmolality is 285 mOsm/kg (275–295). It is based on the concentrations of major solutes in plasma. So sodium concentration contributes mainly to the osmolality.
- Colloidal osmotic pressure is difference in plasma osmotic pressure and interstitial fluid pressure which is normally 25 mm Hg, and is mainly contributed by plasma albumin concentration. Plasma proteins do not go out of capillary wall into the interstitium.

Principles of Fluid Therapy

Indications

- For rapid restoration of fluid and electrolytes in dehydration due to vomiting, diarrhea, shock due to hemorrhage or sepsis or burns.
- Total parenteral nutrition.
- Anaphylaxis, cardiac arrest, hypoxia.
- Post-gastrointestinal surgeries.
- For maintenance, replacement of loss or as a special fluid.

Advantage

Controlled, accurate and adjustable, rapid and predictable.

Problems in fluid therapy

- Needs hospitalization; costly; needs asepsis.
- Fluid overload; pulmonary edema and cardiac failure; infection.
- Thrombophlebitis; hematoma; cellulitis in local area.
- Pyrogenic reaction; air embolism; bacteremia.
- Discomfort; poor patient acceptance.

NUTRITION

Principles of Nutrition

- Malnutrition increases the morbidity and mortality and delays the recovery; there is increased chance of sepsis, poor wound healing, and increased chance of systemic complications. It also reduces the efficacy of radiotherapy and chemotherapy and thereby increasing the chances of complications.
- Timing and type of nutrition is also important.
- Nutrition therapy reduces protein wasting.
- Immunomodulators like glutamine, arginine, omega 3 fatty acids promotes the recovery. Glutamine, a nonessential amino acid is important in cell proliferation, tissue repair, mucosal integrity, immune function, prevention of sepsis. It is usually used as enteral route but intravenous preparations are often considered.

Caloric requirement: Neonatal 100 kcal/kg/day; Adult 40 kcal/kg/day; Adult with catabolism 60 cal/kg/day.

It is given as: Carbohydrates 50%; Fat 30–40%; Protein 10–15%.

Caloric values: Carbohydrate 4 kcal/g; Protein 4 kcal/g; Fat 9 kcal/g.

Indications for Nutritional Support

- Preoperative nutritional depletion.
- Postoperative complications: Sepsis, ileus, fistula.
- Intestinal fistula: High type wherein output is more than 500 mL/day. It may be duodenal, biliary, pancreatic, intestinal.
- Pancreatitis, malabsorption, ulcerative colitis, pyloric stenosis.
- Anorexia nervosa and intractable vomiting.
- Trauma—multiple fractures, fasciomaxillary injuries, head and neck injuries.

*You will never win if you never begin—**Helen Roveland***

- Burns.
- Malignant disease.
- Renal and liver failure.
- Massive bowel resection causing short bowel syndrome.

Assessment
- Bodyweight.
- Mid-arm circumference.
- Triceps skin fold thickness.
- Serum albumin.
- Lymphocyte count.

Nutritional requirements: Carbohydrates, fat, proteins, vitamins (includes fat-soluble vitamins also), minerals, trace elements.

Methods of Feeding

- **Enteral:** By mouth; through nasogastric tube, gastrostomy; jejunostomy.
- **Parenteral** (Total parenteral nutrition/TPN).

Enteral

Gastrointestinal tract is the best route to provide nutrition. Enteral feeding can be delivered by bolus, by gravity or using mechanical pump.
- *By mouth:* Requires—commonsense, cleanliness, compassion.
- *By nasogastric tube:* Confirmation of the tube in the stomach is made by injecting 5 mL of air down the tube and listening with a stethoscope for bubbling entry of air into the stomach. Feeding rate is 30–50 mL/hour. 5 hours gap is given in the night to allow gastric pH to return to normal (Fig. 2.1).
- *By enterostomy:* Gastrostomy; jejunostomy.

Problems with tube feeding
- Blockage.
- Nausea and vomiting, aspiration.
- Hyperosmolarity, diarrhea.
- Tube discomfort.
- Cholestasis.

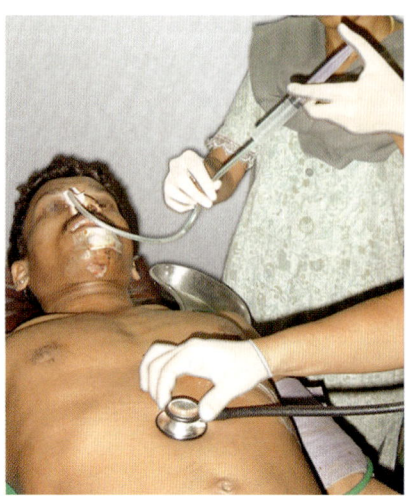

Fig. 2.1: Nasogastric tube passed should be confirmed in place using stethoscope. Tube is used for feeding purpose.

Different preparations and formulas are available for enteral feeding. Soluble fiber containing diets alongwith nutrients are better to prevent diarrhea.

Advantages of enteral nutrition
- Enteral nutrition preserves mucosal protein, digestive enzymes, IgA secretion; prevents mucosal atrophy and bacterial translocation.
- It is more physiological as nutrients pass through liver, the first filter to process and store. Gallstone formation is prevented (unlike long-term TPN) by stimulating gallbladder motility.
- It has got less serious complications. It is cost-effective.
- It supplies glutamine and short chained fatty acids to gut.

Contraindications of enteral nutrition
- Intestinal obstruction, GI bleed, paralytic ileus, severe diarrhea, high output fistula.
- Low cardiac output, hemodynamically unstable patient.

I'd rather attempt to do something great and fail than to attempt to do nothing and succeed—**Robert H Schuller**

- If safe access to enteral feeding is not present.
- Anticipated complications if thought to be present should be avoided.

Complications of enteral feeding
- Aspiration
- Wound infection and leak
- Diarrhea due to rapid feeding or hyperosmolarity.
- Hyperglycemia
- Hypokalemia
- Refeeding syndrome due to severe hypokalemia and hypophosphatemia.

GASTROSTOMY

It is done if feeding is required for more than one month (Fig. 2.2).

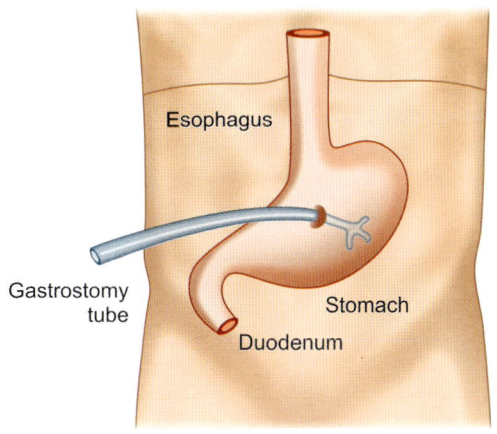

Fig. 2.2: Gastrostomy tube in place for enteral feeding.

Indications
- Severe malnutrition
- Major surgeries
- Severe sepsis
- Trauma
- Head and neck surgeries.

Types

Based on duration of use:
- Temporary
- Permanent

Based on lining:
- Mucus lined (permanent)
- Serosal lined (temporary)

Based on technique:
1. *Stamm's temporary gastrostomy*: After opening the abdomen, anterior wall of the stomach is opened. Feeding tube (Malecot's catheter) is placed in position. Two layers of purse string sutures are put around the tube. Wound is closed.
2. *Kader-Senn temporary gastrostomy.*
3. *Percutaneous endoscopic gastrostomy.*
4. *Janeway's mucus lined permanent gastrostomy* by creating tunnel in stomach wall.

Problems in gastrostomy	Contraindications
• Leak, displacement or blockage of tube • Infection • Aspiration and pneumonia • Diarrhea	• Previous gastric surgeries • Intestinal obstruction • Gastric outlet obstruction

JEJUNOSTOMY

- Jejunostomy for enteral nutrition becoming more popular because of:
  – Its comfort
  – Easy to do
  – Can be kept for long time
  – Lesser complication than gastrostomy.
- Indications are same as gastrostomy.

Types

Witzel jejunostomy: Site of placing jejunostomy is 30 cm from duodenojejunal junction.

Needle jejunostomy using catheter of small gauge (Fig. 2.3).

*Optimism is the faith that leads to achievement. Nothing can be done without hope and confidence—***Hellen Keller**

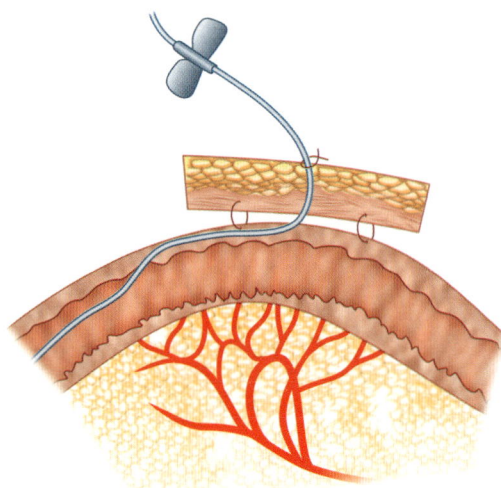

Fig. 2.3: Needle jejunostomy.

TOTAL PARENTERAL NUTRITION (TPN)

Indications
• Failure or contraindication for any enteral nutrition. • High output abdominal fistulas—duodenal, biliary, pancreatic. • Major abdominal surgeries, of liver, pancreas, biliary, colonic • Septicemia, multiple trauma, short bowel syndrome, burns • Acute pancreatitis, bowel ischemia, peritonitis • Massive gastrointestinal bleed.

Note: About 5% of hospital admissions require TPN.

Technique

Using a needle and guidewire a *subclavian vein catheter* is passed just below the clavicle and fixed securely to the skin. TPN is given through *central vein* and not through a peripheral vein. Peripherally inserted central catheter is also used. One should infuse TPN slowly over 24 hours.

The patient should be monitored at regular intervals for body weight, fluid balance, blood glucose, electrolytes, blood urea, LFT, serum calcium, magnesium, phosphate, etc.

Anabolic steroid Durabolin 25 mg IM weekly is given to improve nitrogen balance.

Components used in TPN
• Carbohydrates. • Fat and amino acids. • Vitamins and trace elements. • Electrolytes.

Complications

Technical

- Air embolism, pneumothorax.
- Bleeding, infection, thrombosis.
- Catheter displacement, sepsis, blockage.

Biochemical

- *Electrolyte imbalance*: Hyponatremia, hypoklemia, hypophosphatemia.
- Hyperosmolarity, hyperglycemia.
- Dehydration.
- Altered immunological and reticulo-endothelial function.

Others

- Dermatitis.
- Anemia and increased capillary permeability.
- Cholestatic jaundice—it is quiet common.
- Severe hepatic steatosis.
- Metabolic acidosis.
- Candida infection.

Contraindications

- Cardiac failure.
- Blood dyscrasias.
- Altered fat metabolism.

*The pessimist complains about the wind; the optimist expects it to change; the realist adjusts the sails—**William Arthur Ward***

Home Parenteral Nutrition

- It is becoming popular.
- It is commonly used in western countries.
- It is indicated in short bowel syndrome or any other conditions wherein enteral feeding is not possible but patient can be sent home with provision for home parenteral nutrition.
- Patient himself uses the TPN fluids as advised at home. He will be with TPN catheter.
- Patient should attend TPN clinic weekly for follow up or immediately whenever complications arise.
- Patient will be comfortable psychologically and often can attend his job also.

OBESITY

Definition

Weight more than 20% above the normal. Body Mass Index is weight in kilogram divided by height in meters squared [(wt in kg/ Ht in meters)^2].

Classification

Weight more than the double the expected weight to that age and height of the individual is called as *morbid obesity*.

Nutritional status	BMI (kg/m^2)
Underweight	<18.5
Normal	18.5–24.9
Overweight (Preobesity)	25.0–29.9
Obesity • Class I • Class II (Moderate) • Class III (Severe/Morbid)	>30 • 30.0–34.9 • 35.0–39.9 • >40.0
Super obesity	>50
Super superobesity	>60

Causes of Obesity

- Familial, hyperinsulinism, hyperadrenocorticism, hyogonadism.
- Abnormal eating behavior: Hormones which control eating are—ghrelin from stomach; insulin from pancreas; leptin from fat; PYY 3–36 from colon. Hypothalamus is the center in CNS which controls eating.

Complications of Obesity

- *General:* Difficulty in work, fatigue, depression, back pain, arthritis and gout.
- *Cardiovascular:* Hypertension, stroke, thrombophlebitis, pulmonary embolism.
- *Pulmonary:* Hypoventilation, poor respiratory effort.
- *GIT:* Hiatus hernia with reflux, changes in liver, pancreatitis, gallstones.
- *Endocrine:* Diabetes mellitus.

Obesity and Surgery

- Hernia is more common in obese individual.
- Gallstones are more common.
- Burst abdomen, incisional hernia are more common with obesity.
- Delay in recovering from anesthesia.
- Infertility is more common.

Treatment for Obesity

- Diet restriction, exercise.
- Vertical banded gastroplasty.
- Gastric bypass.
- Laparoscopic gastroplasty or gastric bypass.
- Jaw wiring.
- Biliopancreatic diversion.
- Jejunoileal bypass.

*There is a great difference between worry and concern. A worried person sees a problem, and a concerned person solves a problem—***Harold Stephens**

CHAPTER 3

Wounds, Inflammation, Sinus, Fistula and Ulcer

Chapter Outline

- Wound
- Problems with Wound Healing
- Compartment Syndrome
- Crush Syndrome
- Keloid (Like a 'Claw')
- Hypertrophic Scar
- Sinus
- Fistula
- Median Mental Sinus
- Ulcer
- Trophic Ulcer
- Pressure Sore (Bedsore/Decubitus Ulcer)
- Diabetic Ulcer (Diabetic Foot)
- Meleney's Ulcer
- Traumatic Ulcer
- Arterial/Ischemic Ulcer
- Carcinomatous Ulcer (Epithelioma, Squamous Cell Carcinoma)
- Marjolin's Ulcer
- Rodent Ulcer
- Melanotic Ulcer
- Tropical Ulcer
- Venous Ulcer (Gravitational Ulcer)
- Tuberculous Ulcer
- Lupus Vulgaris
- Ulcer due to Chilblains
- Ulcer due to Frostbite

WOUND

DEFINITION

Wound is disruption of any tissues (soft tissues, organs or bones) structurally and functionally. There is discontinuity or break in the integrity of tissues or organs. Ulcer is disruption or break in the continuity of any lining—may be skin or mucous membrane; ulcer is one of the type of wounds.

I. CLASSIFICATION (Rank and Wakefield)

a. **Tidy wounds**
   They are wounds of surgical incisions and caused by sharp objects.
   Usually primary suturing is done. Healing is by primary intention.

b. **Untidy wounds**
   They are:
   – Crushed
   – Tear
   – Avulsion
   – Devitalized injury
   – Vascular injury
   – Multiple irregular wounds
   – Burns, etc.
   Fracture may be present.
   Wound dehiscence, infection, delayed healing are common.
   Liberal excision of devitalized tissue and allowing to heal by secondary intention is the management.

Worry does not empty tomorrow of its sorrow. It empties today of its strength

II. CLASSIFICATION (Based on Type of Wound)

1. ***Clean incised wound***
   It is a wound caused by sharp objects like knife, glass or blades. Primary suturing is done and it heals by first intention leaving a thin, linear scar (Figs. 3.1 and 3.2).
2. ***Lacerated wound***
   Wound edge is devitalized, crushed and wide. It is treated by wound excision and delayed primary suturing. Scar formed is wide and prone for hypertrophic scar formation (Figs. 3.3A and B).
3. Bruising or contusion.
4. Hematoma (Figs. 3.4 and 3.5).
5. Closed blunt injury.
6. Puncture wounds and bites.
7. ***Abrasion (Fig. 3.6)***
   It is superficial, and is due to shearing of skin in which surface is rubbed off. It heals by epithelialization.
8. Traction and avulsion and degloving injury (Fig. 3.7).
9. ***Crush injury***
   It is caused by war wounds, road traffic accidents, and tourniquet.
   It leads on to:
   – Compartment syndrome

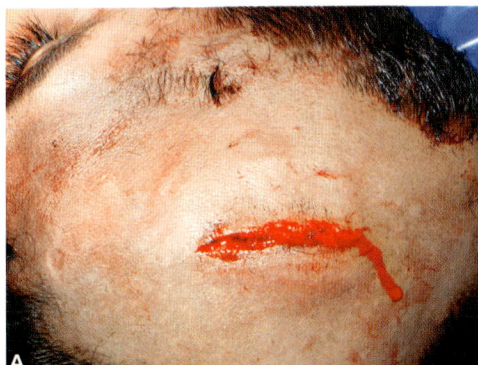

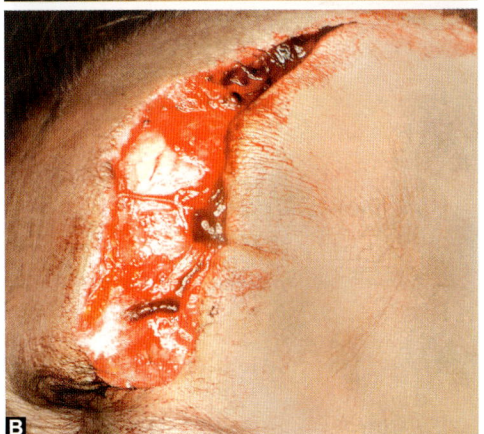

Figs. 3.3A and B: Lacerated wound on the scalp.

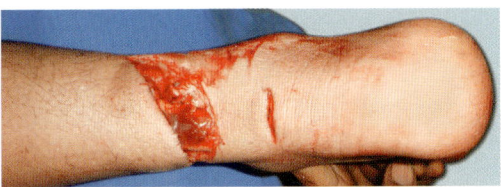

Fig. 3.1: Incised and lacerated wounds in the leg.

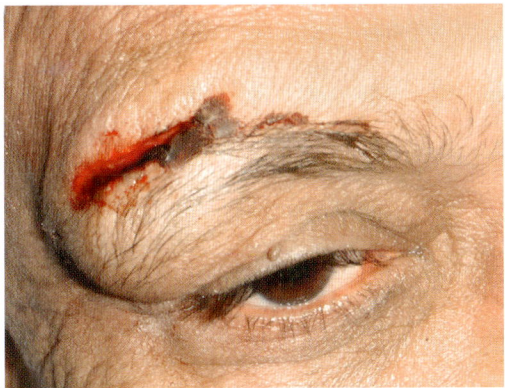

Fig. 3.2: Incised wound over eyebrow.

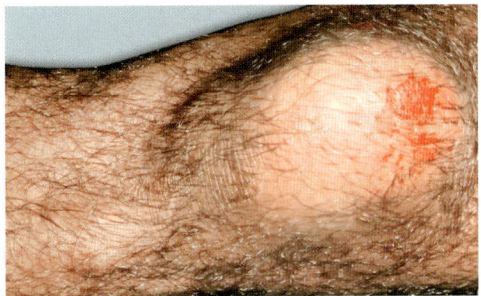

Fig. 3.4: Hematoma leg after trauma.

Always look at what you have left. Never look at what you have lost

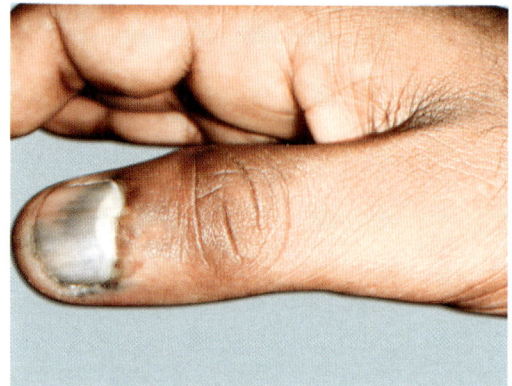

Fig. 3.5: Subungual hematoma.

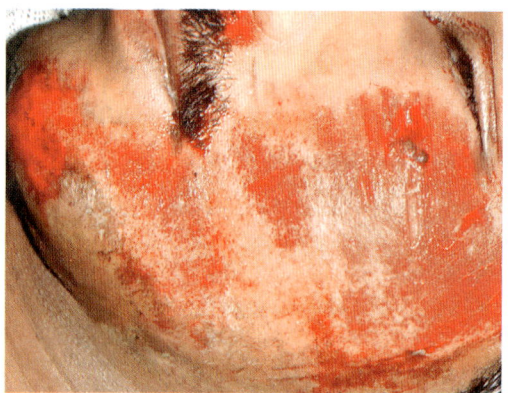

Fig. 3.6: Abrasion over the face due to trauma.

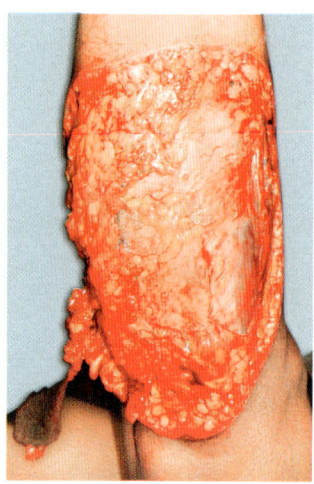

Fig. 3.7: Degloving injury in leg.

- Muscle ischemia
- Gangrene, loss of tissue.
10. War wounds and gunshot injuries.
11. Injuries to **bones** and **joints** may be open or closed.
12. Injuries to **nerves**, either clean cut or crush.
13. Injuries to **arteries** and **veins** (major vessels).
14. Injury to **internal organs** may be penetrating or non-penetrating (blunt) injuries (Figs. 3.8A and B).

III. CLASSIFICATION (Surgical Wounds)

1. **Clean wound**
   - Herniorrhaphy
   - Excisions
   - Surgeries of the brain, joints, heart transplant.
   - Infective rate *is less than 2%* (Fig. 3.9).

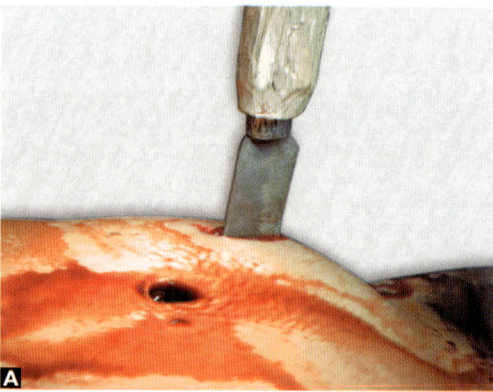

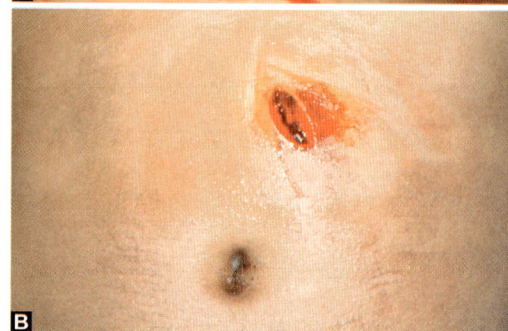

Figs. 3.8A and B: Stab wound in the abdomen using a sharp knife. It is a penetrating trauma.

Always look at what you have left. Never look at what you have lost

Chapter 3 : Wounds, Inflammation, Sinus, Fistula and Ulcer

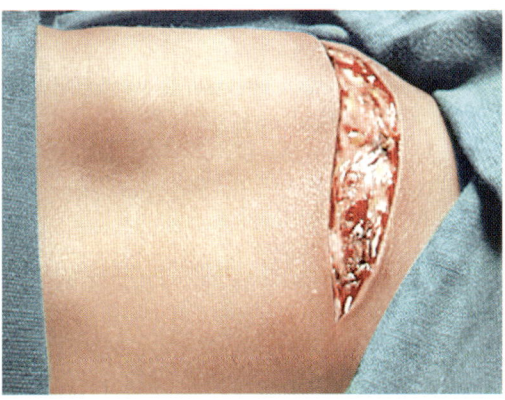

Fig. 3.9: Clean thyroidectomy wound.

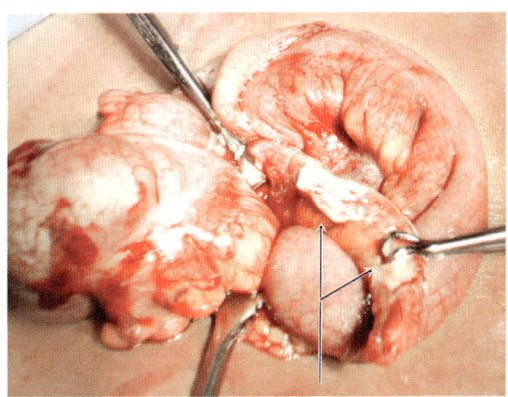

Fig. 3.11: Contaminated wound in suppurative appendicitis.

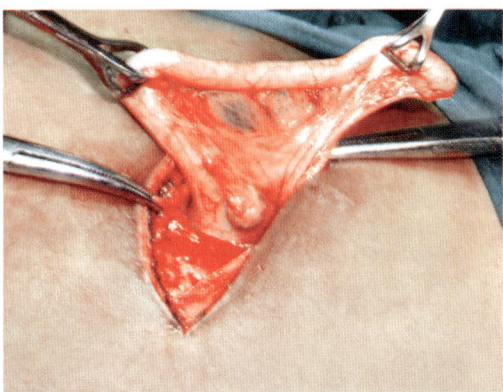

Fig. 3.10: Clean contaminated appendicectomy wound.

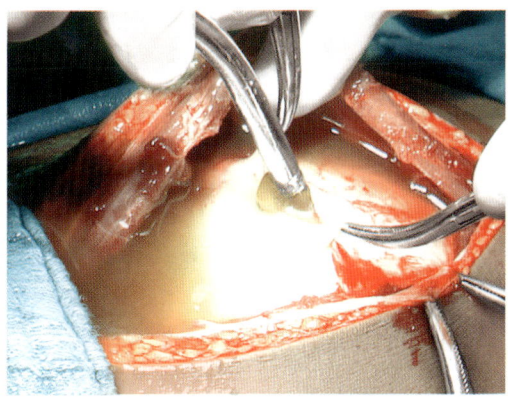

Fig. 3.12: Dirty wound of ileal perforation with peritonitis.

2. **Clean contaminated wound**
   - Appendicectomy (Fig. 3.10).
   - Bowel surgeries.
   - Gallbladder, biliary and pancreatic surgeries.
   - Infective rate is *up to 30%—high*.
3. **Contaminated wound (Fig. 3.11)**
   - Acute abdominal conditions.
   - Open fresh accidental wounds.
   - Infection rate up to 60%.
   - Infection rate >60%.
4. **Dirty infected wound (Fig. 3.12)**
   - Abscess drainage.
   - Pyocele.
   - Empyema gallbladder.
   - Fecal peritonitis.

Wound may be

- **Closed wound** like contusion, abrasion.
- **Open wound** like incised, lacerated, penetrating or crush injury.

INFLAMMATION

It is *response of living tissue to injury*; injury may be of any type—trauma, burns, surgery, infection, chemicals or drugs and so on. Inflammation can be *acute and or chronic*.

Always look at what you have left. Never look at what you have lost

Features of Acute Inflammation

- *Rubor; tumor; calor; dolor and functio laesa.*
- *'Triple response'*: Brief blanching, followed by reddening, flare and wheal.
- *Microscopic features*: Dilatation of vessels; sludging of red cells; fluid leaks into the interstitium with increased permeability of vessels; tissue edema; neutrophil margination and emigration.
- A *transudate* has low protein content, usually caused by alterations in hydrostatic or oncotic pressure; implies a hydrostatic (pressure) problem. An *exudate* has high protein content, caused by increased vascular permeability; implies an inflammatory process.
- White blood cells *margination and emigration*; implies binding to endothelium then directional movement through vessel wall towards injured area.
- *Vasodilatation* increases delivery, increases temperature, removes toxins. *Exudate* delivers immunoglobulins, etc. dilutes toxins, delivers fibrinogen, and increases lymphatic drainage.
- *Increased lymphatic drainage* delivers bugs to phagocytes and antigens to immune system.
- *Cells* remove pathogenic organisms, necrotic debris, etc.
- Pain and loss of function enforces rest, reduces chance of further traumatic damage.
- *Acute phase response* with decreased appetite, altered sleep patterns and changes in plasma concentrations of *acute phase proteins* like—C-reactive protein (CRP), α_1 antitrypsin, haptoglobin, fibrinogen.

Phases of Inflammation

- *Immediate early response:* Histamine is mainly released from mast cells, basophils and platelets, in response to many stimuli. It lasts for half an hour.
- *Immediate sustained response:* It is due to direct damage to endothelium.
- *Delayed response*: It is lasts from 3 hours onwards due to various chemical mediators of inflammation.
- *Resolution of inflammation:* Vessel caliber and permeability becomes normal; neutrophils become normal; fibrin degradation sets in; healing occurs with scarring; tissue regenerate begins.

Chemical mediators of acute inflammation

- *Proteases:* Kinins (bradykinin and kallekrein); Complement system; Coagulation/fibrinolytic system
- *Prostaglandins/leukotrienes*: Numerous metabolites of arachidonic acid; Synthesis blocked by NSAIDS, e.g. aspirin.
- *Cytokines/chemokines*: Interleukins, PAF, TNF alpha, PDGF, TGF beta, MCP.
- Products from platelets: 5-hydroxy tryptamine, histamine, ADP; Platelet-derived growth factor, coagulation proteins.
- Products from neutrophils: Lysosomal constituents; Products released on neutrophil death.
- Products from endothelium: PGI_2 (prostacyclin); Nitric oxide; Endothelin; Plasminogen activators/inhibitors.
- Oxygen derived free radicals: Endothelial damage, inactivation of antiproteases, injury to other cells.

Definitions
- **Phagocytosis:** It involves—Margination; Emigration; Chemotaxis.
- **Neutrophil movement:** Diapedesis and emigration; Chemotaxis

After phagocytosis, lysosomes activate forming phagosomes which kill the agents like bacteria using either oxygen dependent or oxygen independent mechanisms using lysozymes, hydrolases, lactoferrins, cationic proteins.

Factors related to inflammation
- Diabetes mellitus.
- Deficiencies—nutritional; anemia, vitamin deficiencies.
- HIV, steroid therapy.

Contd...

Faith is the basis of every act. You do not run away from the barber though he is armed with sharp scissors

Contd...

- Associated illness like bronchial asthma, tuberculosis, hypertension, cardiac, renal and liver diseases.
- Habits: Smoking, alcohol; tobacco.

Presentations of Inflammation

- *Fever* due to inflammatory and pyrogenic response.
- *Pain*—severity depends on the extent of injury and response.
- *Leukocytosis.*
- *Shock* with tachycardia, hypotension, tachypnea.
- *Effects* on other systems like kidney, liver, lungs, heart, brain.

Problems and Sequelae Caused by Inflammation

- *Local*: Swelling; pain; blockage of tubes like trachea, biliary system, intestine; abscess formation; loss of function.
- *Systemic:* Acute phase response; sepsis; multiorgan failure; spread of bacteria and toxins; SIRS, etc.

Management

- *Evaluation*: Blood count; Peripheral smear; evaluation for specific conditions like liver or kidney function tests, blood sugar, imaging, CRP, other biochemical markers; Blood/urine/fluid cultures.
- *Treatment*: Anti-inflammatory drugs; *Rest*; antibiotics, drainage of an abscess; treating the specific conditions.

WOUND HEALING

Wound healing is complex method to achieve anatomical and functional integrity of disrupted tissue by various components like neutrophils, macrophages, lymphocytes, fibroblasts, collagen; in an organized staged pathways—hemostasis → inflammation → proliferation → matrix synthesis (collagen and proteoglycan ground substance) → maturation → remodeling → epithelialization → wound contraction (by myofibroblasts).

For proper wound healing, wounds must have a minimum oxygen tension of 30 mm Hg for normal cell division, and a minimum of 15 mm Hg for fibroblast proliferation. Phagocytosis of bacteria depends on a high partial oxygen pressure in the tissues. Adequate oxygenation is also required for cell proliferation, angiogenesis, collagen synthesis and reepithelialization.

The following clinical signs indicate poor wound healing: Persistent inflammation for longer than 7 days, malodorous wound and increased exudate and delayed epithelialization, maceration of the surrounding skin, wound dehiscence, and necrotic tissue.

Types of wound healing

- **Healing by primary (first) intention:** It occurs in a clean incised wound which is not contaminated. It leads into thin, linear, clean scar.
- **Healing by secondary (second) intention:** It occurs in a wide wound which is cannot be opposed. Here healing takes longer time; healing leads into wider, poor scar. Infection in the wound is a common factor.
- **Healing by tertiary (third) intention:** Here initially wound is left open to granulate and later is apposed by delayed primary closure using sutures once infection and edema are reduced.

Stages

- Stage of inflammation.
- Stage of granulation tissue formation and organization. Here as the result of fibroblastic activity, synthesis of collagen and ground substance occurs.
- Stage of epithelialization—it occurs in 48 hours.
- Stage of wound contraction and connective tissue formation.

Factors affecting wound healing	
Local factors	**General factors**
1. Infection	Age
2. Presence of necrotic tissue and foreign body	Malnutrition
3. Poor blood supply	Vitamin deficiency (Vitamin C)
4. Venous or lymph stasis	Anemia
5. Tissue tension	Malignancy
6. Hematoma	Uremia
7. Large defect or poor apposition	Jaundice
8. Recurrent trauma	Diabetes
9. X-ray irradiated area	HIV and immunosuppressive diseases
10. Site of wound, e.g. wound over the joint and back has poor healing	Steroids and cytotoxic drugs

- Stage of scar formation and resorption.
- Stage of maturation.

Phases of Wound Healing

Inflammatory Phase (Lag/Substrate/Exudative)

It begins immediately after wound formation lasting for 4–6 days (Rubor, calor, tumor, dolor and loss of function—features of inflammation will develop). Macrophages secrete fibroblastic growth factor, which enhances angiogenesis. Polymorphonuclear leukocytes appear after 48 hours, which secrete inflammatory mediators and bacterial oxygen derived free radicals. Factors involved are—platelet derived growth factor (PDGF), epidermal growth factor (EGF), transforming growth factor (TGF), interleukins, tumor necrosis factor (TNF), prostaglandins, collagenase and elastase.

Proliferative Phase

It begins within 7 days and lasts for 6 weeks. Here, collagen and glycosamines are produced by fibroblasts. Hydroxyproline and hydroxylysine are synthesized by enzymes using iron, alpha ketoglutarate and vitamin C. About 50% of strength is achieved in 30 days.

Remodeling Phase (Maturation Phase)

It begins at 6 weeks and lasts for 6 months to 2 years. There is maturation of collagen by cross-linking and realignment of collagen fibers which is responsible for tensile strength of the scar.

> **Phases of wound healing**
>
> Vascular response → blood coagulation/thrombosis → inflammation → new tissue formation → epithelialization → wound contraction → remodeling.

Management of Wounds

- Wound is inspected and classified as per the type of wound.
- If it is in the vital area, then:
  - The airway should be maintained.
  - The bleeding if present should be controlled.
  - Intravenous fluids are started.
  - Oxygen, if required may be given.
  - Deeper communicating injuries and fractures, etc. should be looked for.
- If it is an incised wound, then primary suturing is done after thorough cleaning.
- If it is a lacerated wound then the wound is excised and primary suturing is done.
- If it is a crushed or devitalized wound, there will be edema and tension in the wound. *Wound debridement* is done by excising all the devitalized tissues and the edema is allowed to subside in 5–6 days. Then, delayed primary suturing is done.
- If it is a deep devitalized wound, after wound debridement, it is allowed to granulate completely. Later, if the wound is small, secondary suturing is done.

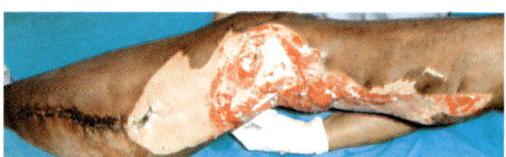

Fig. 3.13: Degloving injury, thigh and leg. It is extensive and needs regular dressing, debridement and later skin grafting.

If the wound is large, a split skin graft (Thiersch graft) is used to cover the defect (Fig. 3.13).
- In a wound with tension, fasciotomy is done so as to prevent the development of compartment syndrome.
- Vascular or nerve injuries are dealt with accordingly. Vessels are sutured with 6-zero polypropylene nonabsorbable suture material. If cut ends of the nerves are having clean-cut, it can be sutured primarily with polypropylene 6-zero or 7-zero suture material. If there is difficulty in identifying cut ends of nerves or if the cut ends of nerves are crushed then a marker stitch using silk is placed at the site and later secondary repair of the nerves are done.
- Internal injuries have to be dealt accordingly (intracranial by craniotomy, intrathoracic by intercostal tube drainage, intra-abdominal by laparotomy). Fractured bones also should be identified and properly dealt with.
- Antibiotics, fluid and electrolyte balance, blood transfusion, tetanus toxoid or antitetanus globulin injection (ATG).

Wound Debridement (Wound toilet, or wound excision) is liberal excision of all devitalized tissues at regular intervals (of 48–72 hours) until healthy, bleeding, vascular tidy wound is created.

Primary suturing means suturing the wound immediately. It is done in clean incised wounds.
Primary suturing after wound excision is done within 6 hours when wound edges are ragged, devitalized or if wound contains foreign bodies. Proper irrigation and excision of devitalized tissues is done and sutured.

Contd...

Contd...

Delayed primary suturing means suturing the wound in 48 hours. It is done in lacerated wounds, wound with edema, hematoma or contamination. This time is allowed for the edema to subside. Wound excision may be added whenever required.

Secondary suturing means suturing the wound in 10–14 days. It is done in infected wounds. Secondary suturing is done once the infection is controlled and healthy granulation tissue appears.

Specific characteristics of the wound healing in oral cavity

Wound healing in the oral cavity is a complex process with high bacterial and viral load with complex anatomy and outcome like speech, swallowing, cosmesis, reconstruction, implants during surgeries.

In the oral cavity, healing process varies in palate, bone, dental epithelium, periodontal region, facial burns, large surgical defects, reconstructed flaps and implants.

There may be excessive bleeding or absence of blood clot formation as seen in alveolitis sicca; the granuloma formation; sinus polyps; fistulas; wound dehiscence; ulcers; perforations; wound necrosis; flap necrosis; pus formation; chronic infections with or without granulation tissue formation; keloid formation; fibrosis, and trismus.

Special factors affecting the oral cavity wound healing
- *Anatomical:* Extent of involvement of soft tissues and bone; skin and mucosal loss; posterior extension; bilateral or unilateral; dentures, implants used; flap reconstruction.
- *Comorbid status:* Diabetes mellitus, steroid therapy, vitamin and protein deficiency, hypoxia, anemia, alcohol intake, smoking and tobacco use, immunosuppression, HIV infection.
- Previous surgery or radiotherapy or chemotherapy.
- Recurrence of the disease; in case of malignancy, stage of the malignant tumor.
- Infection, salivation, aspiration.
- *Trismus due to fibrosis* of the wound is a major problem in oral cavity wounds.

Management of oral cavity wounds
- *Evaluation of the wound for*—its anatomical location, extent, defect, structures involved, cosmetic postulation, functional outcome.

Contd...

Let our advance worrying become advance thinking and planning

Contd...

- Reconstruction using different flaps like pectoralis major, myocutaneous flap, foreheads flap, local flaps (nasolabial), free flaps using microanastomosis (osteomyocutaneous flap).
- *Prevention* of infection, aspiration pneumonia, avoiding wound dehiscence; proper rest to oral cavity by nasogastric tube feeding, interdental wiring; positioning of the area to avoid tension over the flap or kinking.
- *Rehabilitation*, diet, speech therapy, prevention of trismus.

PROBLEMS WITH WOUND HEALING

- *Wound infection* is common in devitalized deep difficult wounds. Diabetes, immunosuppression, cytotoxic drugs, anemia, malnutrition, malignancy increases the chances of wound infection.
- *Wound dehiscence* is common in all the above-mentioned adverse factors. Wound suddenly gives away with pain causing copious serosanguineous discharge. Laparotomy when done especially as an emergency procedure as in trauma, acute abdomen and also in malignancy, abdominal closed wound may burst in 5–7 days. Usually, all layers of abdomen give away causing discharge, occasionally bowel will extrude out. It needs emergency closure of the abdominal wound using specialized sutures or retention sutures.
- *Hypertrophic scar or keloid* formation due to altered collagen synthesis in the wound-healing process. Collagen synthesis is increased *three times* in hypertrophic scar and *20 times* in keloid.
- Deeper wound will cause *specified problems* like paresthesia, ischemia, paralysis, etc.

COMPARTMENT SYNDROME

- It is common in calf and forearm.
- Closed injury causes hematoma leading to increased pressure.
- It is often associated with fracture, which compresses the major vessel further aggravating the ischemia causing **pallor, pulseless, pain, paresthesia, diffuse swelling and cold limb**.
- If allowed to progress, it may eventually lead to **gangrene or chronic ischemic contracture** with deformed, disabled limb.
- **Muscle necrosis** releases myoglobulin, which is excreted in the urine damaging kidneys leading into renal failure.

Treatment

- These patients require longitudinal lengthy, deep incisions, i.e. **fasciotomies** to relieve the pressure and prevent compression (Fig. 3.14).
- Antibiotics.
- Bladder catheterization.
- Mannitol or diuretics to create diuresis so as to flush the kidney.
- Fresh blood transfusion.
- Hyperbaric oxygen.

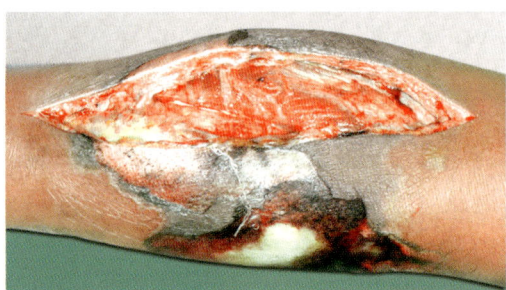

Fig. 3.14: Fasciotomy done for compartment syndrome.

CRUSH SYNDROME

It is due to crushing of muscles causing extravasation of blood and release of myohemoglobin into the circulation, leading to *acute tubular necrosis and acute renal failure*.

Causes

- Earthquakes, road traffic accidents.
- Mining and industrial accidents.

Let our advance worrying become advance thinking and planning

❖ Air crash.
❖ Tourniquet.

Initially tension increases in the **muscle compartment** commonly in the limb, which itself impedes the circulation and increases the **ischemic damage**. In 3 days, urine gets discolored and scanty. Patient becomes restless, apathy and delirious with onset of **uremia**. Crush syndrome is often life-threatening.

Note: Crush injury of small area my not cause crush syndrome (Fig. 3.15).

Effects of crush syndrome

- Renal failure.
- Toxemia; septicemia.
- Disability with extensive tissue loss.
- Gas gangrene.

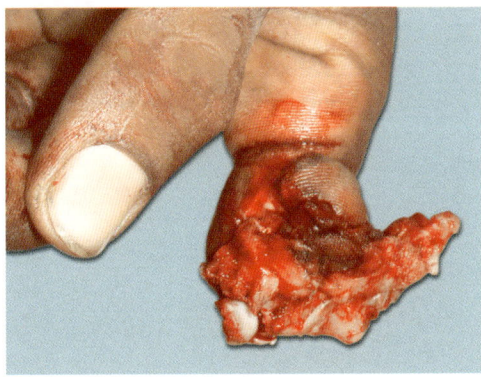

Fig. 3.15: Crush injury of finger.

Treatment

❖ Tension in the muscle compartment is relieved by placing *multiple, parallel, deep incisions* in the limb so as to prevent further damage.
❖ Rheomacrodex, or mannitol is given to improve the urine output by improving the renal function.
❖ Alkalization of the urine is done using sodium citrate or sodium bicarbonate.
❖ Hemodialysis is done sometimes as a life-saving procedure.

❖ Other measures:
  – Bladder catheterization.
  – Oxygen therapy.
  – Antibiotics.
  – Blood transfusion.

KELOID (LIKE A 'CLAW')

❖ Keloid is common in blacks. Common in females. Common in *Negroes*.
❖ Genetically predisposed. Often familial.
❖ There is defect in maturation and stabilization of collagen fibrils.
❖ Keloid continues to grow even after 6 months, may be for many years.
❖ It extends into adjacent normal skin.
❖ It is brownish black in color, painful, tender and sometimes hyperesthetic.

Sites

Common *over sternum*. Other sites are upper arm, chest wall, and lower neck in front (Figs. 3.16A and B, and 3.17A).

Differential diagnosis: Hypertrophic scar.

Treatment

Controversial.

Modes of treatment

❖ Steroid injection: **Triamcinolone** is given **intrakeloidally**, at regular intervals, may be once in 7–10 days, of 6–8 injections.
❖ *Intralesional excision* retaining the scar margin which may prevent recurrence. *It is ideal and better than just excision.*
❖ Steroid injection → Excision → Steroid injection—*not well accepted.*
❖ Methotrexate and vitamin A therapy into the keloid.

Recurrence rate is very high

Note: Excision and primary suturing has got high recurrence rate; hence it is not usually practiced.

A mistake in judgment is never fatal, but too much anxiety about judgment is

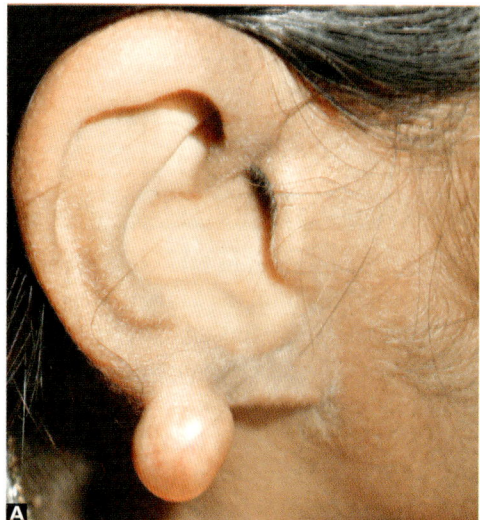

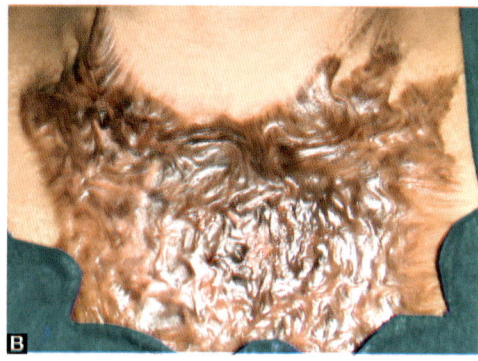

Figs. 3.16A and B: Keloid in ear. Note the keloid at sternum, which is the commonest site.

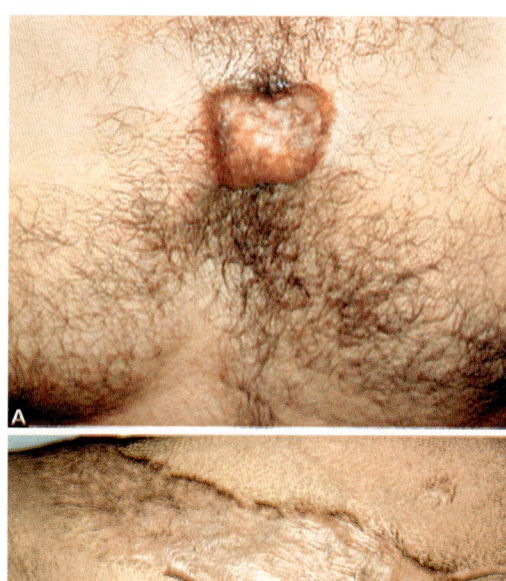

Figs. 3.17A and B: Keloid over sternum and hypertrophic scar over thigh.

HYPERTROPHIC SCAR

- It occurs anywhere in the body (Fig. 3.17B).
- Not genetically predisposed. Not familial.
- Growth usually limits up to 6 months.
- It is limited to scar tissue only. It will not extend to the normal skin.
- It is pale brown in color, not painful, non-tender.
- Often, self-limiting also. It responds very well for **steroid** injection.
- Recurrence is uncommon.
- It is controlled by pressure **garments** or often revision excision of scar and closure, if required with skin graft.

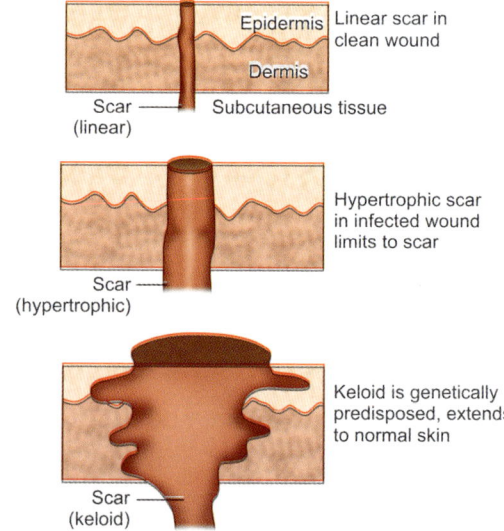

Fig. 3.18: Diagrammatic representation of linear scar, hypertrophic scar and keloid.

A mistake in judgment is never fatal, but too much anxiety about judgment is

Differences between keloid and hypertrophic scar (Fig. 3.18)

	Keloid	Hypertrophic scar
a. Genetic predisposition	Yes	No
b. Site of occurrence	Chest wall, upper arm, lower neck, ear	Anywhere in the body, Common in flexors
c. Growth	Continues to grow without time limit. Extends to normal skin	Growth limits for 6 months. Limited to scar tissue only
d. Treatment	Poor response	Good response to steroids
e. Recurrence	Very high	Is uncommon
f. Collagen synthesis	20 times more than normal skin	6 times more than normal skin
g. Relation of size of injury and lesion	No relation. Small healed scar can form large keloid	Related to size of injury and duration of healing
h. Age	Adolescents, middle age	Children
i. Sex	Common in females	Equal in both
j. Race	More in blacks	No racial relation

Complication

- Repeated breakdown of the scar often occurs causing infection and pain.
- After repeated breakdown it may turn into *Marjolin's ulcer*.

SINUS (FIG. 3.19A)

- "Sinus" means "hollow" or "a bay" (Latin).
- It is a blind track lined by granulation tissue leading from an epithelial surface into the surrounding tissues.
- Sinus sprouts outside and it does not have a floor clinically.

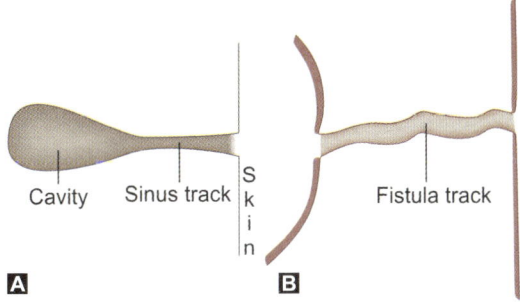

Figs. 3.19A and B: (A) Sinus; (B) Fistula.

- Discharge can be seen on the mouth of the sinus.

Causes of Sinus

- ***Congenital:*** Preauricular sinus.
- ***Acquired:*** Chronic osteomyelitis of bone causing bone spicules and discharge to come out of the sinus opening. *Median mental sinus* in the mentum in lower jaw is due to tooth infection. *Pilonidal sinus* is due to entering of hairs in the interbuttock cleft over the sacrum. *Madura foot* in the foot and leg is due to Nocardia Madurai fungal infection causing multiple discharging sinuses. *Tuberculous sinus* is eventual outcome of cold abscess in neck, groin, etc. discharging cheesy, *caseating*, yellowish material.

FISTULA (FIG. 3.19B)

- It is an abnormal communication between the lumen of one viscus to another or the body surface or between the vessels.
- Fistula means "flute" or "a pipe or tube".

Every exit is an entry somewhere else

Causes of Fistula

- Branchial fistula in neck.
- Thyroglossal fistula.
- Orocutaneous fistula in advanced carcinoma cheek.
- Tracheoesophageal fistula.
- Postoperative gastrointestinal fistula (Fig. 3.20).
- Rectovesical fistula.
- Fistula-in-ano.

Fistula can be

- **External:** Here fistula communicates from skin to hollow viscus inside. For example—parotid fistula, thyroglossal fistula, branchial fistula.
- **Internal:** Here fistula develops between two hollow viscera. Colovesical fistula, aortoenteric fistula.

Fistula also can be

- **Congenital:** Branchial/tracheoesophageal fistula.
- **Acquired:** Thyroglossal fistula, fistula-in-ano, gastrointestinal fistula.

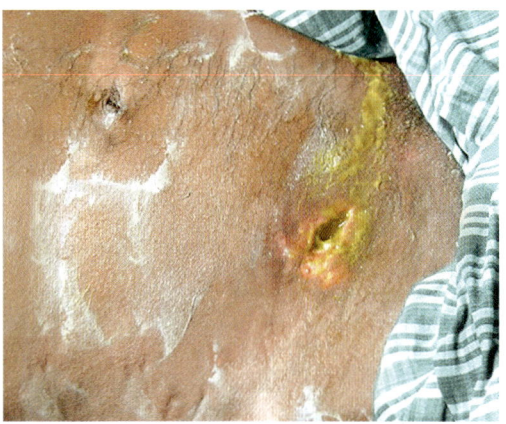

Fig. 3.20: Fecal fistula of abdominal wound.

Types of Sinus/Fistula

Congenital	Acquired
• Preauricular sinus • Branchial fistula • Tracheoesophageal fistula • Congenital AV fistula	• Ruptured abscess • Tuberculosis—common • Actinomycosis • Chronic osteomyelitis • Fistula-in-ano • Acquired AV fistula • Median mental sinus

Clinical Features

- Discharge from the opening of sinus. No floor.
- Raised indurated edge, indurated base, non-mobile.
- Often *sprouting granulation tissue is seen over the sinus opening*.
- Underlying bone may be thickened on palpation if sinus is adherent to bone in osteomyelitis.

Causes of persistence of a sinus or fistula

- A foreign body or necrotic tissue underneath, e.g. suture, sequestrum.
- Insufficient or non-dependent drainage.
- Persistent obstruction in the lumen, e.g. in fecal fistula, biliary fistulas (distal obstruction).
- Lack of rest.
- Walls become lined with epithelium or endothelium.
- Dense fibrosis prevents contraction and healing.
- Specific infections: Tuberculosis, actinomycosis.
- Presence of malignant disease.

Investigations (Fig. 3.21)

- Fistulogram/sinusogram using ultrafluid lipidol or water-soluble iodine dye.
- Discharge from sinus/fistula for culture and sensitivity, AFB, cytology, staining.
- Biopsy from the edge, chest X-ray, ESR.

Every exit is an entry somewhere else

Chapter 3 : Wounds, Inflammation, Sinus, Fistula and Ulcer   41

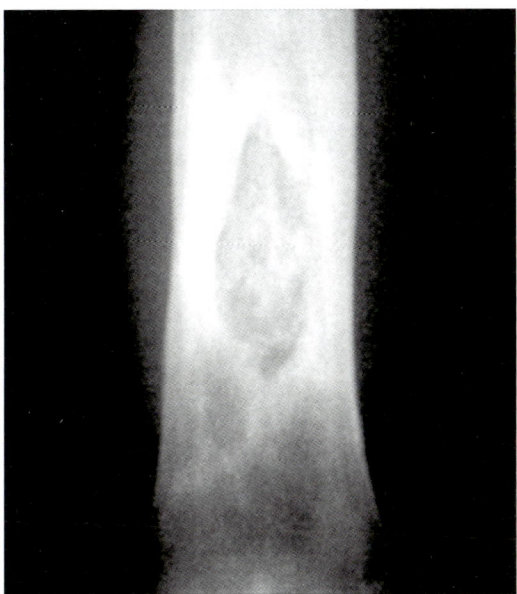

Fig. 3.21: X-ray of femur showing osteomyelitis of the femur with sequestrum and sinus.

Treatment

- The cause is treated—sequestrectomy, foreign body removal, control of tuberculosis.
- *Excision* of sinus or fistulas. Always specimen should be sent for histology.

Different discharges in a sinus/fistula
• Purulent—bacterial infection.
• Caseous—tuberculous.
• Sulfur granules—actinomycosis.
• Mucus—branchial fistula.
• Saliva—parotid fistula.
• Feces—fecal fistula (Figs. 3.22A and B).
• Bile—biliary, duodenal fistula.
• Bone—osteomyelitis sinus.

MEDIAN MENTAL SINUS

It is a chronic infective condition, wherein there is infection of roots of one or both lower incisor teeth forming root abscess, which

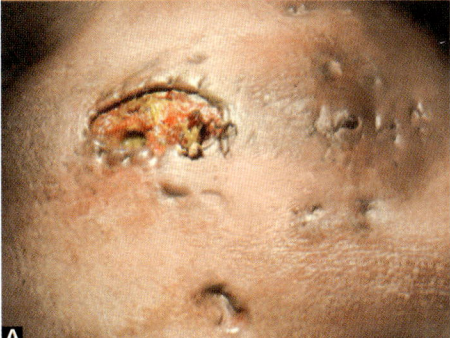

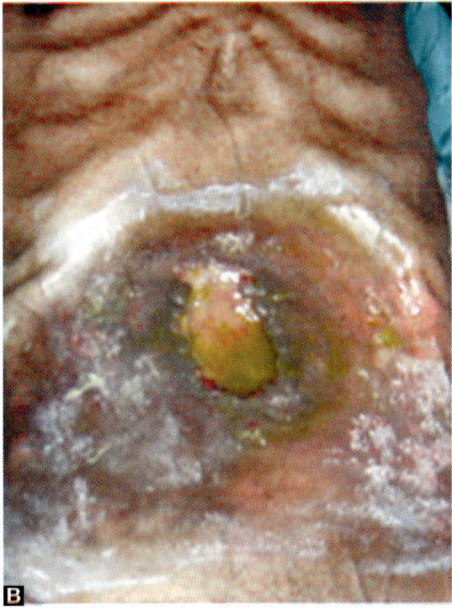

Figs. 3.22A and B: Fecal fistula with discharging fecal matter through the fistulous wound. Note the tension sutures in one of the pictures.

eventually tracks down between two halves of the lower jaw in the midline, presenting as discharging sinus on the point of chin (in midline) (Fig. 3.23).

Clinical Features

- Usually painless discharging sinus in the midline on the point of chin.
- Often infection in incisor may be revealed (in many patients clinically tooth looks

Every oak tree started out as a couple of nuts who stood their ground

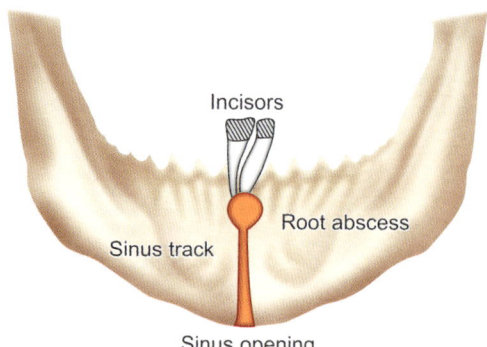

Fig. 3.23: Median mental sinus. Note the origin of the sinus from the root/roots of the lower incisor/incisors.

normal, even though root is infected invariably).
* It is often mistaken for infected sebaceous cyst.
* Osteomyelitis of the mandible is the possible complication.

Differential Diagnosis

* Infected sebaceous cyst.
* Tuberculous sinus.
* Osteomyelitis.

Investigations

* Dental X-ray is diagnostic (plain X-ray mandible may not reveal the disease).
* Discharge study—culture and sensitivity, cytology, AFB.

Treatment

* Antibiotics after doing discharge study (culture and sensitivity).
* Lay opening and excision of the sinus track with *extraction of incisor tooth/teeth*.

ULCER

Definition

An ulcer is a break in the continuity of the covering epithelium, either skin or mucous membrane due to molecular/cell death.

Parts of an Ulcer (Fig. 3.24)

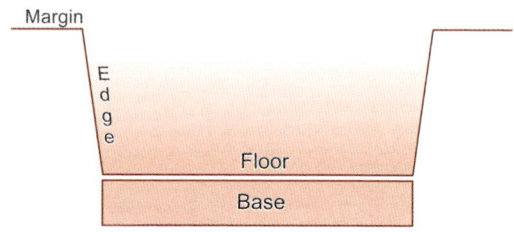

Fig. 3.24: Parts of an ulcer.

Margin
It may be regular or irregular. It may be rounded or oval.

Edge
Edge is the one, which connects floor of the ulcer to the margin.

Different edges are (Fig. 3.25):

Sloping edge: It is seen in healing ulcer. Its inner part is red because of red, healthy granulation tissue.

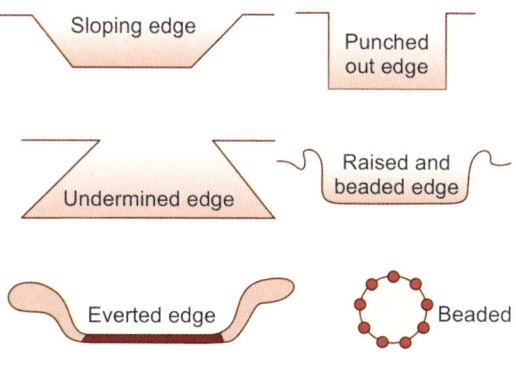

Fig. 3.25: Ulcer edges.

Every oak tree started out as a couple of nuts who stood their ground

Chapter 3 : Wounds, Inflammation, Sinus, Fistula and Ulcer

CLASSIFICATION I (CLINICAL)

Spreading ulcer: Here edge is inflamed and edematous (Fig. 3.28).

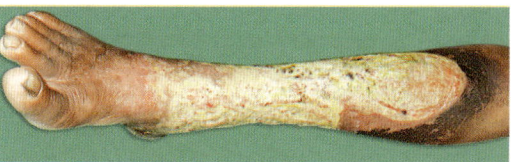

Fig. 3.28: Spreading ulcer.

Healing ulcer: Edge is sloping with healthy pink/red granulation tissue with serous discharge (Fig. 3.29).

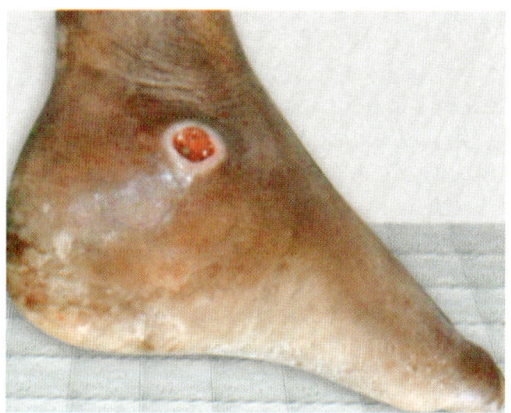

Fig. 3.26: Tuberculous ulcer over the foot. Note the undermined edge.

Undermined edge is seen in tuberculous ulcer (Fig. 3.26).

Punched out edge is seen in gummatous (syphilitic) ulcer, trophic ulcer and pressure sores. It is due to endarteritis.

Raised and beaded edge (pearly white) is seen in rodent ulcer (BCC).

Everted edge (rolled out edge) is seen in carcinomatous ulcer (Fig. 3.27).

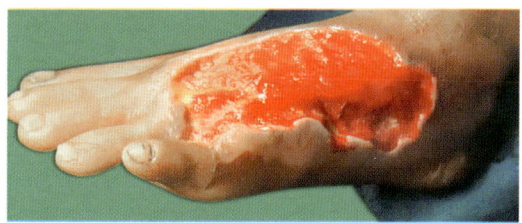

Fig. 3.29: Healing ulcer with healthy granulation tissue.

Nonhealing ulcer: It is chronic ulcer with unhealthy granulation tissue and slough in the floor with purulent or serosanguinous discharge. Edge may be punched out (trophic); undermined (tuberculous); rolled out (carcinomatous); beaded (rodent ulcer). Non-tender regional lymph nodes may be enlarged (Fig. 3.30).

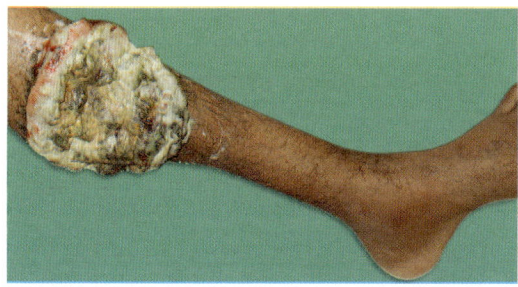

Fig. 3.27: Squamous cell carcinoma leg; note the everted (rolled out) edge.

Floor
It is the one, which is seen. Floor may contain discharge, granulation tissue, or slough.

Base
Base is the one where ulcer rests. It may be bone or soft tissues.

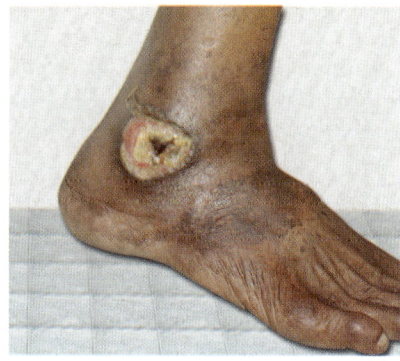

Fig. 3.30: Nonhealing ulcer foot with unhealthy/pale granulation tissue.

Happiness is never found until we have the grace to stop looking for it

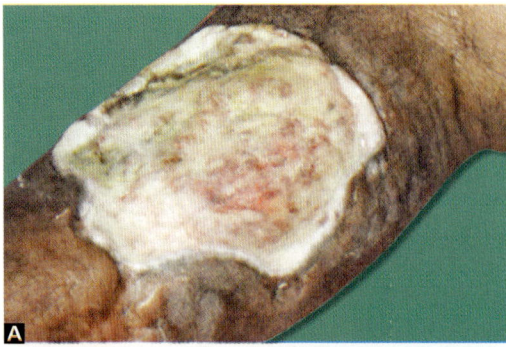

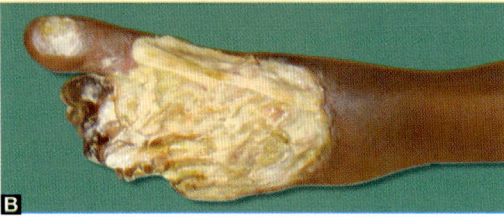

Figs. 3.31A and B: (A) Callous ulcer in the leg. Note the slough on the surface of ulcer with no signs of healing; (B) Callous ulcer leg. Note ulcer floor without any granulation tissue.

Callous ulcer: Floor contains pale unhealthy granulation tissue with indurated edge/base (Figs. 3.31A and B). Ulcer has no tendency to heal. It lasts for many months to years.

CLASSIFICATION II (PATHOLOGICAL)

Specific Ulcers

- Tuberculous ulcer (*see* Fig. 3.25).
- *Syphilitic ulcer:* It is punched out, deep ulcer, with 'wash-leather' slough in the floor and with indurated base.
- Actinomycosis.
- Meleney's ulcer.

Malignant Ulcers

- Carcinomatous ulcer.
- Rodent ulcer.
- Melanotic ulcer.

Nonspecific Ulcers

- *Traumatic ulcer*: It may be due to mechanical, physical, chemical injury.
- *Arterial ulcer:* Atherosclerosis, thromboangiitis obliterans (TAO).
- *Venous ulcer* (gravitational ulcer, postphlebitic ulcer).
- *Trophic ulcer.*
- *Infective ulcers*: Pyogenic ulcer.
- *Tropical ulcers*: It occurs in tropical countries. It is callous type of ulcer, e.g. Vincent's ulcer.
- *Ulcers due to* chilblains and frostbite (*cryopathic ulcer*).
- *Martorell's hypertensive ulcer*: It occurs due to obliteration of end arteries. It is observed in skin over the back of calf region. Ulcer is severely painful with deep, non-healing ischemic look.
- *Bazin's ulcer*: It is seen exclusively in the legs and ankles of young females, as erythematous purplish nodules and nonhealing ulcers. It may be due to ischemic (Fig. 3.32)/hypersensitive/tuberculous etiology. It is treated with antituberculous drugs, dressings, vasodilators and often by sympathectomy. It is also called as *Erythrocyanosis frigida*.

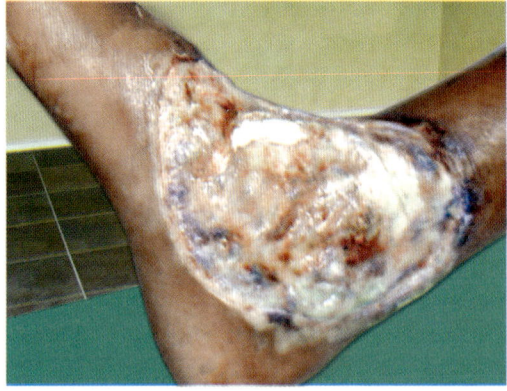

Fig. 3.32: Ischemic ulcer foot is due to poor blood supply due to either, atherosclerosis, thromboangiitis obliterans, diabetes mellitus.

Happiness is never found until we have the grace to stop looking for it

- *Diabetic ulcer.*
- *Ulcers* due to leukemia, polycythemia, jaundice, collagen diseases, lymphedema.
- *Cortisol ulcers* are due to long time application of cortisol (steroid) creams to certain skin diseases. These ulcers are callous ulcers, last for long time and requires excision with skin grafting.

Note: Maggots may form in ulcer and they eat only dead tissues (Fig. 3.33).

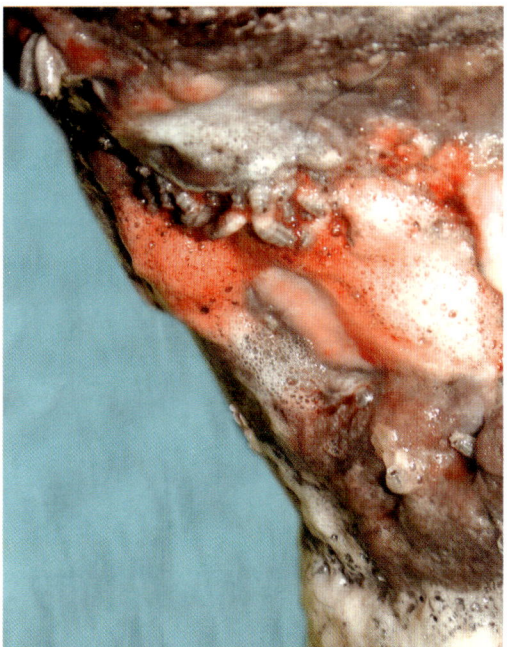

Fig. 3.33: Ulcer showing maggots. Maggots eat only dead tissue.

GRANULATION TISSUE

It is proliferation of new capillaries and fibroblasts intermingled with RBCs and WBCs with thin fibrin cover over it. *Granulation tissue* comprises a dense population of macrophages, fibroblasts, capillary networks, fibronectin, hyaluronic acid and endothelial cells.

Types

Healthy Granulation Tissue

It occurs in a healing ulcer. It has a sloping edge with serous discharge. It bleeds on touch. Skin grafting takes up well with healthy granulation tissue. Streptococci growth in culture should be less than 10^5/gram of tissue before skin grafting (Figs. 3.34A and B).

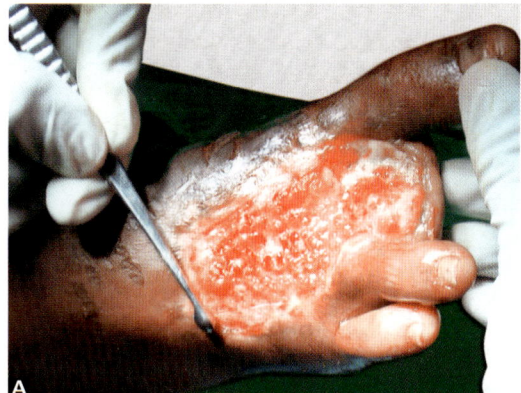

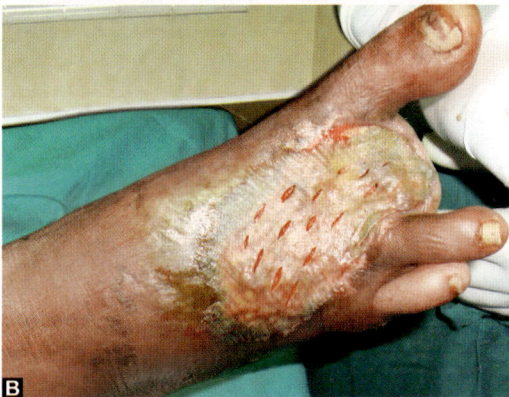

Figs. 3.34A and B: Healthy granulation tissue seen in ulcer bed; it is coverd with split skin graft (SSG).

Unhealthy Granulation Tissue

It is pale with purulent discharge. Its floor is covered with slough. Its edge is inflamed and edematous. It is a spreading ulce.

Unhealthy, Pale, Flat Granulation Tissue

It is seen in chronic nonhealing ulcer (callous ulcer).

Happiness is never found until we have the grace to stop looking for it.

Different discharges in an ulcer (as well as from a sinus)

- *Serous*: In healing ulcer.
- *Purulent*: In infected ulcer.
  - Staphylococci—yellowish and creamy.
  - Streptococci—bloody and opalescent.
- Pseudomonas—greenish color.
- *Bloody*: Malignant ulcer, healing ulcer from healthy granulation tissue.
- *Seropurulent*.
- *Serosanguinous*: Serous and blood.
- *Serous with sulfur granules*: Actinomycosis.
- *Yellowish*: Tuberculous ulcer.

Exuberant Granulation Tissue (Proud Flesh)
It occurs in a sinus wherein granulation tissue protrudes out of the orifice of the sinus like a proliferating mass. It is commonly associated with a retained foreign body in the sinus cavity.

Pyogenic Granuloma
It is a type of exuberant granulation tissue. Here granulation tissue protrudes out from an infected wound or ulcer bed, presenting as well localized, red swelling, which bleeds on touch (Figs. 3.35A and B).

Treatment: Antibiotics, excision and biopsy.

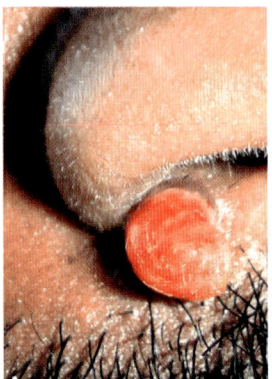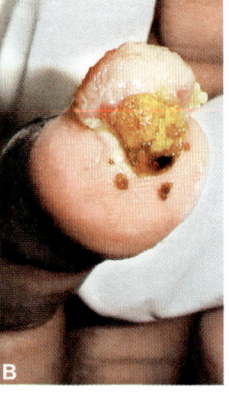

Figs. 3.35A and B: Pyogenic granuloma on the face and finger. They present with pain, bleeding and swelling. It needs excision under local anesthesia.

Investigations for an Ulcer

- *Study of discharge*: Culture and sensitivity, AFB study, cytology.
- *Wedge biopsy*: Biopsy is taken from the edge because edge contains multiplying cells. Usually two biopsies are taken. Biopsy from the center may be inadequate because of necrosis.
- X-ray of the part.
- FNAC of the lymph node.
- Chest X-ray, Mantoux test is done in suspected case of tuberculous ulcer (Figs. 3.36A and B).

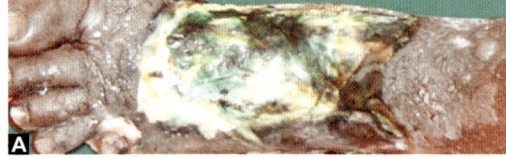
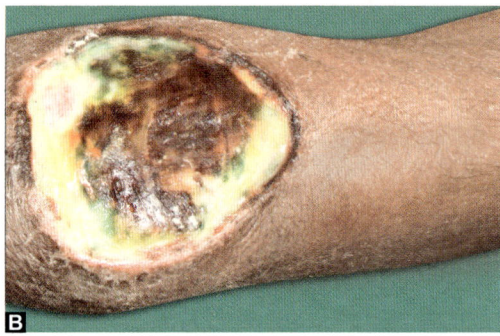

Figs. 3.36A and B: Ulcer with *Pseudomonas* infection. Note the greenish floor.

Induration

- Induration is a feel of hardness in the edge/base or surrounding area of an ulcer/lesion.
- It is observed in squamous cell carcinoma.
- It can also be seen in chronic ulcers like venous ulcer due to long standing fibrosis.
- Brawny induration is typical of an abscess.
- Induration is absent in malignant melanoma/poorly differentiated carcinomas.
- It can be seen in chronic sinus, syphilitic hard chancre.
- Induration is usually absent in tuberculosis.

Happiness is never found until we have the grace to stop looking for it

Treatment of an Ulcer

- Treat the underlying cause like diabetes, anemia, and malnutrition. Often needs blood transfusion.
- Antibiotics are given depending on the culture and sensitivity.
- Regular dressings using EUSOL (Edinburgh University Solution containing calcium hydroxide, boric acid, sodium hypochlorite), H_2O_2, povidone iodine.
- Wound excision/slough excision/debridement of the wound at regular intervals.
- Once wound granulates well, split skin grafting is done to cover the defect (Figs. 3.37A and B).

- If there is no adequate blood supply, or if bone is exposed then flap is needed to close the defect depending on the location of ulcer, either groin flap, pectoralis major flap, etc. is needed.

Management of an ulcer

- Cause should be found and treated.
- Correct the deficiencies like anemia, protein deficiency, vitamins.
- Transfuse blood if required.
- Control the pain.
- Investigate properly.
- Control of infection and rest to the part.
- Care of the ulcer by **debridement, ulcer cleaning and dressing**.
- Removal of the exuberant granulation tissue.
- Topical antibiotics for infected ulcers only like Framycetin, Silver sulphadiazine, Mupirocin, etc.
- Antibiotics are not required once healthy granulation tissues are formed.
- Once granulates, defect is closed with secondary suturing, skin graft or flaps.

Debridement of an ulcer

- It is removal of devitalized tissue.
- Small ulcers are debrided in ward.
- Large ulcers are debrided in operation theater under general anesthesia.
- All dead, devitalized, necrotic tissues are removed.
- Slough should be separated adequately before debridement.
- Often devitalized tissue separates on its own by autolysis.
- Enzymes like collagenase are used for debridement.

Dressing of an ulcer

- To keep ulcer moist.
- To keep surrounding skin dry.
- To reduce pain.
- To soothe the tissues.
- To protect the wound.
- As an absorbent of the discharge.

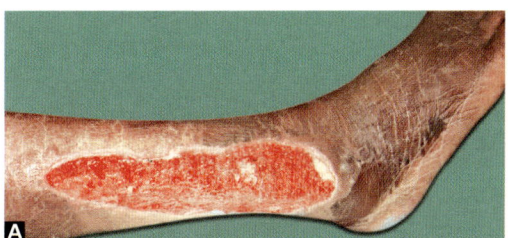
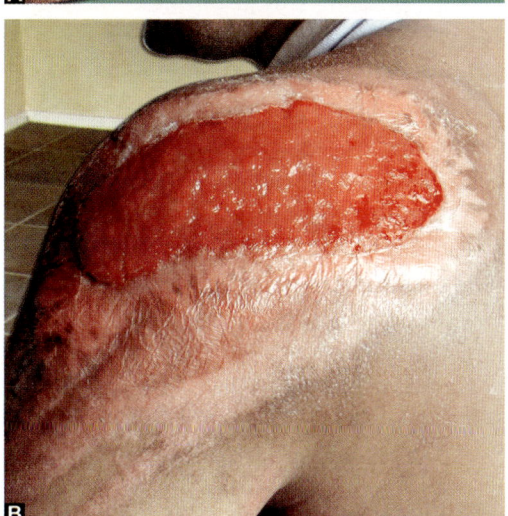

Figs. 3.37A and B: Healing ulcers in leg and shoulder area in different patients. Note the healthy granulation tissue with sloping edge.

Excellence is never granted to man but given as the reward of labour

TROPHIC ULCER (FIG. 3.38)

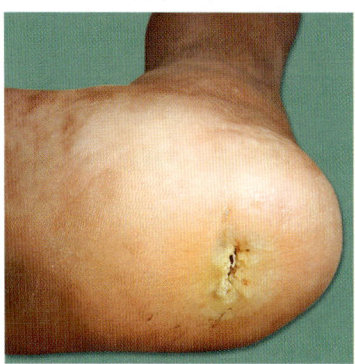

Fig. 3.38: Trophic ulcer heel.

It is due to:
- Impaired nutrition.
- Defective blood supply.
- Neurological deficit.

It usually occurs:
- Over the heel (Fig. 3.38).
- In relation to heads of metatarsals.
- Buttocks.
- Over the ischial tuberosity.
- Sacrum.
- Over the shoulder.
- Occiput.

Because, there is neurological deficit, trophic ulcer is also called as *neurogenic ulcer/neuropathic ulcer*.

Due to repeated trauma and pressure, it initially begins as callosity which suppurates and gives way through a central hole extending into the deeper plane as *perforating ulcer (penetrating ulcer)*.

Neurological causes	
• Diabetic neuropathy. • Peripheral neuritis. • Tabes dorsalis. • Spina bifida. • Leprosy.	• Spinal injury. • Paraplegia. • Peripheral nerve injury. • Syringomyelia. *Bedsores are trophic ulcers.*

Clinical Features

- Painless ulcer, which is punched out.
- Ulcer is non-mobile with base formed by underlying bone.

Investigations

Study of discharge, biopsy from the edge, X-ray of the part, X-ray spine, blood sugar.

Treatment

- Cause should be treated.
- Nutritional supplements.
- Rest, antibiotics, slough excision, regular dressings.
- Once ulcer granulates well, flap cover or skin grafting is done.
- Excision of the ulcer and skin grafting.

PRESSURE SORE (BEDSORE/DECUBITUS ULCER)

Bedsore/pressure sore is a *trophic ulcer* with underlying bone as the base.

It is nonmobile, deep, punched out ulcer.

It is common in:
- Old age.
- Bedridden individuals.
- Tetanus.
- Patients with orthopedic and head injuries.
- Diabetic.
- Paraplegic.
- Comatose.
- Emaciated patient.
- Anemia.
- Prolonged immobilization.

Sites of bedsore are *occiput, heel, sacrum (Fig. 3.39), ischium, scapula*, greater trochanter, spinous process, elbows, and buttocks.

Excellence is never granted to man but given as the reward of labour

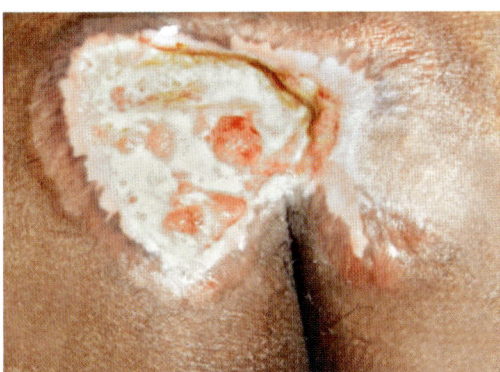

Fig. 3.39: Bedsore over sacral region. It is a trophic ulcer

Predisposing Factors

- Malnutrition, anemia, sensory loss, pressure, moisture.
- Incontinence makes skin moist and septic, so five times more prone for pressure sore.
- Excessive sweating, edema.
- Friction due to foreign body, thick bed sheets, hard and rough cot.

Superficial bedsores are common (75%). They are painful and heal slowly by itself.

Deep bedsores are painless but covered with slough. It requires antibiotics, grafting or flaps to cover it later.

Treatment

- *Change of positions* should always be encouraged.
- Use of waterbed, ripple bed is advised. Bed should be smooth and free from wrinkles and unevenness. Air rings or air cushions are also useful.
- *Moisture* has to be avoided. Skin must be kept clean and dry. It should be washed with soap and water and dried properly. A soothening powder may be beneficial.
- *Ripple bed* has an alternate pressure point pad under the bottom sheet of ordinary mattress. It provides regular automatic frequent redistribution of pressure areas. The pad consists of vinyl plastic pad with alternating sets of air cells. To control the air, an air pump is also present.
- In a patient with urinary incontinence, special silicone bedclothes are used to attain waterproof covering to skin. Indwelling Foley's catheter is placed to drain urine. Thorough washing of the back and drying twice daily is essential. Disposable soft inco-pads are used repeatedly as required.
- Bowker-Davidson special pressure cushions contain foamed cushion with a waterproof polyvinyl chloride bag containing 5 liters of the thixotropic gel.
- Soaking by urine, sweat, pus, and feces has to be taken care off.
- *Good nursing, regular dressing, good nutrition are necessary.*
- Antibiotics, blood transfusions are very essential as per need.
- Excision of dead tissue followed by skin grafting or local rotation flaps may have to be done.

DIABETIC ULCER (FIG. 3.40) (DIABETIC FOOT)

Patients with diabetes are more prone for foot problems like *cellulitis, abscess formation, gangrene, osteomyelitis* of foot. It is due to *neuropathy, more susceptibility for infection, clawing of toes, loss of functioning of foot arch, microangiopathy, bacterial resistance, and decreased body immunity.*

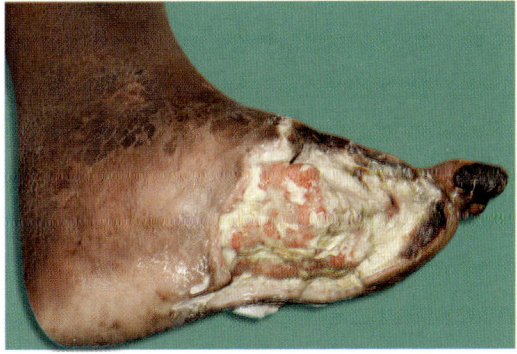

Fig. 3.40: Ulcer foot in diabetic patient.

The drops of rain make a hole in the stone not by violence, but by oft falling

Causes
• Increased glucose in the tissues precipitates infection.
• Diabetic microangiopathy, which affects microcirculation.
• Increased glycosylated hemoglobin decreases the oxygen dissociation.
• Increased glycosylated tissue protein decreases the oxygen dissociation.
• Diabetic neuropathy involving all sensory, motor and autonomous components.
• Associated atherosclerosis.

Sites

❖ Foot-plantar aspect—*is the commonest site.*
❖ Leg.
❖ Upper limb, back, scrotum, perineum.

Diabetic ulcer may be associated with ischemia. Ulcer is spreading and deep.

Investigations

❖ Blood sugar both random and fasting.
❖ Urine ketone bodies.
❖ Discharge for culture and sensitivity.
❖ X-ray of the part.
❖ Arterial Doppler of the limb.

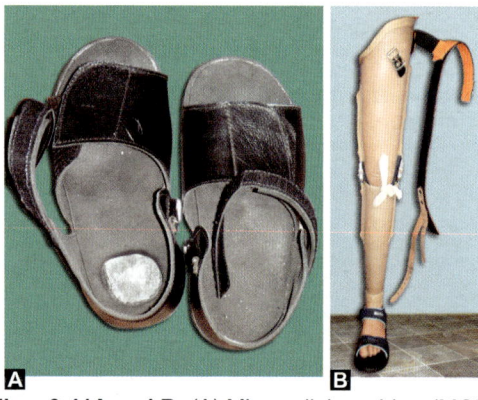

Figs. 3.41A and B: (A) Microcellular rubber (MCR) chappal used in neuropathic diabetic foot; (B) Leg prosthesis used after lower limb amputation for diabetic gangrene.

Treatment

❖ Control of diabetes using insulin. Sliding scale insulin is used depending on the color seen in urine test. Human insulin is the preferred type of insulin. When there is ketosis, intravenous insulin is used in normal saline.
❖ Antibiotics.
❖ Nutritional supplements.

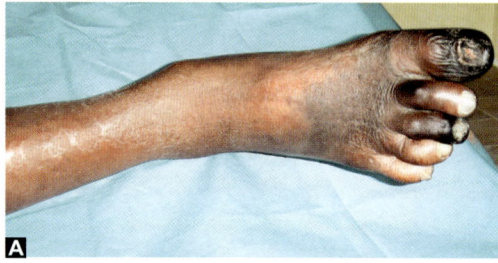

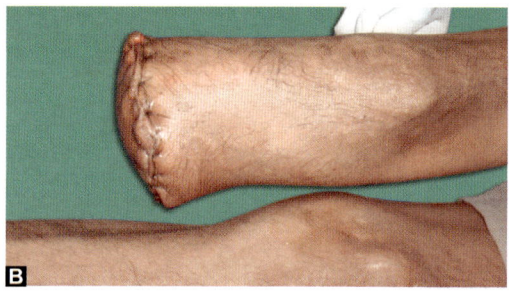

Figs. 3.42A and B: Below knee amputation is done for diabetic gangrene foot.

❖ Regular cleaning, debridement, dressing.
❖ *Microcellular (MCR)* chappals are used to avoid ulcer formation (Fig. 3.41A).
❖ Abscess drainage, toe amputation (Ray amputation), below-knee/above-knee amputations (Figs. 3.42A and B).
❖ Once granulates, the ulcer is covered with skin graft or flap.
❖ Suitable prosthesis to the limb helps the patient to achieve ambulation (Fig. 3.41B).
❖ Patient is prone for *septicemia, ketosis, electrolyte imbalance, silent myocardial infarction* and often all these can be fatal.
❖ *Osteomyelitis* from deeper bone can occur.

The drops of rain make a hole in the stone not by violence, but by oft falling

MELENEY'S ULCER

- It is commonly seen in postoperative wounds in abdomen and chest wall like empyema drainage or after surgery for peritonitis.
- It is common over abdomen and thorax. It begins in wound margin and spreads rapidly. It can also occur in other areas of skin.
- Infection is severe, often with endarteritis of the skin leading to ulcer and destruction.
- It causes severe toxicity and extensive necrosis of the skin and deeper plane, which often needs debridement, antibiotics and later skin grafting.
- Common in old age and immunosuppressed individual.

TRAUMATIC ULCER

- Such ulcer occurs after trauma. It may be *mechanical*—dental ulcer in the margin of the tongue due to tooth injury; *physical* like by electrical burn; *chemical* like by alkali injury.
- Such ulcer is acute, superficial, painful and tender. Secondary infection or poor blood supply of the area makes it chronic and deep.
- *Footballer's ulcer* is a traumatic ulcer occurring over the shin of males due to direct knocks on the shin. It is staphylococcal infection with a chronic and deep ulcer.
- Traumatic ulcers can occur anywhere in the body due to trauma.
- Trauma causes infection, necrosis, fasciitis, crush injury, endarteritis of the skin leading into formation of large/deep non-healing ulcer.
- *Treatment* depends on size and extent of ulcer. Regular dressing, later skin grafting.

ARTERIAL/ISCHEMIC ULCER (FIG. 3.43)

- It is common in toes, feet or legs; often can occur in upper limb digits. It is due to poor blood supply following blockage of the digital or medium sized arteries.
- Atherosclerosis and TAO (thromboangiitis obliterans) are common causes in lower limb.
- Cervical rib, Raynaud's phenomenon and vasculitis are common causes in upper limb.
- Ulcer initially occurs after trauma, soon becomes nonhealing, spreading with scanty granulation tissue.
- Ulcer is very painful, tender and often hyperesthetic. Digits may often be gangrenous. Intermittent claudication, rest pains are common. Other features of ischemia are obvious in the adjacent areas. They are—pallor, dry skin, brittle nail, patchy ulcerations, and loss of hair.
- Ulcer is usually deep, destructs the deep fascia, exposing tendons, muscles and underlying bone. Dead tendons look pale/greenish with pus over it.
- *Management:* Specific investigations like arterial Doppler, angiogram, lipid profile, and blood sugar are done. *Treatment* is done accordingly—drugs like vasodilators; arterial surgeries may be needed.

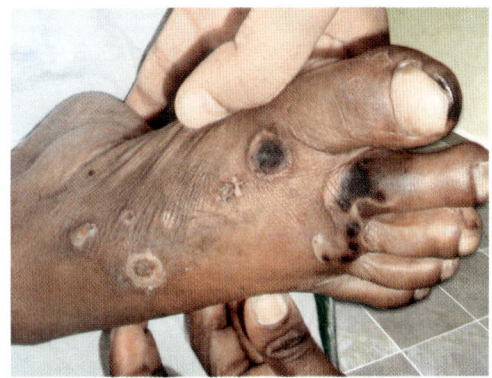

Fig. 3.43: Ischemic ulcer foot and gangrene of toe.

We travel not to find ourselves in the world, but to remember that we have a world inside us

CARCINOMATOUS ULCER (EPITHELIOMA, SQUAMOUS CELL CARCINOMA)

- It arises from prickle cell layer of skin. It may initially begin as a nodule or ulcer; but later forms an ulcerative lesion with *rolled out/everted edge*. Floor contains necrotic content, unhealthy (tumor) granulation tissue and blood (Fig. 3.44).
- Ulcer bleeds on touch and is vascular and friable. *Induration is felt at the base and edge*. It is usually circular or irregular in shape. Initially ulcer is mobile but becomes nonmobile once it infiltrates into deeper tissues. The typical foul smell is due to necrotic material, infection and release of polyamides from the tumor cells.
- *Hard, discrete regional lymph nodes* are often palpable, initially mobile but later become fixed. Lymph nodes can fungate eventually. Ulcer and lymph nodes are initially painless; but becomes painful and tender once there is deeper infiltration or secondary infection. Systemic spread is rare. It is a *locoregional malignant* disease.
- *Verrucous carcinoma* is exophytic, locally malignant well differentiated squamous cell carcinoma without lymphatic spread.
- *Management: Wedge biopsy; FNAC of regional lymph nodes are the investigations.* Treated with wide local excision with skin grafting and regional lymph node block dissection.

MARJOLIN'S ULCER (RENE MARJOLIN, 1828, PARIS)

- It is *slow* growing *locally* malignant lesion—a very well differentiated squamous cell carcinoma occurring in an *unstable scar of long duration*.
- It is commonly seen in chronic venous ulcer scar. Often it is observed in burns scar and scar of previous snake bite. Lesion is ulcerative/proliferative (Fig. 3.45).
- Edge may be everted or may not be. It is painless as scar does not contain nerve fibrils. It *does not* spread into lymphatics as scar is devoid of lymphatics. Induration is felt at the edge and base. There is marked fibrosis also.
- Once lesion spreads into adjacent normal skin, it can spread into regional lymph nodes behaving like squamous cell carcinoma.
- *Managed b*y wedge biopsy and wide local excision and grafting. If large and deep, amputation is needed.

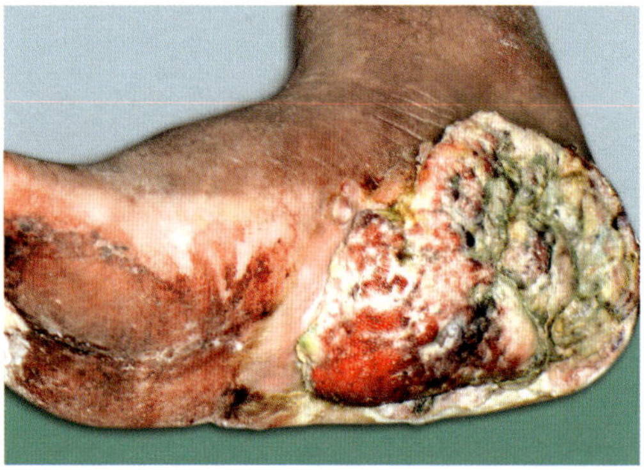

Fig. 3.44: Squamous cell carcinoma heel. It is proliferative ulcer. Note the raised and everted edge.

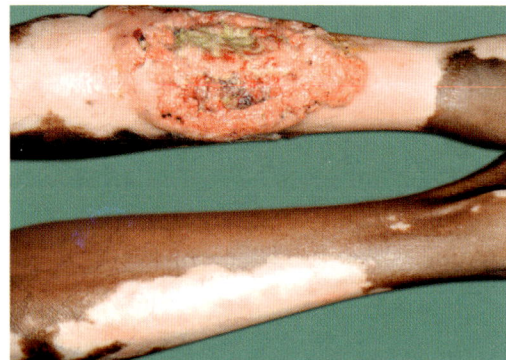

Fig. 3.45: Marjolin's ulcer in a *chronic unstable scar (of long duration)* in the leg. It does not spread through lymphatics.

We travel not to find ourselves in the world, but to remember that we have a world inside us

RODENT ULCER

- It is ulcerative form of basal cell carcinoma, which is common in face with line joining the angle of the mouth to the ear lobule.
- Ulcer shows central area of dry scab with peripheral raised active and *beaded (pearly white)* edge. Often floor is pigmented. It erodes into deeper plane like soft tissues, cartilages and bones hence the name—*rodent ulcer.*
- As lymphatics are blocked early in the disease by large tumor cells, it does not spread to regional lymph nodes. Blood spread is absent. It is only *locally malignant.*
- It is common in face; rarely can it occur over tibia, external genitalia, mucocutaneous junction. It does not occur in mucosa (Fig. 3.46).
- *Management:* Wedge biopsy, CT scan of the part to see the depth, wide excision.

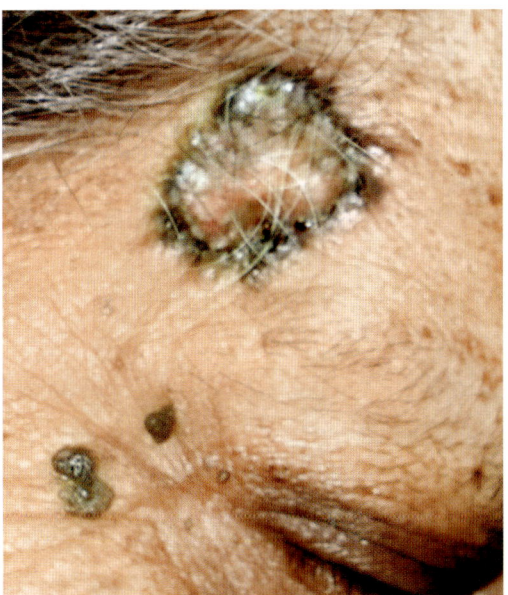

Fig. 3.46: Basal cell carcinoma (BCC/rodent ulcer) face.

MELANOTIC ULCER

- It is ulcerative form of melanoma. It can occur in skin as de novo or in a pre-existing mole. Ulcer is often pigmented with a halo around (Fig. 3.47). *It is the most aggressive skin cancer.*
- Ulcer is rapidly growing, often with satellite nodules and 'in-transit' lesions. It is very aggressive skin tumor arising from melanocytes.
- It spreads rapidly to regional lymph nodes which are pigmented. Blood spread to liver, lungs, brain, and bone is common. It can occur in mucosa, genitalia, and eye. It is a systemic malignant disease.
- *Investigations:* Excision biopsy (usually incision biopsy is not done), FNAC lymph node, US abdomen.
- *Treatment* is wide local excision, regional node block dissection and chemotherapy.

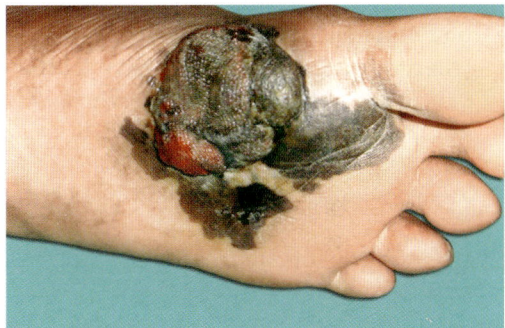

Fig. 3.47: Melanotic ulcer in the foot.

TROPICAL ULCER

- It is endemic in monsoon hit humid tropics with repeated epidemics but sporadic in subtropics. Trauma or insect bite leads into infection exclusively in the lower part of the leg and foot.
- It is an acute ulcerative lesion of the skin observed in tropical regions like Africa, India and South America. It is associated

Judge your success by what you had to give up in order getting it—Dalai Lama

with lower socioeconomic group, anemia, and malnutrition and vitamin deficiency.
- It is commonly caused by *Fusobacterium fusiformis* (vincent's organisms) and *Borrelia vincentii*.
- There are abrasions, redness, papule and pustule formation, acute regional lymphadenitis and severe pain.
- Pustule bursts in 3 days along with necrobiosis and phagedena causing a spreading painful ulcer with an undermined edge, brownish floor and serosanguineous discharge. Spreading stops in few weeks with ulcer persisting for many months to years. Eventually a chronic, large nonhealing/callous ulcer forms with persistent pain, profuse serosanguineous discharge, extremely unpleasant odor, long existing firmly adherent slough in the floor without any obvious constitutional symptoms. During healing it causes a slight pigmented, parchment like round scar.
- Often destruction is progressive without cessation (*phagedena*) to extend into entire soft tissues of foot and leg inviting amputation. **Phagedena** (Greek—to eat) is also seen in chancroid and cancrum oris.
- Occasionally squamous cell carcinoma can develop on it.
- *Treatment*—improvement in nutrition, penicillin, metronidazole, Eusol dressing, skin grafting at a later date.

VENOUS ULCER (GRAVITATIONAL ULCER)

- It is common around ankle (*gaiter's zone*) due to chronic venous hypertension. It is due to *varicose veins* (long saphenous vein/short saphenous vein/perforators) or *postphlebitic* limb.
- Postphlebitic limb consists of veins that is been partially recanalized following deep venous thrombosis, which causes increased venous pressure around ankle through perforators. It is called as **post-thrombotic ulcer**. DVT has to be treated in these patients.
- Varicose veins are common in *females*. 50% of venous ulcer is due to varicose veins; 50% are due to postphlebitic limb (previous DVT). Pain, discomfort, pigmentation, dermatitis, lipodermatosclerosis, ulceration, periostitis, ankle-joint ankylosis, talipes equinovarus deformity and Marjolin's ulcer are the problems of varicose veins and later of venous ulcer (Fig. 3.48).
- Ulcer is initially painful; but once chronicity develops it becomes painless. Ulcer is often vertically *oval*; commonly located on the *medial side*; occasionally on lateral side; often on both sides of the ankle; but *never* above the middle-third of the leg. Floor is covered with pale or often without any granulation tissue. When well granulated, edge is sloping. Induration and tenderness is seen often at the base of an ulcer.
- Inguinal lymph nodes (*vertical* group) are often enlarged. Ulcer often attains very

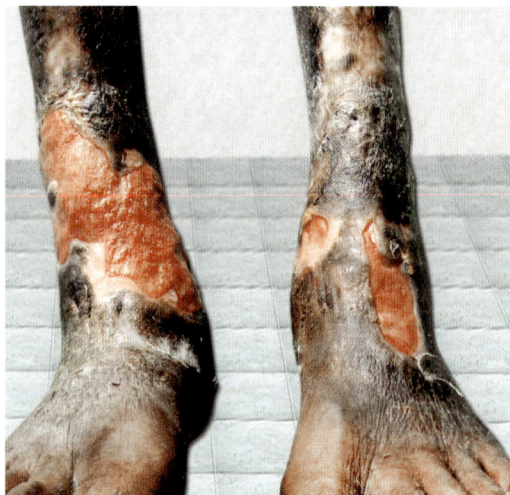

Fig. 3.48: Venous ulcer around ankle with skin changes over surrounding area. It is the commonest site of venous ulcer.

The weak can never forgive. Forgiveness is an attribute of the strong

large size which is nonhealing, indolent and callous.
- Ulcer heals on rest and treatment; but reforms again. Scarring is common due to repeated healing and recurrent ulcer formation. This *unstable scar* of long duration may lead into squamous cell carcinoma (*Marjolin's ulcer*).
- *Management:* Venous Doppler, regular dressing, skin grafting, specific treatment for varicose veins.

TUBERCULOUS ULCER (FIG. 3.49)

- It is due to *Mycobacterium tuberculosis*. It is usually due to cold abscess later forming ulcer in the neck, chest wall, axilla and groin. It can also be primary tuberculosis of the skin (commonly in face). Ulcer can be single or multiple; oval or rounded; *with undermined edge* (due to progression of disease outwards underneath and healing inwards by skin), painful and tender with caseating material on the floor. Ulcer is usually not deep. Regional lymph nodes may be enlarged matted, firm, and nontender.
- *Management:* Discharge study for epithelioid cells (modified histiocytes), AFB; wedge biopsy, antituberculous drugs.

LUPUS VULGARIS

- It is *cutaneous tuberculosis*, which occurs in young age group.
- Commonly seen on face, starts as *typical apple-gelly nodule* with congestion of face around. Eventually ulceration occurs with scarring, necrosis and *undermined edge*.
- Long standing lupus vulgaris can turn into *squamous cell carcinoma.*
- *Investigation:* ESR, discharge study, biopsy, chest X-ray.
- **Treatment:**
  - Antituberculous drugs.
  - If complete healing does not occur, then *excision and skin grafting* is required.

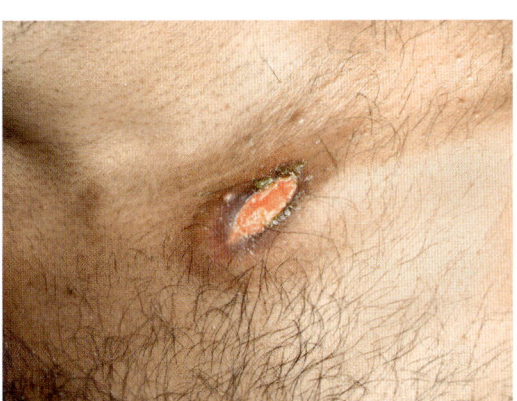

Fig. 3.49: Tuberculous ulcer in the neck. It is typically undermined.

ULCER DUE TO CHILBLAINS

It is due to exposure to intense cold causing blisters, ulceration in the feet. These ulcers are *superficial*. The condition is also called as *perniosis*.

ULCER DUE TO FROSTBITE

- It is due to exposure of the part to wet cold below the freezing point.
- It leads to gangrene of the part. Ulcers, here are always *deep*.

Be yourself; everyone else is taken—Oscar Wilde

CHAPTER 4

Infectious Diseases

Chapter Outline

- Cellulitis
- Lymphangitis
- Erysipelas
- Dangerous Area of Face
- Pyogenic Abscess
- Cold Abscess
- Boil
- Carbuncle
- Pott's Puffy Tumor
- Pyogenic Granuloma
- Pyemia
- Tetanus
- Gas Gangrene
- Tuberculosis
- Leprosy
- Syphilis
- Actinomycosis
- Madura Foot
- Rabies
- Anthrax
- Nosocomial Infection
- Opportunistic Infections
- Necrotizing Fasciitis
- Acute Pyomyositis
- Hepatitis
- HIV Infection and AIDS
- Needle Stick Injury in Surgical Practice
- Gonorrhea
- Surgical Site Infection

CELLULITIS (FIG. 4.1)

It is *spreading inflammation* of subcutaneous tissues and fascial planes. Infection may follow a small scratch or wound or incision or insect/snake/scorpion bites.

- It is more common in patients with diabetes, chronic renal failure, immunosuppressed individuals like patients with HIV infection or on steroid therapy.
- It is common in limbs (lower), face (Fig. 4.1) and perineum and scrotum.

Causative Agents

- Commonly due to *Streptococcus pyogenes* and other Gram +ve organisms.
- Often Gram –ve organisms like *Klebsiella, pseudomonas, E. coli* are also involved (usually Gram –ve organisms cause secondary infection).

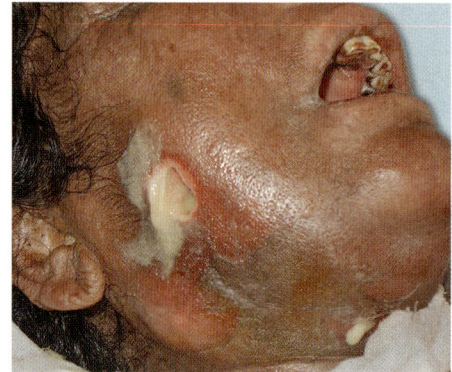

Fig. 4.1: Severe cellulitis face with ulceration and abscess formation.

What the caterpillar calls the end of the world the master calls a butterfly

Sequelae

- Infection can get localized to form **pyogenic abscess**.
- Infection can spread to cause **bacteremia, septicemia, pyemia**.
- Often infection can lead to **local gangrene.**
- Necrotizing fasciitis can occur after *Streptococcus pyogenes* infection.
- Toxic shock syndrome due to release of toxins.

Clinical Features (Fig. 4.2)

- Fever, toxicity (tachycardia, hypotension).
- Swelling is diffuse and spreading in nature.
- Pain and tenderness, red, shiny area with stretched warm skin.
- Cellulitis progresses rapidly in diabetic and immunosuppressed individuals.
- It is diffuse in nature (swelling) without any edge/limit/pus/fluctuation; but often with induration (brawny).
- Tender regional lymph nodes may be palpably enlarged.

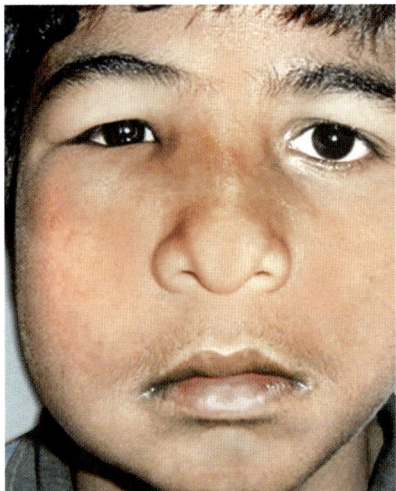

Fig. 4.2: Cellulitis face. Note the diffuse swelling.

Investigations

- Total count raised, differential count, platelet count (decreases) to be done.
- Liver function tests, blood urea and serum creatinine in severe cases.
- Blood sugar estimation, urine test for ketone bodies, glycosylated hemoglobin estimation in diabetic individuals.
- Deep vein thrombosis (DVT) often may mimic cellulitis of lower limb. Venous Doppler and ultrasound of soft tissues of the limb may be required in such situation.

Management

- Elevation of limb or part to reduce edema so as to increase the circulation.
- Antibiotics, penicillins (crystalline penicillin 10 lakh 6th hourly, amoxicillin), quinolones, cephalosporins.
- Dressing (often glycerine magnesium sulphate dressing is used as it reduces the edema because of its hygroscopic action).
- Diabetes to be treated with insulin. Ketosis if present should be confirmed by urine ketone bodies assessment and intravenous insulin.
- Often patient may be in septicemia. Patient in such condition should be treated with higher antibiotics, critical care with fluid management along with maintaining adequate urine output. Catheterization is required; monitoring is done with—renal function tests, hematocrit (platelet count), liver function tests, prothrombin time assay and serum electrolyte estimation.

CELLULITIS OF SPECIAL SITES

Orbital Cellulitis

Cellulitis in orbit causes *proptosis,* leading to impairment of ocular movements and blindness. Infection can spread through ophthalmic veins into cavernous sinus

Persist and persevere, and you will find most things that are attainable, possible.

causing *cavernous sinus thrombosis*. It requires hospitalization and immediate aggressive treatment with higher generation antibiotics (Penicillins, Cephalosporins).

Ludwig's Angina

- It is cellulitis of upper part of the neck involving submandibular region and floor of the mouth along the fascial planes.
- It may be precipitated by tooth extraction, oral cancers, submandibular salivary gland infection, diabetes, chemotherapy, malnutrition (*refer* page 291 and 292 of Chapter 17).

LYMPHANGITIS

- It is an acute *non-suppurative* infection and *spreading* inflammation of lymphatics of skin and subcutaneous tissues due to *beta hemolytic streptococci, staphylococci*, clostridial organisms. It is commonly associated with cellulitis. Erysipelas is a type of lymphangitis.
- In endemic areas, filariasis is the common cause (coastal India). It is caused by *Wuchereria bancrofti*. It is transmitted through bites of *Culex* mosquito. Microfilaria reaches the lymph node forming adult worm which blocks the lymph node causing obstruction, fibrosis and lymphangitis.
- Usually infection occurs following a small trauma with bacterial infectrion. Rapidly warmness and redness develops at the area (Fig. 4.3).

Features

- *Streaky redness* which is spreading, is typical. Area *blanches* on pressure and on release redness reappears.
- Edema of the part, palpable tender *regional lymph nodes* are obvious.
- Fever, tachycardia, features of toxemia.

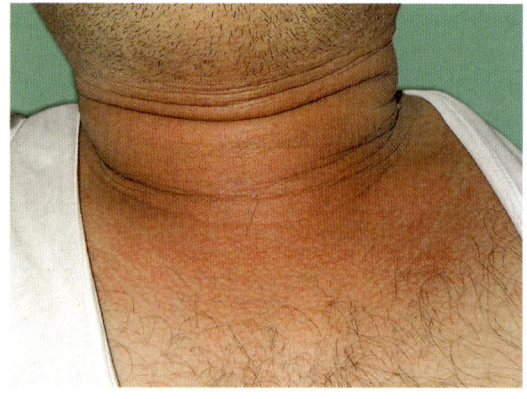

Fig. 4.3: Severe lymphangitis neck.

- Groin lymph nodes are enlarged and tender in *lower limb* lymphangitis (Fig. 4.4). In *upper limb,* as lymphatics are mainly located on the dorsum of hand, edema and redness develops on the dorsum. Infection along the thumb and index finger cause palpable tender axillary nodes; and that along the little and ring fingers causes first tender palpable epitrochlear nodes to appear; infection at middle finger causes deltopectoral nodes to enlarge first.
- Regional lymph nodes (only) may eventually suppurate to form an *abscess*.
- *Toxemia, septicemia* may occur. Rapidity may be more in diabetics and immunosuppressed.
- *Chronic lymphangitis* due to repeated attacks of acute recurrent lymphangitis leads into acquired *lymphedema*.

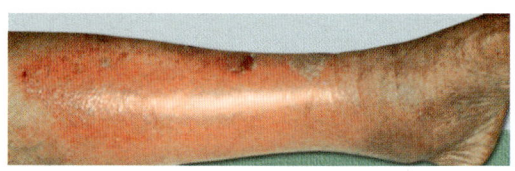

Fig. 4.4: Lymphangitis of the leg. Note typical redness over the lesion.

Success is the ability to go from failure to failure without losing enthusiasm

Management

- *Investigations:* Total and differential count, peripheral smear, serum creatinine, blood culture.
- Antibiotics like penicillin, cloxacillin.
- Elevation, rest, glycerine magnesium sulpha dressing.
- Management of toxemia or septicemia with critical care.

ERYSIPELAS

- It is a *spreading inflammation* of the skin and subcutaneous tissues due to infection caused by *Streptococcus pyogenes*.
- Lesion develops around a skin abrasion or cut leading to cutaneous lymphangitis, with development of *rose pink rash* and cutaneous lymphatic edema. Vesicles form, which eventually ruptures producing serous discharge.
- **Sites:** Orbit; face; scrotum. In the face and orbit, it causes severe edema.
- **Features**
  - *Toxemia* is always a feature.
  - *Rash* is fast spreading and blanches on pressure. It is raised with well demarcated line of advancing margin.
  - *Discharge* is serous *(in cellulitis discharge is purulent)*.
  - **Milian's ear sign** is a clinical sign used to differentiate erysipelas from cellulitis wherein ear lobule is spared. Skin of ear lobule is adherent to the subcutaneous tissue and so cellulitis cannot occur here. Erysipelas being a cutaneous condition can spread into the ear lobule.
  - Disease is common in poorly hygienic debilitated individuals.
- **Treatment:** Penicillin, amoxicillin or cloxacillin.

DANGEROUS AREA OF FACE (FIG. 4.5)

It is in this area, infection from face can spread intracranially causing dangerous cavernous sinus thrombosis.

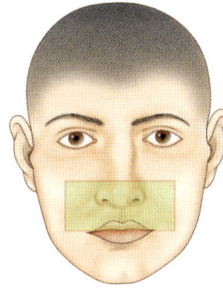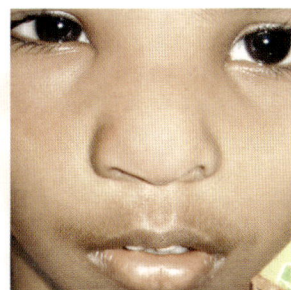

Fig. 4.5: Dangerous area of face—area of upper lip and lower part of nose. Infection from this area spreads through deep facial vein → pterygoid plexus → communicating vein → cavernous sinus causing its life-threatening thrombosis.

PYOGENIC ABSCESS

It is *localized collection* of pus in a cavity lined by granulation tissue, covered by pyogenic membrane. It contains pus in loculi. Pus contains dead WBCs, multiplying bacteria, toxins and necrotic material (Fig. 4.6).

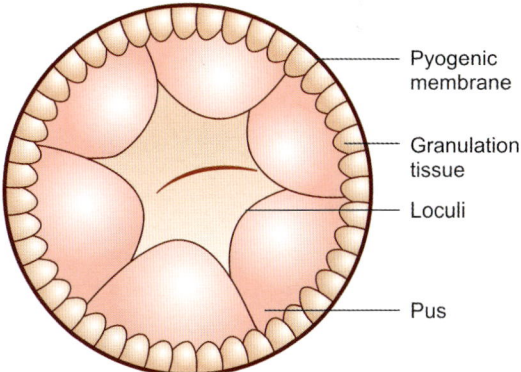

Fig. 4.6: Pyogenic abscess—parts.

Modes of Infection

- Direct.
- Hematogenous.

Learning patience takes a lot of patience!

- Lymphatics.
- Extension from adjacent tissues.

Bacteria Causing Abscess

- *Staphylococcus aureus.*
- *Streptococcus pyogenes.*
- Gram-negative bacteria (*E. coli*, *Pseudomonas*, *Klebsiella*).
- Anaerobes.

Factors Precipitating Abscess Formation

- General condition of the patient: Nutrition, anemia, and age of the patient.
- Associated diseases: Diabetes, human immunodeficiency virus (HIV), immunosuppression.
- Type and virulence of the organism.
- Trauma, hematoma, road traffic accidents.

Clinical Features (Fig. 4.7)

- *Fever* often with chills and rigors.
- *Localized swelling* which is smooth, soft and fluctuant.
- *Visible (pointing) pus.*
- *Throbbing pain* and pointing tenderness.
- *Brawny induration* around.
- *Redness and warmth*, with restricted movement if around a joint.
(Commonly cellulitis occurs first which eventually gets localized to form an abscess).
Visible (pointing) pus, tenderness, fluctuation are the features of *formed abscess.*

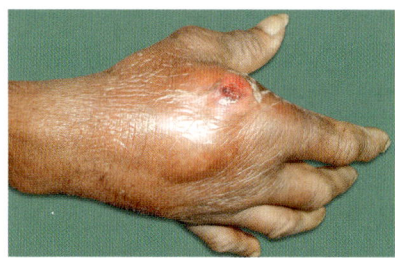

Fig. 4.7: Abscess hand; note the typical features—swelling, redness, pointing pus.

Differences between cellulitis and pyogenic abscess	
Cellulitis	Pyogenic abscess
Diffuse (no edge) and spreading	Well-localized
Pus is not present, only inflammatory fluid	Pus is present
Not fluctuant	Fluctuant
Should not be incised and drained	Should be incised and drained

Sites of Abscess

External Sites (Figs. 4.8 and 4.9)

- Fingers and hand.
- Neck.
- Axilla.
- Breast.
- Foot, thigh—here it is deeply situated with brawny induration.
- Ischiorectal and perianal region.
- Abdominal wall.
- Dental abscess, tonsillar abscess and other abscesses in the oral cavity.

Internal Abscess

- Abdominal: Subphrenic, pelvic, paracolic, amebic liver abscess, pyogenic abscess of liver, splenic abscess, pancreatic abscess.
- Perinephric abscess.
- Retroperitoneal abscess.
- Lung abscess.
- Brain abscess.
- Retropharyngeal abscess.

Investigations

- Total count is raised.
- Urine sugar and blood sugar, to rule out diabetes.
- USG of the part or abdomen or other region when required.
- Chest *X-ray* in case of lung abscess.
- Gallium isotope scan is very useful.

Perfection is the best excuse

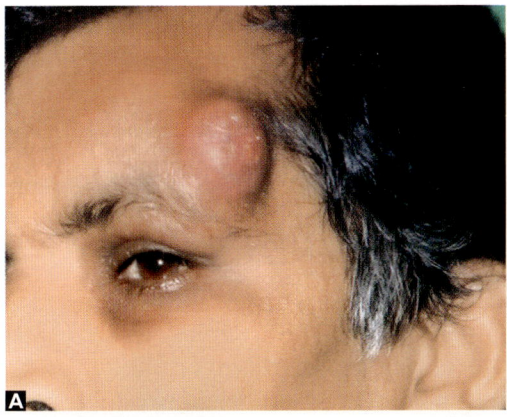
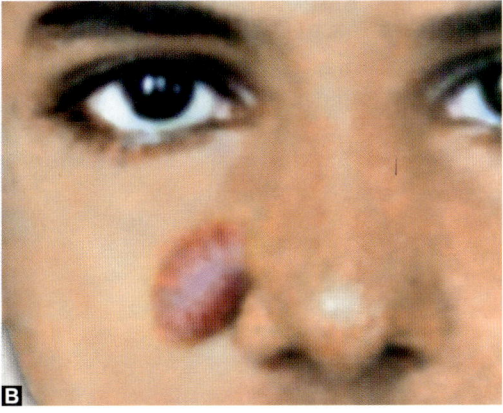

Figs. 4.8A and B: Abscess in the forehead region and face, near right nasolabial groove. Note the well-localized lesion.

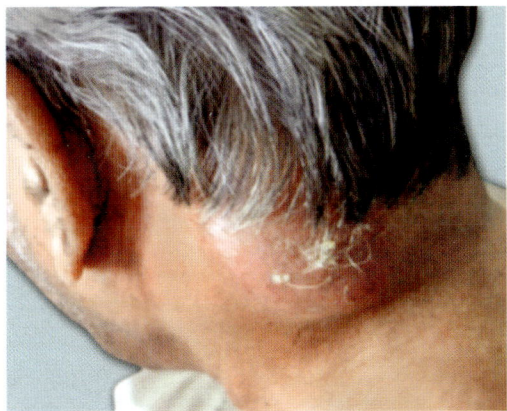

Fig. 4.9: Abscess in suboccipital region, which is a common site in diabetic patient.

- CT scan or MRI in cases of brain and thoracic abscess.
- Investigations relevant to specific types are done: Liver function tests, PO_2 and PCO_2 estimation, blood culture.

Complications of an Abscess

- Bacteremia, septicemia, and pyemia.
- Multiple abscess formation (*Metastatic abscess*).
- Destruction of tissues.
- *Antibioma* (common in breast abscess).
- Sinus and fistula formation.
- Large abscess may erode into adjacent vessels and can cause life-threatening torrential hemorrhage. For example, as in pancreatic abscess.
- Abscess in head and neck region can cause laryngeal edema, stridor and dysphagia.

Specific Complications of Internal Abscess

- Brain abscess can cause intracranial hypertension, epilepsy, and neurological deficit.
- Liver abscess can cause hepatic failure, rupture, and jaundice.
- Lung abscess can lead on to bronchopleural fistula or septicemia or respiratory failure or ARDS.

Treatment of an Abscess

> Abscess should be formed before draining.
> *Exceptions for this rule are:*
> - Parotid abscess.
> - Breast abscess.
> - Axillary abscess.
> - Thigh abscess.
> - Ischiorectal abscess.

Procedure (Figs. 4.10A and B)

- *Hilton's method of draining an abscess* (Fig. 4.11).

Perceive....Conceive....Believe....Achieve!!

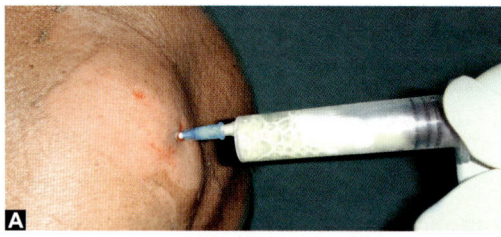

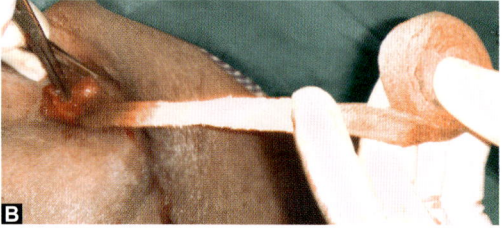

Figs. 4.10A and B: Incision and drainage of pyogenic abscess by Hilton's method. Initial aspiration of abscess is a must; later pack or drain to be placed in the abscess cavity.

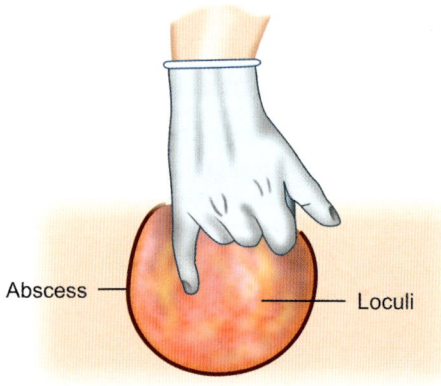

Fig. 4.11: All loculi should be broken with finger or sinus forceps while draining an abscess.

- Initially broad-spectrum antibiotics are started (depending on severity, extent and site of the abscess).
- Under general anesthesia or regional block anesthesia*, after cleaning and draping, abscess is aspirated first and presence of pus is confirmed.
- Skin is incised adequately in the line parallel to the neurovascular bundle, in the most dependent position.
- Next, pyogenic membrane is opened using *sinus forceps*** and all loculi are broken up. Pus is cleared from the abscess cavity and washed with saline.
- A *drain* (either gauze drain or corrugated rubber drain) is placed.
- Wound is *not closed*. Wound is allowed to granulate and heal. Sometimes *secondary suturing or skin grafting* is required.
- Pus is sent for *culture and sensitivity*.
- Antibiotics are continued.
- Treating the *cause* is important.
- Counterincision is necessary in breast abscess and it is placed in upper quadrant.
- Deeper incision is necessary while draining pus in radial and ulnar bursae, palmar spaces and tenosynovitis.

Problems in Drainage

- Improper drainage.
- Bleeding.
- Residual abscess or sinus formation.

Differential Diagnosis for an Abscess

- *Aneurysm,* especially in popliteal, femoral and axillary regions. So aspirating with a needle and confirming the pus is important.
- *Soft tissue tumors*—sarcomas may be smooth, soft and warmer.

Note: Antibioma develops in a pre-existing abscess, if pus not drained and treated only with antibiotics. Here sterile pus is enclosed in a thick fibrous capsule forming a hard lump (common in breast, mimics carcinoma breast).

COLD ABSCESS (TUBERCULOUS ABSCESS)

Cold abscess is common in neck. It can also occur in groin, intercostal space, psoas region,

---

* Local anesthesia is not used as it is not effective, because pus is acidic and local anesthesia will not act.

** Sinus forceps do not have lock and has got serrations in the tip. It is called as sinus forceps because it was initially designed and used to pack sinuses.

Positive attitudes create a chain of positive thoughts

paraspinal region, loin or any site where tuberculous caseating material with *yellowish cheesy* content can get collected and localized.

Sites of Origin

Cold abscess may originate from tuberculosis of spine (thoracic or cervical spines), lymph node, internal organs, bone, etc.

In the neck:

- *Tuberculous lymphadenitis* is common cause. Here cold abscess is commonly seen in *anterior triangle*. It is common in neck; common in upper deep cervical nodes (jugulodigastric—54%); often associated with HIV, lymphoma.
  - In the neck infection begins in tonsils spreading to neck nodes. Infection → lymphadenitis → periadenitis, matting → caseation necrosis → cold abscess formation → collar stud abscess formation → sinus formation.
  - It can be *caseating* (80%, origins from tonsils, matted, poor resistance, drug resistance is common, forms abscess and sinus); *hyperplastic* (20%, blood spread, discrete and firm, no matting, good resistance and response, drug resistance is not common).
  - Nonspecific lymphadenitis, secondaries, branchial cyst, HIV, lymphoma are differential diagnosis.
- *Tuberculosis of cervical spine* is also an important cause. Commonly here cold abscess occurs in *posterior* triangle. Caseating material from the cervical spine collects *in front of* the vertebra behind the prevertebral fascia, which eventually rupture either anteriorly or posteriorly.
  - *Anterior rupture* allows passage of caseating material *below* and behind the prevertebral fascia reaching superior mediastinum; *laterally* behind the prevertebral fascia and carotid sheath to form cold abscess in posterior triangle; in midline upper part, protruding *forwards* from behind the prevertebral fascia in *midline* presenting as chronic retropharyngeal abscess; in midline lower part protrudes into esophagus; caseation runs along the axillary sheath and neurovascular plane to reach axilla and arm to cause cold abscess in axilla and arm/cubital fossa.
  - *Posterior rupture* occurs towards spinal canal facilitating the passage of caseation along the cervical nerves towards posterior triangle and brachial plexus and so axilla and arm.

Features

- It is common in young but can occur in any age group. Equal in both sexes.
- Swelling in the neck, which is smooth, nontender, soft, fluctuant, nontransilluminating, with restricted mobility but is not adherent to skin. Features of acute inflammation is not seen; hence the name—*cold abscess*.
- Neck pain, neck rigidity, restricted cervical spine movements in case of cervical spine tuberculosis. With every change of position and often when patient is seated, he supports his head with his hands and forearm—*Rust's sign* (Jan N Rust, Surgeon, Poland).
- Evening fever, loss of weight and appetite, anemia.
- Features of systemic disease if present like of pulmonary tuberculosis—cough, hemoptysis.
- Matted lymph nodes adjacent to cold abscess may be palpable.
- Oral cavity, tonsils, chest should be examined.

Investigations

- Raised ESR, positive Mantoux test, anemia, lymphocytosis, chest X-ray may show pulmonary tuberculosis, aspiration of cold abscess (FNAC) to see microscopically

Differences between pyogenic abscess and cold abscess	
Pyogenic abscess	**Cold abscess**
Red, warm, tender, with signs of acute inflammation	No signs of acute inflammation
Pyogenic bacteria are nonspecific organisms (Strepto, Staphylo)	Tuberculous bacteria
Dependent incision is used for drainage	Nondependent incision is used
Suturing of the wound is not done	Wound is sutured and curetted
Drain is placed	Drain is not placed (Otherwise sinus will form which is difficult to treat)

epithelioid cells. Acid-fast bacilli may be identified from the aspirated fluid using Ziehl-Neelsen stain.
- X-ray neck in case of tuberculosis cervical spine to identify reduced joint space, vertebral destruction, soft tissue shadow.
- MRI of cervical spine, US/CT scan of neck are needed to confirm the anatomical location, number of lesions.

Sequelae of Cold Abscess
- Secondary infection of the cold abscess—making it tender.
- Formation of collar stud abscess, once pressure increases inside the cold abscess it will give way through the deep fascia to reach the subcutaneous plane to get adherent to skin (Fig. 4.12).
- Sinus formation (Fig. 4.12).
- Spread of disease to multiple lymph nodes and other organs.

Differential Diagnosis
- Branchial cyst and other cystic swellings in neck.
- Secondaries in neck lymph nodes.
- Secondaries in cervical spine.

Treatment
- Antituberculous drugs.
- Nondependent aspiration of the cold abscess.
- Excision of the diseased neck nodes.
- In case of tuberculosis of cervical spine,

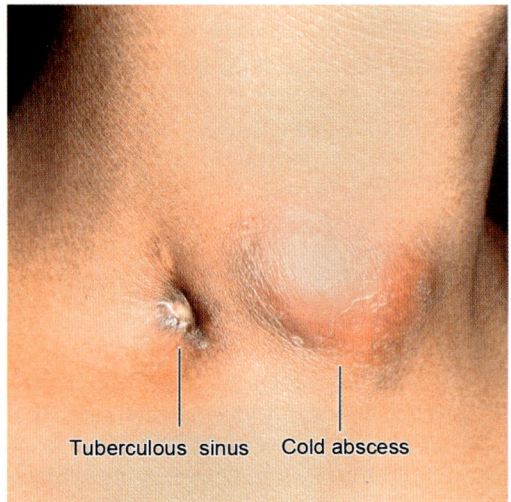

Fig. 4.12: Tuberculous (TB) cold abscess and sinus in the neck.

immobilization of cervical spine by plaster jacket/collar for 4 months. Cervical spine fusion by open surgical method if diseased spine is unstable.

BOIL *(FURUNCLE)* (FIGS. 4.13A AND B)
- It is an *acute staphylococcal infection of a hair follicle with perifolliculitis*, which usually proceeds to suppuration and central necrosis. Often boil opens on its own and subsides.
- Boil or furuncle in external ear is very painful because the skin here is firmly adherent to the perichondrium.
- **Treatment:** Antibiotics; Drainage of boil.

Praise loudly and blame softly

Chapter 4 : Infectious Diseases

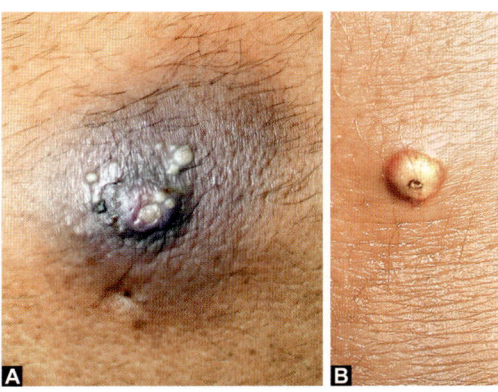

Figs. 4.13A and B: Furuncle/boil is infection of hair follicle with perifolliculitis due to *Staphylococcus aureus*.

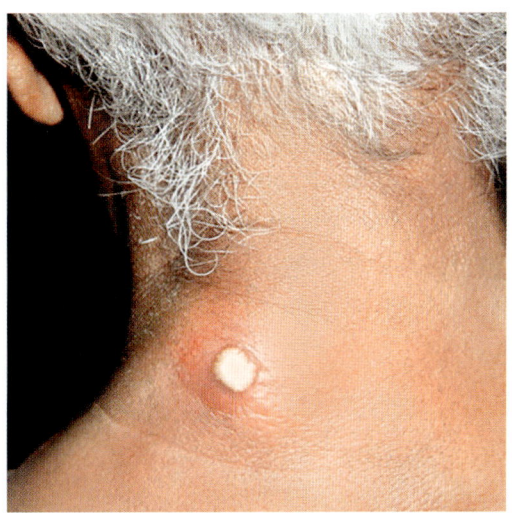

Fig. 4.14: Carbuncle *is an infective gangrene* of skin and subcutaneous tissues. Typical site is nape of the neck.

* **Complications**
  - Cellulitis.
  - Lymphadenitis.
  - Hydradenitis (*Infection of group of hair follicles*).
  - *Cavernous sinus thrombosis* if infection from boil from dangerous area of face extends to cavernous sinuses.

CARBUNCLE

Word meaning carbuncle is charcoal.
* It is *an infective gangrene* of skin and subcutaneous tissue.
* Staphylococcus organism is the main culprit.
* Common site of occurrence is *back and nape of neck* (Fig. 4.14).
* It is common in *diabetics* and after 40 years age.
* It is common in males.
* Patient will be toxic, and in diabetic they are ketotic.
* **Complications:** Extensive necrosis of skin; Septicemia.

Investigations

* Urine sugar and ketone bodies.
* Blood sugar.
* Discharge for culture and sensitivity.

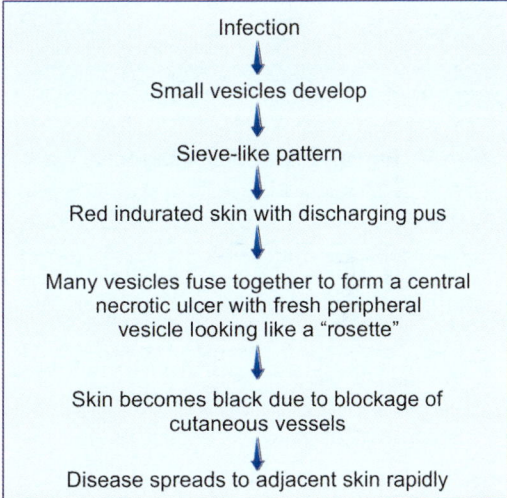

Treatment

* Proper control of diabetes.
* Antibiotics like penicillins, cephalosporins or depending on culture and sensitivity.
* Drainage is done by a *cruciate incision* and debridement of all dead tissues is done. Excision is done later.
* Once wound granulates well, *skin grafting* may be required.

Not in time, place and circumstance, but in man lies success

POTT'S PUFFY TUMOR

- It is formation of diffuse external swelling in the scalp due to *subperiosteal pus formation and scalp edema* (Fig. 4.15).
- It originates commonly in frontal region and may extend into other regions.

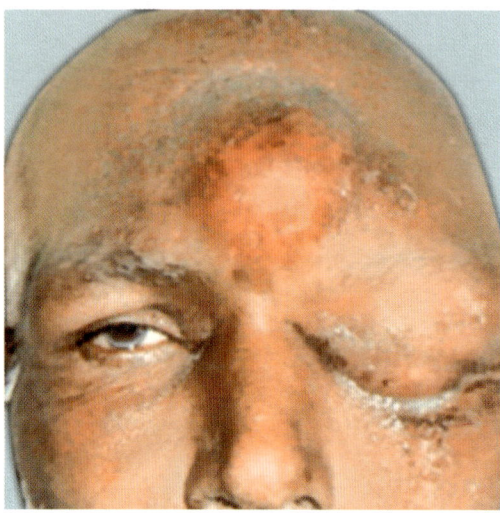

Fig. 4.15: Pott's puffy tumor.

Causes

- Chronic frontal sinusitis which eventually suppurates and extends into subperiosteal region.
- Trauma causing frontal subperiosteal hematoma.
- Chronic otitis media—occasionally.

Clinical Features

- Pain and swelling in frontal region which is warm, tender.
- Toxicity and drowsiness.

Complications

- *Osteomyelitis* of frontal bone.
- Spread of infection into intracranial cavity leading to *intracranial abscess* (extradural or subdural abscess). So may present with features of raised intracranial tension like headache, coning and convulsions.

Investigations

- Total leukocyte count; erythrocyte sedimentation rate (ESR).
- X-ray skull; CT scan.

Differential Diagnosis

Secondaries in skull or in brain.

Treatment

- Antibiotics and drainage under general anesthesia before it spreads into cranial cavity.
- Once it extends into cranial cavity, it is treated accordingly by formal neurosurgical decompression, often using *Dandy's brain cannula*.
- *Osteomyelitic skull bone often needs radical removal with proper reconstruction.*

PYOGENIC GRANULOMA (GRANULOMA PYOGENICUM)

- It is a common condition, which occurs in face, scalp, fingers and toes.
- It may be due to minor trauma or minor infection.
- Infection leads to formation of unhealthy granulation tissue, which protrudes through the wound.
- **Features**
  - Usually single, well-localized, red, firm, nodule, which bleeds on touch (Figs. 4.16A and B).
  - May or may not be tender.
- **Sites:** Face; scalp; fingers; toes.
- **Differential diagnosis:** Hemangioma; papilloma; skin adnexal tumors.
- **Treatment:** Excision; tissue is sent for histopathological study.

Prefer a loss to dishonest gain; the one brings pain at the moment; the other for all the time

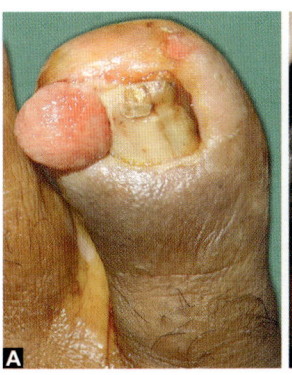 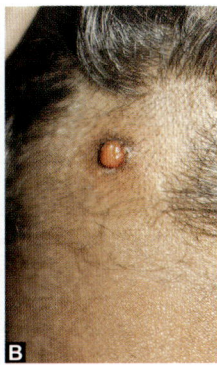

Figs. 4.16A and B: Pyogenic granuloma: (A) Great toe; (B) Scalp.

BACTEREMIA

- It is the presence of bacteria (live) in the blood circulation (sepsis is the host response to bacteria).
- It may be *primary* wherein bacteria are introduced directly into the blood by drug abuse injections, venous catheters or *secondary* wherein bacteria enter blood through some other infection focus like pneumonia, urinary infection, etc.
- Bacteremia may be *transient or intermittent or persistent*. In transient bacteria present in the circulation for only minutes to few hours and gets cleared like in often small procedures and instrumentation. In intermittent type, periodic bacteremia occur—seen in pneumonia or abscess, etc. Persistent is continuous presence of bacteria in blood is seen often in infected heart valve or central line or vessel graft or prosthesis, etc.
- Bacteremia can be *Gram positive or Gram negative*. It is more often seen in meningitis, typhoid, brucellosis, etc. *Risk factors* are HIV, diabetes, transplant, dialysis and immunosuppression.
- *Two blood cultures taken from two separate sites of the body* if show same bacteria it is confirmed bacteremia.

- Condition is treated by effective antibiotic therapy.

SEPTICEMIA

- It is the presence of overwhelming and multiplying bacteria in the blood with toxins causing systemic inflammatory response syndrome (SIRS) or multiorgan dysfunction syndrome (MODS) which later may progress into multiple system organ failure (MSOF). Actually it is sepsis which means body's response to infection eventually causing damage to its own organs. Sepsis is SIRS with infection. Severe sepsis is sepsis syndrome with MODS or MSOF.
- Even though two or more of *SIRS criteria* are used to diagnose sepsis, currently other scoring systems are used. *SOFA score* [Sequential (Sepsis related) Organ Failure Assessment] is ideal using six parameters—respiratory, neurological, cardiovascular, liver, coagulation and renal systems; each having 0,1,2,3,4 scores. *Quick SOFA score* (qSOFA score) is also used based on three parameters—low blood pressure <100 mm Hg; increased respiratory rate >22/minute; altered mentation—GCS <13.
- Septicemia can be Gram positive or Gram negative.
- **Gram positive septicemia** is due to staphylococci, streptococci, pneumococci, etc. infection. It is common in children, old age, diabetes and after splenectomy (*OPSI*—overwhelming post-splenectomy infection).
- **Gram negative septicemia** is common in acute abdomen like peritonitis, abscess, biliary, pancreatic, gastrointestinal or urinary infections, infected wounds and postoperative sepsis. It is commonly seen in malnourished, old age,

immunosuppressed people and diabetics. Common bacteria are *E. coli, Klebsiella, Pseudomonas, Proteus,* etc. Gram negative septicemia causes *endotoxic shock. Initial reversible warm stage* presents with fever, chills and rigors which are due to pyrogenic response; *eventual irreversible cold stage* develops wherein patient goes for complications like acute respiratory distress syndrome (ARDS); renal, liver and multiorgan failure; disseminated intravascular coagulation (DIC); bone marrow suppression (thrombocytopenia).
- **Evaluation of septicemia** is done using clinical assessment; blood parameters (hematocrit, liver and renal function tests, coagulation profile, electrolyte estimation, arterial blood gas analysis, C-reactive protein); culture of urine/pus/discharge/bile/blood; chest X-ray; imaging as per need.
- **Treatment:** Fluid therapy, antibiotics, monitoring (heart rate, respiration, oxygen saturation), urine output (may need to pass Foley's catheter), oxygen supplementation, fresh frozen plasma, or fresh blood transfusion, critical care with ventilator support, electrolyte management. Central venous pressure (CVP) line, parenteral nutrition, management complications (like hemodialysis for renal failure, tracheostomy).

- Jaundice, oliguria, drowsiness.
- Hypotension, peripheral circulatory collapse and later coma with MODS.

Common Causes

- Urinary infection (most common).
- Biliary tract infection.
- Lower respiratory tract infection.
- Abdominal sepsis of any cause.
- Sepsis in diabetic and immunosuppressed individuals like HIV, steroid therapy.

Investigations

- Total leukocyte count.
- Pus; blood; urine culture.
- Blood urea and serum creatinine; liver function test (LFT).

Treatment

- Monitoring of vital parameters.
- Antibiotics (Ceftazidime, Cefoperazone, Ceftriaxone sodium).
- IV fluids, maintenance of urine output.
- Hydrocortisone.
- Blood and plasma transfusion.
- Nasal oxygen, ventilator support, monitoring of pulmonary function.

PYEMIA

It is presence of multiplying bacteria in blood as emboli, which spread and lodge in different organs in the body like liver, lungs, kidneys, spleen, brain causing *metastatic abscess*. This may lead to **Multiorgan Dysfunction Syndrome (MODS)**. It may endanger life if not treated properly.

Clinical Features

- Fever with chills and rigors.

TETANUS

It is an infective condition caused by *Clostridium tetani* organisms leading to reflex muscle spasm, often associated with tonic-clonic convulsions.

Organism

- ***Clostridium tetani*** is a *Gram-positive, anaerobic, motile, noncapsulated,* organism with *peritrichous flagella,* with terminal *spores (Drum stick appearance)*.

Prosperity begins with the state of mind

- Spore is the infective agent. They are found in soil, manure, dust, etc.
- Spore can gain entry through any wound, prick injuries, injuries resulting from road traffic accidents, penetrating injuries, foreign body, anaerobic condition, etc.

Clinical Features

Symptoms

- Jaw stiffness, pain and stiffness in the neck and back muscles.
- Anxiousness, sweating.
- Headache, delirium, sleeplessness.
- Dysphagia; dyspnea.

Signs

- **Trismus**, due to spasm of masseter and pterygoids.
- **Risus sardonicus** (smiling face), due to spasm of the facial muscle—zygomaticus major. Looks as if patient is smiling.
- Neck rigidity.
- Spasm and rigidity of all muscles.
- Hyperreflexia.
- Respiratory changes.
- *Tonic-clonic convulsions*.
- Abdominal wall rigidity often with hematoma formation.
- Severe convulsion may often lead to fractures, joint dislocations and tendon rupture.
- Fever and tachycardia.
- Retention of urine (due to spasm of urinary sphincter), constipation (due to rectal spasm).
- Rarely features of *carditis* are seen due to involvement of the cardiac muscle, which is dangerous, as it often leads to cardiac arrest and death. *Here steroids* are very useful.
- Symptoms will be aggravated by stimuli like light, noise.

Pathogenesis

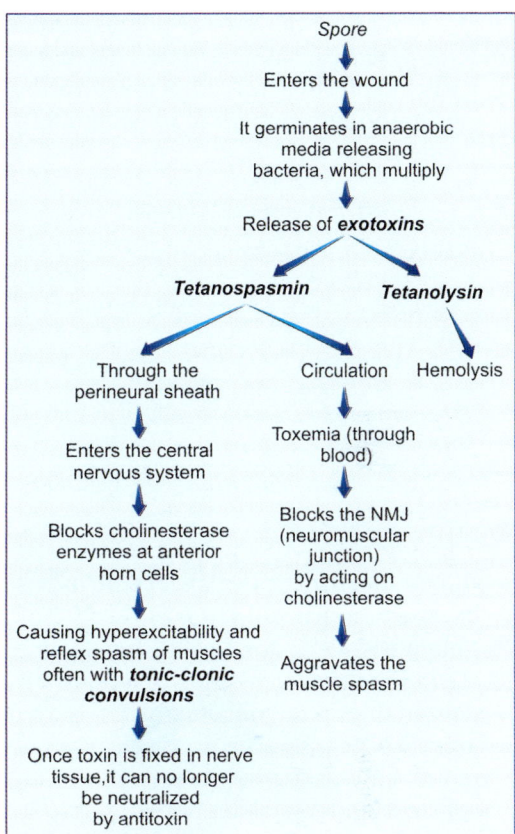

Incubation Period

- Time between the *entry of spore and appearance of first symptom*.
- Usually 7–10 days.
- Shorter the incubation period worser the prognosis and more severe the course of disease.

Period of Onset

- Time between appearance of first symptom and appearance of first sign.

Action, to be effective, must be directed to clearly conceived ends

- Shorter the period of onset worser the prognosis and *vice versa*.

Effects on Respiratory System

Diaphragm and other muscles of respiration undergo spasm causing tachypnea, respiratory distress, respiratory infections, aspiration, cyanosis, and respiratory failure with altered PO_2 and PCO_2 levels.

Different postures in tetanus

- **Opisthotonus**: Posterior muscles are acting more, so *backward bending*.
- **Orthotonus**: *Straight posture*. Both front and back muscles are acting equally.
- **Emprosthotonus**: *Forward bending* as front muscles are acting more.
- **Pleurosthotonus**: *Lateral bending*, as lateral muscles act more.

Types of Tetanus

- ***Early tetanus***: It is a severe form with a short incubation period and poor prognosis.
- ***Latent tetanus***: Wound is healed and forgotten. After a long incubation period, may be years later, under favorable environment, spores release bacteria and cause tetanus. It carries better prognosis.
- ***Late tetanus***: Disease develops many months after injury.
- ***Ascending tetanus:*** Symptoms and signs progress from below upwards.
- ***Descending tetanus***: Symptoms and signs progress from above downwards.
- ***Cephalic tetanus:*** Facial muscles are involved first (3rd, 4th, 6th and 7th cranial nerves can get involved).
- ***Localized tetanus***.
- ***Bulbar tetanus***: Muscles of deglutition and respiration are involved. Highly fatal.
- ***Tetanus neonatorum***: Tetanus occurring in neonates. Spread is through umbilical cord.
- ***Urban tetanus***. Due to repeated injections in IV drug abusers.

Staging of tetanus

- **Mildly ill**: Rigidity, spasm, trismus and different postures.
- **Seriously ill**: Spasm, rigidity, severe respiratory infections.
- **Dangerously ill**: Cyanosis *with respiratory failure and tonic-clonic convulsions.*

Differential Diagnosis

- Strychnine poisoning.
- Trismus due to other causes like—dental, oral, tonsillar sepsis, oral malignancy.
- Meningitis.
- Hydrophobia.
- Convulsive disorders.

Culture media for *Clostridium tetani* are RCM media and nutrient agar.

Treatment

- Patient is admitted and isolated in a dark, quiet room.
- Antitetanus globulin (ATG), 3000/units IM stat. Test dose is not required (it is human immunoglobulin).
  [Antitetanus serum (ATS). When ATG is not available or when patient cannot afford it, as it is expensive ATS is given. After *IV test dose (1000 units of ATS)*, full dose of ATS, i.e. 1, 00,000 units, half of it IM and half of it IV, is given. It is a horse serum, and so possibility of anaphylactic reactions should be kept in mind].
- Wound debridement, drainage of pus, injection of ATG 250–500 units locally to reduce the toxin effect.
- Ryle's tube is passed, initially to decompress, and so as to prevent aspiration, but later for feeding purpose.
- Catheterization.
- IV fluids and electrolyte balance has to be maintained.

The secret of happiness is to admire without desiring

- **Tetanus toxoid** should be given as disease will not give immunity against further infections. To start—first dose; second dose after one month, third dose after 6 months.
- Intravenous (IV) Diazepam 20 mg 4th or 6th hourly. Dose is adjusted depending on severity and convulsions.
- IV Phenobarbitone 30 mg 6th hourly.
- IV Chlorpromazine 25 mg 6th hourly.
- Injection crystalline penicillin 20 lacs 6th hourly, injection gentamicin and metronidazole to prevent secondary infection.
- Regular suction and clearance of respiratory tract.
- Nasal oxygen.
- In *severe cases,* patient is *curarised and placed in ventilator (IPPR).*
- *Endotracheal intubation or tracheostomy* are often *life saving.*
- **Good nursing care**—change of position, prevention of bedsores, prevention of DVT (which is common in tetanus and often requires heparin injection).
- Chest (respiratory) physiotherapy during recovery period.
- *Steroids to be given* when carditis is suspected.
- *Following treatment, patient often gets spasm of different muscles (**ticks**) for a long period of time which can be prevented by giving Methocarbamol for 6 months to one year.*

GAS GANGRENE

It is an infective gangrene caused by clostridial organisms involving mainly skeletal muscle. Earlier, it was called as **malignant edema**.

Organisms

- *Clostridium Welchii (perfringens)*: Gram-positive, central spore bearing, nonmotile, capsulated organisms.
- *Clostridium oedematiens.*
- *Clostridium septicum.*
- *Clostridium histolyticus.*

Clostridium Welchii produce toxins:
- Alpha (commonest): Beta; Epsilon; Iota.
- Various *strains* include—A,B,C,D,E.
- 'A' strain is commonest.

Exotoxins

- **Lecithinase** is important toxin, which is hemolytic, membranolytic and necrotic causing *extensive myositis.*
- **Hemolysin** causes extensive hemolysis.
- **Hyaluronidase** helps in rapid spread of gas gangrene.
- **Proteinase** causes breaking down of proteins in the infected tissue.

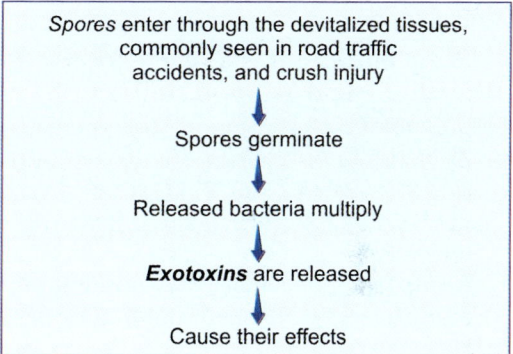

Effects

- Extensive necrosis of muscle with production of H_2S gas, which stains brown or black.
- Usually involves muscle from origin to insertion.
- Often may extend into thoracic and abdominal muscles.
- When it affects the liver it causes necrosis with frothy blood—**foaming liver**, is characteristic.

The fool is never satisfied while the wise man finds wealth in contentment

Clinical Features (Fig. 4.17)

Incubation period is 1–2 days.
- Features of toxemia, fever, tachycardia, pallor.
- Wound is under tension with foul smelling discharge.
- *Khaki brown* colored skin due to hemolysis.
- *Crepitus* can be felt.
- Jaundice may be *ominous sign* and oliguria *signifies renal failure*.

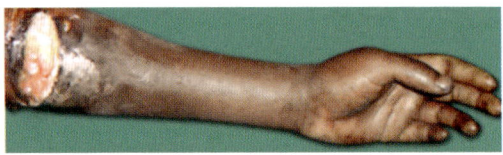

Fig. 4.17: Gas gangrene of forearm and hand after an axe injury. Patient underwent above-elbow amputation and survived.

Clinical Types

- **Fulminant type**—causes rapid progress and often death due to toxemia, renal failure or liver failure or MODS.
- **Massive type**—infection involving whole of one limb containing dark colored gas filled areas.
- **Group type**—infection involving one group of muscles. Extensors of thigh, flexors of leg.
- **Single muscle type**—affecting one single muscle.
- **Subcutaneous type**—of gas gangrene involves only subcutaneous tissues (i.e. superficial involvement).

Investigations

- X-ray shows *gas in muscle plane* or under the skin.
- Liver function tests, blood urea, serum creatinine, total count, PO_2, PCO_2.

Treatment

- Injection Benzyl penicillin 20 lacs 4th hourly + Injection Metronidazole 500 mg 8th hourly + Injection Aminoglycosides (if blood urea is normal).
- **Fresh blood transfusion**.
- **Polyvalent antiserum** 25,000/units given intravenously after a test dose and repeated after 6 hours.
- **Hyperbaric oxygen** is very useful.
- Liberal incisions are given. All dead tissues are **excised** and **debridement** is done until healthy tissue bleeds.
- Rehydration and maintaining optimum urine output (30 mL/hour) {0.5 mL/kg/hour}.
- Electrolyte management.
- In severe *cases amputation* has to be done as a *life-saving procedure*.
- Often ventilator support is required.
- *Once a ward or operation theater is used for a patient with gas gangrene, it should be fumigated for 24–48 hours properly to prevent the risk of spread of infection to other patients.*

TUBERCULOSIS (FIG. 4.18)

It is commonly caused by *Mycobacterium tuberculosis*; occasionally by *Mycobacterium bovis, M. kansasii, M. fortuitum, M. marinum, M. ulcerans*.

M. tuberculosis is *gram neutral, acid-fast and alcohol-fast*, straight or slightly curved rod.

It is prevalent in most of the developing countries and has made its resurgence in the developed countries with the advent of AIDS.

Pathogenesis

The characteristic lesion here is *'tubercle,'* which is an avascular granuloma composed of a central zone containing giant cells, with

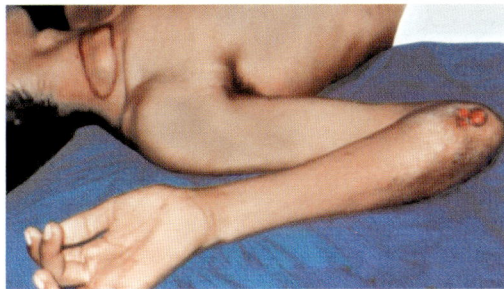

Fig. 4.18: Tuberculous lymphadenitis with tuberculous ulcer.

or without caseation necrosis, surrounded by a rim of **epithelioid cells**, lymphocytes and fibroblasts.

It can occur in almost all organs in the body. Presentation may vary depending on the individual sites.

General Features

- Low-grade fever with evening rise of temperature.
- Loss of appetite and weight loss.

Investigations

- ESR is raised; peripheral smear—lymphocytosis.
- Acid-fast bacillus (AFB) staining using Ziehl-Neelsen stain.
- Chest X-ray to rule out pulmonary tuberculosis.
- Culture of the organism—Löwenstein-Jensen media.
- Mantoux skin test.
- Guinea pig inoculation.
- Relevant investigations depending on the site of the tuberculosis.

Treatment

- Antituberculous drugs are given for 6 months to one year.
- Specific treatment is given depending on the site of the tuberculosis.

LEPROSY (HANSEN'S DISEASE)

It is caused by *Mycobacterium leprae*. It is a Gram-positive, acid-fast bacillus.

It mainly involves *skin, nasal mucosa and peripheral neural tissues.*

It involves only the cooler parts of the body (so axilla, gluteal region are not involved). Testicular involvement is seen but not the ovary. It does not involve the vital organs. Though not acutely fatal, the disease leaves the victim severely deformed and crippled for life.

Types

Multibacillary types
- *Lepromatous leprosy:* Denotes little or no host resistance. Bacilli are seen in large numbers in the superficial nodular lesions and the patient is highly infective.
- Borderline lepromatous.

Paucibacillary types
- Borderline tuberculoid.
- *Tuberculoid leprosy:* Here strong host resistance is observed. The disease is more localized, but it causes more deformities due to early involvement of nerves. Bacilli are scanty in the lesion and so infectivity is minimal.

Investigations

- Regular checking of sensation of the suspected area.
- Split skin smear from lesion or ear lobule.
- Nerve biopsy—sural nerve.

Treatment

- Dapsone 100 mg daily.

*The big lesson in life, baby, is never be scared of anyone or anything—***Frank Sinatra**

- Rifampicin 600 mg once a month.
- Clofazimine 50 mg daily + 300 mg once a month.
- For paucibacillary types treatment is for 6 months.
- For multibacillary types treatment is for 2 years or more.

Surgical Complications in Leprosy

Primary deformities
- *Leonine facies;* multiple facial nodules.
- Collapsed nasal bridge.
- Upper branch facial nerve palsy (causes lagophthalmos).
- Lateral madarosis.
- Keratitis and blindness.
- *Claw hand* either ulnar or combined ulnar and median nerves.
- Radial nerve palsy—*wrist drop* (1%).
- Clawing of toes due to involvement of posterior tibial nerve.
- *Foot drop* due to involvement of lateral popliteal nerve.
  (Medial popliteal nerve, which supplies the tibialis posterior nerve is never involved).

Secondary deformities
- Anesthesia of the part makes it prone to trauma, infection, infective gangrene, destruction, autoamputation and functionless parts.
- Trophic ulcers in the foot are common.

Treatment
Reconstructive surgeries:
- Release of contractures.
- Tendon transfers—Paul Brand's or Stye Bunnel's procedure.
- Arthrodesis.
- Ulcer management.
- Physiotherapy and rehabilitation.

SYPHILIS
(GREAT POX, FRENCH DISEASE)

It is a venereal infection caused by *Treponema pallidum*—spirochaetes.

- **Early syphilis:**
  It lasts for 2 years and the patient is infective during this period.
- **Primary syphilis:**
  It presents as a *'Hunterian chancre.'* It is a shallow, painless, indurated, non-bleeding ulcer usually seen in the genitalia and often on the lips. It occurs in 3–4 weeks after the infection. Lymph nodes are enlarged nontender, discrete, shotty. It is confirmed by dark field microscopic study of the discharge for the organism.
- **Secondary syphilis:** It occurs in 6–12 weeks.
  It presents as:
  - Cutaneous coppery rashes.
  - Snail-track oral ulcers.
  - Fleshy warty lesion in genitalia (condyloma lata).
  - Painless, shotty lymphadenopathy (generalized).
  - Moth eaten alopecia.
  - Hepatitis, arthritis, iritis.
  - Syphilitic osteitis with *'ivory'* sequestrum.
  - Meningitis.
- **Latent syphilis:**
  Untreated early syphilis progress to this next phase. It lasts between 2 years to life time. Serum tests are positive.
  As organisms are seen in lesions of early syphilis and early latent syphilis patient is infective in this period but not in late latent ant late syphilis.

Late (tertiary) syphilis:
- Here vasculitis and obliterative endarteritis occurs.

Always forgive your enemies; nothing annoys them so much—Oscar Wilde

- Painless, punched out, *gummatous ulcers* are seen with *'wash leather base' and silvery tissue paper scar*. Seen in posterior 1/3rd of tongue and sternoclavicular joint. It is a hypersensitivity reaction.
- Develops in 5–15 years.
- *Neurosyphilis.*
- *Cardiovascular syphilis*—dissecting thoracic aortic aneurysm is common.

Investigations

- VDRL test; Kahn test.
- *Treponema pallidum* hemagglutination test (TPHA).
- *Treponema pallidum* immobilization test (TPI).

Treatment

- Penicillin for 15 days is the drug of choice.
- Doxycycline 100 mg can be given thrice daily for 15 days.
- Others: Erythromycin, Tetracycline, Cephalosporins.

Jarisch-Herxheimer reaction is commonly seen after penicillin, which often requires steroid therapy.

CONGENITAL SYPHILIS

Here the infection is transmitted from the mother to fetus through placenta.

Early congenital syphilis:
It is seen in newborn.
Features are:
- Rash, syphilitic snuffles.
- Nasal discharge, weight loss.
- Periostitis, meningitis, hepatosplenomegaly.
- Pneumonia alba.

Late congenital syphilis:

Hutchinson's triad
• Interstitial keratitis. • 8th nerve deafness. • Hutchinson's teeth: Peg-shaped upper incisors, Moon's molar, molars with cusps.

- Hutchinson's triad.
- Congenital neurosyphilis.
- Cutaneous, skeletal or visceral gummas.
- Saddle nose.
- Sabre tibia, Clutton's joint.
- Perforated palate.

Congenital syphilis is treated with penicillins.

ACTINOMYCOSIS

It is caused by *Actinomyces israelii*. It is an anaerobic Gram-positive *fungal like bacterium*, which is a branching filamentous organism. It is called as *'Ray fungus'* because of *sun-ray* appearance. It is present in normal oral flora, may invade the tissues in the presence of *carious teeth* or trauma or poor oral hygiene.

Clinical Types

- **Faciocervical**

Commonest type, lower jaw is more commonly involved. Infection is either from tonsil or from adjacent infected tooth following trauma. Initially an induration develops in the gums. Nodules form with involvement of skin of face and neck. It softens and bursts through the skin forming multiple tortuous *sinuses* which discharge *pus containing sulfur granules (60%).*

Cervical lymph nodes not enlarged.

Differential Diagnosis
Carcinoma in floor of mouth, jaw tumor, osteomyelitis of mandible.

❖ **Thoracic**

Lungs and pleura get infected by direct spread from pharynx or by aspiration. Empyema develops. Later nodules appear over the chest wall leading to discharging sinuses (20%).

❖ **Abdominal**

In right iliac fossa, it presents as a *mass abdomen* with discharging sinus. From the intestine organisms migrate across bowel wall into the pericecal region causing inflammatory reaction and later gets adhered to the anterior abdominal wall causing multiple discharging sinuses in right iliac fossa.

Liver is infected through portal vein from right iliac fossa. Liver is destroyed with multiple abscesses (honeycomb liver).

Pathogenesis

Organism enters through deeper plane of the tissue, causes subacute inflammation with induration and nodule formation. Eventually discharging sinus forms at the surface. Pus collected in a swab or sterile tube will show *sulfur granules*.

Clinical Features

- *Discharging sinus* with induration and nodules.
- *No lymph nodal involvement*.
- Through blood it may cause pyemia and endanger life.

Investigations

- Pus under microscopy shows branching filaments.
- **Gram's staining** shows *Gram-positive mycelia in center* with *Gram-negative radiating peripheral filaments*. These clubs are due to host reaction, which are lipoid material.
- Cultured in brain heart infusion agar and thioglycolate media.

Differential Diagnosis

- Chronic pyogenic osteomyelitis.
- Carcinomas at the site.
- Tuberculous disease.

Treatment

- Injection Crystalline penicillins 10 lacs/day/long-acting penicillins for longer period (6–12 months).
- Tetracyclines and Lincomycin.
- Dapsone and iodides.
- Surgical debridement is occasionally required.

MADURA FOOT *(MYCETOMA PEDIS)*

- It is a chronic granulomatous condition of the foot causing multiple discharging sinuses in the foot (Fig. 4.19).
- It was first identified in *Madurai by Gill*.
- It is common in India and Africa.
- It is common in Tamil Nadu.

Organisms

- *Nocardia madurae* (commonest).
- *Nocardia brasiliensis*.
- *Nocardia asteroides*.
- *Actinomyces israelii*.

Pathogenesis

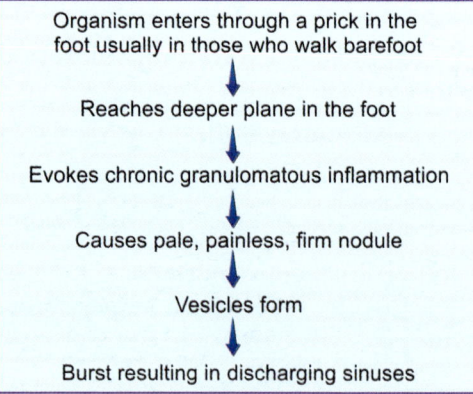

*Life isn't about finding yourself. Life is about creating yourself—**George Bernard Shaw***

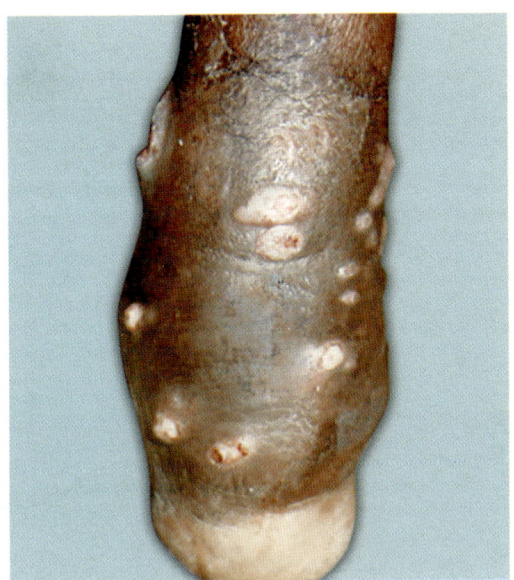

Fig. 4.19: Madura foot. Note the multiple sinuses.

- *Discharging granules* may be *black, red, yellow*.
- In *black type* of Madura foot, infection is mainly subcutaneous.
- In *red and yellow types*, it burrows into the deeper plane including the underlying bone causing bone necrosis (osteomyelitis). Eventually gross swelling of the limb with multiple discharging sinuses with disability occurs.
- Muscles and bones are involved.
- Tendons and nerves are affected.
- Regional lymph nodes are *not involved*.
- Condition deteriorates by secondary bacterial infection.

Clinical Features

- Painless diffuse swelling in the foot of long duration.
- Later multiple discharging sinuses develop in the skin.
- Lymph node involvement will not occur unless there is secondary bacterial infection.
- Significant limb disability is common.

Differential Diagnosis

- Chronic osteomyelitis.
- Tuberculous osteomyelitis.
- Carcinoma.

Investigations

- Discharge study shows branching filamentous appearance **of the organism**.
- Culture in Sabourad's dextrose agar medium.
- Gram stain for actinomycosis shows *sun-ray appearance* with Gram +ve center and Gram –ve clubs.
- X-ray of the foot to look for osteomyelitis.
- FNAC and biopsy is confirmatory.
- USG/MRI are useful.

Treatment

- Antifungal drugs—Amphotericin.
- Long-term penicillins.
- Dapsone.
- Iodides.
- In severe cases amputation may be required.

If infection occurs in the hand it is called as **Madura hand**.

RABIES *(HYDROPHOBIA)*

It is an acute fatal encephalomyelitis caused by *Lyssavirus type 1*.

It is rare in developed countries. It is common in developing countries. It is common in India.

Pathogenesis

- It is commonly due to dog bite. Other animals, which often can cause rabies are cat, jackal, wolf, bat, mongoose, monkey, horse, sheep, goat.
- Transmission is through saliva of the animals. It is commonly through bite or lick.

*Success is how high you bounce when you hit bottom—**George S Patton***

- Asymptomatic carrier stage can occur in animals but they are unlikely to be infective during carrier stage.
- It is considered that only symptomatic animals are infective.
- Street virus of the Lyssavirus type 1 is the infective one (Fixed virus is noninfective and is used for vaccine).
- Virus passes through the peripheral nerve into the central nervous system and develops **Negri bodies** in the brain leading to **fatal encephalomyelitis**.
- It also involves the salivary glands to get secreted in the saliva to cause infection.

Clinical Features

- Incubation period is 3–6 weeks.
- Prodromal symptoms like fever, headache.
- Hyperexcitability and irritability.
- Hydrophobia (fear of water).
- Aerophobia (fear of air).
- Mental instability.
- Once disease starts, patient dies in 72 hours.

Fear of water is seen only in affected human beings not in animals.

Prophylaxis

Postexposure prophylaxis
- The wound is cleaned initially with running water and soap for 5 minutes, and later with povidone iodine or alcohol (40–70%).
- Suturing of the wound should not be done. Because suturing hastens the spread of virus into the deeper plane.
- Local application of antirabies serum into the wound at the earliest is effective in reducing the infection rate.
- Antibiotics: The dog is observed for 10 days. If dog shows symptoms then antirabies vaccine is advised.
- Vaccination: Antirabies serum.

Classification of Wounds

Class I: Touching the diseased animal, lick over intact skin or scratches without oozing of blood.

Class II: Licks on broken skin, scratches with blood ooze, all bites except head, face, palm and fingers. Minor wounds less than five in number.

Class III: All bites over head, face, palm and fingers. Lacerated wounds, wounds more than five in number, wild animal bites.

Indications for antirabies vaccination
• All rabid animal bites.
• If animal is killed or dies during 10 days of observation period.
• Bite by an unidentified animal.
• If laboratory tests in animal show positive for rabies.
• All wild animal bites.

Vaccines for Rabies

Active Immunization

1. **BPL inactivated vaccine**: It is nervous tissue vaccine.

It is 5% emulsion of the infected brain of the sheep containing the inactivated fixed virus.

	Dosage (as recommended by Pasteur Institute, Coonoor)		
	Adult	Children	
Class I	2 mL	1 mL	7 days.
Class II	3 mL	3 mL	10 days.
Class III	5 mL	3 mL	10 days.

Mode of administration: Into the abdominal wall, subcutaneously using long needle.

Antibody develops in 7–30 days. Protection lasts only for 6 months.

Booster doses are given when used along with antirabies serum.

Side effects
- Headache, palpitation, allergic reactions.

*All that we see and seem is but a dream within a dream—**Edgar Allan Poe***

- Redness, tenderness and swelling at the site of the vaccination.
- *Post-vaccinal neuroparalysis*—a dangerous life-threatening complication.
- During therapy patient *should avoid alcohol and steroids.*

2. Nervous tissue vaccine derived from suckling mouse brain.

3. Duck embryo vaccine (DEV) has got less neuroparalytic side effects. It is not available in India.

4. **Cell culture vaccines**: They are more potent and safer.

Human diploid cell vaccine (HDCV): Safest vaccine. But it is costly. It is available in India.

Second-generation tissue culture vaccines: They are potent and cost effective. They are derived from nonhuman base sources. Examples are chick embryo fibroblast, fetal bovine kidney, hamster kidney cells, vero cells.

Dosage: 2.5 IU in one mL. One mL is given daily IM into the deltoid on 0, 3, 7, 14, 28 and 90 (optional) days.

Side effects: Headache, redness at the site, fever. No other serious side effects.

Second generation tissue culture vaccine can also be given intradermally. Intradermal dose is one fifth of the intramuscular dose (0.1 mL).

Passive Immunity/Immunization

It is used in all severe exposures and in all wild animal exposure.

Types

Horse antirabies serum (ARS): It is given on first day with a dose of 40 IU/kg body weight (maximum up to 3000/units). Half is given into the wound and another half given into the gluteal muscle (IM). Single dose.

Human rabies immunoglobulin (HRIG): Dose is 20 units/kg body weight. Part is injected into the wound remaining part into the muscle (IM). Single dose.

Patient should be immunized actively along with serum with additional booster doses.

Side effects: Serum sickness, anaphylaxis.

Pre-exposure prophylaxis is given to veterinarians, animal handlers.

Dose: 1 mL of cell culture vaccine IM or 0.1 mL intradermally on 0, 7, 28 days.

Booster doses are given once in every 2 years.

Post-exposure vaccination is done if individual has been vaccinated earlier: Doses on 0, 3, and 7 days are given. Passive immunity is not given in individuals who had vaccination earlier.

IMMUNIZATION IN ANIMALS

- BPL inactivated nervous tissue vaccine: Single dose 5 mL to dogs. 3 mL to cats. Second dose after 6 months. Then once a year regularly.
- Modified live virus vaccine: Dose—3 mL single dose which is repeated once in 3 years.
- Control of stray dogs and immunization of all dogs will reduce the incidence of rabies.

ANTHRAX

- It is caused by *Bacillus anthracis*, which is a *Gram-positive,* aerobic, spore forming, capsulated, nonmotile, nonacid-fast bacillus. It is *resistant to heat and antiseptics*.
- Disease is common in cattle and seen in people who handle animal hides carcasses, wool, and hairs.
- It is often used in *biological war.*

Types

1. **Cutaneous type**
   - It is the commonest type and occurs within 3–4 days after infection, seen in face, hands and forearm.

If you want to live a happy life, tie it to a goal, not to people or things—**Albert Einstein**

- Indurated papule with black slough surrounded by vesicles—***malignant pustule.*** Pus and pain are absent. Itching is common in papule.
- Regional lymph nodes are involved.
- ***Toxemia*** is common.
2. **Woolsorter's disease**
   - It is respiratory type, and is due to inhalation of spores causing *pneumonia*. It is more dangerous and life-threatening.
3. **Alimentary type**
   - It is due to ingestion of spores.

Diagnosis

Culture of fluid shows *medusa head appearance*. It shows positive M'Fadyean reaction and positive Ascoli's thermoprecipitation test.

Treatment

- ***Penicillins***—drug of choice.
- Ciprofloxacillin.

NOSOCOMIAL INFECTION (HOSPITAL-ACQUIRED INFECTION)

It is an infection acquired because of *hospital stay*.

Sources

- Contaminated infected wounds.
- Urinary tract infections.
- Respiratory tract infections.
- Opportunistic infection.
- Abdominal wounds with severe sepsis.

Spread can occur from one patient to another, through nurses or hospital staff who fail to practice strict asepsis.

It is **more common** in:
- Diabetics.
- Immunosuppressed individuals.

- Patients on steroid therapy and life-supporting machines.
- Instrumentations (indwelling catheter, IV cannula, tracheostomy tube).
- Patients with artificial prosthesis.

Organisms

- *Staphylococcus aureus* is the commonest organism causing wound infection. Others are *Pseudomonas, Klebsiella, E. coli, Proteus*.
- *Streptococcus pneumoniae, Haemophilus, Herpes, Varicella, Aspergillus, Pneumocystis carinii* are the commonest pathogens involved in respiratory tract infection, which spreads through droplets.
- *Klebsiella* is the commonest pathogen involved in hospital-acquired urinary tract infection (UTI), which is highly resistant to drugs.

Management

Most of the time, organisms involved are *multidrug resistant, virulent* and hence, cause *severe sepsis*.
- Antibiotics.
- Isolation.
- Blood, urine, pus for culture and sensitivity to isolate the organisms.
- Blood transfusion, plasma or albumin therapy.
- Ventilator support.
- Maintaining optimum urine output.
- Nutritional support.

Prevention

- Isolation of patients with badly infected open wounds, severe RTI/UTI.
- Following strict aseptic measures in OT and in ward by hospital attendents.
- Proper cleaning and use of disinfectant lotions and sprays for bedpans, toilets, floor.
- The precipitating cause has to be identified and treated, along with taking care of

Only put off until tomorrow what you are willing to die having left undone—**Pablo Picasso**

proper nutrition and improving the anemic status by blood transfusion.

OPPORTUNISTIC INFECTIONS

They are normally *of low pathogenicity,* occur through therapeutic invasive procedures and are common in immune deficiency.
Immune deficiency may be due to:
- Diabetes; HIV.
- Steroid therapy; radiotherapy.
- Immunosuppressive therapy in transplantation.
- Cytotoxic chemotherapy.
- Starvation and old age.

Therapeutic invasive procedures may be in the form of IV cannula, bladder catheterization, tracheostomy and other minor surgical procedures, which permit the skin organisms like *Streptococcus epidermidis* to penetrate the skin and invade the deeper tissues.

Organisms

Bacteria:
- *Gram-negative*: E. coli, Pseudomonas, Klebsiella, Proteus, Serratia.
- *Gram-positive*: Staphylococcus epidermidis, Streptococcus pneumoniae.

Viruses:
Herpes, cytomegalovirus (CMV), varicella zoster, may cause fatal pneumonia.

Fungal:
Candida, *Aspergillus*, yeast.

Protozoal:
Cryptosporidia (causes diarrhea), *Pneumocystis carinii*.

Because there is poor defence mechanism, infection is severe and often life-threatening.

Investigation

Swab; blood; pus culture.

Treatment

- These infections are difficult to treat as they are often *multidrug resistant.*
- Combination of broad-spectrum antibiotics—cephalosporins, aminoglycosides, metronidazole is given.
- Depending on culture and sensitivity appropriate antibiotics are given.
- Often ventilatory support and critical care are required.

NECROTIZING FASCIITIS

- It is *spreading inflammation of the skin, deep fascia and soft tissues with extensive destruction*, and toxemia commonly due to *Streptococcus pyogenes* but often may be due to mixed infections like anaerobes, coliforms, and Gram-negative organisms.
- It is common in old age, diabetics, immunosuppressed, malnourished, obesity, steroid therapy and HIV patients.
- It can occur in limbs (Figs. 4.20A to C), lower abdomen (Meleney's infection), groin, and perineum.
- Muscle is usually not involved in necrotizing fasciitis (Fig. 4.21).

Types

Type I: It is due to mixed infection. It is usually not precipitated by injury.

Type II: It is due to *Streptococcus pyogenes*, usually due to minor trauma like abrasions.

Clinical Features

- Sudden onset of swelling and pain in the part with edema, discoloration, necrotic areas, and ulceration.
- Foul smelling discharge.
- Features of toxemia with high-grade fever and chills, hypotension.
- Oliguria often with acute renal failure due to acute tubular necrosis.

It is our choices that show what we truly are, far more than our abilities—**JK Rowling**

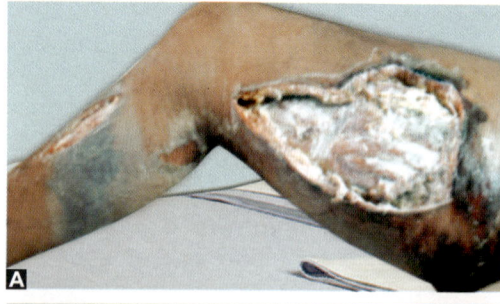
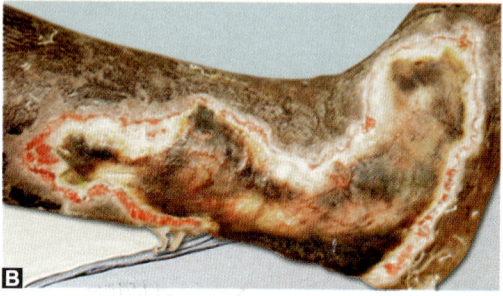
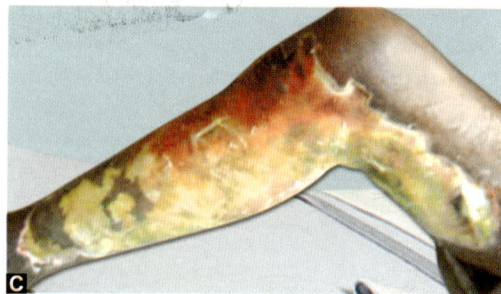

Figs. 4.20A to C: Necrotizing fasciitis of the leg in different patients. Note the extensive involvement of the legs.

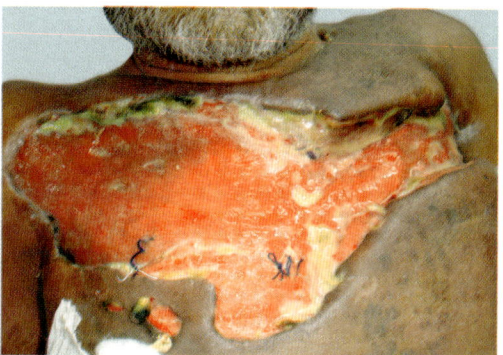

Fig. 4.21: Necrotizing fasciitis on the chest wall and over sternum.

- Jaundice.
- Rapid spread in short period (in few hours).
- Features of SIRS, MODS with drowsy, ill patient.
- Condition may be life-threatening if not treated properly.

Management

- IV fluids, fresh blood transfusion.
- Antibiotics depending on culture and sensitivity or broad-spectrum antibiotics. High dose penicillins are very effective. Clindamycin, third generation cephalosporins, aminoglycosides are also often needed.
- Catheterization and hourly urine output monitor.
- Hematocrit, serum creatinine assessment.
- Pus culture, blood culture.
- Electrolyte management and monitoring.
- Control of diabetes if patient is diabetic.
- Oxygen, ventilator support, dopamine, dobutamine supplements whenever required.
- Radical wound excision of gangrenous skin and necrosed tissues at repeated intervals.
- Once patient recovers and healthy granulation tissue appears, spilt skin grafting is done. As it commonly involves large area, mesh graft (meshing of SSG) is needed.

ACUTE PYOMYOSITIS

- It is infection and suppuration with destruction of skeletal muscles, commonly due to *Staphylococcus aureus* and *Streptococcus pyogenes*, occasionally due to Gram-negative organisms.
- It is common in muscles of thigh, gluteal region, shoulder and arm.
- Precipitating factors are similar to necrotizing fasciitis.

The only impossible journey is the one you never begin—Anthony Robbins

- Creatine phosphokinase will be very high and signifies acute phase.
- Renal failure is common.
- MRI is useful.
- *Creatine phosphokinase* will be very high >50,000 units due to *rhabdomyolysis*.
- Treatment is antibiotics, wound excision and compartment release often with hemodialysis.

HEPATITIS

Hepatitis is inflammation of the liver. Hepatitis may be acute or chronic depending on whether it lasts for less than or more than 6 months.

Causes

Infectious; metabolic; ischemic; autoimmune; genetic; others like neonatal causes.
Infectious hepatitis can be viral; parasitic; bacterial. Viral can be hepatitis A,B,C,D,E,F,G; cytomegalovirus; Epstein-Barr virus; Yellow fever.
Hepatitis viruses: Hepatitis A (HAV)—Picornaviridae (1973); Hepatitis B (HBV)—Hepadnaviridae (1970); Hepatitis C (HCV)—Flaviviridae (1988); Hepatitis D (HDV) (1977); Hepatitis E (HEV) (Caliciviridae) (1983)—Hepeviridae; Hepatitis F—not separate entity —mutant of B virus; Hepatitis G (HGV)—Flaviviridae (1995).
Hepatitis D virus (Delta agent) is a single stranded incomplete RNA virus transmitted parenterally that requires hepatitis B surface antigen to complete its replication and transmission cycle.
Hepatitis E virus: It is unenveloped RNA virus very labile and sensitive. Presents as acute illness; no chronic sequelae. It is more severe in pregnancy. Infection is by feco-oral route through contaminated water.

Hepatitis G virus flavirus: It causes acute, chronic and fulminant hepatitis; transmission is through blood (mother—newborn babies); prevalence is higher in HCV infected people.

Outcome of Hepatitis

- Acute hepatitis can sometimes resolve on its own or progress to chronic hepatitis.
- Often it results in acute fulminant liver failure and death.
- Chronic hepatitis may progress to cirrhosis, liver failure or hepatic insufficiency.
- Liver cancer: Hepatocellular carcinoma (HCC) is more common after hepatitis.

HEPATITIS A VIRUS

- Globally, symptomatic HAV infections are believed to occur in around 1.4 million people a year.
- Hepatitis A is most widespread in parts of the world where standards of sanitation and food hygiene are generally poor, such as parts of Africa, the Indian subcontinent, the Far East, the Middle East, and Central and South America.
- Transmission—fecal-oral. Eating infected food; drinking water in water contaminated with sewage; drinking contaminated water; eating raw or undercooked shellfish from contaminated water; close contact with someone who has hepatitis A.
- Less commonly, through sex, injections, drug abuse.
- Hepatitis A patient is most infectious from around 2 weeks before their symptoms appear and lasts until about a week after the symptoms first develop.

Features

- Incubation period 15–50 days.
- The symptoms of hepatitis A develop, on average, around 4 weeks after becoming infected.

*You only live once, but if you do it right, once is enough—**Mae West***

- **Early features**
  - Feeling tired and generally unwell; joint and muscle pain; mild fever; loss of appetite; lethargy, asthenia; right hypochondriac pain; headache; sore throat and cough; constipation or diarrhea; itching.
  - These symptoms usually last from a few days up to few weeks.
- **Late features**
  - Jaundice; dark urine; pale stools; itchy skin
  - Palpable soft, tender liver.
- **Features in severe cases**
  - Most people make a full recovery within a couple of months, although the symptoms can come and go for up to 6 months.
  - Hepatitis A is not usually a serious illness, but it can cause the liver failure.
  - Sudden, severe vomiting, bruise and bleeding, frequent epistaxis or bleeding gums.
  - Irritability, loss of memory and concentration; drowsiness and confusion.
  - Acute liver failure which can be life-threatening if not treated quickly.

Evaluation

- Immunoglobulin M (IgM) HAV antibody is very useful; immunoglobulin G (IgG) antibody develops later which lasts for longer period.
- Liver function tests; prothrombin time, coagulation factors, hematocrit assessment, renal function status—to be checked.

Treatment

- Hepatitis A vaccine (HAV) is very effective and lasts for >15 years. It is given alone or along with hepatitis B vaccine or with typhoid vaccine.
- Postexposure status immunoglobulin is given along with vaccine.

HEPATITIS B VIRUS

It is a member of hepadnavirus family. It is 42 nm enveloped virion with partially double stranded circular DNA. It contains 4 genes which encode 5 proteins; S gene encodes surface antigen; C gene encodes core and e antigen; P gene encodes polymerase; X gene X protein.

Features

- It is high in blood, serum and wound exudates; moderate in semen, vaginal fluid, saliva; low in urine, feces, tears, sweat, milk.
- Infection occurs through body fluids through transfusions, needle prick or through open wound. Vertical transmission from mother to child can occur.
- The risk of developing clinical hepatitis if the blood was both hepatitis B surface antigen (HBsAg) and HBeAg-positive is 20–30%.
- By comparison, the risk of developing clinical hepatitis from a needle contaminated with HBsAg positive, HBeAg-negative blood was 1–6%.
- Symptoms occur 1 to 3 months after exposure; sometimes symptoms may not be obvious at all.
- **Features are**—fever, joint pain, weakness, jaundice, tender palpable liver, loss of appetite and weight.
- Acute fulminant hepatitis can lead to cholestatic rapidly progressive jaundice with hepatic failure, encephalopathy, coagulopathy and can kill the patient.
- **Complications**: Chronic hepatitis (5–10%); fulminant liver failure (1%); cirrhosis of liver; hepatocellular carcinoma (HCC); glomerulonephritis; polyarteritis nodosa; cryoglobulinemia.

Serology

- Surface antigen (HBsAg) is the first marker to appear and causes the production of

*Those who dare to fail miserably can achieve greatly—**John F Kennedy***

anti-HBs; HBsAg normally implies acute disease (present for 1–6 months); if HBsAg is present for >6 months then this implies chronic disease (i.e. infective).
- Anti-HBsAg implies immunity (either exposure or immunization); it is negative in chronic disease.
- Anti-HBc implies previous (or current) infection; IgM anti-HBc appears during acute or recent hepatitis B infection and is present for about 6 months; IgG anti-HBc persists.
- HbeAg results from breakdown of core antigen from infected liver cells as is therefore a marker of infectivity.
- Previous immunization: Anti-HBs positive, all others negative
- Previous hepatitis B (>6 months ago), not a carrier: Anti-HBc positive, HBsAg negative.
- Previous hepatitis B, now a carrier: Anti-HBc positive, HBsAg positive.

Treatment

- There is no specific treatment in active acute disease stage; immunoglobulins, interferons, symptomatic, nutrition care.
- *Drugs* are useful in chronic stage to delay the onset of complications; it may result in the disappearance of HBsAg, HBV-DNA, and seroconversion to HBeAg. *Alpha-interferon* 2b (original)—alpha-interferon 2a (newer, better); *Antivirals*: Tenofovir; Lamivudine (drug resistance common, relapse can occur); Adefovir (less drug resistance; expensive, toxic); Entecavir (most powerful antiviral known, similar to Adefovir).

Pre-exposure Prophylaxis

It is important that doctors, dentists and all health care workers are vaccinated.

Pre-exposure prophylaxis consists of administration of a 3 dose series of hepatitis B vaccine given over a 6-month period. *Dose*: First is time zero; second is in one month; third is in six months.

Hepatitis B and pregnancy
- All pregnant women are offered screening for hepatitis B.
- Babies born to mothers who are chronically infected with hepatitis B or to mothers who have had acute hepatitis B during pregnancy should receive a complete course of vaccination + hepatitis B immunoglobulin.
- Oral antiviral treatment (e.g. Lamivudine) in the latter part of pregnancy may be useful.
- There is little evidence to suggest cesarean section reduces vertical transmission rates.
- Hepatitis B cannot be transmitted via breast-feeding (in contrast to HIV).

Standard Precautions
They are designed to reduce the risk of transmission of microorganisms from known and unknown sources of infection (blood, body fluids, excretions, secretions, etc). These precautions apply to the care of all patients regardless of their diagnosis or presumed infection status.

The principles of standard precautions:
- Handwashing.
- Protective barriers, i.e. the use, of personal protective clothing, e.g. double gloves, surgical masks, eye protection.
- Management of healthcare waste.
- Correct handling and disposal of needles and sharps.
- Effective cleaning, decontamination and sterilization of equipment, instruments and environment (including blood spillages).
- Use of appropriate disinfectants at the correct working dilution.

Additional measures in a known hepatitis B patient
- Patients should be scheduled at the end of the list.
- Operators and assistants should wear 2 pair of gloves, plastic gown, cap mask, protective eyewear.

*Great minds discuss ideas; average minds discuss events; small minds discuss people—**Eleanor Roosevelt***

- High volume suction should be used; rubber dam should be applied to minimize the formation of aerosols.
- All used instruments should be packed in a labelled plastic wrap.
- After procedure, all equipments and surfaces should be cleaned and decontaminated with disinfectant (0.5% sodium hypochlorite).

Post-exposure Prophylaxis

Two types of products are available for prophylaxis against HBV infection:
- Hepatitis B vaccine, which provides long term protection against HBV infection, is recommended for pre-exposure and post-exposure prophylaxis. Dose: Total 3 doses at zero (start dose), one month and six month.
- HBIG, provides temporary protection (i.e. 3–6 months) and is only indicated in certain post-exposure settings.

Types of Post-exposure Prophylaxis
- *Not vaccinated*: Hepatitis B immune globulin (HBIG) (Dose is 0.06 mL/kg given intramuscularly) and hepatitis vaccine.
- Previously vaccinated:
  - *Responders* if anti-HBS antibody >10 mu/mL: No treatment in needed.
  - *Not responders* if HBS antibody <10 mu/mL: HBIG one dose and hepatitis vaccine; if source is high-risk, then 2 doses of HBIG with one month interval.

HEPATITIS C VIRUS

- Member of RNA flavivirus family.
- Enveloped virion, genome of single-stranded RNA, no virion polymerase.
- It has 6 genotypes and multiple subgenotypes, resulting in a "hypervariable" region in envelope glycoprotein.
- No particular vaccine available.
- HCV is not transmitted efficiently through occupational exposures to blood.

Features

- Incubation period is 6–9 weeks.
- The average incidence of anti-HCV seroconversion after accidental percutaneous exposure from an HCV positive source is 1.8% (range: 0–7%).
- The risk of transmission during a needle stick injury is about 2%.
- The vertical transmission rate from mother to child is about 6%. The risk is higher if there is coexistent HIV.
- Breastfeeding is not contraindicated in mothers with hepatitis C.
- The risk of transmitting the virus during sexual intercourse is probably less than 5%.
- **Complications:** Chronic infection (80–85%)—only 15–20% of patients will clear the virus after an acute infection and hence the majority will develop chronic hepatitis C; cirrhosis (20–30% of those with chronic disease); hepatocellular carcinoma; cryoglobulinemia; porphyria cutanea tarda (PCT) especially if there is alcohol abuse.
- Antibody test confirms that patient had infection earlier. PCR is useful to identify the current infection. Genotyping suggests the prognosis and response for therapy. Genotypes 1 and 4 has got worst prognosis.
- Treatment with antiviral medication is recommended in all people with proven chronic hepatitis C. Drugs are—Pegylated interferon; Ribavirin; Simeprevir or Sofosbuvir—often all three drugs taken together.

Standard precautions—same as for HBV
- No protective antibody response has been identified following HCV infection.

Whatever the mind of man can conceive and believe, it can achieve—**Napoleon Hill**

❖ In the absence of PEP for HCV, recommendations for post-exposure management are intended to achieve early identification of chronic disease and, if present, referral for evaluation of treatment options.

HIV INFECTION AND AIDS

History

❖ 1983: Discovery of the virus. First case of AIDS detected in UK.
❖ 1984: Development of an antibody test.

Definition of AIDS

Confirmed HIV infection with CD_4 T-lymphocyte count $< 0.2 \times 10^6/1$ with symptoms.

Human Immunodeficiency Virus

It was discovered by *Barre-Sinoussi* and *Montagnier* in *1983*.

Types

❖ Human T-lymphocyte virus I
❖ Human T-lymphocyte virus II
❖ Human T-lymphocyte virus III.

They are retroviruses.

Clinical classification of HIV infection

I: Acute infection.
II: Asymptomatic but positive HIV.
III: Persistent generalized lymphadenopathy.
IV: AIDS (HIV related diseases).
   Constitutional diseases like weight loss, fever, diarrhea.
   Neurological diseases—dementia, neuropathy, myelopathy.
   Opportunistic infections.
   Malignancies—Kaposi's sarcoma, non-Hodgkin's lymphomas, primary cerebral lymphomas.
   Other diseases attributable to HIV infection.

Mode of Transmission

❖ Sexual intercourse—vaginal or anal.
❖ Needle pricks—using unsterilized needles for injections, in IV drug abusers, careless handling.
❖ Mother-to-child—during birth through vaginal secretion, transplacental, through breast milk.
❖ Blood transfusions, organ transplantations.

Disease is common in Africa and Asian countries.

HIV mainly harbors in semen, genital secretions, blood, pus, sputum, saliva and other body fluids.

Anti-HIV Antibody

❖ It appears about 3 weeks to 3 months after exposure.
❖ It always indicates infection.
❖ It has got weak neutralizing capacity.
❖ It persists throughout the HIV infection.

Tests for HIV

❖ ELISA test (**screening test**).
❖ Western blot test (**diagnostic test**).
❖ Polymerase chain reaction (PCR).
❖ Anti-HIV detection.
❖ *Viremia quantification*—to start treatment and to see the response of antiviral drugs (useful if it is within $0.5 \log^{10}$).
❖ *CD4+ count*.
   – Normal value $>500/mm^3$.
   – Values between $200–500/mm^3$ is seen in Kaposi's sarcoma, Candida infection,
   – *Mycobacterium tuberculosis*.

Values between $50–200/mm^3$ is seen in *Pneumocystis carinii* and *Toxoplasma* infections.

Values $< 50/mm^3$ is seen in atypical mycobacteria, cytomegalovirus, lymphomas.

After HIV infection, there is a time gap for the patient to become reactive to tests. This time gap is called as *'Window period'*. This

---

I would rather die of passion than of boredom—**Vincent van Gogh**

period is variable. But during this period, the individual is infective.

Pathogenesis

- Envelope glycoprotein of HIV binds with the surface molecule CD_4 of T-lymphocytes, monocytes, macrophages, cutaneous Langerhan's cells, dendritic cells of all tissues.
- CD_4 of lymphocytes—T-helper cells induce and control the normal immune response.
- HIV completely suppresses immune response directly by suppressing 'T' cell, indirectly by suppressing 'B' cell. Finally it dismantles/destroys the immune system making the individual prone for opportunistic infections.
- After HIV infection, antibodies develop to virus envelope and core proteins which persists throughout life.

Pulmonary Problems in HIV Infection

- Pneumonia.
- Tuberculosis.
- Fungal infections.
- *Pneumocystis carinii* pneumonia.
- Cytomegalovirus pneumonia.

General features in HIV

- Weight loss more than 10%.
- Fever more than 1 month.
- Diarrhea more than 1 month.
- Neuralgia, arthralgia, headache.
- Lymphadenopathy.
- Cutaneous rashes, dermatitis, fungal (candida), bacterial, viral (herpes simplex 1 and 2).
- Dental infection, gingivitis, candidiasis of oral cavity and esophagus.
- Varicella zoster infection.
- Opportunistic infections.
- Poor healing after surgery, trauma, infection with more complications. Cold abscess with a discharging sinus in HIV patient can be seen in Figure 4.22.

Tumors in HIV infection

- Kaposi's sarcoma.
- Lymphomas (NHL common).
- Cervical cancer.
- CNS lymphomas.
- Anogenital squamous cell carcinoma.
- Testicular tumors (Germ cell types).
- Lung cancer.
- GIT lymphomas and adenocarcinomas.

Gastrointestinal Problems in HIV Infection

- Gastrointestinal tract (GIT) infections— bacterial, protozoal, viral.
- Kaposi's sarcoma, lymphomas, adenocarcinomas.

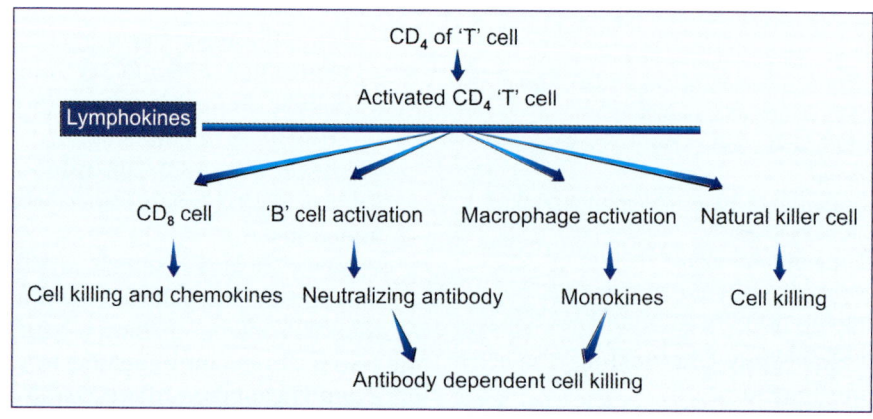

I didn't fail the test. I just found 100 ways to do it wrong—**Benjamin Franklin**

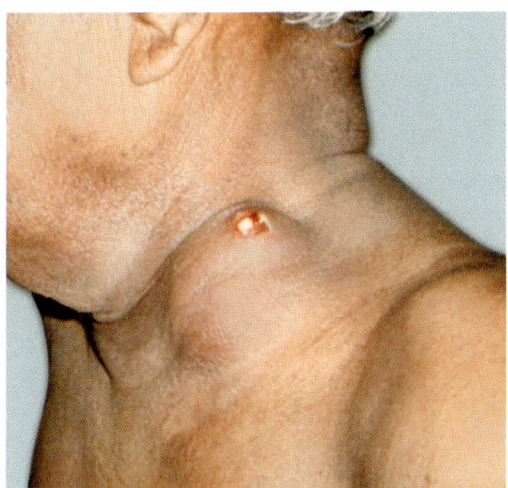

Fig. 4.22: Cold abscess with a discharging sinus in HIV patient.

- Hepatitis ('C' virus), cholestasis.
- Anorectal diseases.
- Abdominal tuberculosis.

Neurological Problems in HIV Infection

- Encephalitis, aseptic meningitis, myelitis.
- Neuropathies with demyelination.
- Opportunistic infections like *Toxoplasma*, *Cryptococcus* causing severe meningitis.
- Primary CNS lymphomas.
- CNS tuberculosis (tuberculomas).
- Visual problems.

Management

Investigations
- Tests for HIV.
- Tests for specific and opportunistic infections.
- Tests relevant for associated tumors.

Treatment

Antiviral therapy

Nucleoside reverse transcriptase inhibitor (NRTI): Zidovudine, Didanosine, Abacavir, Lamivudine, Stavudine.

Non-nucleoside reverse transcriptase inhibitor (NNRTI): Nevirapine, Delavirdine.

Protease inhibitors: Ritonavir, Indinavir, Amprenavir.

Treatment of **opportunistic infections**.
Treatment of **tumors.**

Immunotherapy:
- Alpha and gamma interferons.
- Interleukins.

Bone marrow transplantation.
Anti-CD_3 or IL-2 after **HAART** (**H**ighly **A**ctive **A**nti-**R**etroviral **T**herapy).

Psychotherapy:
- Counseling of HIV patients and their families.
- Life-expectancy after initial HIV infection is 8–10 years.

Prevention

Continues to be our best weapon in combating the menace of HIV infection.

- Safe sex.
- Condom usage reduces the risk of transmission.
- Health education.
- Use of disposable needles to prevent infections.
- Accidental puncture area in surgeon or scrub nurse should be immediately washed with soap and water thoroughly.
- Theater should be fumigated after surgery to HIV patient.

HIV, Hospital and Surgeon

- Isolation *per se* of HIV patient is not required.
- Proper care should be taken to prevent transmission of the virus.
- Open wounds, disposal of excreta, fluids, discharge, pus and other infective materials should be taken care of properly.

It does not matter how slowly you go as long as you do not stop—Confucius

Universal precautions against HIV

- Care in handling sharp objects like needles, blades.
- All cuts and abrasions in a HIV patient should be covered with waterproof dressing.
- Minimal parenteral injections.
- Equipment and areas, which are contaminated with secretions, should be wiped with a sodium hypochlorite solution or 2% glutaraldehyde.
- Contaminated gloves, cottons should be incinerated.
- Equipment should be disinfected with glutaraldehyde.
- Disposable equipment (drapes, scalpels, etc.) should be used for whenever possible.
- Walls and floor should be cleaned properly with soap water.
- Separate operation theater and staff to do surgeries to HIV patients is justifiable.
- Avoid shaving whenever possible before surgery in HIV patients.
- All people inside the theater should wear disposable gowns, plastic aprons, goggles, overshoes and gloves (Figs. 4.23A and B).
- Surgeons, assistants and scrub nurse should wear in addition double gloves.
- Suction bottle should be half filled with freshly prepared glutaraldehyde solution.
- Spilled body fluids should be diluted with glutaraldehyde.

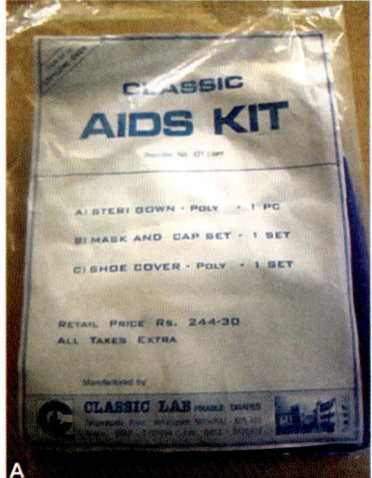

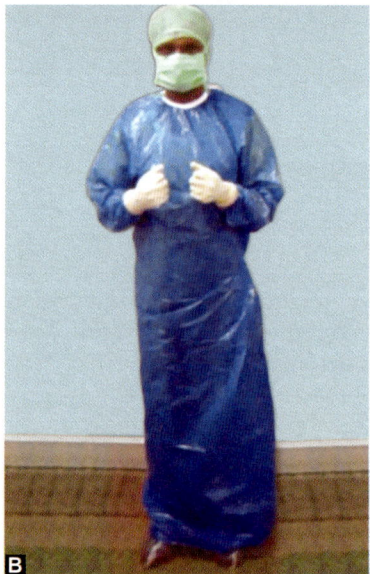

Figs. 4.23A and B: HIV kit should be used while doing any procedure to HIV infected patients. Note the wearing of masks, spectacles, and shoes.

❖ Risk of HIV infection through needle prick is very less (0.03%).

Following measures should be taken while managing HIV patients:
❖ Wearing double gloves.
❖ Wearing proper spectacles (as HIV can get transmitted through eyes directly).
❖ Wearing proper head mask, theater shoes, and apron.
❖ Measures to prevent spread of infection from patient to patient in the hospital.
❖ Disposal of needles through a sharp disposing container.

Disinfection

❖ Autoclave is ideal.
❖ Boiling.

❖ Hypochlorite solution.
❖ 2% glutaraldehyde solution.

NEEDLE STICK INJURY IN SURGICAL PRACTICE

❖ It is the accidental puncture of the skin by a needle during a medical intervention.

Nothing is impossible, the word itself says, 'I'm possible!'—**Audrey Hepburn**

- Accidental contact with blood occurs especially in the following situations: During re-capping; during surgery, especially during wound closure; during biopsy; when an uncapped needle has ended up in bed linen, surgery clothing, etc; when taking an unsheathed used needle to the waste container; during the cleaning up and transporting of waste material; when using more complex collection and injection techniques; in accident and emergency departments; in high-stress interventions—diagnostic or therapeutic.
- The major blood-borne pathogens of concern associated with needle stick injury are: hepatitis B virus (HBV)—6–30%; hepatitis C virus (HCV)—2%; human immunodeficiency virus (HIV)—0.3%.
- Infectious agents who have the potential for transmission through needle stick injury are: hepatitis D virus (HDV or delta agent, which is activated in the presence of HBV) hepatitis G virus (GB virus or GBV-C); cytomegalovirus (CMV); Epstein-Barr virus (EBV); West Nile virus (WNV); malarial parasites.

Prevention of Needle Stick Injury

- Employee training.
- Use devices with safety features to isolate sharps; safe recapping system; do not recap needles or scalpels but dispose them through effective disposal system.
- Plan for safe handling and disposal of sharps before using them.
- Self-sheathing system; retractable technology; add on safety features.

Management

- Report the incident immediately.
- Wash the area immediately under running water or use an eye-washing bottle as appropriate.
- Make the wound bleed for three to four minutes whilst continuing to wash the area. Dry area with paper towel.
- Cover the wound with a water-impermeable sticking plaster and consider double gloving any hand injury if continuing to work.
- The source patient should be identified and arrangements made for a blood sample to be obtained, with informed consent. This should be tested for the presence of the blood borne viruses like hepatitis B, hepatitis C and HIV.
- Arrangements should be made for blood samples to be taken from the staff member (victim) with informed consent. One sample is marked "for storage" and is retained in the relevant laboratory. The other is analyzed to determine the staff member's hepatitis B antibody level.
- Further assessment, treatment and follow up of the staff member are performed in accordance with current best practice. Arrangements should be in place for speedy assessment and treatment.
- Counselling, reassurance and information may be required and arrangements for accessing this should be in place as appropriate.
- Appropriate records must be kept.

GONORRHEA

- It is a sexually transmitted disease caused by *Neisseria gonorrhoeae*.
- It is a *Gram-negative intracellular diplococcus*. It mainly affects epithelium of the urogenital tract, rectum, conjunctivae, pharynx and anterior urethra (in male).
- Incubation period is 2–14 days.

Features

- Dysuria and urethral discharge.
- In women, vaginal discharge, dysuria, bilateral salphingitis and infertility are common.

Life is 10% what happens to me and 90% of how I react to it—**Charles Swindoll**

- After chronic infection gonococcal urethritis causes urethral stricture, usually in the bulbar urethra. It is the commonest cause of stricture urethra along with traumatic cause.
- It also causes recurrent epididymoorchitis, prostatitis and proctitis.
- Gram staining and culture of urine is diagnostic.
- Patient is asked to pass urine in two glasses. Haziness in first glass signifies infection with pus whereas second glass urine is clear.

Treatment

- Penicillins are the antibiotics of choice.
- Ampicillins, Clotrimoxazoles, Ciprofloxacin, Ceftriaxone (single dose IM), Cefixime and Spectinomycin (2 g IM single dose) are also used.
- Gonorrhea is more difficult to diagnose and treat in females than men.
- In complicated gonorrhea, prostatic massage, local irrigation, treatment for stricture urethra, Doxycycline and Gentamicin therapy are indicated.

SURGICAL SITE INFECTION

Surgical site infection (SSI) is the second most common complication following surgical procedures (first being postoperative pneumonia) due to virulent bacterial entry, altered wound microenvironment, and changed host defense. Prevention of SSI can be achieved by better preoperative preparation; proper infection control during surgery; adherence to principles of preventive antibiotic therapy; better surgical techniques to reduce hematoma, tissue injury and foreign bodies within the surgical site; prevention of tissue hypoxia with enhanced oxygen support.

Common Sources of Infection

- Surgical wards, wounds, ulcers, catheters, drains, sputum, urine, faeces, open wounds.
- Operation room without proper ventilation, nurses, surgeons. Operation methods, sterilization of instruments.

Organisms Causing SSI

Commonly *Staphylococcus aureus*. Any organisms like clostridia, Gram-negative bacteria can cause SSI.

Bacteria present in a wound with no signs or symptoms of systemic inflammation is called as *colonization,* usually less than 10^5 cfu/mL. Transient exposure of a wound to bacteria (usually less than 6 hours) is called as *contamination* with varying concentration.

Sequence of Events (in Surgical Wounds)

- *Activation* of inflammation occurs by cuts, incisions, abrasions, burns. This initiates *inflammation* by protein coagulation, platelet aggregation, mast cell activity, release of complements and bradykinin.
- *Phase I of inflammation* begins with vasodilatation, increased bulk flow, increased vascularity.
- Later *Phase II of inflammation* proceeds with phagocytic infiltration and bacterial phagocytosis, removal of dead tissue with release of pro-inflammatory cytokines. Here tissue injury from incision mobilizes phagocytes before bacterial contamination leading into prior preparation against infection. If contamination is controlled monocytes activate to *regulate wound healing* using myofibrocytes and collagen.
- If bacterial *contamination is not controlled*, pro-inflammatory cells release TNF-α to stimulate neutrophils for phagocytosis. It also causes release of reactive oxygen and acid hydrolases from lysosomal vacuoles to resulting in lipid peroxidation, release of interleukins, evoking acute inflammatory response with creation of space containing pus which contains necrotic tissue, neutrophils, bacteria and proteinaceous

An unexamined life is not worth living—**Socrates**

fluid with *all signs of inflammation*—rubor, dolor, calor, tumor. It is *typical surgical site infection* (SSI).

Factors Related to SSI

- *Bacterial entry* (inoculum) into the wound occurs through air in operation room, through instruments, through surgeons and theater staffs, patient's endogenous bacteria like perineum, urine, etc.
- *Bacterial virulence* plays major role in causing SSI.
- *Microenvironment in the wound* like hemoglobin level at surgical site; presence of necrosis which interferes with phagocytosis; presence of dead space and or foreign body in the wound.
- *Host defenses* both natural (innate) and acquired, when altered SSI occurs. Acquired causes are—shock, hypoxia, chronic illness, hypoalbuminemia, malnutrition, hypothermia, hyperglycemia, corticosteroids, HIV infection, malignancy and certain drugs.

Classification of Surgical Wounds

- *Clean wounds*—operative procedure does not enter into normally colonized viscus.
- *Clean-contaminated*—operation enters into a colonized viscus but under elective controlled circumstances.
- *Contaminated wounds*—gross contamination is present at the surgical site in the absence of obvious infection.
- *Dirty wounds*—surgical procedures performed when active infection is present.

Risk Classification and Identification System

It is based on three categories of variables:
1. Those that estimate intrinsic degree of microbial contamination at the surgical site.
2. Those that measure the duration of operation.
3. Host susceptibility markers.

Variables that influence SSI	
Variables that influence SSI	**Point**
1. An abdominal operation.	1
2. Operation lasting more than 2 hours.	1
3. Surgical site classified as contaminated or dirty/infected.	1
4. Operation performed on a patient with more than three discharge diagnosis.	1
Total index	**4**
All variables have equal significance. This index twice better at predicting SSI than wound classification. Disadvantage is that it is not operation specific and variables collected at discharge.	

The National Nosocomial Infections Surveillance (NNIS) system as basic SSI risk index	
NNIS system	**Point**
Operation classified as contaminated or dirty.	1
The patient has an ASA (American Society of Anesthesiology) preoperative assessment score of 3, 4, or 5.	1
Duration exceeds 75th percentile of 'T' point.	1
'T' point defined as length of time in hours that represents 75th percentile of procedures in NNIS survey.	

Note: T point for common surgical procedures are: Coronary artery bypass graft—5; Bile duct, liver or pancreatic surgery, craniotomy, head and neck surgery—4; Colonic surgery, joint, prosthesis surgery, vascular surgery—3; Abdominal or vaginal hysterectomy, ventricular shunt, herniorrhaphy—2; Appendicectomy, limb amputation, cesarean section—1.

Physical Status Classification

Class I — A patient in normal health.
Class II — A patient with mild systemic disease resulting in no functional limitations.

The question isn't who is going to let me; it's who is going to stop me—**Ayn Rand**

Class III — A patient with severe systemic disease that limits activity, but is not incapacitating.
Class IV — A patient with severe systemic disease that is a constant threat to life.
Class V — A moribund patient not likely to survive 24 hours.

Classification of Surgical Site Infection

A. According to the Depth of the Wound Infection (Fig. 4.24)

1. ***Superficial incisional SSI:***
   It occurs within 30 days of operation; involves only skin and subcutaneous tissue; and one of following:
   - Purulent drainage (culture documentation not required), organisms isolated from fluid/tissue of superficial incision, at least 1 sign of inflammation, wound is deliberately opened by the surgeon, surgeon or attending physician declares that the wound is infected.
   - A wound not considered a superficial site infection—if stitch abscess is present; if infection is at episiotomy site; burn wound, SSI extends into the fascia or muscle.

2. ***Deep incisional SSI:***
   It occurs within 30 days of operation or 1 year if an implant is present; involves deep soft tissues of the incision; and at least one of the following:
   - Purulent drainage from the deep incision site without organ/space involvement, fascial dehiscence or deliberate separation by surgeon, deep abscess, identified by—reoperation/histopathology/radiology, surgeon or attending physician declares deep infection present.

3. ***Organ space infection:***
   It occurs within 30 days or 1 year if an implant is present; involves anatomic structures not opened or manipulated during surgery; and one of the following
   - Pus from a drain placed into organ/space, organism isolated by culture, identification of abscess by direct examination, reoperation, histopathology, radiology, diagnosis by surgeon or attending physician.

B. Wound Infections Classification According to the Etiology

1. *Primary infection*—where the wound is the primary site of infection.

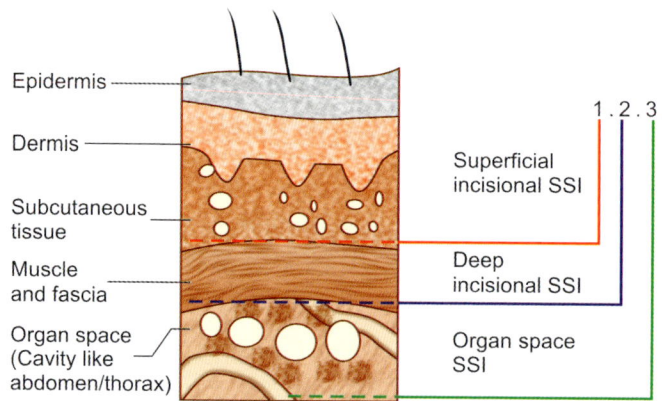

Fig. 4.24: Surgical site infection (SSI) classification as—superficial incisional, deep incisional, organ space.

Winning isn't everything, but wanting to win is—**Vince Lombardi**

2. *Secondary infection*—arises following a complication that is not directly related to the wound.

C. Wound Infections Classification According to the Time

1. An *early infection* presents within 30 days of a surgical procedure.
2. An *intermediate infection* occurs between 1–3 months afterwards.
3. *Late infection* occurs in more than three months after surgery.

D. Wound Infections Classification According to the Severity

1. *Minor* wound infection if there is discharge without cellulitis or deep tissue destruction.
2. *Major* if the discharge of pus is associated with tissue breakdown, partial or total dehiscence of the deep fascial layers of the wound, or if systemic illness is present.

Note: *Southampton wound grading system and Asepsis wound score system is used in assessing the severity of surgical site infection.*

Prevention of SSI

1. **Preoperative**
   - Preoperative cleaning and antiseptic scrub of surgical site. Skin is colonized by various bacteria mainly *Staphylococcus aureus* (50%). Preoperative skin wash using chlorhexidine decreases bacterial colonization by 80% and so wound contamination.
   - Surgical site to be shaved or clipped in the operation theater. Shaving should be done in the theater itself or within 2 hours of beginning of the surgery otherwise infection rate may raise. Clean wound infection after shaving is 2.3%; after clipping it is 1.7%; without shaving or clipping it is 0.9%. However, selective shaving is definitely needed in area like scalp, axilla, groin, and perineum.
   - Surgery should be avoided or postponed if fingers or hand of surgeon has open wounds or infection.
   - Obvious infection in patient if exists should be treated.
   - Prolonged preoperative admission should be avoided for an elective surgery.
2. **Care in the operation theater**
   - One should ensure that caps, masks, gowns and sterile gloves are used.
   - Proper skin cleaning is needed on table after anesthesia using antiseptics like povidone iodine. One should ensure that all drapes are dry throughout the procedure and all instruments are thoroughly sterilized.
   - Unimpregnated plastic drapes are avoided as it is found that it does not have any advantage.
   - Gentle tissue handling, absolute hemostasis, holding tissues using instruments as much as possible, using appropriate suture materials, avoiding dead space during closure are certain essential on table tips to reduce SSI.
   - One should consider leaving wounds open if it is severely contaminated.
3. **Preventive antibiotic therapy**
   - It is used whenever high-risk of infection is associated with the procedure and consequences of infection if possibly severe and if patient has a high NNIS risk index.
   - Antibiotics should be administered as close to the incision time as possible, before induction of anesthesia.
   - Selected antibiotic should have activity against likely pathogens.
   - Postoperative systemic antibiotics for 24 hours (beyond 24 hours not shown to reduce SSI).

*Whether you think you can or you think you can't, you're right—***Henry Ford**

- Benefit of preoperative antibiotics in NNIS risk 0 index is difficult to assess and quantify.
- Proper techniques and wound micro-environment are more important than antibiotics.
- Preventive systemic antibiotics not to be used to prevent nosocomial infections.
- Oral antibiotic bowel preparation with appropriate mechanical bowel preparation.
- If systemic antibiotics are to be used antibiotics of longer half-life are to be chosen.
- Very long procedures should have a redosing strategy during the procedure.
4. **Enhancement of host defences**
    - Increased oxygen delivery facilitates phagocytic eradication of microbes.
    - Optimizing core body temperature is important as warmer patients resist bacteria better.
    - Blood glucose control is essential even to non-diabetics as well.

Management of SSI

- SSI is managed depending on the type of SSI—superficial, deep or organ space.
- All infected material and pus should be removed from the wound site—*debridement.*
- Sutures are removed to allow *free drainage* of infected material.
- Infected fluid is sent for culture and sensitivity and suitable antibiotics are started.

Once wound shows signs of healing by healthy granulation tissue, secondary suturing is done. Often it is allowed to heal by scarring.

Nothing is impossible, the word itself says, 'I'm possible!'—**Audrey Hepburn**

CHAPTER 5

Swellings

Chapter Outline

- Lipoma
- Papilloma
- Cysts
- Dermoids
- Sebaceous Cyst
- Glomus Tumor
- Lymph Cyst
- Neuroma
- Neurofibroma
- Neurilemmoma
- Fibroma
- Ganglion
- Bursae
- Morrant Baker Cyst
- Calcinosis Cutis
- Epignathus
- Chordoma

LIPOMA (FIG. 5.1)

- It is a benign tumor arising from yellow fat.
- Tumor arising from brown fat is called as **hibernoma**.
- It is called as *universal tumor* as it can occur anywhere in the body (except in brain).
- It is the *commonest benign tumor*.
- It can be *diffuse or localized*.
- Diffuse lipomas are not encapsulated, not well-localized. Common in palm, sole, head and neck region, difficult to be removed.
- It can be single or multiple. Multiple lipomas are often associated with many syndromes like **MEN syndrome** (*multiple endocrine neoplasia syndrome*).

Types

- Painful lipomas are called as *neurolipomas*.

Dercum's disease is tender deposition of fat especially on the trunk, is also called as *adiposis dolorosa*. It is basically multiple neurolipomatosis.

- Fibrolipoma.
- Nevolipoma.

Lipomas attain large size in thigh, shoulder, retroperitoneum, back and often may turn into sarcoma (Fig. 5.2).

Sites

1. Subcutaneous—*commonest variety*.
2. Subfascial—difficult to identify because of the overlying fascia.
3. Intramuscular.
4. Intermuscular—common in thigh.
5. Parosteal.
6. Subserosal—beneath pleura/peritoneum.
7. Submucosal—beneath mucous membrane, common in tongue (causes macroglossia), intestine (causes intussusception).

Pursue one great decisive aim with force and determination

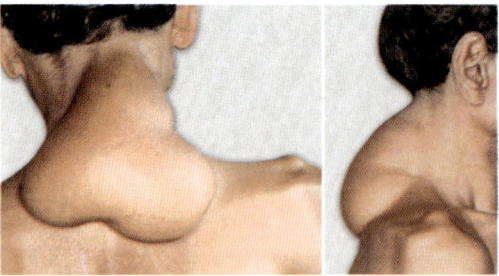

Fig. 5.1: Large lipoma over nape of the neck.

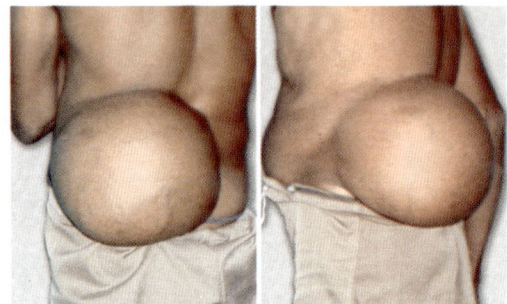

Fig. 5.2: Lipoma in loin region.

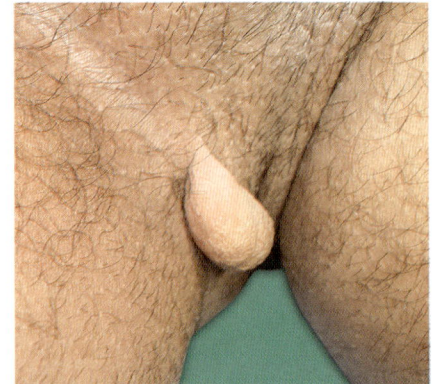

Fig. 5.3: Pedunculated lipoma.

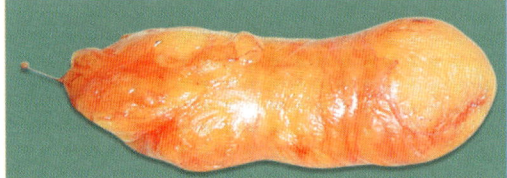

Fig. 5.4: Gross feature of specimen of lipoma.

8. Extradural (not intradural)—rare spinal tumor.
9. Intraglandular—breast, pancreas.

Clinical Features

- Localized swelling, which is lobular, non-tender, semifluctuant, mobile, edge when pressed slips under the palpating fingers *(Slip sign)*, with free skin.
- Lipomas may be pedunculated at times (Fig. 5.3).
- It is not transilluminant.
- Gross features of a specimen of lipoma are shown in Figure 5.4.

Differential Diagnosis

- Neurofibroma.
- Cystic swellings.

Complications

- Myxomatous degeneration.
- Saponification.
- Calcification.
- Submucosal lipoma can cause intussusception and so intestinal obstruction.

Note: Lipoma being a benign soft tissue tumor turning into liposarcoma is disproved now. Liposarcoma starts de novo always—present concept.

Treatment

- **Excision:** Small lipoma is excised under local anesthesia and larger one under general anesthesia (Figs. 5.5A to C).

Liposarcoma
• Rapid growth (commonest type of sarcoma).
• Warm and vascular.
• Dilated veins over the surface.
• Infiltration into deeper plane with restriction of the mobility.
• Skin fixation and fungation.
• Blood spread to lungs.

*To love and be loved is to feel the sun from both sides—**David Viscott***

Chapter 5 : Swellings   99

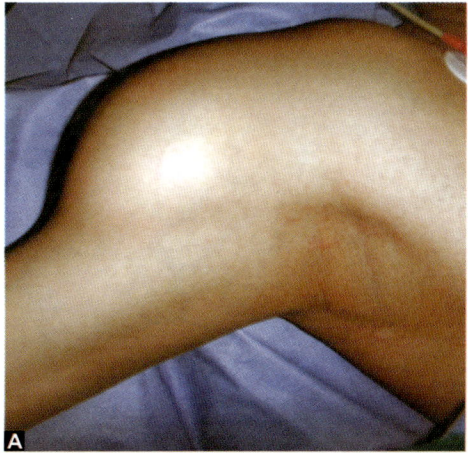
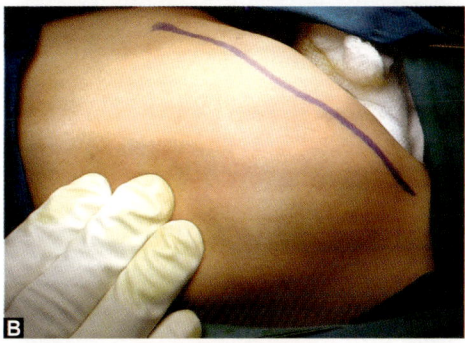
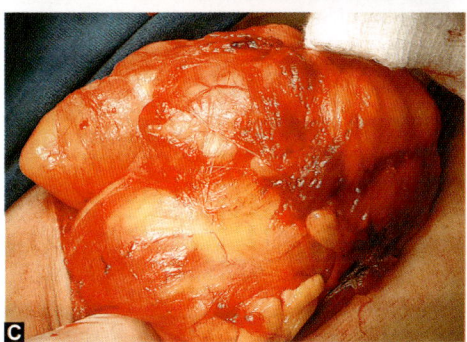

Figs. 5.5A to C: Lipoma over shoulder region. Making incision and excising it.

PAPILLOMA

- It is warty swelling from the skin or often from the mucous membrane.
- It has got a central axis of connective tissue, blood vessels and lymphatics.

- Papilloma can develop *from skin or mucous membrane* (urinary bladder, rectum and gallbladder).
- ***Skin papilloma***:
  - It is often called as skin tag or hamartoma.
  - It can be squamous or basal cell.
  - *Squamous cell papilloma* can be congenital, neoplastic or infective [condyloma (viral)]. It contains *all layers* of skin with sweat and sebaceous glands and hair follicles. It can occur in skin, check, tongue. Soft squamous papilloma can occur over eyelid as *soft* brownish swelling in elderly.
  - *Basal cell papilloma* also called as seborrheic keratosis occurs in elderly in trunk and face as brownish/black elevated skin patch with semitransparent oily appearance.
- ***Infective papilloma*** is a warty lesion due to infection. For example, condyloma acuminata.

True Papilloma (Fig. 5.6A)

- It is a benign tumor with localized overgrowth of the epidermis. It is commonly pedunculated but rarely can be sessile (Fig. 5.6B).
- Pedunculated papilloma is villous with a central axis of connective tissues, blood vessels and lymphatics.
- Papilloma may be single/multiple.
- Papilloma may be pigmented/non-pigmented.
- Surface is usually *warty* (Fig. 5.6C).
- *True papilloma may turn into squamous cell carcinoma occasionally. There will be sudden increase in size, bleeding or ulceration.*
- Papilloma can occur in the breast called as *duct papilloma*, which is the commonest cause of bloody discharge from the nipple.
- Papilloma can occur in mucous membrane like in *oral cavity (Fig. 5.6D), urinary bladder* (transitional papilloma), in the *rectum* (columnar), in the *larynx,* in the *gallbladder* (cuboidal).

Real leaders are ordinary people with extraordinary determination

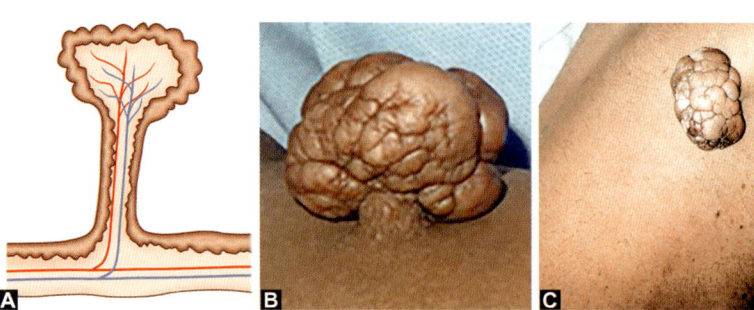

Figs. 5.6A to D: (A) Pedunculated papilloma with its pedicle—diagrammatic look; (B) Pedunculated papilloma; (C) Sessile papilloma; (D) Papilloma tongue. Note the warty surface.

Differential Diagnosis

Amelanotic melanoma, pedunculated lipoma, carcinoma.

Treatment

- *True papilloma* is excised with its base and surrounding 1 cm skin margin.
- *Infective warts* can be treated by excision or CO_2 snow or diathermy coagulation.

Complications of papilloma

- Bleeding.
- Malignant transformation—when occurs in breast, tongue, gallbladder and rectum.
- Ulceration—following infection.
- Mechanical disability like voice change when it occurs in vocal cord.

CYSTS

Cyst is a collection of fluid in a sac lined by epithelium or endothelium. Word meaning of cyst is *'bladder'* (Greek).

TRUE CYST

- Cyst wall is lined by epithelium or endothelium.
- If infection occurs cyst wall will be lined by granulation tissue.
- Fluid is usually serous or mucoid derived from the secretion of the lining.

FALSE CYST

- It does not have epithelial lining.
- Fluid collection is as a result of exudation or degeneration.

Example:
1. Pseudocyst of pancreas.
2. Wall of cystic swelling in tuberculous peritonitis.
3. Cystic degeneration of tumor.
4. In a hematoma after hemorrhage, red blood cells (RBC's) are lysed and get absorbed and fluid remains as a false cyst.
5. ***'Apoplectic Cyst'*** is formed in brain as a result of ischemia causing collection of fluid.
6. Dental/radicular cyst.

Classification

Congenital cysts:
- Dermoids: Sequestration dermoid.
- Tubulodermoids: Thyroglossal cyst, postanal dermoid, ependymal cyst, urachal cyst.
- Cysts of embryonic remnants: Cysts from paramesonephric duct and mesonephric duct. Cysts of urachus and vitellointestinal duct.

Acquired cysts:
- Retention cysts: They are accumulation of secretion of a gland due to obstruction of a duct. For example, sebaceous cyst, Bartholin cyst, cyst of pancreas, cyst of parotid, breast, and epididymis.
- Distention cyst: Lymph cyst, ovarian cyst, colloid goiter.
- Exudation cyst: Bursa, hydrocele.

Contd...

*Love is an irresistible desire to be irresistibly desired—**Robern Frost***

Contd...

Cystic tumors: Dermoid cyst of ovary, cystadenomas.
Traumatic cyst: Due to trauma, hematoma occurs usually in thigh, loin, and shin. It eventually gets lined by endothelium containing brown colored fluid with cholesterol crystals.
Degenerative cyst: Due to cystic degeneration of a solid tumor (due to necrosis of tumor).
Parasitic cyst: Hydatid cyst, trichinosis, cysticercosis.

Clinical Features of a Cyst

Hemispherical swelling which is smooth, fluctuant, nontender, well-localized. Some cysts are transilluminant. Presentation varies depending on its anatomical location.

Effects of a Cyst

- Compression to adjacent structures: Compression over the trachea causing dyspnea, choledochal cyst compressing over the common bile duct (CBD).
- Infection, fever and toxemia.
- Sinus formation.
- Hemorrhage.
- Torsion, e.g. ovarian cyst.
- Calcification.
- Cachexia: In malignant ovarian cyst patient presents with severe cachexia.

Swellings that are brilliantly transilluminant
- Ranula.
- Cystic hygroma and lymph cyst.
- Hydrocele.
- Epididymal cyst (*Chinese-lantern pattern*).
- Meningocele.

DERMOIDS

TYPES

1. *Sequestration Dermoid*

It occurs at the line of embryonic fusion due to inclusion of epithelium beneath the surface, which later gets sequestered forming a cystic swelling in the deeper plane.

Common sites are:
- Forehead.
- External angular dermoid.
- Root of nose.
- Sublingual dermoid.
- Anywhere in midline or in the line of fusion.

Dermoids occurring in the skull may extend into the cranial cavity. When it occurs as external angular dermoid, it extends into the orbital cavity. Or it can extend into any cavity in relation to its anatomical location (e.g. thorax, abdomen).

Dermoid cyst contains putty-like desquamated material. It is lined by both dermal and epidermal components.

Types of angular dermoid (Figs. 5.7A and B)
- *External angular dermoid*: It is a sequestration dermoid situated over the external angular process of the frontal bone. Outer extremity of the eyebrow extends over some part of the swelling. This typical feature differentiates it from the swelling arising from the lacrimal gland. It may extend into the orbital cavity also (Fig. 5.8).
- *Internal angular dermoid*: It is a sequestration dermoid cyst near central position at the root of the nose.

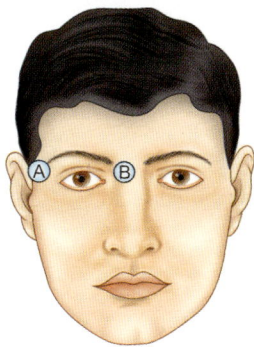
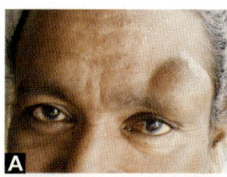
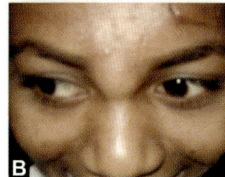

Figs. 5.7A and B: Types of angular dermoid: (A) External angular dermoid; (B) Internal angular dermoid.

Money is like manure, if you spread it around it does a lot of good.
But if you pile it up in one place, it stinks like hell

Clinical features

- Painless swelling in the line of embryonic fusion, presents in the second or third decade onwards, which is smooth, soft, nontender, fluctuant (*Paget's test positive*, i.e. swelling is fixed with two fingers and summit is indented to get sensation of yielding due to fluid), nontransilluminating, with free skin often adherent into the deeper plane (Fig. 5.9).
- There will be *resorption and indentation* of the bone beneath.

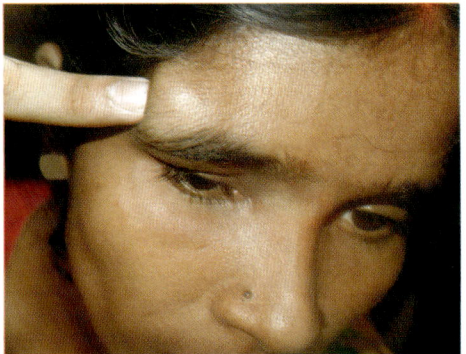

Fig. 5.8: External angular dermoid. Indentation using finger is done to identify bone erosion due to intracranial extension.

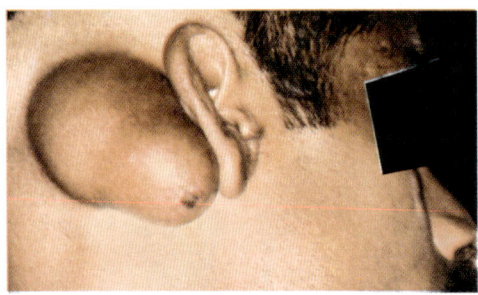

Fig. 5.9: Postauricular dermoid.

Differential diagnosis
- Sebaceous cyst—*Punctum* is seen over the summit and cyst is adherent to skin.
- Lipoma.

Investigations
- X-ray skull or part.
- CT scan head or part.

Treatment
Excision is done under general anesthesia. Often, formal neurosurgical approach is required by raising cranial osteocutaneous flaps.

2. Tubulodermoids

It arises from the embryonic tubular structures. Examples include:
- Thyroglossal cyst.
- Ependymal cyst.
- Postanal dermoid.

3. Implantation Dermoid (Figs. 5.10A and B)

- Due to minor pricks or trauma (often forgotten), epidermis gets buried under the deeper subcutaneous tissue, which causes reaction and cyst formation.

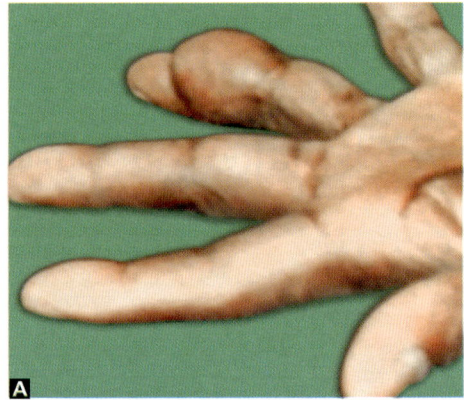

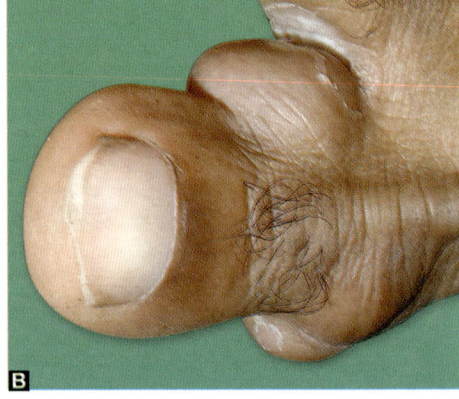

Figs. 5.10A and B: Implantation dermoid in (A) hand and (B) great toe (foot).

Life would be tragic if it weren't funny—**Stephen Hawking**

* It is common in fingers (common in tailors), toes and feet.

Clinical features
* Swelling which is painless, observed after minor trauma, slowly progressing in fingers or toes.
* It is smooth, soft, mobile, tensely cystic, nontransilluminating and is adherent to skin.

Differential diagnosis
* Lipoma.
* Bursa.

Treatment
* Excision.

4. *Teratomatous Dermoid*

* It arises from all germinal layers ecto, meso and endoderms.
* It occurs in ovary, testis, retroperitoneum, mediastinum.
* It contains hairs, teeth, cartilage, muscle.
* It can be benign or malignant.

SEBACEOUS CYST (WEN, EPIDERMAL CYST)

* It is a *retention cyst* that occurs due to obstruction to the mouth of a sebaceous duct.
* It is common in face, scalp, and scrotum (Figs. 5.11 and 5.12).
* *It is not seen in palms and plantar aspect of foot (sole) as there are no sebaceous glands.*
* Sebaceous cyst contains yellowish material with fat, and epithelium, has *putty-like* consistency, with a parasite in the wall—*demodex folliculorum*. It is lined by only epidermal layer of squamous epithelium (epidermoid cyst).

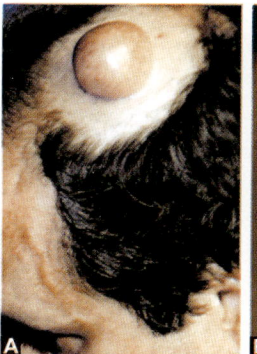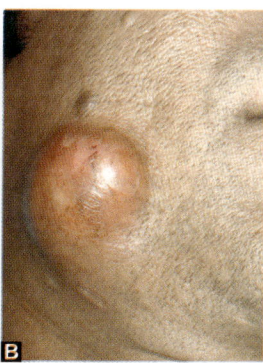

Figs. 5.11A and B: Sebaceous cyst: (A) Scalp; (B) Infected sebaceous cyst.

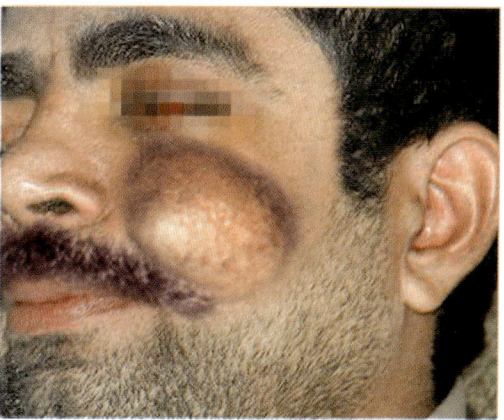

Fig. 5.12: Large sebaceous cyst in face.

Clinical Features

* Painless slow growing swelling, which is smooth, soft, nontender, freely mobile, adherent to skin especially over the summit, fluctuant *(positive Paget's test)*, nontransilluminating *with punctum over the summit.*
* It moulds on finger indentation.
* In 70% of cases, **punctum** is present over the summit because here the sebaceous duct that directly opens into the skin is been blocked. Punctum is depressed black colored spot over the summit of the sebaceous cyst. Because of the denuded

*Victory has thousand fathers but defeat is an orphan—**John F Kennedy*** squamous epithelium (keratin) it is black in color. In 30%, sebaceous duct opens into the hair follicle and so punctum is not seen.

Multiple sebaceous cysts may be associated with syndromes like Gardner's syndrome.

Complications

- Infection and abscess formation.
- Surface gets ulcerated with discharge and is called as **Cock's peculiar tumor**—often resembles epithelioma.
- Sebaceous horn (Figs. 5.13A and B).

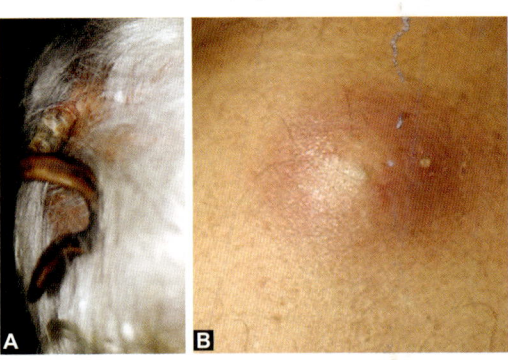

Figs. 5.13A and B: (A) Sebaceous horn scalp; (B) Infected sebaceous cyst.

Treatment (Fig. 5.14)

- Excision including skin adjacent to punctum.
- Incision and avulsion.
- If abscess is formed, then initially drainage, later excision.
- The cyst recurs if capsule is not removed properly.

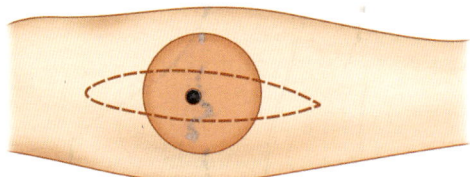

Fig. 5.14: Incision for sebaceous cyst is elliptical which includes punctum.

GLOMUS TUMOR

- It is also called as *glomangioma*.
- It arises from a cutaneous glomus composed of a tortuous arteriole that communicates directly into the venule and these vessels being surrounded by network of small nerves.
- They are often seen in limbs and common in nailbeds.
- They regulate the temperature of the skin.
- The tumor is commonly seen under the nailbed, 2–3 mm in size.
- Tumor consists of a mixture of blood spaces, nerve tissues, muscle fibers derived from the wall of the arteriole, with large cuboidal glomal cells—*angiomyoneuroma*.
- It does not turn into malignancy.

Features

- *Severe burning sensation and pain, out of proportionate to the size.*
- It is compressible and pain aggravates when the limb is exposed to sudden changes of temperature.
- **Treatment:** Excision.

LYMPH CYST (LYMPHATIC CYST)

- It is an *acquired type of distension cyst* wherein lymphatics form a localized swelling with a capsule around it.
- It usually occurs in subcutaneous plane, which is smooth, soft, nontender, mobile, and brilliantly transilluminant (Fig. 5.15). It is not usually adherent to the skin.
- **Common sites**—neck and limbs.
- It can get infected and form an abscess.
- **Differential diagnosis**—cold abscess, dermoid cyst.
- **Treatment**—excision.

Every child is an artist; the problem is staying an artist when you grow up—**Pablo Picasso**

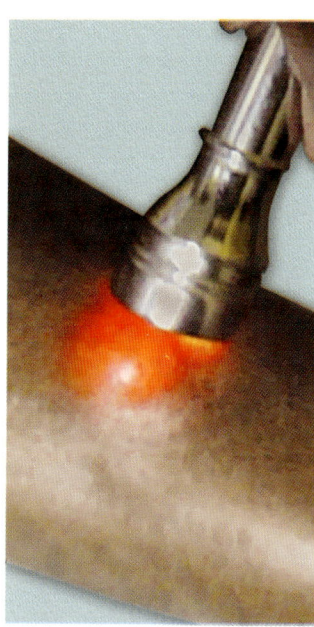

Fig. 5.15: Lymph cyst, which is transilluminant. It is an acquired condition.

NEUROMA

It is swelling arising in relation to the nerve fiber. It can be false or true neuroma.

True neuroma is a *rare* tumor. It usually develops in relation to sympathetic nervous system. *Ganglioneuroma* type contains ganglion cells and nerve fibers; it arises from sympathetic chain; it presents as mass in the neck, thorax, retroperitoneum or adrenal medulla. It is benign but attains large size. It is treated by complete excision. Rare *myelinic neuroma* type contains only nerve fibers without ganglion cells which is seen in spinal cord and pia mater.

False neuroma is *common* which occurs due to injury to nerve by trauma or during surgery like amputation; it arises from connective tissue of the nerve sheath. It contains fibrous tissue with coiled nerve fibers. It can be **end neuroma** (Fig. 5.16A), commonly seen in a amputation stump as tender, localized, firm, swelling which is adherent to scar underneath.

It causes stump neuralgia; troubles the proper usage of prosthesis. It can be prevented during amputation by cutting the nerve after pulling down for significant length so that nerve end gets retracted adequately proximally. ***Lateral (side) neuroma*** (Fig. 5.16B) is seen after traumatic partial nerve injury; presents as tender, firm swelling along the line of peripheral nerve.

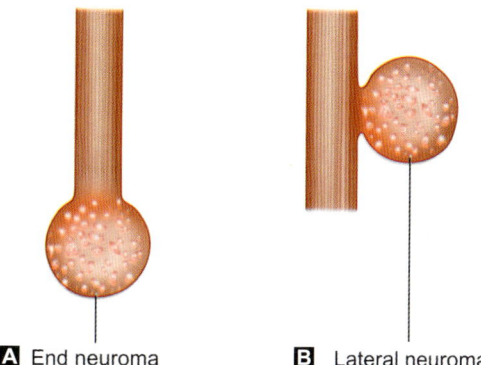

A End neuroma   **B** Lateral neuroma

Figs. 5.16A and B: Types of false neuromas: (A) End neuroma; (B) Side neuroma.

NEUROFIBROMA

- *It is a benign tumor arising from (connective tissue of) the nerve containing ectodermal neural and mesodermal connective tissue components.*
- It can be single or multiple. Neurofibromas may be associated with pheochromocytomas, hypertension and few syndromes.
- **Sites:** *Cranial; spinal; peripheral.*

Types

- ***Nodular neurofibroma***
  Presents as a single smooth, firm, tender (often) swelling, which moves horizontally or perpendicular to the direction of the nerve, but not in the direction of the nerve. There is pain and hyperesthesia in the distribution of the nerve.

*You will live once; but if you live it right, once is enough—**Adam Marhshall***

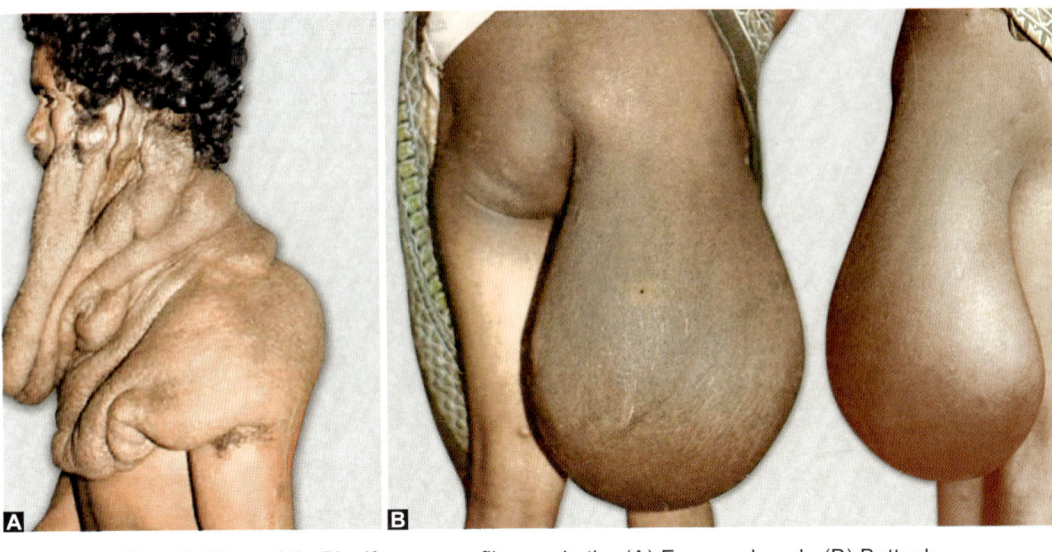

Figs. 5.17A and B: Plexiform neurofibroma in the (A) Face and neck; (B) Buttock.

- ❖ **Plexiform neurofibroma**
  Commonly occurs along the distribution of 5th cranial nerve in the skin of the face. It often occurs in the cutaneous distribution of the peripheral nerve. It attains enormous size with thick edematous pigmented skin, which hang downwards as pedunculated folds in front of neck (Figs. 5.17A and B). *It causes erosion into the bone, orbit and deeper structure.* The hanging skin fold can obstruct the vision. *It may also undergo myxomatous degeneration. It causes cosmetic problem.*
  - **Pachydermatocele** is a variant of plexiform neurofibroma involving the neck as thickened edematous pigmented skin with thrombosed veins with enormous proliferation of subcutaneous nerve fibers causing folded pendulous hanging thickened skin. It is common in trigeminal (5th cranial) nerve.
- ❖ **Generalized neurofibromatosis** (*von Recklinghausen's disease*):
  - It is an inherited autosomal dominant disease wherein there are multiple neurofibromas all over the body presenting as widespread soft, nontender, cutaneous nodules (over face, neck and limb).
  - It may involve cranial, spinal or peripheral.
  - It is associated with pigmented spots (coffee colored) in the skin, commonly seen on the back, abdomen, and thigh *(café au lait spots)* (Fig. 5.18).
- ❖ **Elephantiatic neurofibromatosis**
  It is of congenital origin. Often over the lower limb. Skin of the limb is greatly thickened coarse dry. Subcutaneous tissue is thickened and replaced by fibrous tissue.

Complications

1. *Sarcomatous changes*: When it occurs it shows rapid enlargement, warmness, and more vascularity with dilated veins. Secondaries in lungs occur through blood spread.
2. *Hemorrhage* into the tissues.
3. Spinal and cranial neurofibromas can cause neurological deficits.
4. Erosion into deeper planes, bone, and orbit.

Have no fear of perfection, you'll never reach it—**Salvador Dali**

FIBROMA

It is a benign tumor arising from fibrous tissue. It is capsulated.

Classification of True Fibroma

1. *Soft fibroma*—contains immature fibrous tissue. Common in face, presents as a soft brown swelling.
2. *Hard fibroma*—contains well-formed fibrous tissue.

Treatment of true fibroma is excision.

Note:
- True fibroma is rare and cannot be diagnosed clinically. It is mostly combined with mesodermal tissues like nerve sheath (neurofibroma), fat (fibrolipoma), muscle (fibromyoma).
- An entity called **aggressive fibromatosis** is known to occur as unencapsulated proliferation of fibrous tissue, common in abdominal wall and chest wall. It is considered presently *as locally malignant* condition. It does not spread through lymphatics or blood. *But recurrence is common.*
- **Desmoid tumor** is a variant of aggressive fibromatosis seen in females, often associated with Gardner's syndrome. (Desmos = tendon, eidos = appearance).
- **Recurrent fibroid of Paget's** is a rare type of fibrosarcoma occurring in scar tissue after many years.

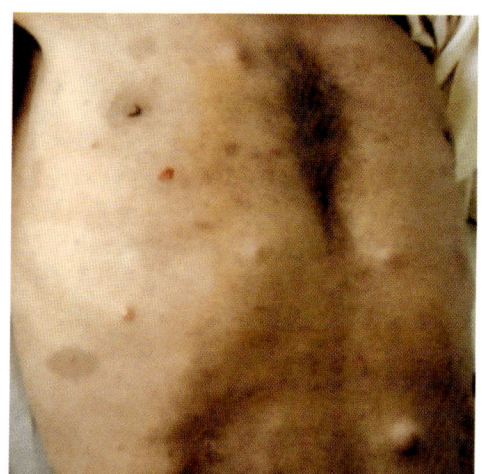

Fig. 5.18: Multiple neurofibromas with café au lait spots in the skin.

Note: Familial type of neurofibroma may be associated with scoliosis.

Treatment

Excision
Indications:
- Symptomatic neurofibroma.
- Cosmetically problematic lesion.
- Recent increase in size.
- Malignant transformation.

NEURILEMMOMA (SCHWANNOMA)

- It arises from Schwann (neurilemmal) cells. They are lobulated, encapsulated, soft, and whitish in appearance. They displace the nerve from which they arise and can be removed. They are common in acoustic nerve but can also occur in a peripheral nerve. Often they are multiple.
- Presentation is pain along the distribution of the nerve, hyperesthesia, and tenderness.
- **Treatment:** Excision.

Note: Recurrent schwannoma could be malignant.

GANGLION

It is a cystic swelling occurring in relation to tendon sheath or synovial sheath or joint capsule. It contains clear gel-like fluid.

Common Sites

- Dorsum of wrist (Fig. 5.19).
- Flexor aspect of wrist.
- Around ankle joint—occasionally.

Those who don't study the past will repeat its errors. Those who study it, will find other ways to err!!—**Charles Wolf**

Pathogenesis

- Cystic degeneration of the tendon sheath.
- Leakage of synovial fluid through joint capsule.
- There are small islets of microspaces in synovial sheath, which often fuses together or one of them get enlarged to form ganglion. Small ganglion is often mistaken for sesamoid bone or exostoses.

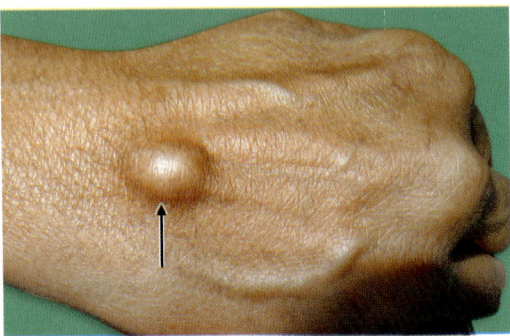

Fig. 5.19: Ganglion over the wrist (commonest site).

Features

- Well-localized, smooth, soft, cystic, or tensely cystic (Paget's test is + ve), nontender, transilluminant, swelling which is mobile but mobility is restricted when tendon is contracted against resistance.
- Occasionally it is communicating with joint capsule.
- Often pain, tenderness and restricted joint movement may be the presentation (but rare).
- **Differential diagnosis:** Lipoma; lymph cyst; sebaceous cyst.
- **Treatment:**
  - Excision, usually under local anesthesia (lignocaine plain 2%).
  - Patient should be explained of *high recurrence* rate (30%).
  - After excision it should always be sent for histopathology.

BURSAE

- Bursa is a sac-like cavity containing fluid within, which in normal location prevents friction between tendon and bone.
- Minor injuries and pressure leads to bursitis.
- Inflammation of this bursa due to friction causes **bursitis**, which commonly presents as swelling, pain, and restricted movements.

Different Types

- Anatomical (Fig. 5.20).
- Adventitious.

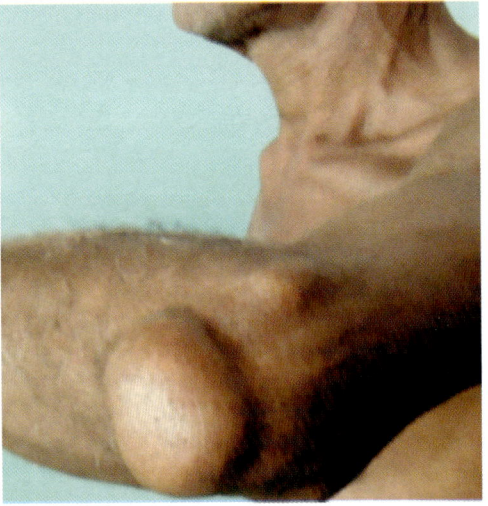

Fig. 5.20: Bursa near elbow joint.

Anatomical

- *Subhyoid bursa*—an horizontally oval swelling situated below the hyoid bone, in front of the thyrohyoid membrane.
- *Subacromial bursitis*—located in front and lateral to humeral head in relation to supraspinatus tendon between acromion and greater tuberosity of humerus
- *Bicipitoradial bursitis.*
- *Olecranon bursitis* (*Student's elbow*) (*Miner's elbow*) (Fig. 5.21).

Life is not a problem to be solved, but a reality to be experienced—**Søren Kierkegaard**

Adventitious Bursa

- Occurs in an unusual site like in hallux valgus (**bunion**) **(Fig. 5.23A)**, over first metatarsal, over lateral malleolus (***tailor's bursa***) **(Fig. 5.23B)**, between tendo-Achilis and skin (***retro-Achilis bursitis***) or over gluteal tuberosity. It occurs due to friction or pressure.

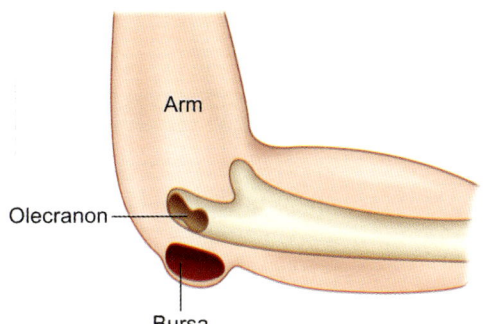

Fig. 5.21: Olecranon bursa location (student's elbow).

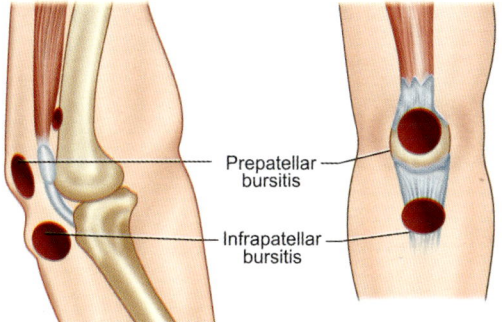

Fig. 5.22: Prepatellar (housemaid's knee) and infrapatellar bursae (Clergyman's knee).

- *Psoas bursa*—a tensely cystic swelling beneath and below the inguinal ligament in the lateral aspect of the femoral triangle. But it will not extend above the inguinal ligament into the iliac region (unlike in psoas abscess which extends above and is cross fluctuant).
- *Prepatellar bursitis (housemaid's knee) (Fig. 5.22).*
- *Infrapatellar bursitis (Clergyman's knee) (Fig. 5.22).*
- *Semimembranosus bursitis.*
- *Bursa anserina*—located under the tendons of Guy ropes (sartorius, gracilis and semitendinosus tendons—*goose's foot*).
- *Retrocalcaneum bursitis*—between calcaneum and tendo-Achilis.

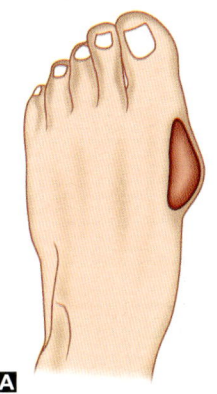 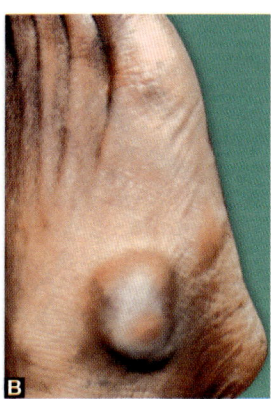

Figs. 5.23A and B: (A and B) Adventitious bursa in the foot (Bunion)—common site.

- **Differential diagnosis:**
  - Soft tissue tumor.
  - Cold abscess.
- **Management:**
  - X-ray of the part and often fine needle aspiration cytology (FNAC) are required.
  - Excision of the bursa.

SEMIMEMBRANOSUS BURSA

It is a cystic swelling in the upper medial aspect of the popliteal fossa under the semimembranosus tendon. It is said to be due to friction under the tendon causing bursitis.

Features

- Common in young individuals.
- Soft, smooth, cystic, often transilluminant and nontender swelling located in

*A lifetime of happiness! No man alive could bear it; it would be hell on earth—**Bernard Shaw***

upper and medial aspect of the popliteal fossa.
* On knee flexion swelling becomes flaccid but cannot be reduced completely; on knee extension swelling becomes tenser.
* Swelling does not communicate into knee joint cavity.
* Knee joint is normal.

Treatment

* Ultrasound of popliteal fossa shows the cystic swelling under semimembranosus tendon.
* X-ray knee joint is normal.
* Excision is done under general anesthesia using tourniquet. Complete excision of the sac is needed to prevent recurrence.

MORRANT BAKER CYST

It is a cystic swelling containing gel-like fluid in the *lower midline of the popliteal fossa*. It occurs due to herniation of the synovial membrane of the knee joint as a result of chronic arthritis.

Features

* It is common in middle-aged individuals.
* It is smooth, soft and cystic, often tender swelling located below and in midline of the popliteal fossa.
* On flexion swelling decreases and on extension it increases in size.
* Pain and tenderness are present in knee joint with effusion showing *positive patellar tap*.
* The knee joint movements are painful and restricted.
* **Management:** X-ray of joint shows arthritic changes; MRI may be needed occasionally.

* **Treatment:** Arthritis is treated and Baker's cyst is excised under general anesthesia in prone position.

CALCINOSIS CUTIS

* It is circumscribed foci of calcification (dystrophic) in or under the skin.
* Commonly seen in females. Common site is in the waist (Fig. 5.24).

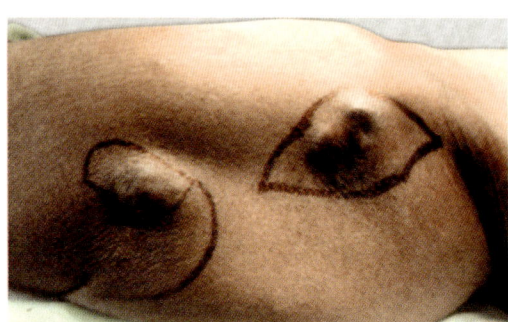

Fig. 5.24: Calcinosis cutis near waist is a common site. It is common in females.

* Usually bilateral.
* It is said to be due to friction causing degeneration of skin and immediate deeper structure with increased local alkalinity of the tissues causing precipitation of the calcium leading to solid, hard, swelling in the skin. Cut section shows hard, yellowish material.
* It may mimic calcified lipoma or neurofibroma.
* **Treatment:** Excision and closure of defect often with local flaps.

EPIGNATHUS (FIG. 5.25)

This is a type of anomaly seen in neonates wherein growth from the base of skull protrudes through the mouth.

Be yourself; everyone else is already taken—Oscar Wilde

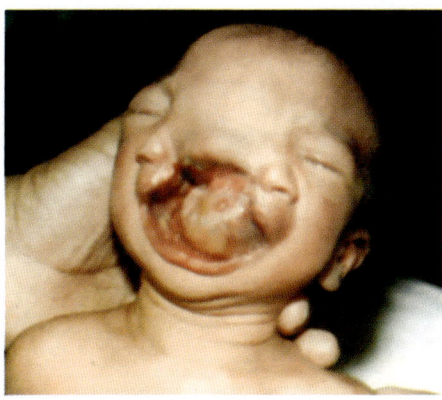

Fig. 5.25: Epignathus.

CHORDOMA

- It is the tumor arising from remnants of notochord.
- It is seen in sacrococcygeal/sphenoid sinus region and around the foramen magnum.
- It invades the surrounding structures like nerves.
- It is radioresistant.
- Resection is difficult.

CHAPTER 6

Shock, Hemorrhage and Blood Transfusion

CHAPTER OUTLINE

- Shock
- Cardiogenic Shock
- Central Venous Pressure
- Pulmonary Capillary Wedge Pressure
- Systemic Inflammatory Response Syndrome
- Oxygen Therapy
- Hyperbaric Oxygen
- Cardiac Arrest
- Mechanism of Blood Coagulation
- Hemorrhage
- Blood Transfusion
- Blood Fractions
- Massive Blood Transfusion
- Blood Substitutes
- Autologous Blood Transfusion
- Recycled Blood
- Artificial Blood
- Tourniquets

SHOCK

DEFINITION

Shock is defined as a state of cellular and tissue hypoxia with either reduced oxygen delivery or poor oxygen utilization or increased oxygen consumption with circulatory failure (collapse) and poor perfusion.

CAUSES OF SHOCK

1. **Hypovolemic shock:**
   Due to reduction in total blood volume.
   It may be due to:
   a. *Hemorrhage*
      - External from wounds, open fractures.
      - Internal from injury to spleen, liver, mesentery or pelvis.
   b. *Severe burns*, which results in loss of plasma.
   c. Peritonitis, intestinal obstruction.
   d. Vomiting and diarrhea due to any cause.
2. **Cardiac causes:**
   A. *Cardiogenic shock:*
      It results due to intrinsic problem within the cardiac muscle or valve causing decreased cardiac function.
      a. Acute myocardial infarction, acute carditis.
      b. Acute pulmonary embolism, wherein embolus blocks the bifurcation of pulmonary artery or one of the major branches. Air embolism (50 mL of

Nothing stands in front of a willing heart and strong determination.

air) also can cause shock due to pulmonary embolism.
   c. Drug induced.
   d. Toxemia of any causes.
   e. Cardiac surgical conditions like valvular diseases, congenital heart diseases.
  B. *Cardiac compression causes*:
   i. Cardiac tamponade due to collection of blood, pus, fluid in the pericardial space, which prevents the heart to expand leading to shock.
   ii. Trauma to heart.
3. **Septic shock:**
   It is due to bacterial infection, which release toxins leading to shock.
4. **Neurogenic shock:**
   Sudden anxious or painful stimuli cause sympathetic failure leading to severe splanchnic vessel vasodilatation. It leads to cerebral hypoperfusion, cerebral hypoxia, and unconsciousness. Here patient either goes for sudden cardiac arrest and dies or recovers fully spontaneously.
   Causes: Injury to spinal cord, dental extraction done with ineffective local anesthesia.
   Treatment: Patient is made to lie down immediately; foot end elevation is done to improve cerebral perfusion; rapid infusion of fluids; vasopressin if hypotension persists.
5. **Anaphylactic shock:**
   It is due to type I hypersensitivity reaction. It presents with skin rash, bronchospasm, laryngeal edema, which leads into breathing difficulty, hypotension and unconsciousness.
6. **Respiratory causes:**
   a. Atelectasis (collapse) of lung.
   b. Thoracic injuries.
   c. Tension pneumothorax.
   d. Anesthetic complications.
7. **Other causes:**
   a. Acute adrenal insufficiency (Addison's disease).
   b. Myxedema.

Pathophysiology of Shock

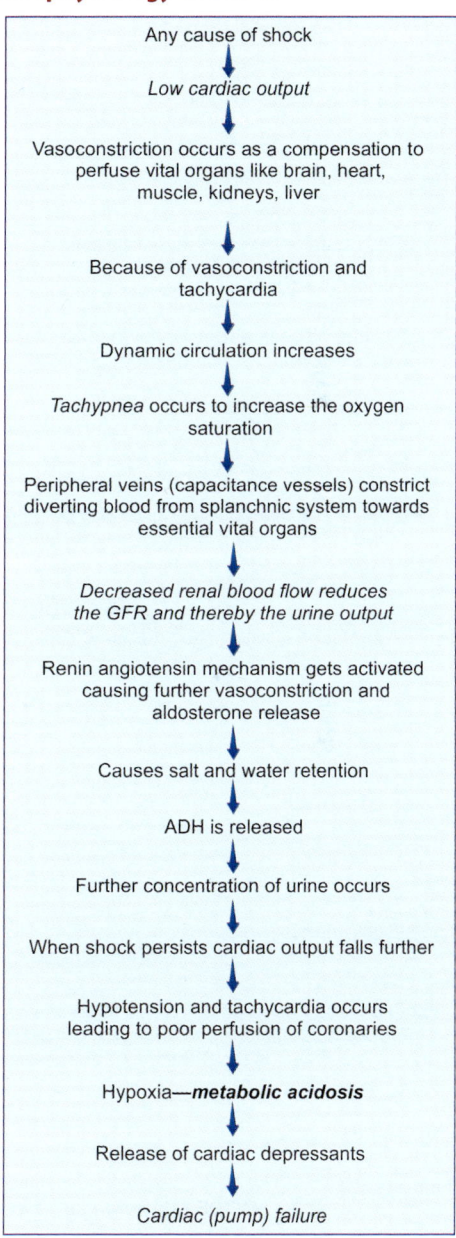

*May you live every day of your life—**Jonathan Swift***

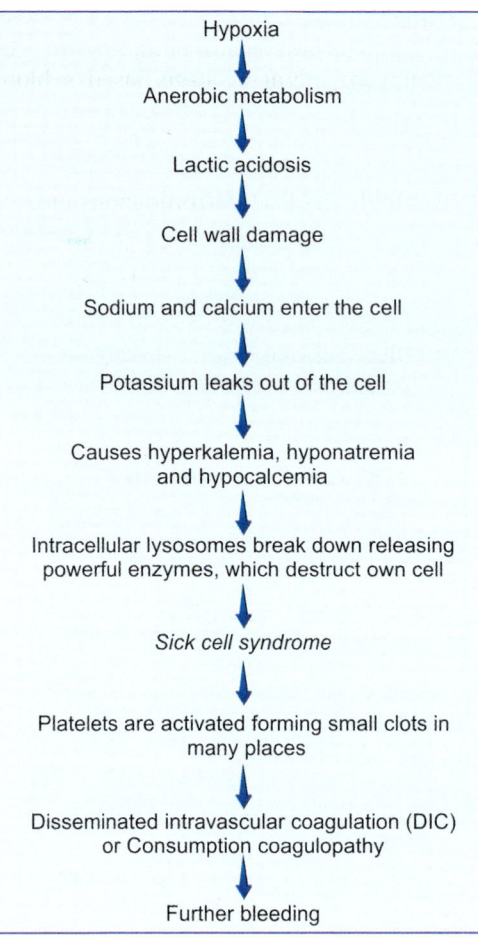

Effects of Shock

Heart: Low perfusion → low venous return → decreased cardiac output → hypotension → tachycardia. Persistent shock causes hypoxia and release of myocardial depressants leading to further cardiac damage.

Lung: Interstitial edema → decreased gaseous exchange → pulmonary arteriovenous shunting → tachypnea → *Adult respiratory distress syndrome (ARDS)* and pulmonary edema.

Metabolic: Shock leads to hypoxia, which activates anaerobic metabolism leading to lactic acidosis. Antidiuretic hormone (ADH) is released which increases the reabsorption of water from renal tubules. Other hormones released are adrenocorticotropic hormone (ACTH), prostaglandins, histamine, bradykinin, serotonin to compensate the effects of shock to increase the perfusion of vital organs like heart, brain, and lungs.

Cellular changes occur in persistent shock due to release of lysosomal enzymes, which alters the cell membrane permeability causing cell death—*sick cell syndrome.*

Sympathetic overactivity alters the microcirculation leading to capillary dysfunction.

Stages of Shock

Causes
(Infection, trauma, burns, hemorrhage, hypovolemia)
↓
Hypoxia and its effects
↓
Systemic inflammatory response syndrome (SIRS) is due to vasodilatation, increased endothelial permeability, thrombosis, leukocyte migration and activation
↓
All these leads to altered cytokines level, abnormal NO (nitric oxide) synthesis, abnormal arachidonic acid metabolism, neutrophil activation, free radical formation, altered complement activation, failure to have a localization of inflammation. It is severe type of reversible shock
↓
Which leads to established microvascular occlusion, cellular dysfunction, sick cell syndrome, DIC, and PUMP failure
↓
MODS *(Multiorgan dysfunction syndrome)* *(Irreversible shock)*

Nothing is impossible to a willing heart

Brain perfusion once decreases and the patient becomes drowsy. Brain is the last organ to get underperfused in shock.

Kidneys: Glomerular filtration rate (GFR) decreases and tubular reabsorption of salt and water increases for compensatory response. But in severe cases, tubular necrosis sets in leading to irreversible damage.

Blood: Alteration in cellular components including platelets leads to *disseminated intravascular thrombosis (DIC)*. It causes bleeding from all organs.

Gastrointestinal tract (GIT): Mucosal ischemia develops causing bleeding from GIT with hematemesis and melena. It is aggravated by DIC. Hepatic ischemia leads into increased enzyme levels.

Types of hypovolemia

a. **Covert compensated hypovolemia**: When blood volume is reduced by 10–15%, there will not be significant change in heart rate, cardiac output and splanchnic blood compensates for the same.
b. **Overt compensated hypovolemia**: Here patient has cold periphery, tachycardia, a wide arterial pressure, tachypnea, confusion, hyponatremia, metabolic acidosis, but systolic pressure is well-maintained.
c. **Decompensated hypovolemia**: Here all features of hypovolemia is present. Hypotension, tachycardia, sweating, tachypnea, oliguria, drowsiness, eventually features of SIRS appears, and often if not treated on time leads to MODS, i.e. irreversible shock.

Septic Shock

Also called as **endotoxic shock**. It occurs due to Gram-negative bacterial infections, often seen in cases of strangulated intestines, peritonitis, GIT fistulas, biliary sepsis, urinary sepsis, etc.

Stages of Septic Shock

1. *Hyperdynamic (warm) shock*: This stage is **reversible stage**. Patient is still having inflammatory response and so presents with fever, tachycardia, tachypnea, etc. Pyrogenic response is still intact. Patient should be treated properly at this stage. Based on blood culture, urine culture (depending on focus of infection), combination of higher antibiotics like third generation Cephalosporins, Aminoglycosides, Metronidazole, etc. are started. The underlying cause is treated like draining the abscess if any, laparotomy for peritonitis, etc. Ventilatory support with proper ICU monitoring may prevent the patient going for the next *cold stage of sepsis*.
2. *Hypodynamic hypovolemic septic shock (Cold septic shock)*: Here pyrogenic response is lost. Patient is in decompensated shock. It is an **irreversible stage** along with multiorgan dysfunction syndrome (MODS) patient presents with anuria, respiratory failure (cyanosis), jaundice (liver failure), cardiac depression, pulmonary edema, hypoxia, drowsiness. Eventually coma and death occurs.

Common organisms involved are *E. coli, Klebsiella, Pseudomonas, Proteus*.

Septic shock

- Common causes are biliary, urinary, GIT sepsis (peritonitis, strangulation).
- Common bacteria are *E.coli, Klebsiella, Pseudomonas*.
- Common pathophysiologies are release of toxins, neutrophil activation, cytokine release, sick cell syndrome, SIRS, MODS.
- Clinical stages are hyperdynamic and hypodynamic.
- Find out the source of the infection by ultrasound CT scan.
- Do pus/blood/urine culture.
- Start antibiotics of high generations like ceftazidime, amikacin, cefoperazone.
- Dopamine/dobutamine infusion (slow).
- Monitoring by pulse, BP, respiration, urine output, level of consciousness.
- Blood transfusion may be required.
- Ventilator support, ICU management.
- *Treat the cause like peritonitis, abscess drainage.*

Note:
❖ Sepsis is life-threatening organ dysfunction caused by a dysregulated host response to

---

*You may be disappointed if you fail, but you are doomed if you don't try—***Beverly Sills**

infection identified by the presence of 2 or more SOFA points (scores) [Sequential (sepsis related) organ failure assessment]. Quick SOFA (qSOFA) score is also used—low blood pressure <100 mm Hg; increased respiratory rate >22/minute; altered mentation—GCS <13.
- Mean arterial pressure (MAP) is an average blood pressure during single phase of cardiac cycle. It is measured by = Diastolic pressure + 1/3rd of pulse pressure.

Anaphylactic Shock

Injections—Penicillins, anesthetics, stings, shellfish, etc. may be having antigens which combines with IgE of mast cells and basophils, releasing histamine and large amount of *SRS-A* (Slow Releasing Substance of Anaphylaxis). They cause bronchospasm, laryngeal edema, respiratory distress, hypotension and shock. Mortality is 10%.

Anaphylactic shock
- Sudden onset.
- Distributive shock.
- Bronchospasm, laryngeal edema.
- Generalized rashes and edema.
- Hypotension, feeble pulse.
- Mortality 10%.
- To start Adrenaline 100 μg IV, steroids, IV fluids, oxygen with foot end elevation.
- Ventilator in severe cases.
- Cardiac massage, defibrillation.

Clinical Features of Shock
- In early stage, tachycardia, sweating, cold periphery, hypotension, restlessness, air hunger, tachypnea, oliguria, collapsed veins.
- In late stage, cyanosis, anuria, jaundice, drowsiness occurs.

Investigations
- Regular monitoring of BP, pulse.
- Heart rate.
- Respiratory rate.
- Central venous pressure line (CVP).
- Pulmonary capillary wedge pressure (PCWP).
- Measurement of urine output.
- Arterial PO_2 and PCO_2 analysis.
- Serum electrolyte estimation.

Treatment of Shock

Guidelines:
- *To treat the cause.*
- *To improve cardiac function.*
- *To improve tissue perfusion.*

- Treat the cause, e.g. arrest hemorrhage, drain pus.
- Fluid replacement: A large bore cannula is inserted into the forearm vein for infusion. Plasma, normal saline, dextrose, Ringer lactate, plasma expander (*Haemaccel*—maximum 1 liter can be given in 24 hours). Blood transfusion in case of blood loss.
- Inotropic agents: Dopamine, Dobutamine, Adrenaline infusions. To improve myocardial contractility.
- Correction of acid base balance.
- *Steroids* is often life-saving. 500–1,000 mg of hydrocortisone can be given. It improves the perfusion, reduces the capillary leakage and systemic inflammatory effects.
- Antibiotics in patients with sepsis; proper control of blood sugar and ketosis in diabetic patients.
- Catheterization to measure urine output (normal output—30–50 mL/hour or >0.5 mL/kg/hour).
- Nasal oxygen to improve oxygenation or monitoring in intensive care unit with ventilator support has to be done.
- CVP line to perfuse adequately and to monitor fluid balance. Total parenteral nutrition (TPN) can be given when required. Brain perfusion can also be improved by using Trendelenburg position (Fig. 6.1).
- PCWP to monitor very critical patient.
- Hemodialysis may be necessary when kidneys are not functioning.

A misty morning does not signify a cloudy day.

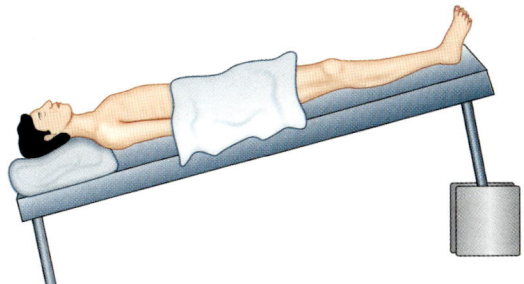

Fig. 6.1: Trendelenburg position is used in all patients in shock to improve the brain perfusion.

CARDIOGENIC SHOCK

Cardiogenic shock is defined as circulatory failure causing diminished forward flow leading into tissue hypoxia in the setting of adequate intravascular volume with systolic blood pressure <90 mm Hg for 30 minutes; cardiac index <2.2 L/minute/sq meter; raised PCWP >15 mm Hg. It is commonly seen in acute myocardial infarction (MI) with a mortality >50%. Cardiogenic shock develops within 24 hours of MI. It occurs when 50% of left ventricular wall is damaged by infarction. It leads to pulmonary edema and severe hypoxia. Ischemic necrosis of left ventricular wall causes failure of pump thereby decreasing stroke volume.

Diagnosis is established by *ECG* (echocardiography), arterial blood gas analysis, *cardiac enzymes, PCWP* and electrolyte estimation (hypokalemia and hypomagnesemia are common) are the essential investigations.

Management

- Proper oxygenation with intubation, ventilator support, cardioversion, pacing, antiarrhythmic drugs, correction of electrolytes, avoiding fluid overload, prevention of pulmonary edema as immediate measures.
- Dobutamine (β_1 receptor agonist) is used to raise cardiac output provided there is adequate preload and intravascular volume (it is peripheral vasodilator and reduces BP). Dopamine is preferred in patients with hypotension. But it may increase peripheral resistance and heart rate worsening cardiac ischemia. Often both Dopamine and Dobutamine combination may be required.
- Careful judicial use of Epinephrine, Norepinephrine, Phosphodiesterase inhibitors (Amrinone, Milrinone) are often needed. Anticoagulants and Aspirin are given. Thrombolytics can be used. β blockers, nitrates (nitroglycerin causes coronary arterial dilatation), ACE inhibitors are also used.
- *Intra-aortic balloon pump (IABP)* may need to be introduced transfemorally as a mechanical circulatory support to raise cardiac output and coronary blood flow.
- Relief of pain, preserving of remaining myocardium and its function, maintaining adequate preload, oxygenation, minimizing sympathetic stimulation, correction of electrolytes should be the priorities.
- Percutaneous transluminal coronary angioplasty *(PTCA)* and coronary artery bypass graft *(CABG)* are the final choices.

CENTRAL VENOUS PRESSURE

Central venous pressure (CVP) is a method to measure the right atrial pressure by placing a venous catheter (20 cm) into the SVC. Commonly for CVP monitoring, a venous catheter is passed through right internal jugular vein or infraclavicular subclavian vein to the superior vena cava (SVC) (used for TPN purpose). Or occasionally a long catheter (60 cm) can be passed through basilic vein (not commonly done). Under radiological guidance, initially a needle is passed 3 cm above the medial end of the clavicle, in the hollow between the two heads of sternomastoid muscles, directing towards the suprasternal notch into the right internal jugular vein. Then through a guidewire, a venous catheter is passed into the SVC through right internal jugular vein, which can also be confirmed by changes in flow during inspiration and expiration.

*The most difficult thing is the decision to act, the rest is merely tenacity—**Amelia Earhart***

Catheter is connected to saline manometer, taking manubriosternal angle (*angle of Louis*) as zero point (Figs. 6.2A and B).

Normal value is 2–10 cm of saline.

Complications of CVP

- Pneumothorax.
- Hemothorax.
- Injury to brachial plexus and vessels.
- Bleeding.
- Sepsis.
- Catheter displacement.

If less than 2 cm, more fluid is infused.

If more than 10 cm, fluid infusion should be restricted.

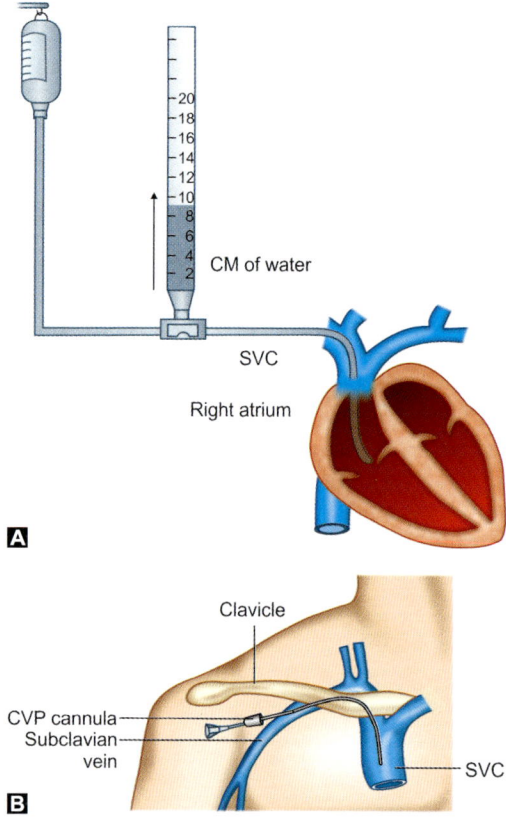

Figs. 6.2A and B: Central venous pressure (CVP) is used to monitor the patient. Note the location of the central venous catheter.

PULMONARY CAPILLARY WEDGE PRESSURE

It is a better indicator of circulating blood volume and left ventricular function.

Catheter used is *Swan Ganz* triple channel pulmonary artery balloon catheter.

It is used to differentiate right and left ventricular failure, pulmonary embolus, and septic shock. To measure cardiac output, to monitor fluid therapy, inotropic agents, vasodilators.

Procedure (Fig. 6.3)

Under strict aseptic precaution, using cannula and guidewire, catheter is passed through internal jugular vein, into the right atrium. Balloon is inflated by 1.5 mL of air and then negotiated into pulmonary artery, until it reaches a small branch and wedges it. Pressure at this point is called as *pulmonary capillary wedge pressure*.

PCWP normally is 8–12 mm Hg, considering midaxillary point as zero reference point.

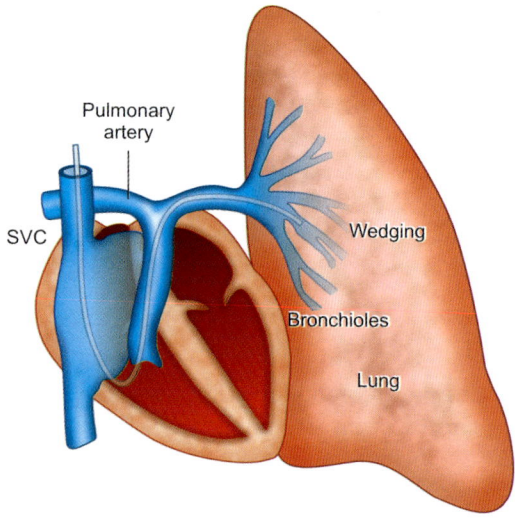

Fig. 6.3: Pulmonary capillary wedge pressure (PCWP) is better index of shock. But it is technically difficult and cannot be kept for more than 72 hours. It cannot be used for perfusion purpose unlike CVP line.

Not in time, place, or circumstance, but in the man lies success

Differences between CVP and PCWP	
CVP	**PCWP**
• Technically easier.	• Requires skilled experts.
• Normal pressure is 2–10 cm of saline.	• 8–12 mm Hg.
• Gives gross idea about fluid balance.	• Better and specific.
• Left ventricular function is not assessed.	• Left ventricular function is very well-assessed
• Not used to differentiate between right and left ventricular function.	• Very well-differentiates.
• Can be kept in situ as long as required.	• Cannot be kept in situ for more than 72 hours.
• Catheter tip is in SVC.	• Catheter tip is in pulmonary capillary with wedging
• Plain tip catheter.	• 1.5 mL air filled balloon tip.
• Can be used for TPN, fluid infusion, etc.	• Cannot be used for TPN, or fluid infusion.
• Complications are easy to tackle.	• Often difficult to tackle.
• Not as sensitive and specific as PCWP.	• Sensitive and specific.

After that, balloon is deflated to get pulmonary artery pressure which is normally 25 mm Hg systolic and 10 mm Hg diastolic.

PCWP catheter can be kept in situ only for 72 hours.

Complications of PCWP

- Arrhythmias.
- Pulmonary artery rupture. Balloon rupture.
- Pulmonary infarction.
- Pneumothorax.
- Hemothorax.
- Bleeding, sepsis, thrombosis.

SYSTEMIC INFLAMMATORY RESPONSE SYNDROME

❖ It is final common pathway in shock due to any cause (trauma, sepsis, endotoxemia, burns), where there is failure of inflammatory localization with vasodilatation, increased endothelial permeability with damage, thrombosis, leukoctye migration and activation.
❖ It is associated with release of free radicals, abnormal arachidonic acid release, cytokine release, neutrophil sequestration, abnormal NO synthesis, complement activation, and DIC.
❖ **SIRS** is systemic manifestations of inflammation due to variety of causes like infection, pancreatitis, polytrauma, burns, transfusion reaction, and malignancy. So it is often categorized as infectious cause SIRS or noninfectious cause SIRS. It causes either *hyperthermia (>38°C) or hypothermia (<36°C); tachycardia (pulse >90/minute); tachypnea (>20/minute); total white cell count >12,000/cu mm, or count <4000/cu mm.*
❖ It is a part of severely decompensated *reversible shock,* which eventually leads to MODS (multiorgan dysfunction syndrome), a state of *irreversible shock* wherein patient is anuric, drowsy, cold and terminally ill.
❖ SIRS carries poor prognosis.

OXYGEN THERAPY

Indications

❖ Chest injuries, any severe hemorrhage.
❖ Gas gangrene with toxic hemolysis.
❖ Coal gas poisoning.
❖ Over morphinization.
❖ Pulmonary embolism and fat embolism.
❖ Spontaneous pneumothorax, pulmonary edema, cardiac infarction, pneumonia, cor pulmonale.
❖ Cardiogenic shock and acute bronchitis.

*Before anything else, preparation is the key to success—**Alexander Graham Bell***

About 27% oxygen is delivered through ventimask (disposable polythene mask) at a rate of 4–6 liters per minute. Oxygen is also given along with positive pressure ventilation.

HYPERBARIC OXYGEN

It is administration of oxygen 1 or 2 atmospheres above the atmospheric pressure in a compression chamber. It increases the arterial oxygen saturation so that oxygen perfusion of tissues will be increased.

Indications

- Carbon monoxide poisoning.
- Tetanus, gas gangrene infections.
- Bedsores, frostbites.
- Drenching in paralytic ileus to reduce the nitrogen gas in distended bowel.
- As a radiosensitizer in the treatment of cancer.

Complications of hyperbaric oxygen: CO_2 narcosis, respiratory depression.

CARDIAC ARREST

It is the cessation of the heart. Heart stops contracting.

Causes: All causes for shock.

Features of cardiac arrest
• No palpable pulse.
• Heart sounds not heard.
• Cessation of respiration—cyanosis occurs.
• Development of unconsciousness.
• Pupils start dilating.

Critical period: Once heart and lungs stop, *brain death occurs in 3 minutes.*

Immediate measures
• **A**irway.
• **B**reathing.
• **C**ardiac compression.
• **D**rugs and **D**efibrillator.
• **E**CG, **E**ndotracheal tube and monitor.

- **External cardiac compression (massage):** Patient is laid flat on a *hard surface (never on soft surface)*. Manual compression is exerted over the lower sternum, using both hands one over other without bending the elbow at a rate of 60 to 70 per minute. Rib cage damage during procedure can be very well ignored. (Heel of right hand is placed over the sternum 8 cm above xiphoid process and left hand is placed over it) (Fig. 6.4).
- At the same time, another person should give *mouth-to-mouth breathing* at a rate of 20 to 30 per minute after clearing the airway by removing froth, dentures if present. A bag with mask can be used to ventilate using air or oxygen (Fig. 6.5).
- Endotracheal intubation and ventilator support.
- Injection of 1:10,000 Adrenaline and 10% Calcium chloride intravenously.

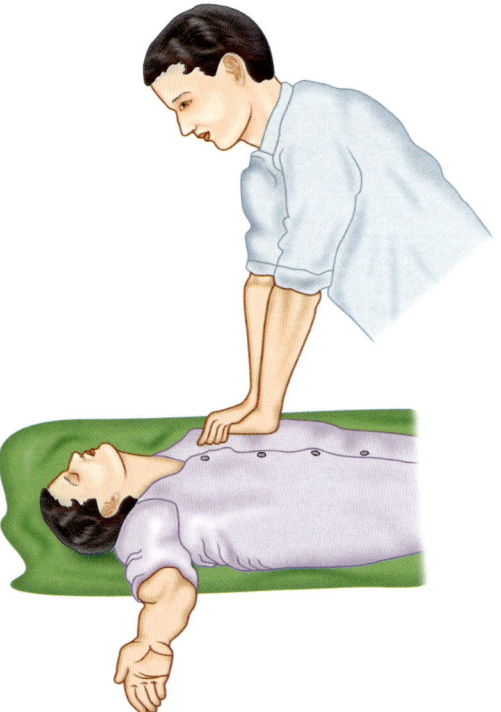

Fig. 6.4: Technique of cardiac massage.

Kindness is the golden chain by which society is bound together.

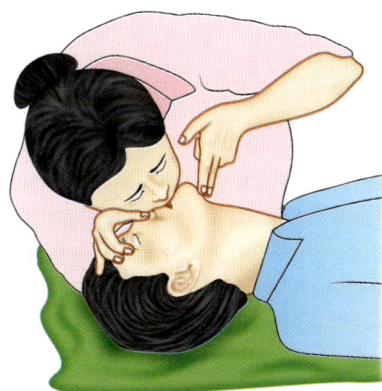

Fig. 6.5: Technique of mouth-to-mouth respiration. Note patient's nose should be held closed with right hand of the doctor/assistant and with left hand lower jaw should be pushed forward.

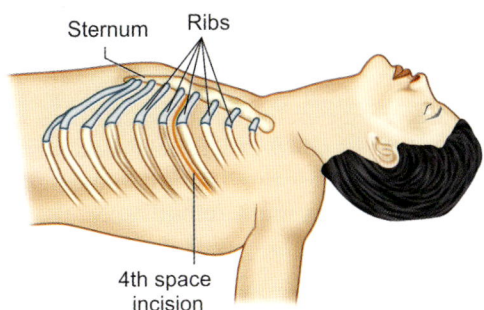

Fig. 6.6: Left thoracotomy for open internal cardiac massage.

- Sodium bicarbonate 8.4% injection, Hydrocortisone injection.
- Defibrillation, if there is ventricular fibrillation.
- Analysis of blood gas (PCO_2 and PO_2), and serum electrolytes assessment at repeated intervals.
- Urinary catheterization, Ryle's tube insertion.
- Monitoring the patient with BP, pulse, respiration, and temperature chart.

Observations to be made are
- Groin pulse.
- Respiration and breath sounds.
- Blood pressure.
- Pupillary reaction.
- ECG activity.

Once patient recovers, the cause and sequelae has to be managed properly.

Sequelae are due to hypoxia and circulatory collapse
- Cerebral edema and permanent brain damage.
- Adult respiratory distress syndrome (ARDS).
- Renal failure.

Internal Open Cardiac Massage (Fig. 6.6)

This method is used when cardiac arrest occurs in the operation theater during surgery, acute tamponade, and acute bilateral pneumothorax.

Left side thorax is opened through a lengthy incision along 4th or 5th intercostal space. Initially heart with intact pericardium is rhythmically compressed and relaxed using left hand against sternum. Meantime costal cartilages above and below are cut with a knife to have a better exposure. Pericardium is opened in front of the phrenic nerve. Direct cardiac massage is undertaken until heart regains its function and later shifted to ventilatory support and critical care.

Defibrillation Technique (Fig. 6.7)

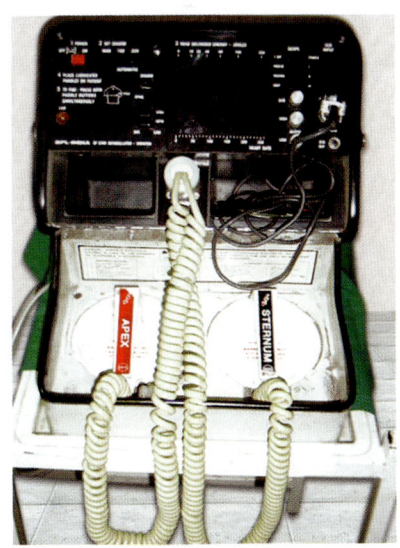

Fig. 6.7: Defibrillator used in case of cardiac arrest.

Success is walking from failure to failure with no loss of enthusiasm—**Winston Churchill**

Gelly is applied to the site of electrodes. One electrode is placed at the base of heart to the right of the sternum, other over the estimated area of the apex of the heart. **Ensure that nobody is in contact with the patient**. The defibrillator is activated. Ventilation and ECG monitoring is resumed immediately. After that continuous monitoring is done, acidosis is corrected, bladder is catheterized and urine output is observed. Patient is kept in ICU.

MECHANISM OF BLOOD COAGULATION

Hemostasis is the spontaneous arrest of bleeding. When an injury occurs **platelet adhesion** occurs to injured vessel/capillary wall which activates the release of ADP (Adenosine diphosphate) which makes more platelet to aggregate (**platelet aggregation**). These activated platelets release thromboxane A2 which further increases the adhesion and aggregation of platelets. Circulating fibrinogen binds to an activated platelet receptors glycoprotein IIb and IIIa and fibrinogen gets converted into fibrin.

Clotting factors are proteins synthesized by the liver which with a series of cascade method activates clotting factors and achieves blood coagulation by a complex mechanism. Factor II, VII, IX and X are vitamin K dependent for their synthesis in liver (carboxylation of glutamic acid). In the process of coagulation, each factor gets activated to an enzyme by partial proteolysis which in turn activates other needed coagulation factors. Eventually, fibrinogen gets converted into soluble fibrin and later into insoluble *fibrin*.

Two types coagulation system are there:
- Intrinsic pathway.
- Extrinsic pathway.

In vitro coagulation occurs by intrinsic coagulation system. Cascade gets activated by vessel wall injury, shear stress of vessel or other factors. It activates the cascade to get the final result—prekallikreine, kininogen.

Coagulation Cascade System

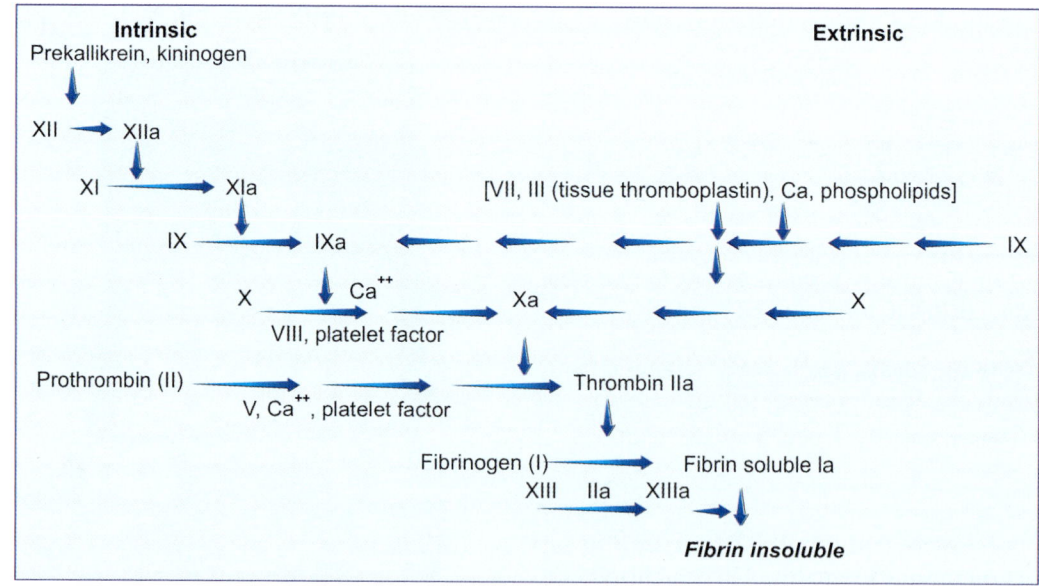

Everything takes practice, except being born.

Blood Clotting Factors

Factor no.	Common name
I	Fibrinogen
II	Prothrombin
III	Thromboplastin
IV	Ionic calcium
V	Hereditary labile factor, activator (AC) globulin, proaccelerin
VI	Accelerin, supposed to be active form of factor V
VII	Proconvertin; serum prothrombin—conversion accelerator (SPCA)
VIII	Antihemophilic factor (AHF)
IX	Plasma thromboplastin component (PTC; Christmas factor)
X	Stuart-Prower factor
XI	Plasma thromboplastin antecedent (PTA)
XII	Hageman factor
XIII	Fibrin stabilizing factor, fibrinase
XIV	Prekallikrein
XV	Kallikrein
XVI	Platelet factor

Hemophilia and *von Willebrand's disease* are the two most common inherited bleeding disorders due to deficiency of factor VIII.

Factor VIII has two components; smaller one—factor VIII C is needed for activation of factor X in intrinsic coagulation pathway; its deficiency leads to *classic hemophilia*. It is inherited as an X-linked recessive trait, thus it occurs in males and homozygous females. The larger component of factor VIII called *von Willebrand's factor,* facilitates the adhesion of platelets to subendothelial collagen, hence crucial for hemostasis, its absence leads to *von Willebrand's disease.*

1. **Classic hemophilia:**
   It is called hemophilia A, is caused by deficiency of factor *VIII C* with X-linked *recessive* trait. It occurs in males or homozygous females. APTT is raised (↑); PT is normal. Recurrent hemarthroses are common presentation. Petechiae and ecchymoses are absent. Bleeding time is normal but coagulation time is prolonged. Treatment is cryoprecipitate, VIII hemophilic factor replacement. After dental extraction, patient may go for a life-threatening bleeding, if proper history/precaution is not taken.

   von Willebrand's disease:
   It is deficiency of larger component (99%) of the factor VIII—vWF. It is autosomal *dominant* disease with normal bleeding time and normal platelet count. Common presentations are spontaneous bleeding from mucous membrane, excessive bleeding from wounds and severe menorrhagia. APTT ↑; BT ↑; PT is normal. Hemarthroses are not common in von Willebrand's disease. Treatment is replacement of specific factors.

   Treatment—administration of DDAVP; cryoprecipitate infusion.

2. **Hemophilia B:**
   Also called as *Christmas disease* is due to factor IX deficiency and is inherited as X-linked autosomal recessive trait.

HEMORRHAGE

Classification I

1. *Arterial*:
   It is bright red in color, spurt like jet along with rhythm of pulse of the patient.
2. *Venous*:
   It is dark red, steady and continuous flow. Blood loss may be severe and rapid when bleeding is from femoral vein, jugular vein, other major veins, varicose veins, portal vein, and esophageal varices.
   Note—Pulmonary arterial blood is dark red in color and pulmonary venous blood is bright red in color.
3. *Capillary*:
   Here bleeding is rapid and bright red. It is often torrential due to continuous ooze.

I hear : I forget/I see : I remember/I do : I understand—**Chinese Proverb**

Classification II

1. ***Primary:***
   Occurs at the time of injury or operation.
2. ***Reactionary:***
   It occurs within 24 hours after surgery or after injury (commonly in 4–6 hours).

Precipitating factors	Causes
• Coughing	• Thyroid surgery
• Vomiting	• Cholecystectomy
• Straining	• Major abdominal surgeries
• Rise of blood pressure	• Circumcision
• Restlessness	• Hydrocele surgery
• Venous refilling during recovery from anesthesia	• Tonsillectomy
• Slipping of ligature	
• Clot dislodgement	

3. ***Secondary:***
   It occurs in 7–14 days after surgery.

Factors	Causes
• Infection	• Erosion of carotid artery by cancer (secondaries in the neck)
• Pressure by drain or bone	• Hemorrhoidectomy
• Malignancy	• Inguinal block dissection

Classification III

Revealed hemorrhage	Concealed hemorrhage	Initially concealed but later revealed
• It is visible external hemorrhage	• It constitutes internal hemorrhage	• Hematemesis
	• Liver injury	• Melena
	• Spleen injury	• Hematuria
		• Fracture femur
		• Ruptured ectopic gestation
		• Cerebral hemorrhage
		• Hemothorax

Classification IV

1. **Acute hemorrhage:**
   It is sudden, severe hemorrhage after trauma, surgery.
2. **Chronic hemorrhage:**
   It is chronic repeated bleeding for long time like in hemorrhoids, bleeding peptic ulcer, carcinoma cecum, etc. They present with chronic anemia with hyperdynamic cardiac failure. They are in a state of chronic hypoxia. It is corrected by *packed cell transfusion* not by whole blood itself. Cause has to be treated accordingly.
3. **Acute on chronic hemorrage:**
   It is more dangerous as the bleeding occurs in individuals who are already hypoxic, which may get worsened faster.

Classification of Hemorrhagic Shock (Circulatory Failure)

Class	Blood loss	Features
I.	Up to 15% (<750 mL)	Normal
II.	Blood loss 15–30% (750–1500 mL)	Pallor, thirsty, tachycardia
III.	Blood loss 30–40% (1500–2000 mL)	Hypotension, tachycardia, oliguria, confusion
IV.	Blood loss >40% (>2000 mL)	Rapid pulse, low BP, anuria, unconsciousness, MODS

Effects of hemorrhage
• Acute renal shut down.
• Liver cell dysfunction.
• Cardiac depression.
• Hypoxic effect.
• Metabolic acidosis.
• GIT mucosal ischemia.
• Sepsis.
• Interstitial edema, A-V shunting in lung— ARDS.
• Hypovolemic shock MODS.

Most problems have either many answers or no answer. Only few problems have a single answer.

Clinical Features of Hemorrhage

- Pallor; cyanosis; tachycardia.
- Tachypnea.
- Cold clammy skin due to vasoconstriction.
- Dry face, dry mouth and goose skin appearance (due to contraction of errector pilorum)
- Rapid thready pulse; hypotension; oliguria.
- Features related to specific causes.

Signs of significant blood loss

- Pulse >100/minute.
- Systolic BP<100 mm Hg.

Signs of significant blood loss

- Diastolic BP drop on sitting or standing >10 mm Hg.
- Pallor/sweating.
- Shock index >1.

Measurement of Blood Loss

- Clot size of a clenched fist is 500 mL.
- Blood loss in a closed tibial fracture is 500–1500 mL; in a fracture femur is 500–2000 mL.
- Weighing the swab before and after use is an important method of on-table assessment of blood loss.
- Hb% and PCV estimation.
- Blood volume estimation.
- Measurement of CVP or PCWP.

Pathophysiology of Hemorrhage

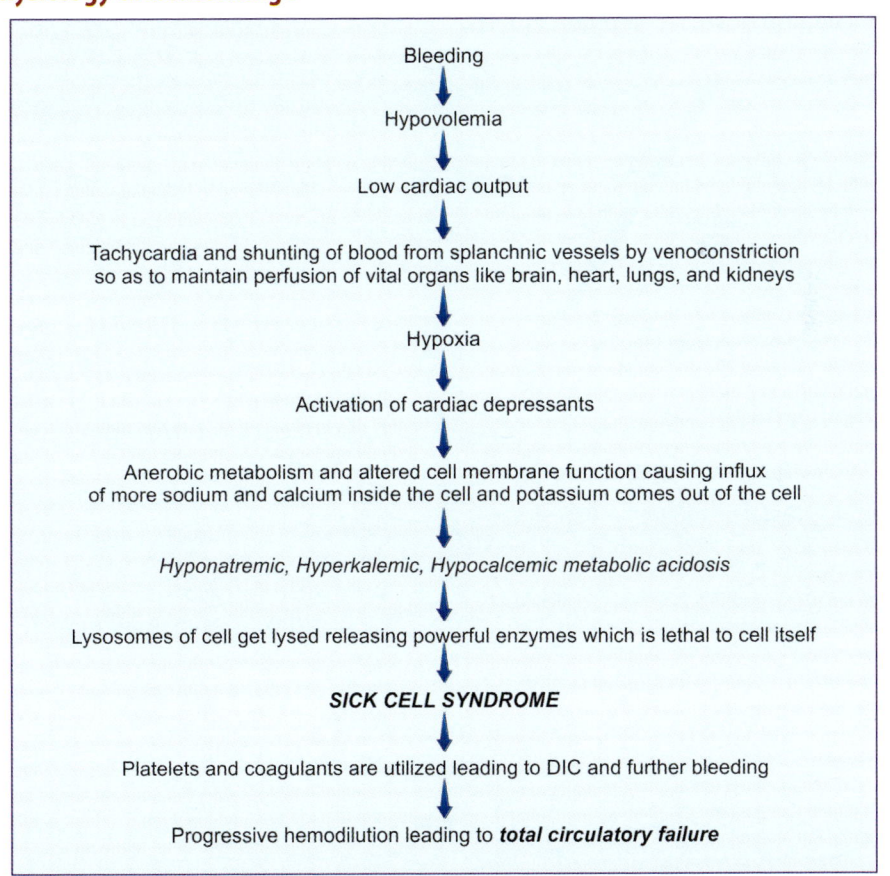

The only place where success comes before work is in the dictionary—**Vidal Sassoon**

Rains factor

Total amount of blood loss =
Total difference in swab weight × 1.5
or
Total difference in swab weight × 2
(For larger wounds and larger operations)

- Investigations specific for cause: Ultrasound abdomen, Doppler study in vascular injury and often angiogram, chest X-ray in hemothorax, CT scan in major injuries, CT head in head injuries.

Lethal Triad

Hypothermia (temperature <36°; Clotting factor and platelet function will reduce severely), *Metabolic acidosis, Progressive coagulopathy*. Coagulation is affected when factors are below 25%. *Lactic acidosis* is lactic acid level >4 mmol/L with metabolic acidosis.

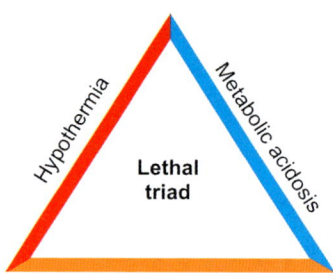

Progressive coagulopathy

Treatment of Hemorrhage

Immediate resuscitation

- *Airway; Breathing; Circulation (ABC).* Oxygen should be started (15 liters/minute). Correction of hypotension by *fluid therapy* by *fresh warm whole blood transfusion or packed cell, fresh frozen plasma, platelet as 1:1:1 ratio* (two wide bore IV cannulas should be placed and blood is drawn for blood grouping and cross matching and essential investigations).

Contd...

Contd...

- Warm normal saline or Ringer lactate infusion should be started until blood is ready. Unwarmed fluid infusion causes *hypothermia*.
- Isotonic, hypotonic and colloid solutions cause leak of fluid into interstitial space and edema with only a part remaining within the intravascular system. Haemaccel, SAG-M blood and dextran can also be used initially until blood products are available.
- *Damage control resuscitation (DCR)* approaches by earlier and more aggressive correction of coagulopathy and metabolic derangement with—permissive hypotension; the use of blood products over isotonic fluid for volume replacement; and the rapid and early correction of coagulopathy with component therapy.

End points of resuscitation

- Keeping patient *warm* (prevention of hypothermia; temperature below 32°C is lethal).
- Correction and prevention of further *coagulopathy* (TIC)—fibrinogen infusion 4 grams as initial dose then 50 mg/Kg; Fibrinogen and *prothrombin complex concentrate* (PCC) transfusion; cryoprecipitate and recombinant activated factor VIIa transfusion.
- *Fluid and electrolyte* management, sepsis control (antibiotics).
- *Further monitoring* by hourly urine output, hemodynamic stability, respiration, and estimation of lactic acid, base deficit, fibrinogen, platelet, prothrombin INR, APTT, hematocrit, arterial blood gas (ABG), liver and renal functions.

Control of Hemorrhage and Other Measures

- Restoration of blood loss: By blood transfusion, albumin 4.5%, SAG-M blood, saline, haemaccel (gelatin), dextran, plasma infusions.
- Catheterization, foot end elevation, monitoring.
- Pressure and packing.
- Wound exploration and proceeding, i.e. ligation of the small vessel, suturing the part, vessel suturing (anastomosis), excision of the tissues.
- Absolute rest, analgesics, morphine 10–20 mg IM/IV to relieve pain, sedation.

The specialist learns more and more of less and less, finally he knows everything about nothing; whereas generalist learns less and less about more and more until, finally he knows nothing about everything

- Intercostal tube (ICT) placing for hemothorax.
- Laparotomy for liver or spleen or mesentery or bowel injuries.
- Topical applications for local ooze—oxycel, gauze soaked with adrenaline, bone wax for oozing from bone and other local hemostatic agents (Figs. 6.8 and 6.9).
- In venous hemorrhage limb elevation, ligation of vein or suturing of venous wall in case of large vein, pressure bandaging, and packing will be helpful.
- Tourniquet is often useful in operation theater for control of hemorrhage in limbs. But it is not advisable as a first aid measure.
- TPN, CVP monitoring, electrolyte management are all equally important.
- Steroid injection, antibiotics, ventilator support is often required.

BLOOD TRANSFUSION

Indications

- After trauma with severe blood loss, e.g. liver, spleen, kidney, GIT injuries, fractures, hemothorax, perineal injuries.
- During major surgeries: Abdominoperineal surgery, thoracic surgery, hepatobiliary surgery.
- Following burns.
- In septicemia.
- Packed cells are given in chronic anemia, blood fractions are given in idiopathic thrombocytopenic purpura (ITP), hemophilias.
- As a prophylactic measure prior to surgery.

Donor Criteria

- Donor should be fit without any serious diseases like HIV I/HIV II/hepatitis.
- Weight of donor should be more than 45 kg.

Collection of Blood

About 410 mL blood is collected from antecubital vein in a sterile sac containing 75 mL of CPD (Citrate Phosphate Dextrose) solution constantly mixed during collection

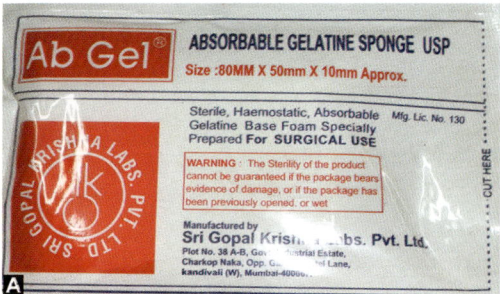

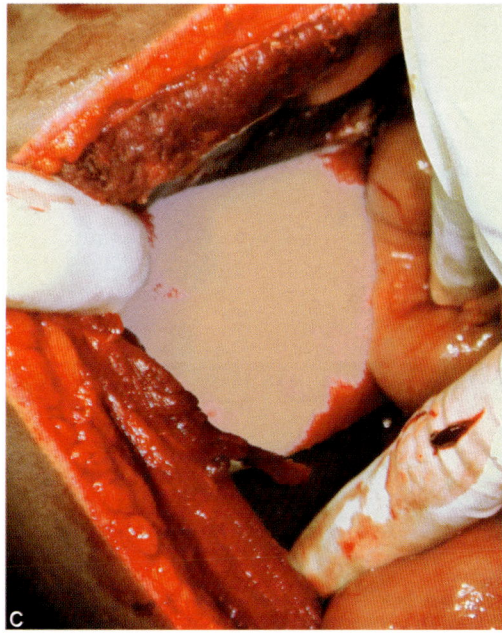

Figs. 6.8A to C: Gel foam (gelatin sponge) is a good hemostatic agent in oozing surface like gallbladder bed after cholecystectomy.

*If you are not willing to risk the usual, you will have to settle for the ordinary—**Jim Rohn***

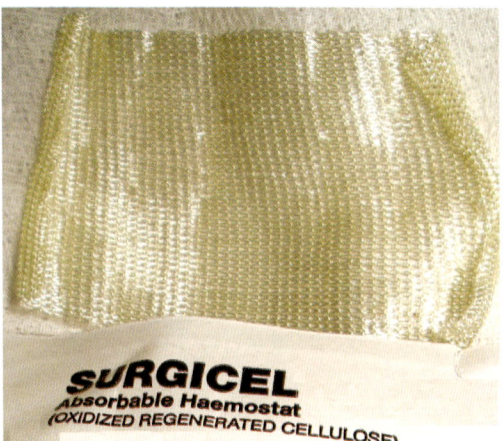

Fig. 6.9: Oxidized regenerated cellulose is very good local hemostatic agent; but it is much costlier than gelatin sponge.

to prevent coagulation and stored in special refrigerators at 4°C. CPD blood lasts for 3 weeks.

In Stored Blood

- Red blood cells (RBC's) last for 3 weeks.
- White blood cells (WBC's) are destroyed rapidly.
- Platelets also get reduced in 24 hours.
- Clotting factors are labile and so their levels fall quickly.

BLOOD FRACTIONS

a. **Packed cells:**
   - It is obtained by centrifuging whole blood at 2000–2300 g for 15–20 minutes.
   - It is used in chronic anemias, in old age, in children.
   - It minimizes the cardiac overload due to transfusion.
b. **Plasma**:
   - This is obtained in the same way as packed cells by centrifugation.
   - It is indicated in *burns, hypoalbuminemia, severe protein loss*.
   - It can be fractionalized into different fragments.
c. **Human albumin 4.5%** is obtained after repeated fractionations and can be stored for several months in liquid form at 4°C.
d. **Fresh frozen plasma:** Fresh plasma obtained is rapidly frozen and stored at –40 °C. It contains all coagulant factors and is the choice for severe liver disease with abnormal coagulation function.
e. **Cryoprecipitate:** When fresh frozen plasma is allowed to thaw at 4°C, visible white supernatant layer develops and is called as cryoprecipitate, which is rich in Factor VIII and fibrinogen. It is stored at –40°C.
f. **Fibrinogen** is obtained by organic liquid fractionation of plasma and is stored in dried form. It is very useful in DIC and afibrinogenemia. It has got risk of transmitting hepatitis.
g. **Platelet rich plasma:** It is obtained by centrifugation of freshly donated blood at 150–200 g for 15–20 minutes.
h. **Platelet concentrate:** It is prepared by centrifugation of platelet rich plasma at 1,200–1,500 g for 15–20 minutes.

SAG-M Blood

A proportion of donations will have plasma removed and will be replaced by crystalloid solution of SAG-M.

    S—Sodium chloride.
    A—Adenine.
    G—Glucose anhydrate.
    M—Mannitol.

Advantages

- This allows good viability of cells.
- But it is devoid of any protein.
- It is very useful in anemias.

Precautions

- For every four units of SAG-M blood, one whole blood has to be given.

His heart cannot be pure whose tongue is not clean

Chapter 6 : Shock, Hemorrhage and Blood Transfusion

❖ Later for every two units of SAG-M blood, one unit (400 mL) of 4.5% human albumin has to be given.
❖ Coagulation status and platelet count should be checked regularly.

After grouping and cross matching, 540 mL of blood is transfused in 4 hours (40 drops per minute), using a filtered drip set.

Complications of Blood Transfusion

1. Congestive cardiac failure.
2. Transfusion reactions:
   – Incompatibility—major and minor reactions with fever, rigors, pain, hypotension.
   – Pyrexial reactions due to pyrogenic ingredients in the blood.
   Allergic reactions.
   Sensitization to leukocytes and platelets.
   Immunological sensitization.
3. Infections:
   – Serum hepatitis.
   – HIV infection.
   – Bacterial infection.
   – Malaria transmission
   – Epstein-Barr virus infection.
   – Cytomegalovirus infection.
   – Syphilis, Yersinia.
   – *Babesia microti* infection.
   – *Trypanosoma cruzi* infection.
4. Air embolism.
5. Thrombophlebitis.
6. Coagulation failure:
   – Dilution of clotting factors.
   – DIC.
7. Hemochromatosis in repeated transfusions like in chronic renal failure.
8. Citrate intoxication causing bradycardia and hypocalcemia
9. Congestive cardiac failure (CCF)—due to rapid infusion of blood in anesthesia.
10. Immunosuppression.

MASSIVE BLOOD TRANSFUSION

❖ It is defined as replacement or transfusion of blood equivalent to patient's blood volume in 24 hours corresponding to that particular age or single transfusion of blood more than 2,500 mL continuously (in adult, it is 5–6 liters, in infants, it is 85 mL/kg body weight).
❖ Massive transfusion causes severe electrolyte imbalance (hypocalcemia, hyperkalemia), altered platelet and coagulation factors. They require proper monitoring and management.
❖ Massive transfusion is used in severe trauma associated with liver, vessel, cardiac, pulmonary, and pelvic injuries. Often it is required during surgical bleeding (primary hemorrhage on table) of major surgeries.

Massive transfusion

- Transfusion of blood in 24 hours equivalent to patients blood volume.
- Single transfusion of blood of 2,500 mL or more in 6 hours.
- Indicated in class IV hemorrhages like injuries to major vessels, liver and spleen
- Causes citrate toxicity, hyperkalemia, hypocalcemia, thrombocytopenia, sepsis, DIC, etc.

BLOOD SUBSTITUTES

❖ ***Human albumin 4.5%***
There is no risk of transmitting hepatitis.
❖ ***Dextrans***—are useful to improve plasma volume. They are polysaccharides of varying molecular weights.
   a. *Low molecular weight dextran* (40,000 mol wt) (*Dextran 40, Rheomacrodex*): Dextran 40 is very effective in restoring blood volume immediately. But small molecules are readily excreted in kidney and so effect is transitory. It may be useful in prevention of sludging in kidney and hence renal shut down.

If you genuinely want something, don't wait for it—teach yourself to be impatient—**Gurbaksh Chahal**

b. *High molecular weight dextran* (*Dextran 110 and Dextran 70*): Less effective, but long acting and so useful to have prolonged effect.

Precautions

1. Blood samples for blood group and cross matching should be taken before giving dextrans as it interferes with rouleaux formation of red cells.
2. Dextrans also interfere with platelet function and so may precipitate abnormal bleeding.
3. Total volume of Dextrans should not exceed 1000 mL.

Gelatin—in a degraded form of molecular weight 30,000S, is used as a plasma expander. Up to 1000 mL of 3.4–4% solution containing anions and cations is given intravenously—Haemaccel.

AUTOLOGOUS BLOOD TRANSFUSION

- A healthy individual with no infection and hematocrit of ≥30% can predonate blood few weeks prior to any elective surgeries, which in turn can be used at the time of elective surgery to the same individual.
- It is used in orthopedic/gynecological/urologic surgeries.
- Patient donates one unit of blood weekly; last one if at all 72 hours prior to procedure but not later.

RECYCLED BLOOD

- In major surgeries, if there is significant blood loss, then patient's bled blood is carefully sucked out through a sterile system and is filtered and reused again to the patient.
- This will reduce the number of transfusions.

ARTIFICIAL BLOOD

- *Perfluorocarbon*—an abiotic RBC substitute as synthetic oxygen carrier. Its half-life is 7 days. It is inert, odorless, dense, poorly soluble biocompatible liquid.
- *Stroma free hemoglobin.*
- *Chelates,* which reverse bound oxygen.

TOURNIQUETS

Uses

- To attain blood less field in limb surgeries— upper and lower limbs, orthopedic surgeries, soft tissue tumors, amputations.
- It is used (rubber tourniquet) to get assess to veins for IV injections and IV sampling.
- Tourniquet is used in diagnostic tests for varicose veins, purpura (ITP), etc.
- It is used as a first aid in bleeding conditions of limbs, snake bite (it is controversial).
- Tourniquets are also often used for small procedures in fingers and toes.

Types

- *Rubber tourniquet*—simple red rubber catheter is used for drawing blood, to have access to veins.
- *Pneumatic tourniquet*—used in limbs, will give the arterial pressure and also acts as a tourniquet. (Sphygmomanometer cuff is a simple and easily available type).
- Esmarch rubber *elastic bandage tourniquet (Fig. 6.10)*.
- Specialized sophisticated tourniquets are available, which gauge pressure, timing accurately.

Don't be afraid to give up the good to go for the great—**John D Rockefeller**

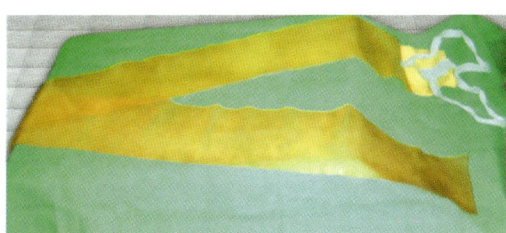

Fig. 6.10: Esmarch rubber tourniquet.

Contraindications

In all peripheral vascular diseases and atherosclerosis.

Complications

- Crushing effect on muscles in thigh may lead to crush syndrome.
- Tourniquet palsy in upper limb.
- Infection.
- Improper application of tourniquet leads to more bleeding.
- Forgetting the removal of tourniquet or using more time to release may compromise the blood supply of the limb leading to severe ischemia and gangrene.

Tourniquet time for upper limb is one hour and for lower limb is two hours.

---

*I don't know the key to success, but the key to failure is trying to please everybody—**Bill Cosby***

CHAPTER 7

Burns

CHAPTER OUTLINE

- Burns
- Management of Burns
- Eschar
- Burns Contracture
- Electrical Burns
- Inhalation Burns
- Chemical Burns

BURNS

Types of burns

- Thermal injury
  - Scald—spillage of hot liquids
  - Flame burns
  - Flash burns due to exposure of natural gas, alcohol, combustible liquids
  - Contact burns—contact with hot metals/objects/materials
- Electrical injury
- Chemical burns—acid/alkali
- Cold injury—frost bite
- Ionizing radiation
- Sun burns

Classification of Burns

1. *Depending on the Percentage of Burns*

❖ **Mild** *(Minor)*:
  - Partial thickness burns <15% in adult or <10% in children.
  - Full thickness burns less than 2%.
  - Can be treated as outpatient basis.

❖ **Moderate:**
  - Second degree of 15-25% burns (10-20% in children).
  - Third degree between 2-10% burns.
  - Burns, which are not involving eyes, ears, face, hand, feet, and perineum.

❖ **Major** *(Severe)*:
  - Second degree burns more than 25% in adults, more than 20% in children.
  - All third degree burns of 10% or more.
  - Burns involving eyes, ears, feet, hands, perineum.
  - All inhalation and electrical burns.
  - Burns with fractures or major mechanical trauma.

Extensive burns, more than 50% are shown in Figure 7.1.

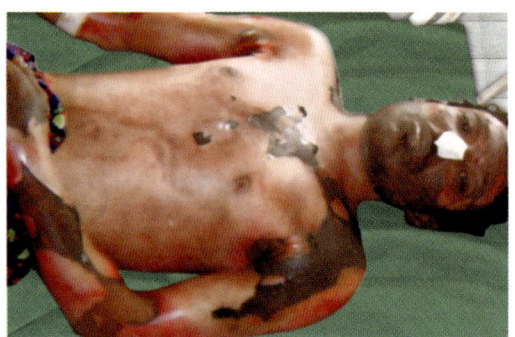

Fig. 7.1: Extensive burns more than 50%.

Try not to become a man of success. Rather become a man of value—**Albert Einstein**

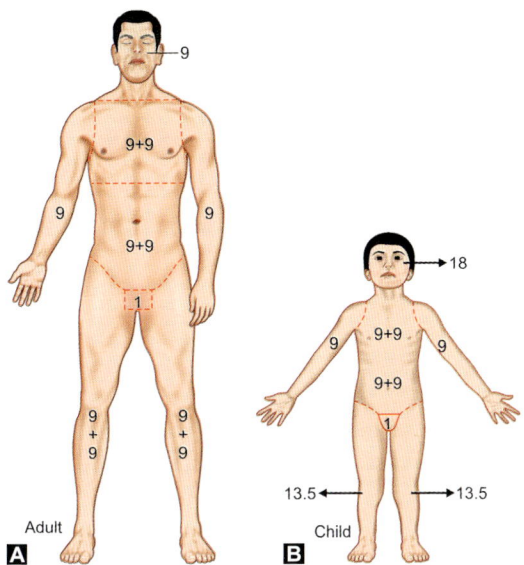

Figs. 7.2A and B: Percentage of burns in (A) Adults; (B) Children.

> **Rule of Nine (Wallace's rule of '9') (Figs. 7.2A and B)**
> - Head and neck 9%.
> - Front of chest and abdominal wall—9 × 2 = 18%.
> - Back of chest and abdominal wall—9 × 2 = 18%.
> - Lower limb each is 18% and so both—18 × 2 = 36%.
> - Upper limb each is 9% and so both—9 × 2 = 18%.
> - Perineum 01%.

2. *Depending on Thickness of Skin Involved (Fig. 7.3)*

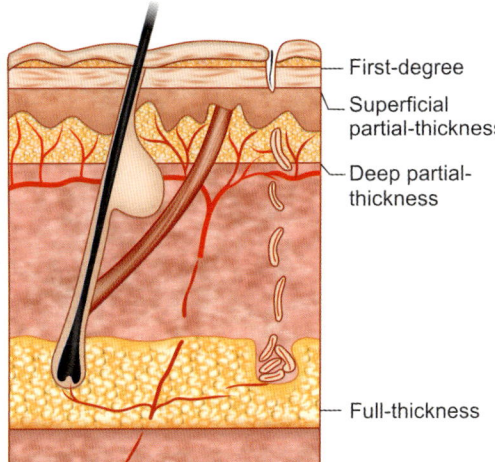

Fig. 7.3: Degree's of burn.

❖ ***First degree (Fig. 7.4):***
Epidermis looks red, painful, no blisters, heals rapidly in 5–7 days by epithelialization without scarring.

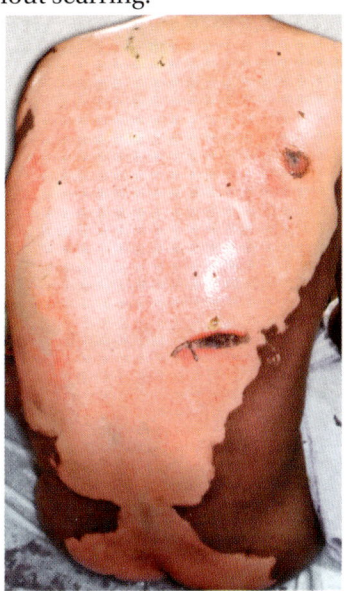

Fig. 7.4: First degree burn.

❖ ***Second degree:***
Mottled red, painful, with blisters, heals by epithelialization in 14–21 days (Fig. 7.5).
  – Superficial second degree burn heals, causing pigmentation.
  – Deep second degree burn heals, causing scarring, and pigmentation.

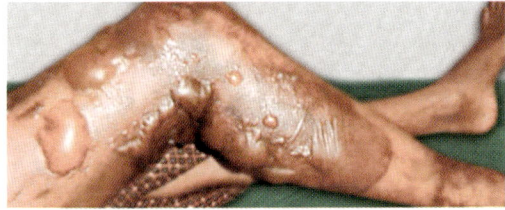

Fig. 7.5: Second degree burns with blisters.

❖ ***Third degree:***
Charred, parchment like, with thrombosis of superficial vessels, painless and insensitive surface. It requires grafting. Charred, denatured, insensitive, contracted full thickness burn is called as *eschar*.

*Things work out best for those who make the best of how things work out—**John Wooden***

It is also classified as:
- **Partial thickness burns**: It is either first or second degree burn which is red and painful, often with blisters.
- **Full thickness burns**: It is third degree burn which is charred, insensitive, deep involving all layers of the skin.

Clinical Features
- History of burn (Fig. 7.6).
- Pain, burning, anxious status, tachycardia, tachypnea, fluid loss.
- In severe degrees, features of shock.

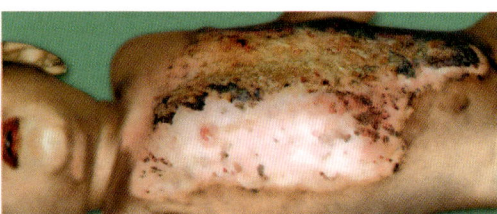

Fig. 7.6: Burns in a child.

Pathophysiology

Tolerable temperature to human skin is 40°C for brief period.

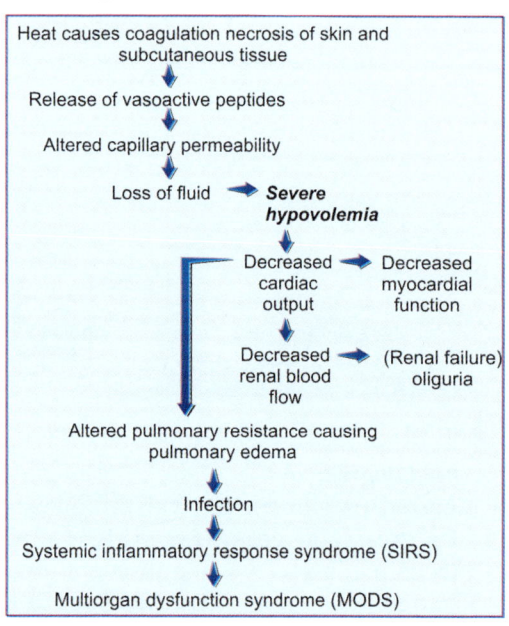

Massive edema in the body is due to altered pressure gradient because of the injury to basement membrane.

Cardiac dysfunction is due to:
- Hypovolemia.
- Release of cardiac depressants.
- Hormonal causes like catecholamines, vasopressin, angiotensins, etc.

Renal changes are due to:
- Release of antidiuretic hormone (ADH) from posterior pituitary to cause maximum water reabsorption.
- Release of aldosterone from adrenals to cause maximum sodium reabsorption.
- Toxins released from the burn wound and also sepsis cause acute tubular necrosis.
- Myoglobin released from muscles in case of electric injury or often from eschar, which is most injurious to kidneys.

Pulmonary changes are due to:
- Altered ventilation-perfusion ratio.
- Pulmonary edema due to burn injury, fluid overload, inhalation injury.
- Acute respiratory distress syndrome (ARDS); aspiration; Septicemia.

Gastrointestinal tract (GIT) changes are due to:
- *Acute gastric dilatation,* which occurs in 2–4 days.
- Paralytic ileus.
- Curling's ulcer in the stomach in burns more than 35%.
- Cholestasis and hepatic damage.

Metabolic changes:
- Hypermetabolic rate (BMR).
- Negative nitrogen balance.
- Electrolyte imbalance.
- Deficiencies of vitamins, essential elements.
- Metabolic acidosis due to hypoxia and lactic acid.

Common infections are:
- Staphylococci and streptococci.
- Pseudomonas.
- *Candida albicans.*

An ounce of application is worth a ton of abstraction

Effects of burn injury

1. **Shock** due to hypovolemia.
2. Renal failure.
3. Pulmonary edema, respiratory infection, adult respiratory distress syndrome (ARDS), respiratory failure.
4. Infection by *Staphylococcus aureus,* beta hemolytic *Streptococcus, Pseudomonas, Klebsiella* results in bacteremia, septicemia, etc. Fungal and viral infections of dangerous types can also occur.
5. GIT: Hypovolemia, ischemia of mucosa, erosive gastritis—**Curling's ulcer**.
6. Fluid and electrolyte imbalance.
7. Post-burn immunosuppression predisposes to severe opportunistic infection of different bacterial, fungal and viral types.
8. Eschar formation and its problems like defective circulation, ischemia.
9. Electrical injuries often cause fractures, major internal organ injury, and convulsions.
10. Development of contracture is a late problem. It can cause ectropion, microstomia, disability of different joints, defective hand functions, and growth retardation causing shortening.
11. Inhalation burn causes pulmonary edema, respiratory arrest, ARDS.
12. Chemical injury causes severe GIT disturbances like erosions, perforation, stricture esophagus (**alkali**), pyloric stenosis (**acid**), mediastinal injury.
13. Other problems like deep vein thrombosis (DVT), pulmonary embolism, urinary infection, bedsores, severe malnutrition with catabolic status.
14. Complications of burn contracture itself like hypertrophic scar, keloid formation.
15. **Toxic shock syndrome**: It is a life-threatening exotoxin mediated disease caused by *Staph. aureus*, is common in children with rashes, myalgia, diarrhea, vomiting, and multiorgan failure with high mortality.
16. Other problems like catheter-induced infections, bedsores, respiratory infection.

Sepsis in Burn Patient

- Focus may be at the burn site, catheter site, cannula/central venous pressure (CVP) line site, or respiratory infection.
- Low immunity, loss of proteins and immunoglobulins, loss of barrier causes sepsis. Opportunistic infection is also common.
- Associated conditions like diabetes, HIV infection, old age, respiratory diseases worsen the sepsis in burn injury.
- It may be *local infection commonly* by *Staphylococcus aureus* in early period, *Pseudomonas, Candida, Aspergillus,* herpes simplex virus in partial thickness nasolabial burns. It may be suppurative thrombophlebitis also.
- *Systemic infection* like pneumonia, bacteremia, septicemia can occur.
- Burns itself *creates* immunosuppression.
- Sepsis is identified by fever, lethargy, *leukocytosis*, and *thrombocytopenia*.

Causes of Death in Burns

- Hypovolemia; renal failure.
- Pulmonary edema and ARDS.
- Septicemia; multiorgan failure.

MANAGEMENT OF BURNS

First Aid

- Stop the burning process and keep the patient away from the burning area.
- Cool the area with **tap water** by continuous irrigation for 20 minutes (**not cold water** which can cause hypothermia).

Definitive Treatment

- Admit the patient.
- Maintain **A**irway, **B**reathing, **C**irculation.
- Assess the percentage, degree, and type of burn.
- Keep the patient in a clean environment.
- Sedation.

The only person you are destined to become is the person you decide to be—**Ralph Waldo Emerson**

Fluid Resuscitation

Parkland regime
4 mL/% burn/kg body weight/24 hours.
Maximum percentage considered is 50%.
Half the volume is infused in first 8 hours, rest given in 16 hours.

Muir and Burclay regime

$$\frac{\% \text{ Burns} \times \text{Body weight in kg}}{2} = 1 \text{ Ration}$$

3 Rations in first 12 hours.
2 Rations in second 12 hours.
1 Ration in third 12 hours.

Fluids used are normal saline, Ringer lactate, Hartmann fluid, plasma, etc. Blood is used in later period (after 48 hours).

In first 24 hours crystalloids should be given (crystalloids are one which can pass through capillary wall) like saline—either hypo, iso or hypertonic, dextrose saline, Ringer lactate.

Sodium is assessed by formula: $0.52 \text{ mmol} \times \text{kg body weight} \times \%$ body burns given at a rate of 4.0 to 4.4 mL/kg/hour.

After 24 hours up to 30–48 hours, *colloids* should be given to compensate plasma loss. (colloids are one, which retain in intravascular compartment). Plasma, haemaccel (gelatin), dextrans, hetastarch are used. Usually used at a rate of 0.35–0.5 mL/kg/% burns in 24 hours.

- Urinary catheterization to monitor urine output; 30–50 mL/hour should be the urine output.
- Monitoring the patient: Hourly pulse, BP, PO_2, PCO_2, electrolyte analysis, blood urea, serum creatinine.
- Nasal oxygen, often intubation is required.
- IV Ranitidine 50 mg 8th hourly.
- **Ryle's tube initially for aspiration purpose later for feeding purpose** *(Enteral feeding)*.
- Antibiotics: Penicillins, Aminoglycosides, Cephalosporins, Metronidazole.
- In burns of oral cavity, tracheostomy may be required to maintain the airway.
- ***Total Parenteral Nutrition (TPN)*** is required for faster recovery using carbohydrates, lipids, vitamins ***(Through a CVP line)***.

Local Management

- ***Dressing*** at regular intervals under GA using paraffin gauze, hydrocolloids, plastic films.
- Slough excision is done regularly.
- After cleaning with povidone iodine, *Silver sulfadiazine* ointment is used. It is an antiseptic and soothening agent. Other agents used are *Sulfamylon* (**Mafenide acetate**) and *Silver nitrate*. Sulfamylon is antipseudomonal, anticlostridial and it penetrates well into the tissues but it is an irritant. Silver nitrate causes staining of burn area.
  Regular culture and sensitivity for bacteria is required—to see streptococcal growth, which should be less than *1,00,000/- (10^5) per gram of tissue.*
- Once the area granulates well, in 3 weeks usually, split skin grafting is done (SSG, Thiersch graft).
- For wider area mesh split skin graft is used.
- If there is eschar, *escharotomy* is required to prevent compression of vessels.
- In certain areas like face and ear full thickness graft (Wolfe graft) or flap is required.

Treatment of burns

- Fluid management and resuscitation.
- Cleaning the wound and debridement.
- Open method using silver sulfadiazine ointment.
- Closed method after applying ointment dressing and bandaging.
- Tangential excision and skin grafting (split skin graft/mesh graft).

There is something wrong if you are always right—**Arnold Glasow**

Synthetic Dressings in Burn Wound

- Vaseline impregnated gauze dressing prevents stiffness of eschar.
- Hydrocolloid dressing (*duoderm*) helps moist environment, proper epithelialization. It is useful in mixed deep burns. It is changed once in 3 days.
- *Opsite* is less expensive, with less pain, creates moist barrier. But it does not have antimicrobial effect and it causes accumulation of exudates.
- *Biobrane* is collagen coated silicone sheet which gets adherent to wound acting as barrier without any pain. But it does not have antimicrobial effect and it causes accumulation of exudates. It is used for second degree burns.
- *Transcyte* has similar features of biobrane. It contains growth factor derived from cultured fibroblasts which promotes wound healing.
- *Integra* contains deeper collagen matrix as dermal substitute; outer silicone sheet as epidermal substitute. Inner collagen matrix acts as dermis whereas outer silicone sheet is removed 2 weeks after dressing and additional autograft should be placed. It provides complete wound cover. Scarring after healing is reduced significantly.

Biologic Dressings for Burn Wound

It is used to cover the wound temporarily as a barrier and also to have some immunologic function. Eventually, graft will slough. Later, wound is covered with auto skin graft. It is used for massive burn injuries more than 50%. Possible problem is transmission of viral diseases.

Xenograft is of pig skin. *Allograft* is of cadaver skin (homograft)—it gives all existing normal skin function for temporary period. It may leave a dermal equivalent in the wound later.

ESCHAR

- It is charred; denatured, full thickness deep burns with contracted dermis.
- It is insensitive, with thrombosed superficial veins (Figs. 7.7A and B).

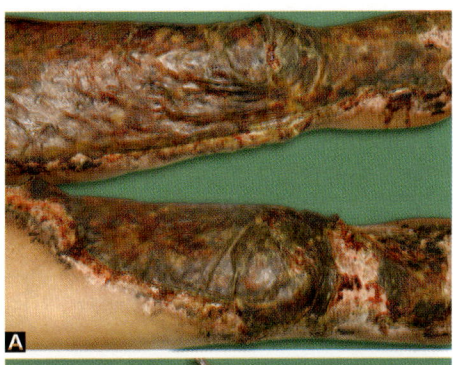

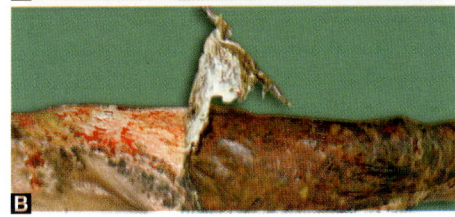

Figs. 7.7A and B: (A) Typical eschar. (B) Note the escharotomy being done.

- **Circumferential eschar** in the upper limb, lower limb, neck, thorax can cause more edema which initially causes venous compression but later arterial compression causing ischemia, gangrene of the distal part. So distal area should be monitored for circulation.
  - If required, deep tangential full thickness incisions are made in different areas, so as to prevent collection of edema fluid and also to prevent compression over the vessels. This is called as **escharotomy**.
- Early rapid separation of eschar indicates severe sepsis underneath.
- Eschar should be excised eventually, the area is allowed to granulate and later skin grafting should be done.

I failed my way to success—**Thomas Edison**

BURNS CONTRACTURE

During healing process of burns, if skin grafting or coverage is not done, healing takes place with fibrosis. This leads to development of contracture, thereby different deformities and complications depending on the location of burns.

Complications of Burns Contracture

- Ectropion of eyelid causing keratitis and corneal ulcer.
- Disfigurement of face.
- Narrowing of mouth opening—*microstomia*.
- Contracture in the neck causes restricted neck movements (Fig. 7.8).

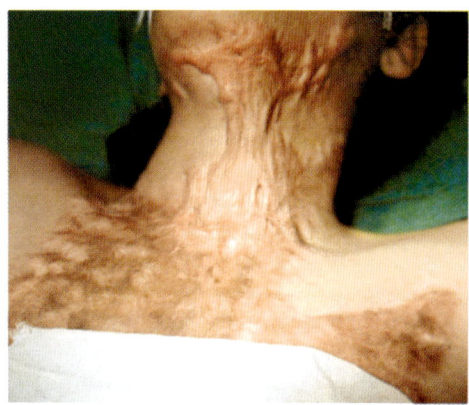

Fig. 7.8: Hypertrophic burn scar with contracture neck in a female.

- Disability and nonfunctioning of joints due to contracture (Fig. 7.9).

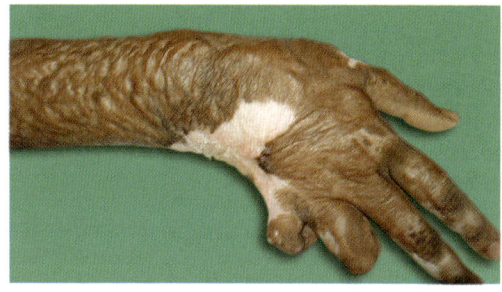

Fig. 7.9: Burn contracture of hand and fingers.

- Hypertrophic scar and keloid formation.
- Repeated breaking of scar, infection, ulcer, and cellulitis.
- Pain and tenderness in the scar contracture.
- *Marjolin's ulcer*: It is a very well-differentiated squamous cell carcinoma occurring in a scar ulcer due to repeated breakdown. It is locally malignant. As there are no lymphatics in the scar, there is no spread to lymph nodes. It is painless as there are no nerves in the scar.

Treatment for Contracture

- Release of contracture surgically and use of Z plasty or skin grafting or different flaps.
- Proper physiotherapy and rehabilitation is essential.

Prevention of Development of Contracture

- Encourage joint exercise in full range during recovery period of burns.
- Use of pressure garments for long period.
- Topical silicon sheeting.
- Saline expanders for scars.

Problems in Managing Burn Contracture

- Giving proper anesthesia is challenging.
- Scar excision can cause significant bleeding.
- Identifying major structures in the area and safeguarding vascular and other structure is often worrisome.
- Need for repeated surgeries as staged one.
- Maintaining the position with skeletal traction, fixation, collar, plaster of Paris (POP) cast, etc.
- Psychological problems and needs counseling.
- Prolonged hospital stay, cost factors.

ELECTRICAL BURNS

- It is always a deep burn (***Always a major burn***).

If a thing is done wrong often enough, it becomes right—**Richard A Leahy**

Electrical burns

Types	Treatment	Complications	Monitoring and prevention
High voltage: • Can cause ventricular fibrillation, cardiac arrest, death. Extensive organ and surface injuries with fractures. **Low voltage:** • Deep burn at the site of wound of entry.	• Emergency resuscitation • Assessment of burn • Prevention of renal failure by hydration, dialysis, alkalization of urine to clear myoglobin, Mannitol therapy, IV sodium bicarbonate. • Extensive fasciotomy, debridement. • Infection control. • Reconstruction.	• Neurological like epilepsy, hemiplegia, aphasia, memory loss, headache. • Cardiac—arrhythmias. • Vascular injuries—major vessels, bleeding. • Compartment syndromes. • Ischemia, gangrene of limbs. • Contracture development. • Bronchopneumonia, pleural effusion. • Abdominal—ileus, erosive gastritis, Curling ulcer, injury to liver, pancreas, spleen, GIT. • Bone and joint injuries. • Cataract can occur in high voltage burn. • Severe potassium deficiency is common.	**Monitoring:** • ECG, echocardiography. • Relevant investigations like X-ray, ultrasound, CT, electrolytes, urine analysis, LFT, renal function tests. **Prevention:** • Care during electrical work and with electrical system. • Unused outlets should be sealed with plastic. • Electrical system should be away from water source.

❖ There will be *wound of entry (Figs. 7.10 and 7.11) and wound of exit*.
❖ Patient may be having major internal organ injury, GIT, thoracic injuries.
❖ Often convulsions can develop.
❖ Death may occur due to cardiac arrhythmias. (***Instant death due to ventricular fibrillation***).
❖ **Gas gangrene** is common after electric injury.
❖ Release of myoglobin can cause renal tubular damage and **renal failure**.
❖ Patient should *always be admitted* and should be assessed by ECG, cardiac monitor, ultrasound abdomen, chest X-ray, sometimes even CT scan head.

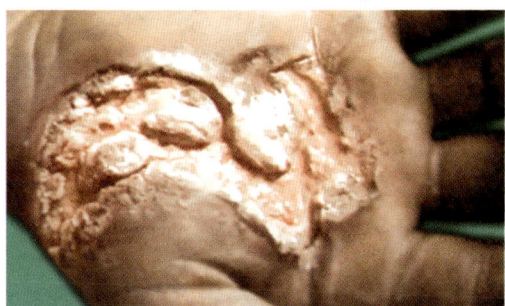

Fig. 7.10: Wound of entry in an electric burn.

❖ Depending on the injury it is managed accordingly.
❖ Fractures and dislocations are common in electric injuries, which is treated accordingly.

The road to success and the road to failure are almost exactly the same—**Colin R Davis**

* Pulmonary embolism; pulmonary edema; pneumothorax.

Clinical Features

* They will have low oxygen saturation.
* Charring of mouth, oropharynx with facial burns.
* Carbon sputum.
* Change in the voice with singed facial and nasal hair.
* Decreased level of consciousness with stridor or dyspnea.

Management

* Replacing the patient from the site earliest.
* Ventilator support; bronchoscopy.
* Antibiotics.
* Tracheostomy whenever required.

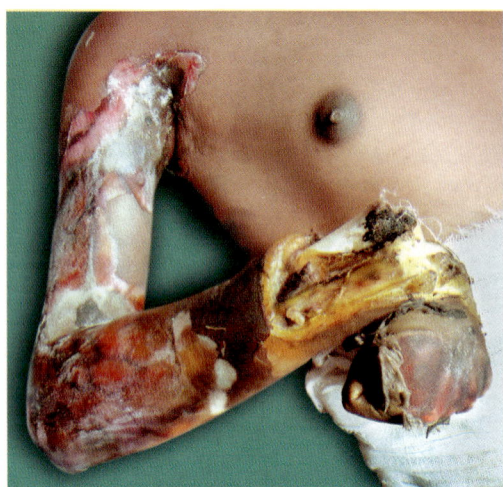

Fig. 7.11: High voltage electric burn, wound of entry in the hand with extensive destruction.

* *Mafenide acetate* is better agent as it penetrates well and it is useful against clostridial infection.
* *Mannitol* should be used to prevent myoglobin-induced renal failure.

INHALATION BURNS

* It occurs after major fire burns.
* It is due to:
  - Inhalation of heat.
  - Noxious gases and incomplete products of combustion.
* At the site of fire, oxygen concentration is less than 2%, which can cause death in 45 seconds due to hypoxia.
* Inhaled carbon monoxide binds with Hb immediately to form carboxyhemoglobin causing severe anoxia and death.
* Smoke contains hydrocyanide, which causes tissue hypoxia and profound acidosis; laryngeal edema and laryngospasm; bronchial edema and bronchospasm.

Later Problems

* ARDS; pneumonia; atelectasis.

CHEMICAL BURNS

* In chemical burns, tissue destruction is more and progressive. It is always a deep burn.
* **Acid** burn occurs in skin, soft tissues and GIT. In GIT, it is common in **stomach** due to either nitric acid or sulfuric acid, which may lead to severe gastritis or pyloric stenosis. Acids commonly involved—Formic acid, hydrofluoric acid, nitric acid, and sulfuric acid. They cause metabolic acidosis, renal failure, ARDS, hemolysis. Acidemia should be corrected by IV sodium bicarbonate.
* **Alkali** burns occur in oral cavity and *esophagus*, which leads to multiple esophageal strictures. Common alkalis involved are—Sodium hydroxide, lime, potassium hydroxide and bleach. They cause saponification of fat, fluid loss, release of alkali proteinates and hydroxide ions which are toxic.
* **External chemical burns** are always deep and cause extensive disfigurement with cosmetic problems.

Anybody can win—unless there happens to be a second entry—George Ade

- *Initial treatment* is dilution with water (**Hydrotherapy**).
- *Neutralization with antidote should never be done at initial phase* of treatment as it creates exothermic reaction, which aggravates the tissue damage. Neutralizing agents are used later.
- Treatment should be always with hospitalization.
- Mannitol diuresis, hemodialysis, IV calcium gluconate, pain relief, serum electrolyte management, TPN, ventilator support are the initial systemic management required.
- Late treatment is reconstruction of the face, esophageal dilatation or colonic transposition for esophageal alkali burn, gastrojejunostomy for acid-induced pyloric stenosis.

*You talk when you cease to be at peace with your thoughts—**Kalil Gibran***

CHAPTER 8

Reconstruction and Transplantation

CHAPTER OUTLINE

- Skin Grafting
- Flaps
- Transplantation
- Renal Transplantation
- Liver Transplantation
- Bone Marrow Transplantation
- Graft Rejection
- Cimino Fistula
- Immunosuppressive Agents

Flaps: These are transfer of tissues from one area to another with their blood supply (with pedicle).

Graft: It is transfer of tissues from one area to another without its blood supply or nerve supply.

> *Autograft* is transfer of tissue from one location to another on the same patient.
> *Isograft* is transfer of tissue between two genetically identical individuals, i.e. between two identical twins.
> *Allograft* is transfer of tissue between two genetically different members, e.g. kidney transplantation.
> *Xenograft* is transfer of tissue from a donor of one species to a recipient of another species.

SKIN GRAFTING

It is transfer of skin from one area (donor area) to the required defective area (recipient area). It is an *autograft*.

TYPES

Partial Thickness Graft (Split Skin Graft—SSG)

Also called as *Thiersch graft*. It is removal of full epidermis + part of the dermis from the donor area.

Depending on the amount of thickness of dermis taken, it may be:
- Thin SSG.
- Intermediate SSG.
- Thick SSG.

Indications
- Well-granulated ulcer.
- Clean wound or defect, which cannot be apposed.
- After surgery to cover and close the defect created. For example:
    - After wide excision in malignancy.
    - After mastectomy.
    - After wide excision of squamous cell carcinoma, etc.

People will believe anything if you whisper it

Graft can survive over periosteum or paratenon or perichondrium.

Pre-requisite

- Healthy granulation area.
- Streptococci load <10^5 per gram of tissue, otherwise graft failure occurs.

Contraindications

- SSG cannot be done over bone, tendon cartilage or joint or on avascular surface.
- Unhealthy granulation tissue.
- Presence of beta hemolytic streptococcal infection in recipient bed.

Donor area
Commonly thigh, occasionally arm, leg, forearm.
Knife used is Humby's knife.
Blade is Eschmann blade, Down's blade, Power dermatome is also used.

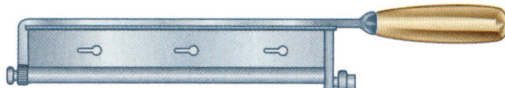

Fig. 8.1: Humby's knife with Eschmann blade to take split skin graft.

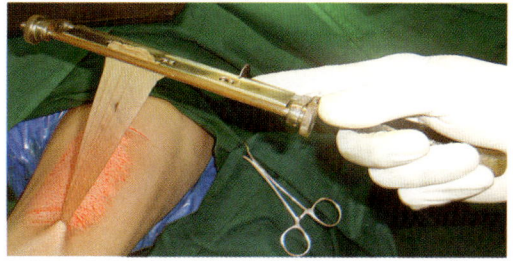

Fig. 8.2: Split skin graft—Humby's knife showing SSG harvesting.

- Using Humby's knife graft is taken from the donor area. Punctate bleeding from the graft is observed which says that proper graft has been obtained (Figs. 8.1 to 8.3).
- Donor area is dressed and dressing is opened *after 10 days*, not earlier than that (Fig. 8.4).

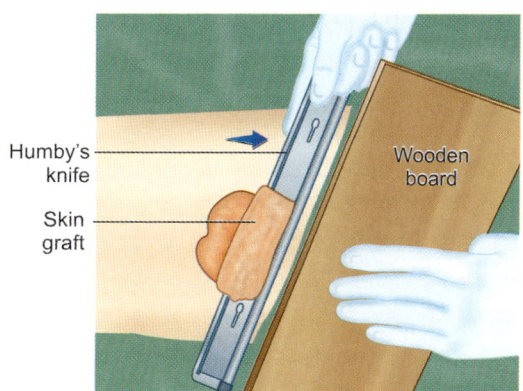

Fig. 8.3: Harvesting a skin graft.

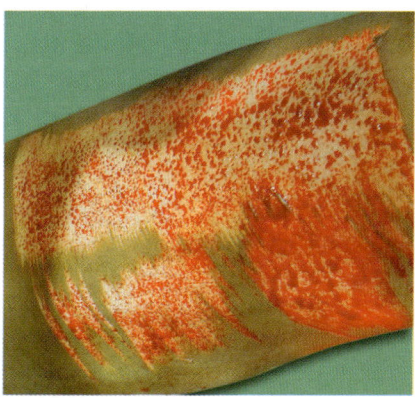

Fig. 8.4: Punctate hemorrhage is typical look after harvesting the split skin graft from the thigh.

- ***Recipient area*** is scraped well and graft is placed after making window cuts in it in order to avoid the development of seroma. Graft is fixed and *tie-over* dressing is placed. If graft is near a joint, then the part is immobilized to prevent friction, which may separate the graft. On *5th day* dressing is opened and observed for graft intake (Fig. 8.5).

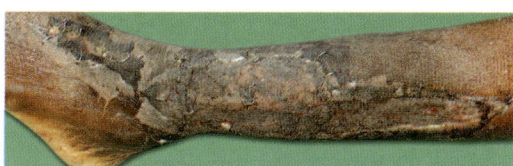

Fig. 8.5: Graft has taken up well in the leg which was a large area defect/ulcer.

*Life is really simple, but we insist on making it complicated—**Confucius***

Stages of Graft Intake

1. *Stage of plasmatic imbibition*: Thin, uniform, layer of plasma forms between recipient bed and graft.
2. *Stage of inosculation*: Linking of host and graft, which is temporary.
3. *Stage of neovascularization*: New capillaries proliferate into graft from the recipient bed, which later attains circulation.

Disadvantages of SSG

- **Contracture of graft.**
  Two types:
  - *Primary contracture* means SSG contracts significantly once graft is taken from donor area (20–30%). Thicker the graft more is the primary contracture.
  - *Secondary contracture* occurs after graft has been taken up to recipient bed during healing period, due to fibrosis. Thinner the graft more is the secondary contracture.
- Seroma and hematoma formation will prevent graft take up.
- Infection.
- Loss of hair growth, blunting of sensation.
- Dry, scaling of skin due to nonfunctioning of sebaceous glands. So after healing oil (coconut oil) should be applied over the area.
- Graft failure (Fig. 8.6).

Advantages

- Technically easier.
- Wide area of recipient can be covered. To cover large areas like in burns wound, graft size is increased by passing the graft through a **Mesher** which gives multiple openings to the graft which can be stretched over the wider area like a net (Figs. 8.7 and 8.8).
- Graft take up is better.
- Donor area heals on its own.

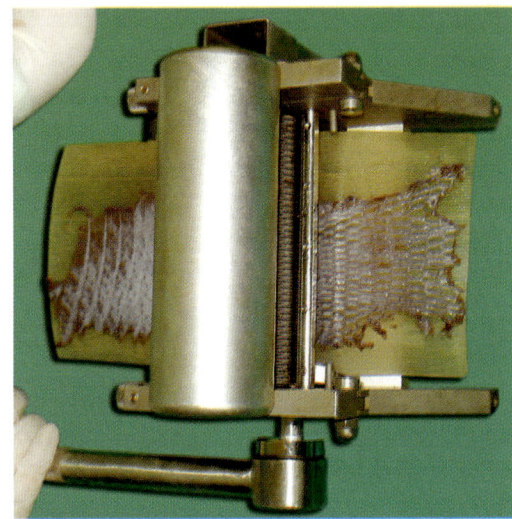

Fig. 8.7: Mesher is used to increase the size of the donor skin graft.

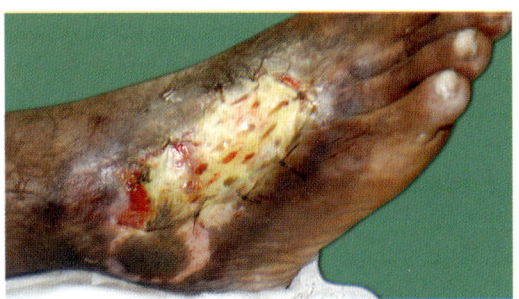

Fig. 8.6: Typical look of graft failure.

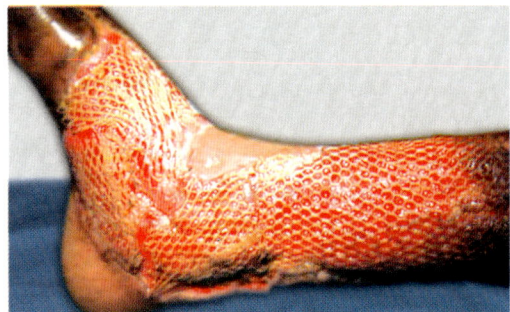

Fig. 8.8: Mesh graft. Split skin graft is passed through a mesher to get a wide mesh graft which can be used over to cover a wider area like of burns.

*The universe is not only stranger than we imagine, it is stranger than we can imagine—**JBS Haldane***

Full Thickness Graft (Wolfe Graft)

- It includes both epidermis + full dermis.
- It is used over the face, hands, fingers, and over the joints.
- It is removed using scalpel blade. Deeper raw area is closed by primary suturing. If a large full thickness graft is taken, then that donor area has to be covered with SSG, which is a disadvantage in full thickness graft.

Common sites of donor area:
- Postauricular area.
- Supraclavicular area.

Advantages
- Color match is good. Especially for face.
- No contracture (unlike in SSG).
- Sensation, functions of sebaceous glands, hair follicles are retained better compared to SSG.

Disadvantages
- Only for small area it can be used.
- Wider donor area has to be covered with SSG to close the defect.
- Cannot be used to cover ulcers.

Other grafts
• Composite graft where skin + fat + other tissues like cartilage.
• Tendon graft.
• Bone graft.
• Nerve graft.
• Venous graft.
• Corneal graft.

FLAPS

It is transfer of donor tissue with its blood supply to the recipient area.

Parts of flaps: Base, pedicle, tip of flap.

Vasculature is usually through the pedicle in the center of the flap. Tip is the place where often flap goes for necrosis (Figs. 8.9 and 8.10).

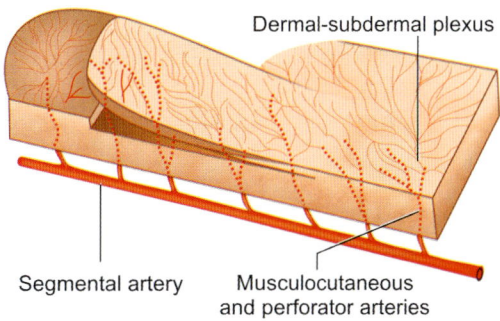

Fig. 8.9: Anatomy and blood supply of a skin flap.

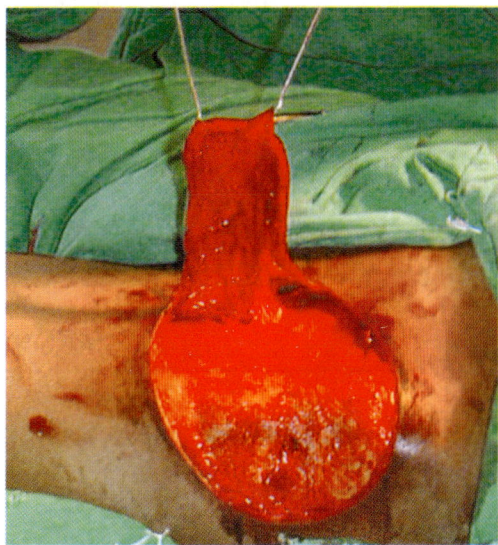

Fig. 8.10: Raising the skin flap. Note the different parts—base/pedicle/tip.

Indications

- To cover a wider, deeper defects.
- To cover over bone, tendon, cartilage.
- If skin graft repeatedly fails.

*Life is a long lesson in humility—**James M Barrie***

Types

1. *Random pattern flaps*: Here vascular basis is subdermal plexus of blood vessels.
2. *Axial pattern flaps*: Here superficial vascular pedicles pass along their long axes, e.g. forehead flap, deltopectoral flap, groin flap.

Anatomical types depending on the types of tissue in the flap:

- *Cutaneous flap*: Forehead flap, deltopectoral flap.
- *Faciocutaneous flap*: Radial forearm flap, scapular flap, lateral arm flap.
- *Muscle flap*: Gluteus maximus muscle flap, gracilis flap, tensor fascia lata muscle flap.
- *Myocutaneous flap*: Pectoralis major myocutaneous flap, latissimus dorsi flap (Fig. 8.11).

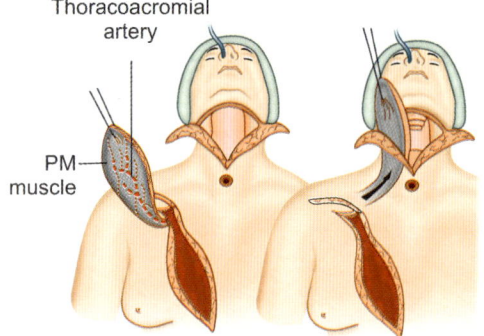

Fig. 8.11: Pectoralis major (PM) myocutaneous flap.

- *Osteomyocutaneous flaps*: Radius with brachioradialis and skin, rib with intercostal muscles and skin.
- *Local rotation flaps.*
- *'Z' plasty.*
- *Rhomboid flap* (Figs. 8.12A and B).
- *Free flaps*: Vascular pedicle of the flap, both artery and vein are anastomosed to recipient vessels using operating binocular microscopes.
- Omental flaps.
- Island flap.

Areas where commonly flaps are used:
- Oral cavity, neck, breast, limbs (leg), buttock, bedsores, etc.

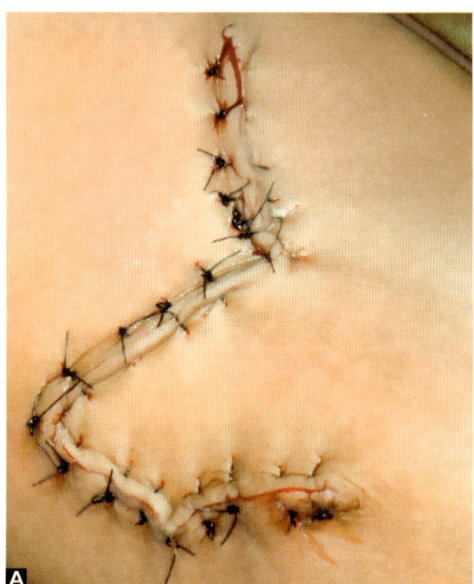

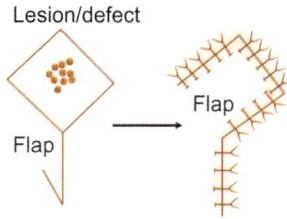

Figs. 8.12A and B: Rhomboid flap is used to cover the defect.

Note:
- Flaps mobilized from donor area with its pedicle is placed and sutured to recipient area. Once flap gets taken up usually in 3–6 weeks, base of the flap is cut and sutured to recipient area.
- **Saltatory flap** is mobilizing the flaps in stages from distant donor area towards

*He travels fast who travels alone-----but he hasn't anything to do when he gets there—**Finagle***

recipient area. It requires many staged surgeries and long-term hospitalization.

Advantages

- Good blood supply, good take up.
- Gives bulk, texture, color to the area.
- Allowing the required movements in the recipient area, e.g. jaw movements following pectoralis major flap after wide excision with hemimandibulectomy for carcinoma cheek.
- Cosmetically better.

Disadvantages

- Long-term hospitalization.
- Infection.
- Kinking, rotation and flap necrosis.
- Staged procedure.
- Positioning of the patient for long time is important to have a good flap take up which is a real discomfort to the patient.

DIFFERENT FLAPS

Forehead Flap

- It is fasciocutaneous flap from forehead based on *anterior branch of superficial temporal artery*. Superficial temporal artery is terminal smaller branch of external carotid artery. It begins under the parotid behind the neck of mandible, runs vertically upwards, crossing the root of zygoma at preauricular point; 5 cm above the zygoma it divides into anterior and posterior branches. Anterior branch anastomose with supraorbital and supratrochlear branches of ophthalmic artery. Artery supplies scalp of temple region and side, parotid, ear, facial muscles. Superficial temporal artery gives transverse facial artery which runs from anterior margin of parotid, and middle temporal artery which runs deep to temporalis muscle.
- It used for cheek defects (carcinoma, cancrum oris) and nasal reconstruction.
- *Standard forehead flap* is taken from above the eyebrow level starting from the opposite side of the midline with base at just above the zygoma. Width of the flap is usually of about 3–4 cm. Flap is dissected from the distal end of the marked area going deep up to epicranium, raising the flaps using scissor dissection. Flap is held up using skin hooks. Flap is rotated towards the cheek defect area. Inner area of the flap is covered with split skin graft. Donor flap area is covered with another split skin graft. After 3 weeks, base of the flap is disconnected; remaining proximal part of the flap can be replaced into forehead donor area. SSG over donor flap area takes up well. This flap often can be rotated under (deep to) the zygoma also (Fig. 8.13).

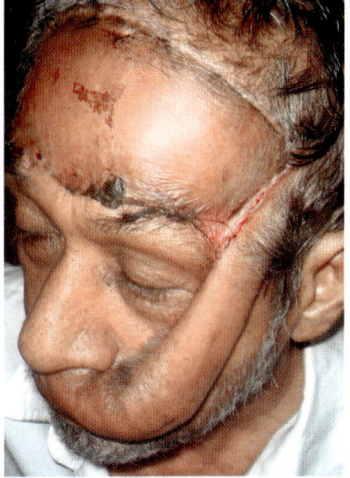

Fig. 8.13: Forehead flap based on superficial temporal artery. It is fasciocutaneous flap.

Deltopectoral Flap (Bakamjian Flap)

- It is a fasciocutaneous flap (axial pattern) based on first three perforating branches of the internal mammary artery (mainly 2nd perforator). Flap runs horizontally across the chest wall anteriorly towards shoulder tip from its base over the sternal

Love the life you live. Live the life you love.—Bob Marley

border. Its upper border is along the line of the clavicle; its lower border is along the line of anterior axillary fold line. Raw area often requires a spilt skin grafting. It is usually rotated upwards often with waltzing. It is tubed and attached above. Tube is drained to prevent any collection to occur.
- Rotation angle is important to prevent any kinking in the pedicle. It is usually used to cover the defects in cheek, chin, mastoid and parotid region. *Pivot point* of rotation is located in upper medial aspect. Often flap is delayed to get adequate length. Upper medial point is rotating pivot point. It moves a *quarter circle* (Fig. 8.14).

from femoral artery, over the medial border of sartorius and ends at anterior superior iliac spine. Deep branch is at the margin of the sartorius and superficial branch continues towards anterior superior iliac spine. 1:1 rectangular flap with deep fascia is used.
- Dissection of raising the flap is done up to the medial border of the sartorius. Secondary defect can usually be closed with sutures. It is used mainly for defects in wrist/forearm where positioning is easier. Often tubed groin flap can be transferred to cheek or leg using wrist as carrier (Fig. 8.15).

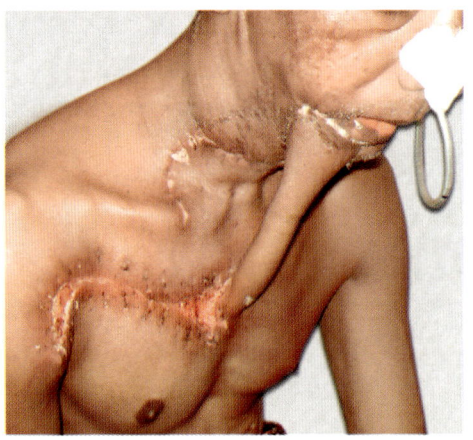

Fig. 8.14: Deltopectoral cutaneous flap (Bakamjian flap).

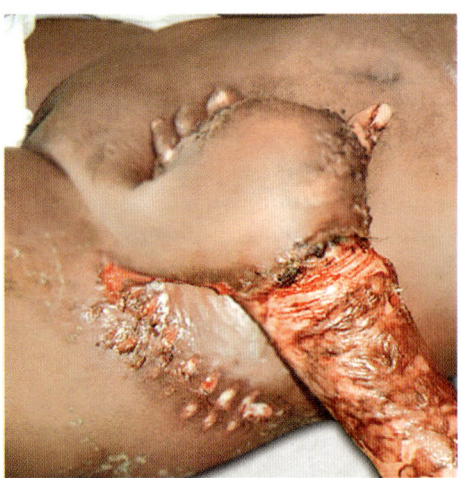

Fig. 8.15: Groin flap is used for burns defect in hand.

Pectoralis Major Myocutaneous Flap

- Pectoralis major myocutaneous flap (PMMF) is based on the pectoral branches of *thoracoacromial artery*. Usually, skin below and medial to nipple over the muscle is used. Muscle pedicle is made as broad as skin. It is used to cover the defect over the cheek/neck/pharynx/intraoral lesions after wide excision with removal of skin over the tumor. Vessel marking is 2 cm medial to coracoid process, obliquely below the clavicle at the junction between middle third and outer third. Line runs

- Flap can be reached as high as defect over the zygomatic region, as rotating lower border of the flap slack and lax (as it is near anterior axillary fold which is lax). Occasionally, it is also used to transfer below to the chest or abdomen.

Groin Flap

- It is a cutaneous flap (axial pattern) based medially on superficial circumflex iliac artery, which is 2–3 cm below and parallel to the inguinal ligament. Artery originates

Don't judge each day by the harvest you reap but by the seeds you plant

towards the xiphoid process. Oblique downwards incision is placed encroaching the ellipse of the needed skin in the flap. Often skin incision begins below the line of 3rd rib to retain the deltopectoral flap area in case for future need. Lower border of the muscle is raised by dissecting beneath the pectoral fascia.

❖ While raising the flap of the chest wall thoracoacromial vessels can be visualized. Enough care should be taken not to injure it. Flap is raised over the medial and lateral margins of the pectoralis major muscle. In front, it is dissected off from the deep fascia. Skin with muscle is dissected from the deeper structures like ribs, intercostal muscles and pectoralis minor. Flap is raised upwards up to the coracoid.

❖ Lateral pectoral vessels if possible are retained, otherwise can be sacrificed. Pectoral nerves should be retained. Defect below is usually closed primarily with sutures. Often it needs spilt skin grafting. Flap is tunneled in subcutaneous plane towards neck or oral cavity.

❖ Postoperatively flap is observed for color changes, seroma, and infection. Neck is flexed towards the flap side during postoperative period to prevent tension. Suction drain should be placed, which is removed once drainage stops or in 72 hours.

❖ In the neck, flap covers the carotid vessels thereby protecting it. In oral cavity, if flap is of large size, its skin can be split into half to cover both inner and outer aspect of the oral cavity. It gives bulk and adequate movements of the jaw.

❖ Pectoralis major flap can be used along with deltopectoral flap with proper planning (Figs. 8.16A and B).

Cross Leg Flap

❖ It is commonly used to cover the defect on the opposite foot/leg. It is random pattern flap.

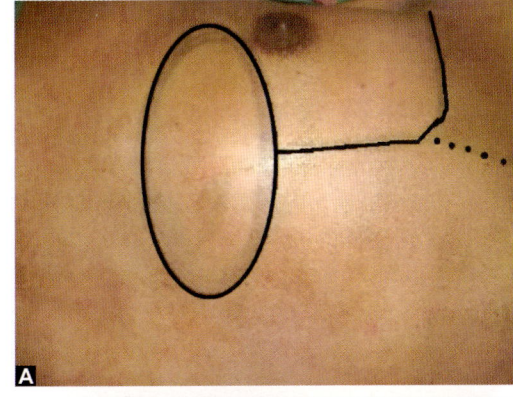
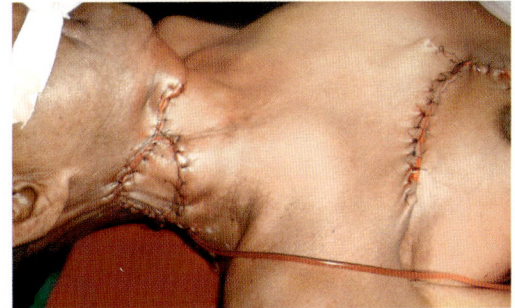
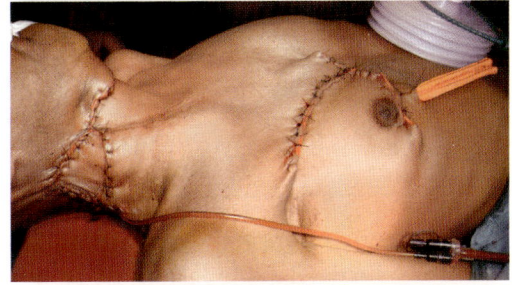
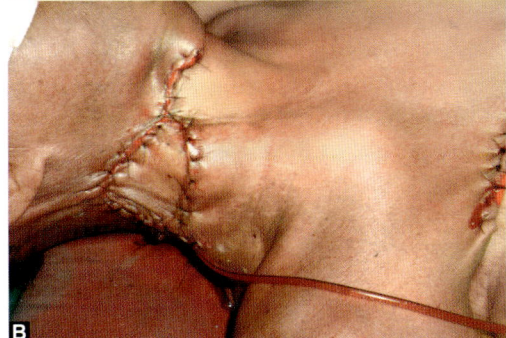

Figs. 8.16A and B: Pectoralis major myocutaneous flap used for a defect in the neck (after radical neck dissection with skin removal).

*Life is ours to be spent, not to be saved—**DH Lawrence***

- Limb should be immobilized for 3 weeks by plaster of Paris or external fixation. Raw donor flap area needs split skin graft cover.
- It is direct flap with 1:1 length to breadth ratio.
- It is commonly used in post-trauma defects in younger individuals. Joint stiffness due to immobilization may be a problem (Fig. 8.17).

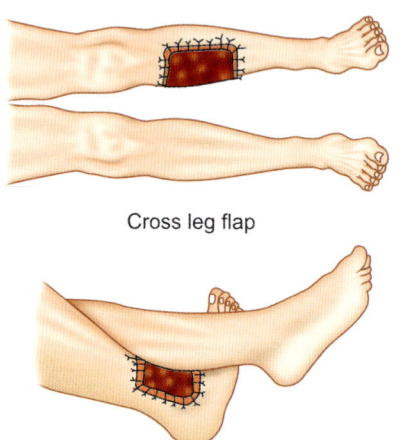

Fig. 8.17: Cross leg flap.

Free Flaps

- Flap with a single lengthy wide calibered arteriovenous system is transferred with its vascular pedicle. Here vascular pedicle is transected with flap and both artery and vein of the flap is anastomosed to the specific artery and vein at recipient area to reattain its perfusion through new blood vessel. *Length and caliber of the vessels* are deciding factors here. Often associated nerves either motor or sensory are also anastomosed. *Healthy vessel wall and adequate pulse volume* are essential in recipient vessel. Presence of *infection* in recipient area is *absolute contraindication*. It can cause thrombosis of the vessel and flap necrosis. Vein ideally should be as large as artery. Often, if possible a second vein is also anastomosed. Caliber of the vessels of both recipient and donor parts should be reasonably corresponding. Recipient bed and vessel preparation and donor flap raising should be done simultaneously. *The ischemic time* (time between division of the donor vessel and restoration of perfusion at recipient) should be kept minimum as much as possible.
- Anastomosis is done *end to end or side to end* to the flap vessel from recipient vessel (side of the recipient vessel to end of flap vessel). When diameters of the both vessels are equal end to end anastomosis is done. When diameter is unequal, then side to end anastomosis is done. End to end in such situation may cause turbulence in blood flow due to unequal diameter leading into thrombosis of the vessel.
- Instruments used for anastomosis are: spring handled needle holder; spring handled scissors; fine dissecting and cutting scissors; blunt tipped forceps as vessel dilator; microclamps.

Radial Forearm Flap

- It is perfused from the radial vessels and raised on the flexor aspect of the forearm. Perforating branches of these vessels supply deep fascia and skin over it. Flap can be fasciocutaneous or osteofasciocutaneous/osteomyofasciocutaneous if radial bone is also used as part of the flap.
- Radial forearm free flap is commonly used for mandible defects. It is technically easier and safer. Flap is raised along with skin, segment of the radius along its intermuscular septum through which vessels pass and brachioradialis as components.
- Care is taken in dissecting vessels of the bed and not to injure the radial nerve. In free flap artery is sutured to the recipient artery like facial artery using microscope. Other similar flaps are—ulnar forearm flap, scapular flaps, and vascularized fibular transfer.

Have, goals, they give direction, purpose and meaning to lofe.

TRANSPLANTATION

Preoperative evaluation of the patient for transplantation.
* General evaluation about pulmonary, cardiac, gastrointestinal tract (GIT), renal and cancer screening.
* Immunologic evaluation, serology for hepatitis, human immunodeficiency virus (HIV), cytomegalovirus.

Placing the organ in the same position is called as *orthotopic transplantation*, e.g. liver.

Placing the organ in new position is called as *heterotopic transplantation*.

Donor Criteria

Cadaver Donor

Individuals with severe brain injury resulting in brain death.

Brain death is defined as '*Complete irreversible cessation of all brain functions*' along with:
* Absence of reflexes.
* Absence of spontaneous movements.
* Unresponsiveness.

Other criteria for cadaver donor:
* Normothermic patient.
* No respiratory effort by the patient.
* No depressant drugs should be there while evaluating the patient.
* Individual should not have any sepsis, cancer.

Living Donor

* Living unrelated donor.
* Living related donor.
* Individual should have normal health.

Requirements

* ABO typing.
* Serology tests.
* Angiogram.
* Intravenous urography.
* Human leukocyte antigen (HLA) typing.

RENAL TRANSPLANTATION

Two types of donors:
1. Living related donors.
2. Cadaver donors.

Compatibility should be checked by tissue typing, i.e. ABO blood group system and major histocompatibility complex.

Usually *left kidney is taken for transplantation* because of long *left renal vein*.

It is placed in right iliac fossa with ureter connected to the urinary bladder; renal artery to internal iliac artery (end to end); renal vein to external iliac vein (Fig. 8.18).

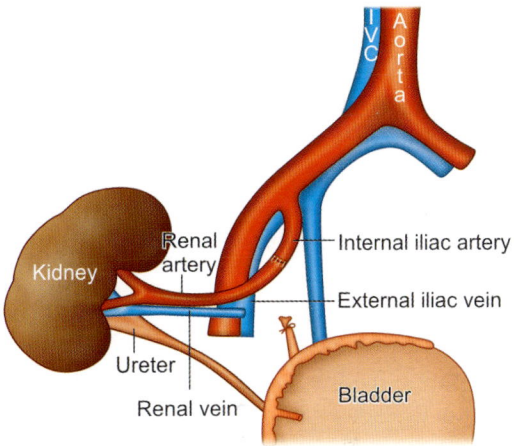

Fig. 8.18: Renal transplantation.

Postoperative Management

* Immunosuppression: By Cyclosporine, Azathioprine, Prednisolone, Antithymocytic globulin and Antilymphocytic serum.
* Proper fluid balance has to be taken care off.

Complications

* Acute tubular necrosis.
* Rejection.
* Obstruction of the collecting system.
* Infection.

*If you really look closely, most overnight successes took a long time—***Steve Jobs**

- Urine leakage.
- Secondary hemorrhage.
- Renal infarction.
- Hazards of immunosuppression:
  - Infection by unusual organisms like cytomegalovirus, herpes, *Pneumocystis carinii*, varicella and other bacterial infections, candidial infection.
  - Changes in the cellular component of blood.
  - Uncommon malignancies of CNS and skin.
  - Nephrotoxicity, GIT bleeding and perforation.
  - Hirsutism, delayed wound healing, cataract formation.

LIVER TRANSPLANTATION

INDICATIONS

- Primary biliary atresia.
- Cirrhosis.
- Malignant diseases of the liver.

Children respond better for liver transplantation. Tissue typing and cross-matching are not that necessary as they do not influence the results.

If the transplantation is done at the same place after doing hepatectomy, it is called as **orthotopic liver transplantation**. If it is placed in a different place it is called as **ectopic or heterotopic liver transplantation**. Success rate in liver transplantation is better.

BONE MARROW TRANSPLANTATION

Indication

- Leukemias.
- Aplastic anemias.
- Immune deficiencies, etc.

Recipients are initially treated with total body irradiation. As bone marrow is an active immune system, *proper tissue typing* is essential. *Infant bone marrow* is better marrow as a *donor*. Marrow aspirated from donor's bone is transplanted by *intravenous injection* to the recipient.

Immunosuppression with Cyclosporin-A is always needed. It will take few weeks to show the response.

Problems

- Graft rejection.
- *Graft-versus-host* disease (GVH) is more dangerous.

GRAFT REJECTION

Types

1. **Hyperacute** rejection is due to antibody reaction, which occurs within minutes of vascularization of the graft.
2. **Acute** rejection results due to cell-mediated immunity, occurring in a few days to first 3 months of transplant. It responds well to steroids and immunosuppressants.
3. **Chronic rejection** occurs in 12 months after transplant. It is not very common. It is due to late vasculitis. When it occurs, it responds very poorly to steroids or other drugs.

CIMINO FISTULA

- It is an arteriovenous fistula created for *hemodialysis*. Usually at wrist, radial artery is anastomosed side-to-side to cephalic vein.
- A good created fistula shows continuous thrill and bruit, with increased venous engorgement along with hyperdynamic circulation.
- At the ankle, fistula is created between posterior tibial artery and saphenous vein or in the thigh between femoral artery and long saphenous vein.

Courage is fear that has said its prayers

- Distal gangrene is not common.
- **Complications:** Infection, bleeding, hyperdynamic circulation.

IMMUNOSUPPRESSIVE AGENTS

Induction therapy: It is used immediately after transplantation up to 3 weeks. Anti-lymphocytic globulin (ALG) acts against T cells. Monoclonal antibody (OKT3) acts at TCR complex affecting the cell-mediated immunity. Interleukin 2 receptor inhibitors like basiliximab and daclizumab are used along with other immunosuppressants. Rituximab, an anti-CD20 monoclonal antibody, alemtuzumab, an anti-CD52 monoclonal antibody and intravenous immunoglobulin (IVIG) are other drugs used.

Maintenance therapy: It is for prolonged period. Drugs are—Prednisolone, Antiprolifrating agents like azathioprine, mycophenolate mofetil, leflunomide, T cell directed immunosuppressants like cyclosporine, tacrolimus, sirolimus—are the drugs used.

Risks related to immunosuppression
Infection like cytomegalovirus, *Pneumocystis carinii*, pneumonia, pancreatitis, hepatitis can occur.

Malignancy: It is 10 times more common; skin cancers and carcinoma cervix, human papilloma virus (HPV), Kaposi's sarcoma, lymphomas are common.

Cyclosporin A

- *Cyclosporine* (Borel, 1972) is extracted from fungus *Tolypocladium inflatum*. It contains 11 amino acids with molecular weight 1202.6 gram/mol. It is metabolized in the liver by cytochrome P-450.
- It is selective inhibitor of TCR mediated activation suppressing T cells. It inhibits formation of mature CD4 and CD8 T cells in thymus.
- It is a very good immunosuppressant. But it does not cause myelosuppression.
- It is used to prevent transplant rejection as maintenance therapy.
- *Dose*: IV dose given initially is 4 mg/kg in 500 mL of saline; later changed to oral therapy as 12 mg/kg daily; after few weeks dose is tapered to 5 mg/kg/day. Regular serum cyclosporine estimation twice weekly with estimation of hematocrit, blood urea and serum creatinine is needed. It is commonly given along with prednisolone and azathioprine.
- *Side/toxic effects are—nephrotoxicity*, hypertension, hirsuitism, gingival hyperplasia, hyperkalemia, neurotoxicity, tremor, hepatotoxicity, risk of infections (CMV, *Candida, Pneumocystis carinii*, secondary infections) and malignancy (lymphoma, skin and CNS).

CHAPTER 9

Hand and Foot

Chapter Outline

- Surgical Anatomy of the Hand
- Hand Infections
- Acute Paronychia
- Chronic Paronychia
- Terminal Pulp Space Infection (Felon)
- Infection of Webspaces
- Deep Palmar Space Infection
- Acute Suppurative Tenosynovitis
- Hand Injuries
- Compound Palmar Ganglion
- Dupuytren's Contracture
- Syndactyly
- Mallet Finger (Base Ball Finger)
- Heberden's Nodes
- Spina Ventosa
- Callosity
- Corn
- Plantar Fasciitis (Policeman's Heel)
- Ingrowing Toe Nail (Onychocryptosis)

HAND

SURGICAL ANATOMY OF THE HAND

Flexor Retinaculum

- It extends medially from pisiform and hook of hamate laterally to scaphoid tubercle and trapezium crest as strong fibrous band so as to bridge carpus to create carpal tunnel.
- Ulnar nerve and vessels, palmar cutaneous branches of median and ulnar nerves, palmaris longus muscle are superficial to the carpal tunnel.
- Median nerve, tendons of flexor digitorum superficialis, profundus and pollicis longus, radial and ulnar bursa are deep to flexor retinaculum.

Palmar Aponeurosis

It is thickened, modified deep fascia in the palm with its apex pointing proximally (as continuation of palmaris longus) and base towards distal part with four parts. They extend over deep transverse ligament into lumbrical tunnel.

Blood Supply of the Hand

- *Superficial palmar arch* is mainly formed by ulnar artery and is completed by superficial palmar branch of radial artery. It gives four digital branches to medial three fingers.
- Deep palmar arch is formed by radial artery and is completed by deep branch of ulnar artery. It gives three palmar metacarpal arteries, which communicate with superficial palmar arch. It also gives

*The journey of a thousand miles begins with one step—**Lao Tzu***

communicating, perforating branches to dorsal metacarpal arteries.

Muscles of the Hand

- **Thenar muscles:** Abductor pollicis brevis, flexor policis brevis, opponens pollicis and adductor pollicis.
- **Hypothenar muscles:** Palmaris brevis, abductor digiti minimi, flexor digiti minimi and opponens digiti minimi.
- **Lumbricals** are four in number—named from lateral to medial.
- Four **palmar interossei**.
- Four **dorsal interossei**.

Nerve Supply

- Abductor pollicis brevis, flexor pollicis brevis, opponens pollicis and 1st and 2nd lumbricals are supplied by median nerve (5 muscles).
- Rest of the muscles (15 muscles) in hand are supplied by ulnar nerve.

HAND INFECTIONS

- Hand is a compact actively functioning unit. It contains neurovascular bundles, muscles, bones and ligaments.
- Infection can occur due to minor injuries and hematogenous spread.

Precipitating causes
• Diabetes.
• Immunosuppression.
• Trauma.
• HIV infection.
• Steroid therapy.

Common organisms
• *Staphylococcus*.
• *Streptococcus*.
• Gram-negative organisms like *E. coli, Klebsiella, Pseudomonas*.
• Occasionally fungal infection causing chronic paronychia, Madura hand due to nocardia group of fungi, viral infection like *ORF* can occur.

General Features of Hand Infection

- Infection spreads faster in all areas.
- Causes edema over the dorsum of hand due to lax skin and more lymphatic network even though infection per se is more over the volar aspect. It looks like *frog hand* (Figs. 9.1A and B).
- Restricted movements of fingers and hand. The hand functions like *hook, pinch, grip, grasp* are lost.
- Severe pain and tenderness, with fever.
- Tender palpable axillary lymph nodes are often present.

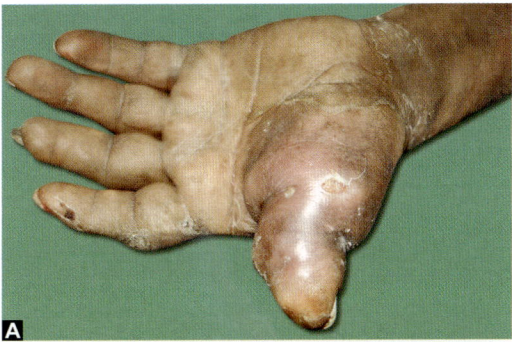
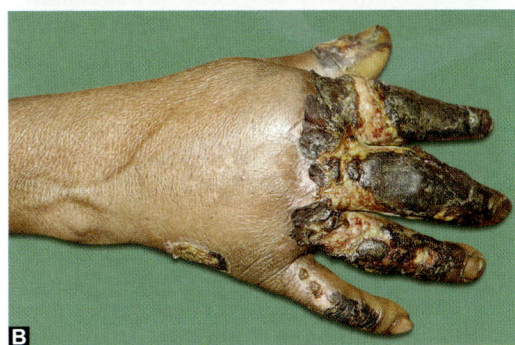

Figs. 9.1A and B: Typical hand infection in two different patients.

Different Types of Hand Infections

- Acute paronychia.
- Chronic paronychia.
- Terminal pulp space infection (***felon***).
- Subungual infection.
- Web space infection.

Failure is the condiment that gives success its flavor

- Midpalmar space infection.
- Thenar space infection.
- Deep palmar abscess.
- Acute suppurative tenosynovitis.
- Chronic tenosynovitis of flexor tendon sheath of palm and forearm—*Compound palmar ganglion*.
- Lymphangitis of the hand.

Investigations
- Pus for culture and sensitivity.
- Blood sugar.
- Urine sugar and ketone bodies.
- X-ray of the part.

General Principles of Managing Hand Infections
- ***Antibiotic therapy:*** Amoxycillin, cloxacillin are used commonly; later depending on culture report appropriate antibiotics are given.
- ***Position of rest*** with wrist slightly abducted and extended, thumb and index fingers away (glass holding position). Position of function is, when thumb and index fingers are pinching firmly with wrist extension.
- ***Elevation of hand*** reduces the edema, increases perfusion, and promotes healing.
  Early recognition of localized pus. Once localized, ***incision and drainage*** must be done ideally under general anesthesia or regional block (*not local anesthesia*). Draining incision should not cross the palmar crease. Incision should have adequate length and depth (deep to palmar fascia, otherwise evacuation of pus is inadequate). Care should be taken not to injure neurovascular bundles. Pus should be sent for culture and sensitivity. Slough if present should be excised thoroughly. Gauze drain is placed. Regular dressings are done with continuation of antibiotics. Communications into other areas of hand should also be drained.
- ***Bloodless field*** (using tourniquet) is better to drain pus from hand.
- Proper care must be taken after treatment. Initial rest, elevation of hand, later proper physiotherapy and regular exercise of hand and fingers should be done to restore normal function.

Complications of hand infections
- Stiffness of digits and hand (ankylosis).
- Deformity and disability.
- Bacteremia and septicemia.
- Osteomyelitis of bones depending on location of abscess like metacarpal bones, terminal phalanx.
- Suppurative arthritis of joints.
- Paralysis of median nerve.

ACUTE PARONYCHIA

- It is the most common hand infection.
- It occurs in subcuticular area under the *eponychium*.
- Minor injury to finger is the common cause.
- Suppuration occurs very rapidly.
- It tracks around the skin margin and spreads under the nail causing *hang nail or floating nail*.
- Organisms are *Staphylococcus aureus* and *Streptococcus pyogenes*.

Features
Presents with severe throbbing pain and tenderness (dependent throbbing), with pus visible under the nail root (Fig. 9.2). Nail on touch is very tender (paronychia means '***run around***').

Treatment
- Pus is sent for culture and sensitivity.
- Antibiotics like Cloxacillin, Amoxicillin.
- Analgesics.
- The pus is drained by making an incision over the eponychium.
- If there is a *floating nail*, then the nail is dead, it has to be removed.
- Recovery is fast.

What you do speaks so loudly that I cannot hear what you say—**Ralph Waldo Emerson**

Chapter 9 : Hand and Foot

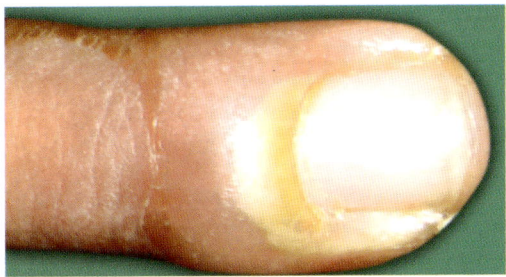

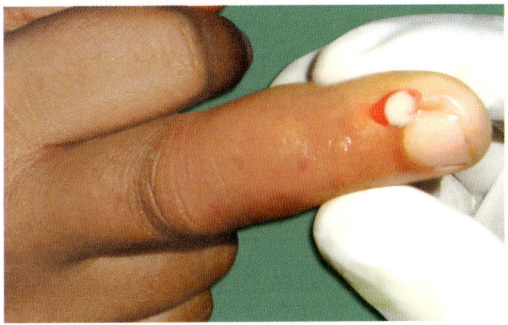

Fig. 9.2: Acute paronychia showing pointing/visible pus.

CHRONIC PARONYCHIA

It is commonly due to fungal infection.

Features

- Itching in the nailbed.
- Recurrent pain; discharge.
- Secondary bacterial infection may supervene.
- **Investigations:** Culture of scrapings for fungus and other causative agents.

Treatment

- Long-term antifungal therapy.
- Antibiotics for secondary infection.
- In severe cases, removal of nail is required.

TERMINAL PULP SPACE INFECTION (FELON)

- It is the second most common hand infection (25%).

- Index and thumb are commonly affected.
- Usually by a minor injury like finger prick.

Surgical Anatomy (Fig. 9.3)

Terminal pulp space contains fat and is partitioned by septae, which is attached from periosteum of terminal phalanx to skin.

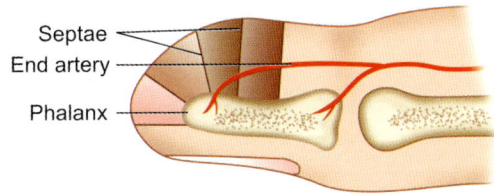

Fig. 9.3: Anatomy of the terminal pulp space.

Proximally deep fascia is attached to the periosteum distal to the base of terminal phalanx, i.e. distal to the attachment of flexor tendon.

So, terminal space is a closed compartment which causes increased pressure when there is infection, compresses terminal artery leading to thrombosis resulting in osteomyelitis of terminal phalanx.

Bacteria
• *Staphylococcus*.
• *Streptococcus*.
• Gram-negative organisms.

Features

- Pain, tenderness, swelling in the terminal phalanx; fever.
- Tender axillary lymph nodes.

Often suppuration is severe, forming **collar stud abscess**, which eventually may burst.

Causes of collar-stud abscess
• Tuberculous cold abscess.
• Terminal pulp space infection (Felon).
• Deep palmar space infection.

*You must be the change you wish to see in the world—**Gandhi***

* **Investigation:**
    – X-ray of the part is often required to rule out osteomyelitis of terminal phalanx.
    – Pus for culture and sensitivity.
* **Treatment (Fig. 9.4)**
    – Antibiotics and analgesics.
    – **Drainage** of pus from terminal pulp space by an oblique deep incision.
    – If osteomyelitis sets in, then the terminal phalanx may have to be amputated.

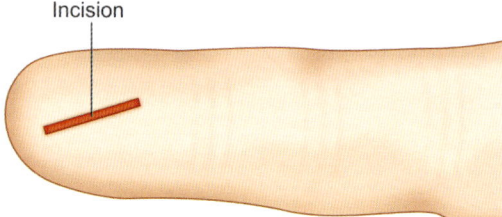

Fig. 9.4: Incision for pulp space drainage.

* **Complications**
    – Osteomyelitis of the terminal phalanx.
    – Septicemia.

INFECTION OF WEBSPACES

Surgical Anatomy

There are three triangular webspaces filled with fat between the dorsal and volar skin. When the space is filled with pus it straddles the deep transverse ligament. Even though pus is on volar aspect, it points out dorsally.

It originates from:
* Abrasion.
* Infection of proximal volar space of finger.
* Callosities.
* Infection of proximal spaces.

Bacteria

* *Staphylococcus.*
* *Streptococcus.*
* *Gram-negative organisms.*

Clinical Features

* Fever; pain and tenderness.
* Edema of dorsum of hand.
* Maximum tenderness is on the volar aspect.
* **'V' sign**—separation of fingers.
* If untreated, infection may spread into other webspaces and hand spaces.

Treatment

* Elevation of hand
* Antibiotics and analgesics
* **Drainage of pus** under regional or general anesthesia. A horizontal incision is made on volar skin of the web, and deepened to reach the space by dividing fibers of palmar fascia (Fig. 9.5). Pus has to be sent for culture and sensitivity. If other webspaces are involved they should be drained through a separate incision. Edges of the wound are cut to leave a diamond shaped opening in front. Often counter-incision over dorsal skin of web is needed.

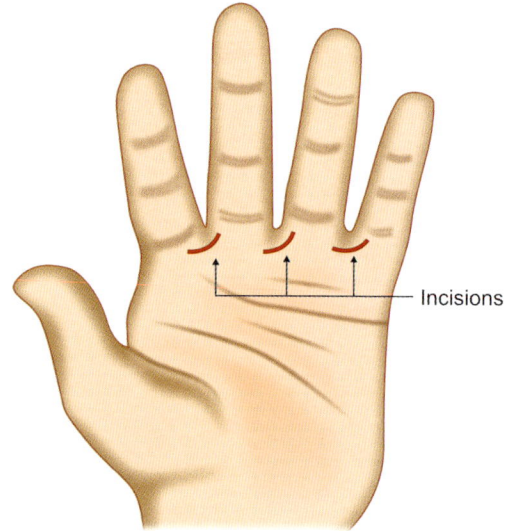

Fig. 9.5: Incision for webspace drainage.

The most vital test of a man's character is not how he behaves after success, but how he sustains defeat

DEEP PALMAR SPACE INFECTION

Surgical Anatomy
Two deep palmar spaces are present
- *Midpalmar space*
- *Thenar space.*

Midpalmar space:
It is bound in front by palmar aponeurosis, behind by medial three metacarpals, laterally by a vertical line from lateral margin of the middle finger. It contains flexor tendons, neurovascular bundles and lumbricals. It is the common site of the infection.

Thenar space:
It is located anterior to lateral two metacarpals. Infection here is usually due to extension from midpalmar space.

Causes
- Trauma.
- Spread from infection of finger spaces and webspaces.
- Hematogenous spread.
- Spread from tenosynovitis.

Clinical features
• Pain and tenderness in the palm.
• Edema of dorsum of hand (**frog hand**).
• Loss of concavity of palm.
• Painful movement of metacarpophalangeal joint (but movements of interphalangeal joint are normal and painfree).
• Fever.
• Palpable tender axillary lymph nodes.
• Eventually pus may come out of palmar aponeurosis forming collar-stud abscess and later with formation of sinus.

X-ray of the part is required.

Treatment
- Elevation of the affected limb.
- Antibiotics and analgesics.
- **Drainage of pus** under general anesthesia. A horizontal incision is placed on the volar aspect without crossing the palmar crease and should be extended deep to palmar aponeurosis. A drain is placed. Pus should be sent for culture and sensitivity and appropriate antibiotics are continued.

Complications
• Osteomyelitis of metacarpals.
• Stiffness of hand.
• Suppurative arthritis.
• Extension of infection into other spaces.

ACUTE SUPPURATIVE TENOSYNOVITIS

It is the bacterial infection of flexor tendon sheaths.

Surgical Anatomy
- **Radial bursa** is flexor sheath of flexor tendon of thumb, which extends to the digit.
- **Ulnar bursa** is flexor sheaths of medial four flexor tendons, which extends into the digit of the fifth (little) finger.

Common bacteria:
Staphylococcus aureus, Streptococcus pyogenes.

Clinical features
• Symmetrical swelling of entire finger.
• Flexion of finger—**Hook sign**.
• Severe pain on extension.
• Tenderness over the sheath.
• Edema of whole hand, both palm and dorsum (due to lymphatic spread).
• As ulnar bursa extends into the little finger, pain and tenderness extends into little finger but not much to other fingers.
Kanavel signs
• Swollen finger held in flexion.
• Exquisite pain on passive extension.
• Tenderness precisely over the tendon sheath.
• Area of greatest tenderness is over the part of ulnar bursa lying between transverse palmar creases.

In infection of radial bursa, thumb is swollen with pain and tenderness over the sheath of the flexor pollicis longus along with inextensibility of interphalangeal joint.

Keep your face to the sunshine and you can never see the shadow—**Helen Keller**

Swelling just above the flexor retinaculum is common.

Treatment

- Elevation of the affected limb.
- Antibiotics and analgesics.
- Position of rest.
- **Drainage of pus** under general anesthesia. Incisions are placed over the site of maximum tenderness and flexor sheath should be opened up. Many a times multiple incisions are required.

Complications

- Spread of infection proximally into forearm.
- Stiffness of fingers and hand.
- Suppurative arthritis.
- Osteomyelitis.
- Median nerve palsy.
- Bacteremia and septicemia.

In hand	
Do's	**Dont's**
• Examine hand carefully.	• Incise every infected digit.
• Think of other diagnosis.	• Make puncture incisions or over pads.
• Wait for abscess to localize.	• Injure the digital nerves or vessels.
• Place adequate length and depth of incisions.	• Place incisions crossing the crease line.
• Immobilize, elevate the hand.	• Close human bites or lacerated wounds.
• Give antibiotics and proper dressings.	• Forget to send pus for culture and sensitivity.

Parona's space is space in the forearm to which infection can occur as extension from the hand.

HAND INJURIES (FIG. 9.6)

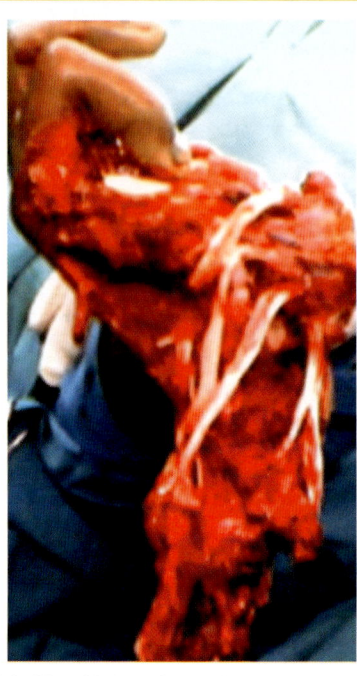

Fig. 9.6: Hand injury. Note the severity of injury. Hand injuries are tidy/indeterminate/untidy injuries.

Classifications

Tidy injuries:
They are clean incised wounds and are usually treated by primary suturing; depend on the tissues involved like nerves, tendons and muscles.

Untidy injuries:
They are lacerated wounds and are treated by debridement and later by delayed primary or secondary suturing.

Compartment injuries:
It is deep injury causing increased pressure within the deep fascia causing vascular compromise of muscles leading to arterial block; muscle necrosis and Volkmann's ischemic contracture as a late effect. Often it may cause renal failure due to myoglobulinuria

*The will to win the desire to succeed, the urge to reach your full potential....
will unlock the door to personal excellence.*

and septicemia. It may be life-threatening unless immediate surgical intervention is done.

Degloving injuries (Figs. 9.7A and B):
It is avulsion of the large part of skin and fascia exposing wide part of deeper structures like muscles, vessels and bones without coverage. It needs proper debridement and later skin coverage by skin grafting or flaps. It may cause extensive tissue loss; infection, neurological deficit; gas gangrene, etc.

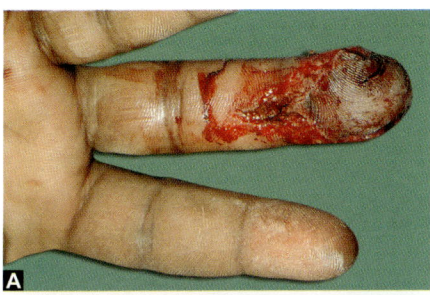
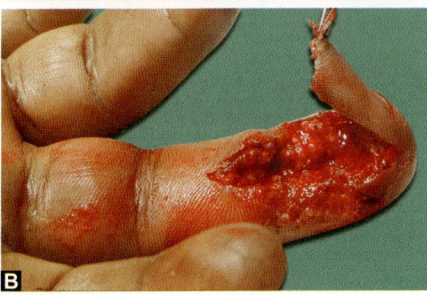

Figs. 9.7A and B: Crush and degloving injury of finger.

Indetermined injuries
It could not be assessed.

Assessment of injury:
Should include:
Number, extent, depth, deformity and disability, neurovascular injuries, tendon injuries, muscle injuries, bone and joint injuries.

Complications and morbidity of hand injuries
• Infection.
• Osteomyelitis.
• Arthritis of joints.
• Stiffness.
• Loss of function due to disability.

Principles of treatment
• Hemostasis.
• Use of tourniquet.
• Wound debridement and cleaning.
• Antibiotics and antitetanus treatment (toxoid and antitetanus globulin).
• Primary suturing if it is incised wound or delayed primary suturing if there is edema.
• Skin grafting or flaps for skin loss.
• Tendon suturing or tendon graft.
• Rest and elevation of the affected parts.
• Management of fractures by splint, wiring.
• Nerve repair.
• Immobilization up to 21 days.
• Later physiotherapy with warm, exercise, active movements.
• Microsurgical restoration of digits.

COMPOUND PALMAR GANGLION

❖ It is chronic tenosynovitis of flexor tendon sheaths due to tuberculosis (tuberculous tenosynovitis) or rheumatoid arthritis.
❖ It can be unilateral or bilateral.

Pathology

❖ Flexor tendon sheath on either side of the wrist is involved, i.e. both in the volar surface of palm and lower forearm.
❖ Swelling contains fluid with typical ***melon seed bodies***.
❖ Condition is often bilateral in case of rheumatoid arthritis.

Features

❖ Swelling in the palm and lower forearm, which is smooth, soft, nontender, non-transilluminating, fluctuant and cross fluctuant across flexor retinaculum.
❖ Wasting of hand and forearm muscles.
❖ Matted axillary lymph nodes may be palpable.
❖ Primary focus may be there in lungs.
❖ **Investigations:** Erythrocyte sedimentation rate (ESR); chest X-ray; fine needle

*The best way out is always through—**Robern Frost***

aspiration cytology (FNAC) of axillary lymph node and swelling itself.
- **Treatment:**
  - Start antituberculous drugs: Isoniazid (INH), Rifampicin, Ethambutol and Pyrazinamide for 9 months.
  - Excision of flexor tendon sheath with caseating material, tubercles, melon seed bodies.
  - Care should be taken not to injure median and ulnar nerves.

DUPUYTREN'S CONTRACTURE

- It refers to localized thickening of palmar aponeurosis and later formation of nodules with severe permanent changes in metacarpophalangeal (MCP) and interphalangeal (IP) joints (Fig. 9.8).
- It starts in ring and little fingers, with flexion of ring and little fingers. Later involving all fingers.
- There is thickening and nodule formation in the palm with adherent skin.
- It is often familial and bilateral.
- Pads (of fat) develop in knuckles and are called as *Garron's pads*.

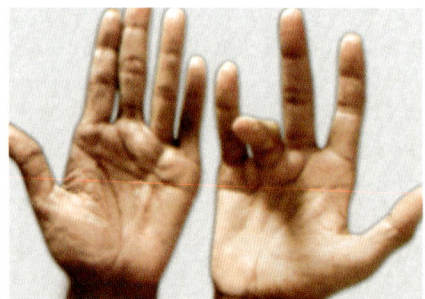

Fig. 9.8: Dupuytren's contracture in the hands. Note the involvement of the ring finger.

Condition often is associated with:
- Plantar fasciitis.
- Mediastinal and retroperitoneal fibrosis.
- Peyronie's disease of penis.
- Nodules in the face and ear.

- **Etiology**
  - Repeated minor trauma.
  - Cirrhosis.
  - Epileptics on treatment with phenytoin sodium.
  - Diabetics; other metabolic conditions.
  - Familial.
- **Complications**
  - Restriction of hand function and so disability.
  - Arthritis of MCP and IP joints.
- **Treatment**
  - Fasciotomy of palmar aponeurosis and later physiotherapy (Fig. 9.9).
  - In severe cases fasciectomy.
  - Treatment for the cause.

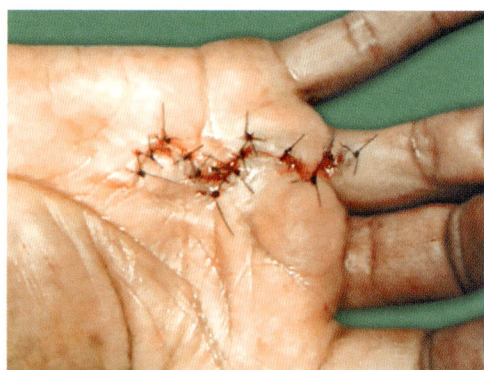

Fig. 9.9: Z plasty done for Dupuytren's contracture.

SYNDACTYLY

It is *webbing or fusion* of fingers (Fig. 9.10).

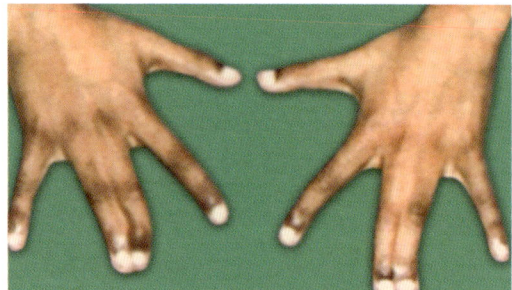

Fig. 9.10: Syndactyly in both hands. It can be bony or fibrous.

When work is a pleasure, life is a joy! When work is a duty, life is slavery.

Causes

- Congenital and hereditary—common.
- Traumatic like burns.

Types

- Cutaneous.
- Fibrous.
- Bony.
- It can be unilateral or bilateral.
  Often there will be webbing of toes also (Fig. 9.11).
  If bony type is suspected X-ray of the part should be taken.

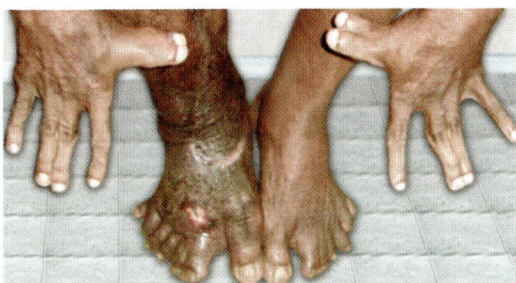

Fig. 9.11: Syndactyly and polydactyly of both hands and both feet.

Treatment

- If cutaneous, release of web is done in staged procedure with 'Z' plasty or skin grafting.
- If fibrous, release can be done.
- If bony type release is difficult because blood supply will be compromised which will lead to gangrene of digit.

MALLET FINGER (BASE BALL FINGER)

The terminal phalanx cannot be extended because of tear at insertion of extensor tendon or avulsion fracture of the base of the terminal phalanx.

HEBERDEN'S NODES

These are seen in osteoarthritis occurring behind the distal interphalangeal joints of *index*, middle, little and ring fingers.

SPINA VENTOSA

Refers to phalangeal tuberculosis (*tuberculous dactylitis*). It is called as spina ventosa because of its appearance as 'air filled balloon'.

FOOT

CALLOSITY (FIG. 9.12)

It is a hard, thickened skin occurring as a protective measure seen in wider area usually over heel and heads of metatarsals.

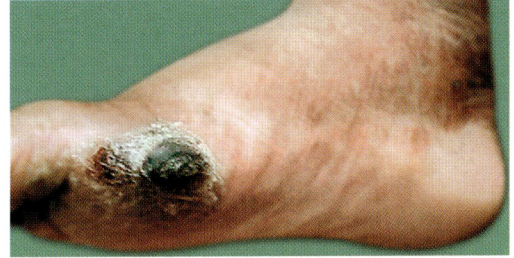

Fig. 9.12: Callosity in the foot.

CORN (FIG. 9.13)

Types

- Hard corn.
- Soft corn.

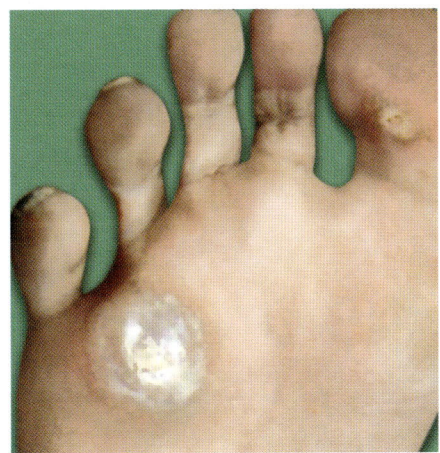

Fig. 9.13: Corns in the plantar aspect of the foot.

*People are just as happy as they make up their minds to be—**Abraham Lincoln***

Hard Corn

- It is localized area of thickening over bony projections like heads of metatarsals.
- Histologically, it differs from callosity by having severe keratoses with a central core of degenerated cells and cholesterol.
- It presses over the adjacent nerves causing pain. It can get infected causing severe pain and tenderness with inability to walk.
- **Treatment**: Excision.

Soft Corn

It usually occurs between 4th and 5th toes due to friction of bases of adjacent proximal phalanges.

PLANTAR FASCIITIS (POLICEMAN'S HEEL)

- It occurs due to friction of the ossified posterior insertion of the plantar fascia, which is common in people who stand or walk for long time.
- **Treatment:** Analgesics, rest, steroid injections to the site.

INGROWING TOE NAIL (FIG. 9.14) (ONYCHOCRYPTOSIS)

- It is also called as *embedded toe nail*.
- It is due to curling of side of the nail inwards causing it to form a lateral spike, which results in repeated irritation and infection of overhanging tissues in the nail fold.
- **Causes:** Tight shoes; improper cutting of nails (very short and convexly curved).

Features

- It is common in *great toe* and is often *bilateral*.
- Both medial and lateral sides of the toe can be involved.
- Pain, tenderness, swelling of margins of the toe, often with foul smelling discharge.

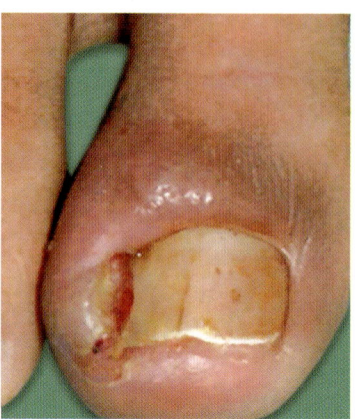

Fig. 9.14: Ingrowing toe nail. Note the granuloma caused by repeated infection and inflammation.

Treatment (Fig. 9.15)

- Regular dressing and packing.
- Antibiotics.
- Discharge should be sent for culture.
- Nails should be cut concavely without leaving lateral spikes.

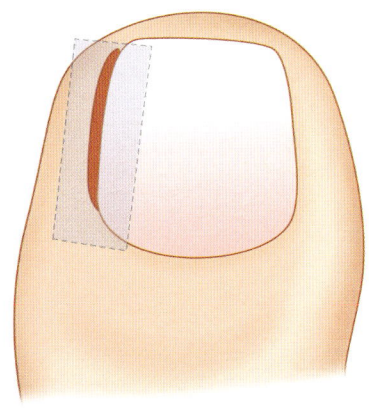

Fig. 9.15: Zadik's or Fowler's operation.

Zadik's or Fowler's operation: Skin in lateral margin and root is incised so as to expose the lateral spike and germinal matrix. ***Infected tissues with pus and germinal matrix of ingrown part are excised.***

Often excision of entire nail with its root is required.

One only gets to the top rung of the ladder by steadily climbing up one at a time.

CHAPTER 10

Trauma

CHAPTER OUTLINE

- Triage
- Spinal Injury
- Neck Injuries
- Bullet Injuries
- Blast Injuries
- Penetrating Injury
- Abdominal Trauma
- Duodenal Injury
- Pancreatic Injury
- Small Bowel Injury
- Colonic Injury
- Liver Injury
- Splenic Injury
- Renal Injury
- Urinary Bladder Injury
- Abdominal Compartment Syndrome

Trauma is the major public health problem in all countries (Fig. 10.1).

TRIAGE

Triage means *'To sort' in French*.

Triage was a system to attend patients with trauma formulated by a *committee of Trauma of the American College of Surgeons*.

Assessing Four Components

1. Physiologic response.
2. Anatomical injury.
3. Biomechanical injury.
4. Comorbid factors.

TRIAGE ALGORITHM

Step one (Assess physiological impact)
Measure vital signs and level of consciousness:

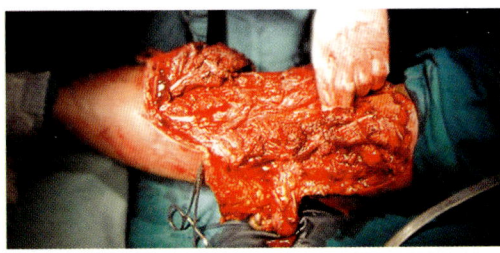

Fig. 10.1: Crush injury leg due to road traffic accident.

- By Glasgow Coma Scale.
- Systolic blood pressure.
- Respiratory rate.
- Revised trauma score. It is based on airway, laryngeal injury, spine injury, maxillofacial injury.

Step two (Assess anatomical impact)
All penetrating injuries to head, neck, thorax, major burns, fracture bones, pelvic fractures, paralysis.

Nobody is worth your tears and the one who is, will never make you cry

Step three (Assess mechanism)
- Automobile accidents, crash or blast injuries, high-energy injuries, fall from more than 20 feet.
- Bullet injury.

Step four (Assess history)
- Patient's age below 5 years or age more than 55 years.
- Cardiac diseases, respiratory and metabolic diseases.
- Pregnancy.
- Patients with bleeding disorders.
- Immunosuppressed individuals.

Based on the step, consider to shift the patient to trauma center and trauma team should be kept alert.

(It is important in multiple and mass casualities (fire, blasts, automobile accidents, train accidents).

MANAGEMENT
- Initial evaluation of the patient.
- Physiologic stabilization.
- Control of hemorrhage.
- Management of thoracic and abdominal injury.
- Management of cranial injury.

Tag the patient accordingly
- **Red color:** Immediate treatment is required.
- **Yellow color:** Urgent treatment is required.
- **Green color:** Delayed treatment is required.
- **Blue color:** Expectant treatment is required.
- **Black color:** Deceased.

I. PRIMARY MANAGEMENT
- **A**irway management.
- **B**reathing.
- **C**irculation.
- **D**isability and assessment of level of consciousness by Glasgow coma scale.
- **E**xposure of the patient from head to toe for final assessment.
- **F**ingers and tubes: Finger evaluation, Foley's catheterization.

Goals
- Identify life-threatening conditions.
- Decide and implement appropriate treatment to the area of trauma.
- First think of salvage of life, then think of salvage of limb.
- Rapid assessment, rapid resuscitation, rapid stabilization.
- Optimum, complete care.
- Transport efficiently to higher trauma center.

Airway
- Chin lift.
- Jaw thrust.
- Nasal airway.
- Oral airway.
- Endotracheal intubation.
- Tracheostomy [assess airway patency].

Breathing
- 100% oxygen.
- Assess bilateral chest raise.
- Assess breath sounds.
- Use pulse oximetry.
- Treat flail chest, pneumothorax.
- Intercostal tube drainage.

Circulation
- Monitor vitals.
- Heart sounds.
- ECG.
- IV fluids.
- Blood transfusion.
- Treatment of shock.
- Control of external bleed.
- Use two IV lines— 14G/16G.

Disability evaluation
- Neurological examination.
- Glasgow coma scale.
- Pupillary reaction.

Expose the patient fully
- Undress the patient.
- Hypothermia assessment.
- Assess injuries.
- Examine joints, bones, abdomen,
- and other systems.
- Look for identification marks.

Fingers and tubes
- Examine all orifices like P/R, P/V, etc.
- Use required tubes like catheter, Ryle's tube.

Categorize the patient:
- I: Deceased.
- II: Walking wounded.
- III: Immobile wounded.
- IV: Trapped wounded.

---

*Sing like no one's listening, love like you've never been hurt, dance like nobody's watching, and live like it's heaven on earth—**Mark Twain***

II. INVESTIGATIONS

- X-ray spine, chest, pelvis, extremities.
- CT scan.
- Blood group and cross matching.
- Arterial blood gas analysis.
- Serum electrolytes.
- US abdomen.

Abbreviated injury scale (AIS)
It is an anatomical scoring system. Injuries are ranked on a scale of 1 to 6, with 1 being minor, 5 severe and 6 a nonsurvivable injury. This assesses the 'threat to life' of an injury and is not a measure of severity.

Injury	AIS score
1	Minor
2	Moderate
3	Serious
4	Severe
5	Critical
6	Unsurvivable

Injury severity score (ISS)
It is an anatomical scoring system that provides an overall score for patients with multiple injuries. Each injury is assigned with AIS with one of the six body regions—head, face, chest, abdomen, extremities including pelvis, external. The highest AIS score in each body region is used. The *3 most severely injured body regions have their score squared and added together to produce the ISS score*. A major trauma is defined as the Injury Severity Score being greater than 15; it is associated with mortality of 10% or more. ISS ranges from 1 to 75.

Note:
- ***Values indicative of critical physiologic derangement include***—Temperature <35°C; pH < 7.2; base excess > –6; lactate > 4 mmol/L; ionized calcium <1.1 mmol/L; platelet count <50,000/; PT-INR >1.5; APTT >1.5 × normal; fibrinogen level <1.0 g/L.
- Major trauma is ISS >15; 15% of injured patients will have major trauma.

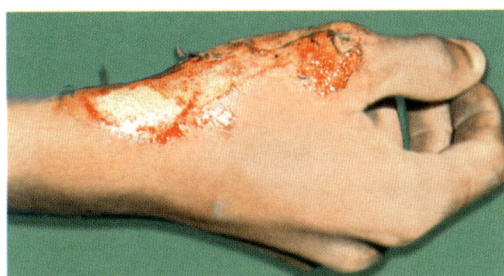

Fig. 10.2: Abrasion hand.

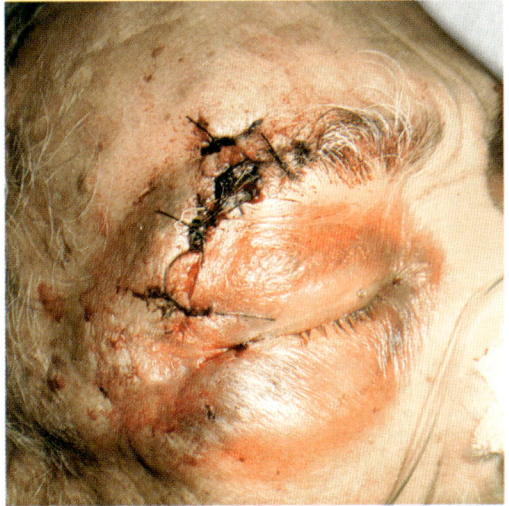

Fig. 10.3: Face injury. Note the edema, abrasions over eyelid.

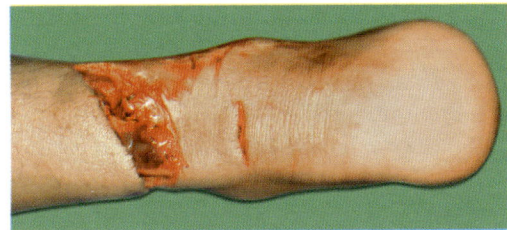

Fig. 10.4: Lacerated deep wound leg. Tendo-Achilis injury in deeper plane should be suspected.

III. SECONDARY SURVEY

- Re-evaluate the patient completely again.
- Assess the external wound properly now—abrasions, lacerations, combined wounds, etc. (Figs. 10.2 to 10.4).

IV. DEFINITIVE CARE (FIGS. 10.5 AND 10.6)

Definitive care means management of individual trauma in detail like abdomen by laparotomy; thoracic by chest tube insertion or thoracotomy; cranial injury by carniotomy, etc.

Life is not always as it appears, you have the power to alter yours and make the difference

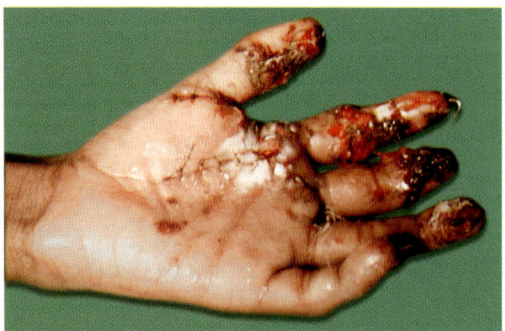

Fig. 10.5: Hand injury involving all fingers.

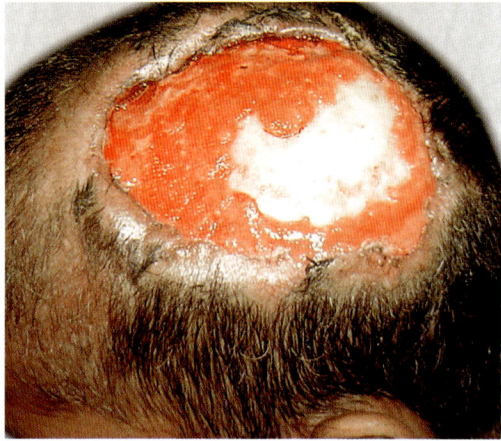

Fig. 10.6: Degloving scalp trauma and exposed bone is granulating well.

DAMAGE CONTROL SURGERY

- Resuscitation and early therapy in operation theater itself.
- Minimum but essential surgery to control bleeding and prevent contamination.
- Secondary definitive surgery at a later period to have final control.
- **Damage control surgery** is done when there is inability to control bleeding, complex abdominal injuries like of liver or pancreas, major vascular injuries with or without bowel injuries, retrohepatic inferior vena cava (IVC) injury which is not accessible; decline in physiological reserve like temperature, pH, prothrombin time, serum lactate, systolic blood pressure less than 90 mm Hg for 60 minutes; if operating time expected is more than one hour, inability to close the wound or whenever reopening the cavity is needed.
- Principles of damage control surgery apply to injuries of the abdomen, thorax and extremities equally.

Concepts of managing the trauma

- Primary management using **ABCDEF**; assessment of patient as stable or unstable with defined parameters.
- One should follow *ATLS* (Advanced Trauma Life Support) or other guidelines.
- *"Timeline principle/concept"* in which clinician should act within the *'critical time window'* in the compensatory stage only patient should be addressed properly to prevent the patient from going to decompensatory stage. We have to look everywhere and focused exclusion of specified anatomical regions; check for hidden injuries.
- Patient should be taken up for *damage control surgery (DCS)* with following criteria— hypothermia <34°C; pH <7.2; serum lactate >4 mmol/L; coagulopathy; blood pressure <70 mm Hg or MAP <65 mm Hg; transfusion of blood of 15 units; ISS >36%.
- *"Early Total Care" (ETC)* approach is done if patient is stable with definitive procedures. Criteria for ETC are—stable hemodynamically; no inotropics; no hypoxemia; no hypercarbia; normothermia; serum lactate <2 mmol/L; urine output >1 mL/hour/kg.

SPINAL INJURY

- Assess the type, extent and severity of the injury.
- Careful first aid and transfer to prevent further damage to the spinal cord.
- Assess the sensory loss or motor loss properly.
- Assess fractures clinically by X-ray and MRI.
- *Central cord syndrome* is common and is due to hyperflexion or hyperextension

of the neck in an injured patient causing ischemia of spinal column due to interfering of spinal artery blood flow.
- *Brown-Séquard syndrome:* It is due to partial transection of the cord causing ipsilateral motor function loss and contralateral sensory function loss.
- High-dose of steroid is very useful to prevent further damage.
- Rest, traction to neck.
- Decompression of spinal canal surgically is useful by removing bone, disk, hematoma.
- Spinal stabilization.

NECK INJURIES

Neck is divided into zones for managing neck injuries.
- *Zone I*—from clavicle to cricoid cartilage.
- *Zone II*—from cricoid cartilage to angle of the mandible.
- *Zone III*—above the angle of the mandible.

Indications for Exploration in Neck Injuries

- Expanding hematoma.
- Uncontrolled external hemorrhage.
- Decreased carotid pulse.
- Stridor, hoarseness, dysphonia, hemoptysis.
- Severe dysphagia, odynophagia.
- Blood in oropharynx.

Treatment

- Explore the neck with adequate incision under general anesthesia.
- Suture the injured structures like carotid, esophagus, trachea, muscles, etc.
- Antibiotics.
- Blood transfusion as required.
- Ryle's tube for 5–7 days.

Other injuries like of head, thorax, maxillofacial region are discussed in respective chapters.

BULLET INJURIES

Bullet injury has got *wound of entry and wound of exit*. Extent of damage is not related to the external wound. It is related to the travel of bullet inside, extent of blast or cavitation effect inside caused by the bullet. It causes burn damage.

It can damage vessels, organs like liver, spleen, kidneys, bowel, lungs, heart, cranial structures, soft tissues, bone and joints.

Management

- The wound is explored properly under general anesthesia.
- All dead tissues and dead muscles are excised.
- Skin is incised generously and adequately.
- Injured nerves are cleaned and silk marker stitches are placed to identify for later secondary suturing (should not be closed primarily).
- All foreign bodies are removed.
- Tendon repair should not be done primarily.
- Wound should not be closed. It should be left open.
- Adequate blood transfusion and antibiotics coverage is given.
- Major artery or vein should be sutured. Vein graft can be used. But *synthetic graft should never be used*.
- Thorough inspection, irrigation and debridement of injured joints is done.
- Immobilization.
- Tetanus toxoid, antitetanus globulin (3000 units IM), antigas gangrene serum is given.
- Second look surgeries are done at a later period once patient has been stabilized.
- Delayed primary closure in 7 days or secondary closure in 14 days is done.
- Depending on extent of defect, skin grafting or flaps is used.
- Laparotomy, thoracotomy or craniotomy is done depending on the site of the injury.

*Doing the best at this moment puts you in the best place for the next moment—***Oprah Winfrey**

BLAST INJURIES

Here extent of damage is much more than bullet injuries.

It creates **complex blast wave,** which contains **blast pressure wave** and **mass movement of air**.

This explosion pressure wave is more than 1000 pounds per square inch. This pressure wave has got incident pressure and reflected pressure. Both will cause severe damage.

Factors causing the damage

- High pressure wave.
- Chemical injury.
- Mechanical injury.
- Thermal injury.
- Inhalation of toxic gases and smoke.

Organs affected:
- Ear drums.
- Lungs.
- Gastrointestinal tract (GIT).
- Brain.
- Skeletal system.

Individual becomes **deaf** after blast and so rescue work may be delayed.

Management

- Critical trauma care.
- Management of shock and triage primary management.
- Urgent surgeries like laparotomy, thoracotomy, craniotomy.
- Massive blood transfusion.
- Antibiotics.
- Ventilator support.
- Management of specific organs like eye, ear.

PENETRATING INJURY

- It can occur in abdomen, thorax or cranial cavity (Fig. 10.7).
- It causes hemorrhage, damage to internal organs like liver, bowel, vessels, lung, pericardium and heart, brain, etc.
- It is life-threatening and immediate surgical intervention is the only treatment (Fig. 10.8). Patient requires adequate number of blood transfusion, antibiotics, and shock management.

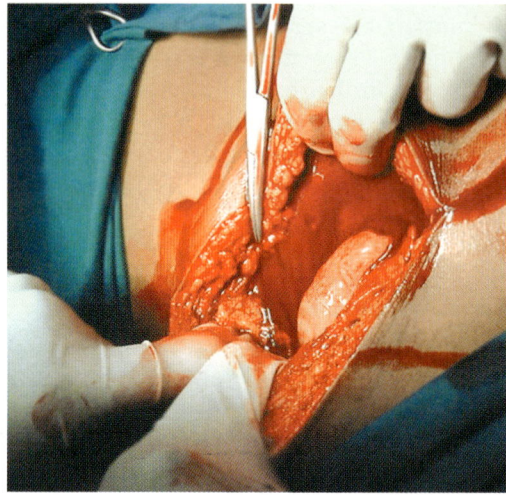

Fig. 10.7: Traumatic hemoperitoneum.

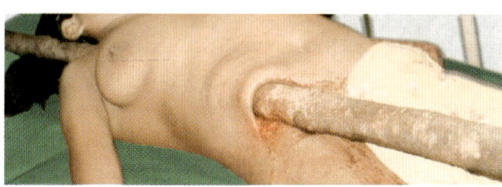

Fig. 10.8: Penetrating injury. Pole missed all the major vessels. Miraculously the patient survived, after a Marathon surgery to tell her tale to her children.

ABDOMINAL TRAUMA

It can be:
- Blunt trauma.
- Stab injury.
- Abdominal wall injury.

Types

- Liver injury.
- Spleen injury.
- Gastric/small bowel/colonic injuries.

Love means sharing the same road, wherever it leads.

- Duodenal injuries.
- Pancreatic injuries.
- Injuries to kidney/bladder/urethra.
- Mesenteric injury.
- Vascular injuries.
- Associated injuries like of diaphragm, lungs.
- Abdominal compartment syndrome.
- Gunshot or blast injuries.

General Clinical Features

- Features of shock—pallor, tachycardia, hypotension, cold periphery, sweating, oliguria.
- Abdominal distension.
- Pain, tenderness, rebound tenderness, guarding and rigidity, dullness in the flank on percussion.
- Respiratory distress, cyanosis depending on the amount of blood loss.
- Bruising over the skin of the abdominal wall.
- Features specific of individual organ injuries.

Investigations

- Ultrasound abdomen.
- **Diagnostic peritoneal lavage** (DPL): It is done in case of blunt injury abdomen. Through a subumbilical lavage catheter, one liter of normal saline is infused into the peritoneal cavity. Patient is made to lie in different positions. Fluid content is aspirated from the abdomen for assessment.

One of the criterias signifies the positive lavage

- About 10 mL or more of gross blood.
- RBC count more than 1,00,000/ cu mm.
- WBC count more than 500/ cu mm.
- Amylase level in the fluid more than 175 IU/dL.
- Presence of bile, bacteria, food particles or foreign body.

Contraindications for DPL

- When laparotomy is definitely indicated.
- Previous laparotomy.
- Pregnancy.
- Obesity.

CT scan is indicated in assessing retroperitoneum, solid organ injuries. It is noninvasive and highly specific.

Treatment

Emergency Laparotomy

Indications:
- Frank hemoperitoneum.
- Significant diagnostic peritoneal lavage.
- Hemodynamically unstable patient.
- Ultrasound or CT scan shows significant intra-abdominal injuries.

DUODENAL INJURY

Its severity depends on the type and extent of the injury.

It can be hematoma or lacerations.

Lacerations can be duodenal disruption which may be <50% or >50% or 75% or more.

Laceration may extend into the ampulla, distal CBD, pancreas or with duodenal devascularization.

Management

- CT scan is more relevant investigation.
- Associated other injuries should be managed accordingly.
- Hematoma without extension is managed conservatively with nasogastric aspiration, antibiotics and IV fluids.
- Lacerations are sutured surgically with stenting or often with bypass like gastrojejunostomy.
- Endoscopic retrograde cholangiopancreatography (ERCP) stenting or com-

*Originality is nothing but judicious imitation—**Voltaire***

mon bile duct (CBD) bypass is also often required.

Complications of duodenal injury

- Infection.
- Duodenal leak.
- Peritonitis.
- Hemorrhage.

PANCREATIC INJURY

It can be in the head or body and tail of the pancreas.

It may be associated with injury to duodenum or portal or superior mesenteric veins.

It can be contusion or severe lacerations.

Management

- High resolution CT scan is diagnostic.
- Distal pancreatectomy is done for distal injuries.
- Conservative treatment is useful with antibiotics, IV fluids.
- Whipple's operation or total pancreatectomy is done as a last resort.
- Drainage of the pancreatic bed is simple and often useful method.

Complications of pancreatic injury

- Pancreatitis.
- Septicemia.
- Pancreatic fistula.
- Pancreatic abscess formation.

Pancreatic injury has got high mortality (>45%).

SMALL BOWEL INJURY

- It can be blunt injury or stab injury.
- Blunt injury causes disruption of either duodenojejunal region or ileocecal region.
- Presentation is like hemoperitoneum or with features of peritonitis.
- *Monks localizing zones* in the abdomen signify the location of the small bowel injury.
- Site and the 'pattern' bruising over the abdominal wall signifies the small bowel injury and its site. It is called as *London's sign*.

Management

- Plain X-ray abdomen shows gas under abdomen with ground-glass appearance.
- Ultrasound abdomen is useful.
- Laparotomy and closure of the perforation is done if it is small.
- If there is extensive bowel injury or multiple injuries, then resection and anastomosis is done.
- Any associated injuries should be dealt with accordingly.

COLONIC INJURY

- Left sided injury, if it is small, it is treated with proximal colostomy with closure of the wound and if wide area is involved resection and anastomosis is done. Closure of colostomy is done at later stages after 3–6 months.
- Small wound over right-sided colon can be sutured primarily.
- Ileostomy alone or ileostomy with ileotransverse anastomosis or right hemicolectomy with ileostomy is indicated in following situations:
    - Extensive peritoneal contamination.
    - Colonic vascular injuries.
    - Hemodynamically unstable patients.
    - Long-term hypotension after trauma.

LIVER INJURY

It can be subcapsular hematoma, lacerations, deeper injuries, and lacerations with disruption of hepatic lobes or segments or liver injury with vascular injuries like of inferior vena cava or hepatic veins.

Presentation is of hemorrhagic shock, distension of the abdomen, tenderness, rebound tenderness, guarding, rigidity.

In life, let us from the past, to profit by the present, and to live better for the future

Management

- Small tear is sutured.
- For larger tears:
  - Deep sutures.
  - Packing.
  - Debridement.
  - Hemocoagulants.
- Liver resection is not done (not advisable) usually for injuries.
- **Pringle maneuver** is compressing the porta near foramen of Winslow.
- Blood transfusions.
- Treatment of associated injuries like of diaphragm, lung, duodenum, colon.
- Antibiotics.

Complications of liver injury
- Hemorrhage.
- Septicemia.
- Bile leak.
- Liver failure.
- Hemobilia.
- Subphrenic abscess.
- Common bile duct (CBD) stricture.

SPLENIC INJURY

It can be subcapsular hematoma, laceration or hilar injury.

It can be associated with other organ injuries like left kidney, left lobe of the liver, splenic flexure of the colon or pancreas.

It can cause torrential hemorrhage and shock.

Management

- Ultrasound abdomen and diagnostic peritoneal lavage are the investigations.
- Blood transfusions.
- Splenorrhaphy in selected patients so as to save the spleen.
- Splenectomy.
- Management of associated injuries.

Complications of splenectomy
- Left lung atelectasis.
- Overwhelming postsplenectomy infection (OPSI).
- Pancreatitis and pancreatic fistula.
- Gastric bleeding.
- Subphrenic abscess.

RENAL INJURY

- It is often managed conservatively.
- Intravenous urography (IVU) is the investigation of choice in renal injury.
- Surgery is indicated when there is hilar injury, progressive bleeding, failure of conservative treatment or perinephric abscess formation.

URINARY BLADDER INJURY

Intraperitoneal bladder injury occurs in distended bladder. It is treated always by surgical exploration through transabdominal approach. Bladder tear is sutured with keeping a suprapubic cystostomy using Malecot's catheter.

Extraperitoneal injury can be treated conservatively by placing a Foley's catheter for 2–3 weeks.

ABDOMINAL COMPARTMENT SYNDROME

- There is sudden increase in intra-abdominal pressure which causes decreased venous return to heart.
- It causes increased respiratory pressure, hypoxia, hypotension and decreased venous return.
- Measurement of bladder pressure is diagnostic.
- Rapid decompression by opening the abdominal wound is the treatment of choice.

*Love is like the wind, you can't see it, but you can feel it—**Nicholas Sparks***

CHAPTER 11

Arterial Diseases

Chapter Outline

- Surgical Anatomy of Thoracic Outlet
- Arteries of Upper Limb
- Upper Limb Ischemia
- Raynaud's Phenomenon
- Acrocyanosis
- Polyarteritis Nodosa
- Scleroderma/Systemic Sclerosis
- Thakayasu's Pulseless Arteritis
- Temporal Arteritis
- Erythromelalgia/Erythralgia
- Livedo Reticularis
- Subclavian Steal Syndrome
- Arteries of Lower Limb
- Arterial Diseases
- Atherosclerosis
- Thromboangiitis Obliterans
- Acute Arterial Occlusion
- Compartment Syndrome
- Reperfusion Injury
- Embolism
- Caisson's Disease or Decompression Disease
- Aneurysms
- Carotid Artery Aneurysm
- Gangrene
- Diabetic Foot and Diabetic Gangrene
- Ainhum
- Vascular Anomalies
- Cirsoid Aneurysm
- Arteriovenous Fistula

SURGICAL ANATOMY OF THORACIC OUTLET

- Thoracic outlet is bounded by manubrium sternum in front, spine posteriorly, and the first rib laterally. At the superior aperture of thorax subclavian vessels, brachial plexus traverse the cervicoaxillary canal to reach the upper limb.
- *Cervicoaxillary canal* is divided into proximal *costoclavicular space and distal axilla* (divided by first rib).
- Costoclavicular space is bounded superiorly by clavicle, inferiorly by first rib, anteromedially by the costoclavicular ligament, and posterolaterally by scalenus medius muscle along with long thoracic nerve.
- Scalenus anticus muscle divides the costoclavicular space into two compartments, the anterior one containing subclavian vein and the posterior one containing subclavian artery and brachial plexus.
- This posterior compartment is called as *scalene triangle* bounded by scalenus anticus anteriorly, scalenus medius posteriorly, and the first rib inferiorly.
- Cervical rib narrows this triangle and causes compressive features of C_8, T_1 nerve roots and subclavian artery. Anything that narrows costoclavicular space causes *Thoracic outlet syndrome*.

Life is made of ever so many partings welded together—**Charles Dickens**

ARTERIES OF UPPER LIMB

- *Right subclavian artery* begins from brachiocephalic trunk (innominate artery) whereas left subclavian artery directly from the arch of aorta. From underneath the sternoclavicular joint, subclavian artery arches over the pleura and apex of lung about 2.5 cm above the clavicle and then reaches the lateral border of first rib to continue as axillary artery. Subclavian artery is divided into three parts by scalenus anterior muscle.
- *Axillary artery* is divided into three parts by pectoralis minor muscle. At the lower border of teres major muscle, it enters the arm and continues as *brachial artery*. About 2.5 cm below the crease of the elbow joint, it bifurcates into *radial and ulnar arteries*, which run in the forearm.
- *Ulnar artery* forms the superficial palmar arch, which is completed by superficial palmar branch of radial artery.
- *Radial artery* after passing through the anatomical snuffbox enters the dorsum of hand and first intermetacarpal space to form deep palmar arch. It is completed by deep palmar branch of ulnar artery and is 1 cm proximal to superficial palmar arch.

UPPER LIMB ISCHEMIA (FIGS. 11.1A AND B)

- It is a rare uncommon entity compared to lower limb ischemia but important because of its difficulty in managing. *Higher-level amputations are rare in upper limb ischemia.*
- Its incidence is rare (5%) due to abundant collateral supply, infrequency of atherosclerosis, decreased metabolic demand and smaller muscle mass.
- It mostly affects distal small arteries (90%).
- Symptoms are usually delayed.

TYPES OF UPPER LIMB ISCHEMIA

1. Acute.   2. Chronic.

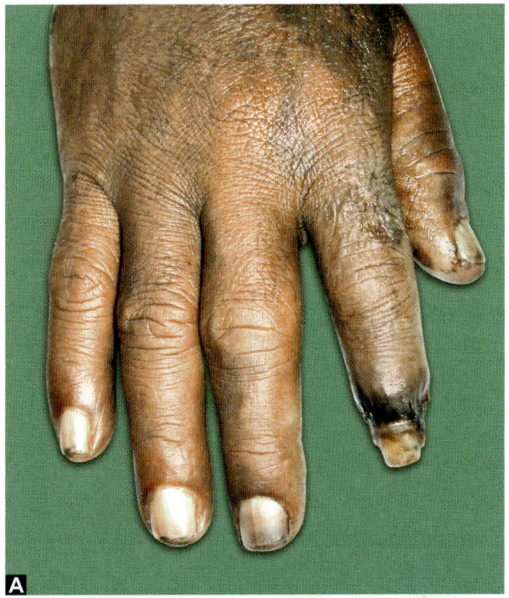
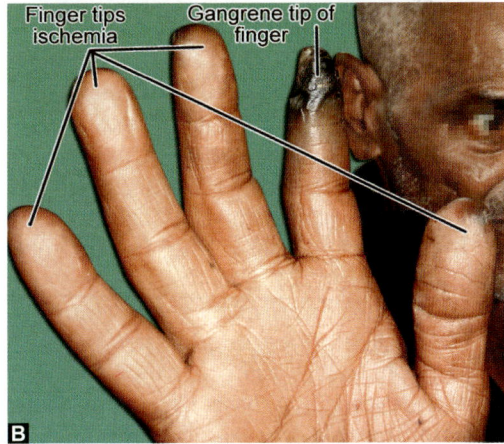

Figs. 11.1A and B: Gangrene of finger in upper limb ischemia. Note the other fingers which are showing ischemic features.

Acute Type

Causes

- **Embolism—common.** 30% of the peripheral emboli lodge in upper extremity. Commonest site is at the bifurcation of brachial artery (40%); next common is at axillary artery (12%). Embolism is due to:

- Cardiac origin (70%): Valvular lesions (atrial fibrillation, endocarditis), ischemic heart disease (IHD), paradoxical.
- Others: Aneurysms, *thoracic outlet syndrome*, plaque.
❖ **Trauma—commonest.** Brachial artery injury is seen in 30% of civilian trauma with arterial injuries, blunt injuries, fractures and dislocations, penetrating injuries.
❖ Iatrogenic.
❖ Post AV fistula 'Steal syndrome'.
❖ Aortic dissection.

Symptoms of Acute Ischemia

Pain, pallor, poikilothermia, paresthesia, paralysis.

Chronic Type

Causes

❖ Arteritis: Aortoarteritis, Takayasu arteritis, giant cell arteritis, connective tissue disease/vasculitis—scleroderma, systemic lupus erythematosus (SLE), rheumatoid arthritis (RA), polyarteritis nodosa (PAN), etc.
❖ Atherosclerosis: Commonest cause in USA.
❖ Thromboangiitis obliterans (TAO) of upper limb.
❖ Others: Fibromuscular dysplasia; Raynaud's phenomenon; post-irradiation—lung, breast; occupational injuries; vibration injury, hypothenar hammer syndrome; hypercoagulable states; APLA, polycythemia, cold agglutinins.

Symptoms of Chronic Ischemia

❖ Upper limb 'Claudication'.
❖ Weakness and wasting.
❖ Digital ischemia—ulcer, gangrene in finger tips.
❖ Raynaud's phenomenon.

Signs of Chronic Ischemia (Fig. 11.2)

❖ Wasting of arm, forearm and hand muscles.
❖ Ischemic changes in skin; tapering of finger tips.

❖ Drop in systolic pressure >20 mm Hg.
❖ Proximal thrill or bruit.
❖ Mass in the neck, thrill and bruit in the neck in supraclavicular region.
❖ Adson test, hyperabduction (Halsted) test, Roos test, Allen's tests are important.

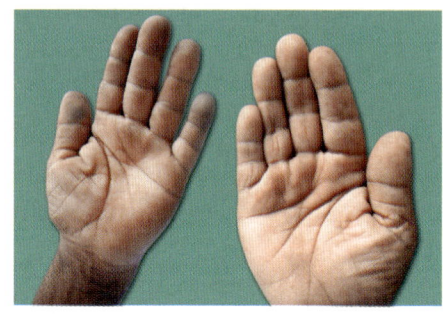

Fig. 11.2: Upper limb ischemia. Note the ischemic features in left hand—color changes, wasting.

INVESTIGATIONS IN UPPER LIMB ISCHEMIA

❖ Laboratory tests for vasculitis, hypercoagulable states, and atherosclerotic risk factors.
❖ X-rays—for cervical rib; clavicular and first rib fractures; fractures and dislocations in extremity; pulmonary lesions of connective tissue disorders.
❖ Arterial Doppler study.
❖ Angiogram (subclavian angiogram)—CT/MR (conventional) (Fig. 11.3).
❖ CT scan neck and thorax.
❖ Blood sugar, lipid profile, cardiac evaluation.

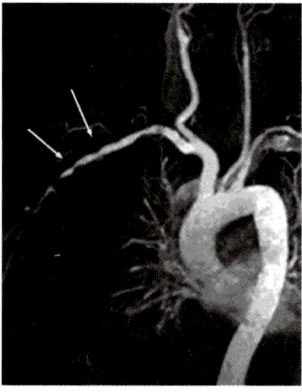

Fig. 11.3: Upper limb angiogram showing blocks in subclavian artery.

*Be happy for this moment. This moment is your life—**Omar Khayyam***

MANAGEMENT OF UPPER LIMB ISCHEMIA

Treatment of the cause.

Treatment of Embolus

* Time since the first symptom is very important.
* Clinical assessment of extent of ischemia, immediate anticoagulation with heparin, Doppler study and angiogram of the arterial system, evaluation for the source of embolus—are the protocols.
* Embolectomy (Fig. 11.4)
    - *Brachial embolectomy:* Local/regional/general anesthesia is used. Longitudinal incision in the arm is used for proximal embolus; Lazy S-shaped incision across the elbow is done for embolus extending into the bifurcation and to expose the branches.

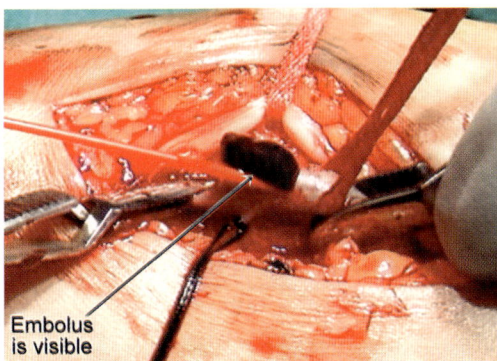

Fig. 11.4: Brachial embolectomy (upper limb)—open method.

Treatment in Trauma

* General evaluation and resuscitation.
* Control of bleeding in open wound—pressure bandage/manual compression (DO NOT USE TOURNIQUET).
* Time since the event and clinical assessment of limb perfusion.
* Stabilization of fractures and dislocations.
* Doppler study of arterial system, angiogram if required.
* Arterial repair; bypass graft either venous or synthetic.

Treatment of Chronic Ischemia

* *Medical management*
    - Risk modification—diabetes, hypertension, dyslipidemia, smoking, homocystinemia, exercise training.
    - Antiplatelets—Aspirin/Ticlopidine/Clopidogrel.
    - Anticoagulants—Heparin/warfarin.
    - Xanthines/Pentoxiphylline/Cilostazol.
    Cilastozol—suppresses cyclic adenosine monophosphate (cAMP) phosphodiesterase III rise in cAMP levels with antiplatelet, antithrombotic effects; induces vasodilatation; increases plasma high-density lipoprotein (HDL) cholesterol; decreases plasma triglycerides.
* *Catheter-based interventions*
    - Atherectomy
    - Angioplasty ± stenting by conventional or subintimal approach.
    - Stent grafts.
    - Cryoplasty.
* *Surgery*
    - Endarterectomy.
    - Bypass surgery.
    - Sympathectomy, extraperiosteal resection of the cervical rib.

Bypass Surgeries in Upper Limb Ischemia

* Conventional bypass
    - Aorto—subclavian/axillary bypass.
    - Subclavian—axillary/brachial bypass.
    - Brachiodistal bypass.
* Extra-anatomical bypass
    - ***Carotid—subclavian/axillary bypass.***
    - Subclavian—subclavian bypass.
    - Axillary—axillary bypass.
* Subclavian carotid transposition.

Obstacles are those frightful things you see, when you take your eyes off your goals

Treatment of Raynaud's Phenomenon
* Avoiding triggering agents
* Drugs—vasodilators—calcium channel blockers, angiotensin II receptor blockers, alpha-1 adrenergic blockers, sildenafil, prostaglandin E1.
* Surgery—sympathectomy.

THORACIC OUTLET SYNDROME
* Thoracic outlet syndrome (TOS) is syndrome complex due to compression of neurovascular bundle in the thoracic outlet.
* *Thoracic outlet has got two main spaces:*
  - *Scalene triangle* is bound by scalenus anterior, scalenus medius and first rib. It contains subclavian artery and brachial plexus.
  - *Costoclavicular space* is bound by clavicle, first rib, costoclavicular ligament and scalenus medius. It contains subclavian artery and vein and brachial plexus.

Causes
* Cervical rib.
* Long C_7 transverse process.
* Anomalous insertion of scalene muscles.
* Scalene muscle hypertrophy.
* Scalene minimus.
* Abnormal bands and ligaments.
* Fracture clavicle or first rib.
* Exostosis.
* Tumors in the region.
* Brachial plexus trauma and diseases.

Differential diagnosis of TOS

* Carpal tunnel syndrome.
* Cervical spondylosis.
* Spinal canal tumors.
* Shoulder myositis.
* Angina.
* Raynaud's disease.
* Spinal stenosis.
* Ulnar nerve compression.
* Epicondylitis.

Clinical Features
Neurological
* Paresthesia.
* Pain in shoulder, arm, forearm and fingers.
* Occipital headache as referred pain from tight scalene muscles.
* Limb weakness in forearm, hand.

Vascular
Claudication, ischemic ulcers, gangrene.

Signs
* Scalene muscle tenderness.
* Pulsatile swelling in supraclavicular region with thrill and bruit (25%).
* Bony mass above clavicle.
* Positive Adson's test.
* Positive Roos test.
* Positive elevated arm stress test.
* Costoclavicular compression maneuver—radial pulse becomes feeble or absent.
* Hyperabduction maneuver—radial pulse becomes feeble or absent.
* Poor capillary refilling.
* Absence or feeble pulse.

Investigations
* X-ray neck and cervical spine.
* Doppler.
* Subclavian angiogram, CT angiogram, CT neck.
* Nerve conduction studies, electromyography.

Treatment
* Conservative.

Conservative treatment for TOS

* Exercises—neck stretching, postural and breathing exercises.
* Drugs—analgesics, muscle relaxants, antidepressants.
* Avoid weight lifting.
* Physiotherapy.
---

* Surgical.

Surgical treatment of TOS

* Transaxillary (Roos)—mainly for first rib excision and also cervical rib.
* Supraclavicular approach for cervical rib and soft tissue excision, scalenotomy, neurolysis, arterial reconstruction.
* Cervical sympathectomy may be needed.

It takes a minute to have a crush on someone, an hour to like someone, and a day to love someone... but it takes a lifetime to forget someone—**Kahlil Gibran**

CERVICAL RIB

Definition

- It is an extension of transverse process of C_7 vertebra more than 2.5 cm (normal).
- Syndrome caused by it, is called as *cervical rib syndrome, thoracic inlet syndrome, thoracic outlet syndrome, scalene syndrome.*
- It is 0.46% common, common in females, more frequently seen on right side.
- It can be *unilateral or bilateral;* can be *asymptomatic or symptomatic.*

Types

1. *Complete bony*: Cervical rib is radiopaque, anteriorly ends over the first rib or manubrium.
2. *Fibrous*: Cannot be demonstrated radiologically.
3. *Combined*: Partly bony partly fibrous.
4. *Partial bony*: With free end expanding as bony mass.

Pathology (Figs. 11.5A and B)

Cervical rib narrows the scalene triangle (bounded by scalenus anterior, scalenus medius and first thoracic rib below)
↓
Compression of subclavian artery; C_8 and T_1 nerve roots due to cervical rib
↓
Angulation of subclavian artery occurs
↓
Causes constriction of artery at the site where artery crosses the cervical rib
↓
'Eddie's current' created in the blood flow causes sudden release of pressure distal to the narrowing
↓
Poststenotic dilation → Venturi phenomenon
↓
Stasis of blood occur
↓
Thrombosis → Embolus
↓
Features of ischemia in the hand and forearm. Later digital gangrene occur

Compression of C_8 and T_1 will cause tingling and numbness along its distribution, i.e. in the little finger, medial side of hand and forearm.

Clinical Features

- Majority of patients are asymptomatic.
  Vascular manifestations:
  Pain is due to ischemia in the muscle. It is aggravated by work, exercise and is relieved by rest.
- *Roos test* is raising the arm above the shoulder. The side where cervical rib is present, patient cannot continue and so drops the hand down.
- EAST—Elevated Arm Stress Test (*Modified Roos test*): Arm is elevated above the shoulder, with elbow stretched fully. Rapid movements of fingers cause fatigue on the side where cervical rib is present.
- *Adson's test*: The hand is raised above after feeling the radial pulse. The patient is asked to take a deep inspiration and turn the head to the same side. Any change in pulse, i.e. either becoming feeble or absent is noted.
- *Modified Adson's test* is same as Adson's, but neck is turned towards the opposite side.
- *Wasting* of thenar, hypothenar and forearm muscles, often *digital gangrene.*
- Limb is *colder and paler* than the opposite side.
- *Neurological features*: Is due to compression of T_1 and C_8 causing tingling and numbness in the little finger, medial side of hand and forearm.

Features in the neck

- Hard, fixed, bony mass in the supraclavicular region.
- *Palpable thrill* above the clavicle in the subclavian artery.
- *Bruit* on auscultation.

Differential Diagnosis

1. Cervical spondylosis—to differentiate, X-ray neck—lateral view should be taken (Fig. 11.5C).

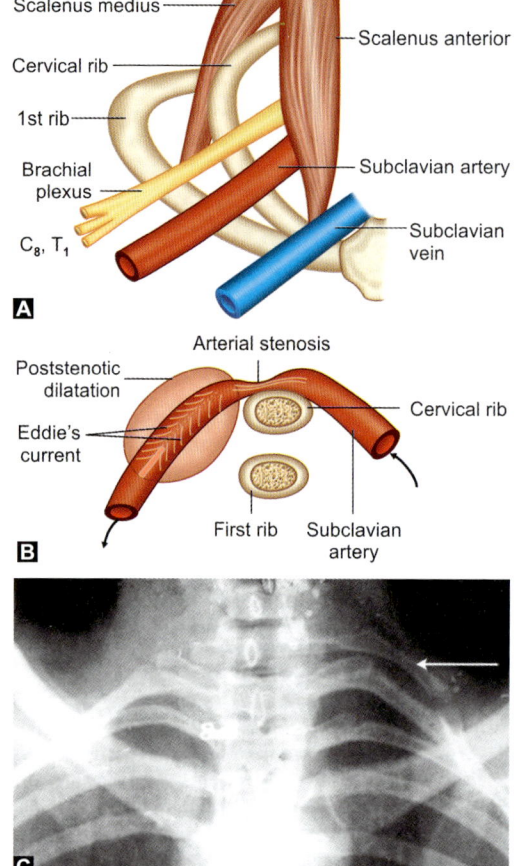

Figs. 11.5A to C: Anatomy of cervical rib and its relation to subclavian artery and vein and brachial plexus. Note the Eddie's current, poststenotic dilatation due to arterial compression by cervical rib. X-ray picture shows left sided complete cervical rib.

2. Carpal tunnel syndrome.
3. Tumors or swellings compressing over the vessel or nerves in the neck.
4. Raynaud's phenomenon.

Investigations

- Chest X-ray—PA view and lateral view including neck—only (radiopaque) bony rib can be identified.
- Nerve conduction studies to confirm neurological compression and also to rule out carpal tunnel syndrome or cervical spondylosis.
- Arterial Doppler of subclavian artery and of the upper limb.
- Subclavian angiogram.

Treatment

- In symptomatic cervical rib without arterial compression (subclavian artery), along with scalenotomy (cutting scalenus anterior muscle), extraperiosteal resection of cervical rib and often resection of first rib is done to increase the thoracoaxillary channel and therefore to reduce arterial compression.
- In symptomatic cervical rib with significant subclavian artery compression along with scalenotomy, extraperiosteal resection of cervical rib, resection of first rib, subclavian artery reconstruction with or without a graft has to be done.
- Along with scalenotomy, extraperiosteal resection of cervical rib, resection of first rib, reconstruction of subclavian artery, cervical sympathectomy has to be done to improve the circulation to the ischemic upper limb.

Approaches

- *Supraclavicular approach*—mainly when there is need for vascular reconstruction.
- *Transaxillary approach*—through axillary crease, rib is approached and removed.
- *Thoracotomy approach*.

RAYNAUD'S PHENOMENON

It is *an episodic, localized, vasospasm* of small vessels of hands and feet, i.e. arteriolar spasm. It is common in upper limb.

> **Raynaud's syndrome:** It is sequence of clinical features due to arteriolar spasm.
> 1. *Local syncope*: It is due to vasospasm, causing white and cold palm and digits along with tingling and numbness.
>
> *Contd...*

*I AM IGNORANT of absolute truth. But I am humble before my ignorance and therein lies my honor and my reward—***Khalil Gibran**

Contd...

2. *Local asphyxia*: It is due to accumulation of deoxygenated blood as the result of vasospasm causing bluish discoloration of palm and digits with burning sensation (due to accumulated metabolites).
3. *Local recovery*: It is due to relief of spasm in the arteriole, leading to return of blood to the circulation causing flushing and pain in digits and palm (pain is due to increased tissue tension).
4. *Local gangrene*: If spasm persists more than ischemic time (more than one hour in upper limb), then digits go for ulceration and gangrene. Does not occur regularly but is an occasional phenomenon in the cycle.

Causes for Raynaud's Phenomenon

Raynaud's disease:
- It is seen in females, usually bilateral.
- It occurs in upper limb with normal peripheral pulses.
- It is due to upper limb (hand) arteriolar spasm due to abnormal sensitivity to cold. Patient develops blanching, cyanosis and later flushing as Raynaud's syndrome. Occasionally, if spasm persists it result in gangrene. Symptoms can be precipitated and observed by placing hands in cold water.
- Working with *vibrating tools*: Like pneumatic road drills, chain saws, wood cutting, fishermen traveling in machine boats.

Collagen vascular diseases:
Like scleroderma, rheumatoid diseases causing vasculitis (all autoimmune diseases), SLE.

Other causes:
Cervical rib, Buerger's disease, scalene syndrome. It is often associated with CREST syndrome. (**C**alcinosis cutis, **R**aynaud's phenomenon, **E**sophageal defects, **S**clerodactyly, **T**elangiectasia).

Types of Raynaud's phenomenon	
1. *Vasospastic.*	2. *Obliterative.*

Pathology of Raynaud's Phenomenon

Exaggerated vasomotor response to stress; more common in females; no structural changes in vessels except in late stages; recurrent attacks can lead into atrophy of skin, subcutaneous tissue and muscles, with often ischemic ulcers and gangrene.

Investigations

- Type is identified by angiogram of palm, Doppler, duplex scan.
- Other investigations required are X-ray of the part, specific tests for autoimmune diseases.

Treatment

- Treat the cause.
- Avoid the precipitating factors.
- Vasodilators, Pentoxiphylline.
- Small dose of Aspirin (100 mg daily).
- Cervical sympathectomy.

CERVICAL SYMPATHECTOMY

Indications
• Cervical rib with vascular manifestations—useful.
• Raynaud's phenomenon—useful.
• Hyperhidrosis—very useful.
• Upper limb vasospasm due to other causes—useful.
• Acrocyanosis—useful.
• Causalgia—very useful.
• Sudeck's osteodystrophy.

Approaches

a. ***Supraclavicular approach:*** Through a incision in supraclavicular region, sternomastoid, omohyoid, scalenus anterior muscles are divided. Phrenic nerve is displaced medially; subclavian artery is pushed downwards; suprapleural membrane is depressed, stellate ganglion is identified in the neck of the first rib. All

One ought, every day at least, to hear a little song, read a good poem, see a fine picture, and if possible to speak a few reasonable words.

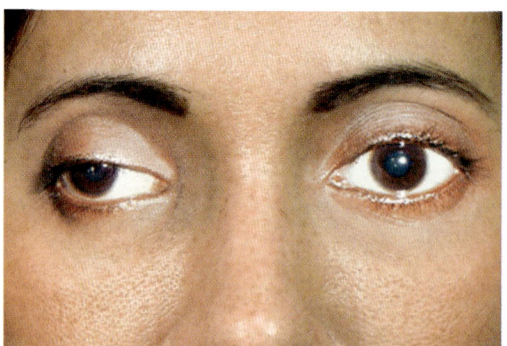

Fig. 11.6: Ptosis right eye in Horner's syndrome.

rami communicanting from second and third ganglia are divided. Gray ramus from second ganglion to first thoracic nerve called as *Kuntz nerve* is also divided.
Complications (Fig. 11.6):
- Bleeding.
- Injury to subclavian artery and nerves.
- Pneumothorax and hemopneumothorax.
- Horner's syndrome with ptosis, miosis, anhydrosis, enophthalmos (Fig. 11.6).

b. ***Transthoracic approach:*** This gives better visibility and easier removal of rami, compared to supraclavicular approach.

c. ***Thoracoscopic sympathectomy:*** It is the choice, and popular approach at present. Advantages are better visibility with magnification, less trauma of access (wound), faster recovery, and precise (thoracoscopic).

ACROCYANOSIS

- It is persistent, painless cyanosis seen in fingers and often in legs with paresthesia and chilblains affecting young females.
- It is chronic persistent arteriolar constriction with slow rate of blood flow.
- Trophic changes, ulcerations are not seen.
- Cyanosis, *which is persisting* may aggravate by exposure to cold.
- It may be associated with endocrine dysfunction.

- **Treatment:** Vasodilators; cervical sympathectomy (effective).

Raynaud's phenomenon	*Acrocyanosis*
• Episodic.	• Persistent.
• Painful.	• Painless.
• Acute arteriolar spasm.	• Chronic constriction.
• Ischemic changes are common.	• Ischemic changes are not seen.

POLYARTERITIS NODOSA

- Polyarteritis nodosa (PAN) is a necrotizing inflammatory reaction with commonly microscopic polyarteritis and nodule formation, often of small and medium sized arteries (not capillaries), causing ischemia of lower and upper limb.
- Visceral arterial (mesenteric) involvement (70%) can cause abdominal pain, GI bleed; mucosal ulceration and perforation of small bowel can occur. Massive hepatic infarction, cholecystitis can develop.
- Renal artery involvement can cause loin pain, hematuria, and renal hypertension.
- Coronary artery also can get involved causing myocardial infarction.
- Disease is common at bifurcation of medium/small sized arteries leading to localized aneurysms.
- It is common in males (3:1); fever, weakness, myalgia, arthralgia are early features.
- Presents with localized small aneurysms, like multiple 5–10 mm nodules, palpable along the course of the artery.
- In late stage presents with myocardial infarction, renal failure, sepsis, GI bleed.
- HBsAg is positive in 40% patients of polyarteritis nodosa.
- Angiogram of renal, mesenteric, peripheral arteries will show aneurysms at branching points.
- Biopsy of tender nodule, tender muscle is useful for diagnosis.

We choose our joys and sorrows long before we experience them—**Kahlil Gibran**

- *Treatment* is prednisolone 60 mg daily with cytotoxic drugs.
- *Prognosis* is poor with rapid death in early years.

SCLERODERMA/SYSTEMIC SCLEROSIS

- It is *a progressive* disease causing fibrosis of skin, GI tract, lungs, heart and kidney.
- It is common in females (4:1) at 4th/5th decades.
- It is considered as vasculitis even though earlier considered as collagen disease.
- Pathology consists of cytotoxic endothelial injury causing interstitial edema, severe fibroblast proliferation causing fibrosis of affected vessels, and dilatation and proliferation of remaining capillaries as telangiectasis.
- Thin epidermis, thick dermis with more collagen along with absence of appendages and rete pegs are typical.
- Lower 2/3rd esophagus is sclerosed (50%) with increased collagen in submucosa with atrophied mucosa and muscularis. Dysphagia is common.
- Diffuse interstitial fibrosis, thickening of alveolar membrane and pulmonary hypertension occurs.
- Synovial thickening causes arthritis; fibrosis of skeletal muscles; interstitial myocardial fibrosis causes bundle branch block, pericardial effusion.
- Glomerulosclerosis in kidney is common (50%). Renal failure is common.
- Fibrosis of thyroid, periodontal membrane can occur. Malabsorption syndrome is common due to small bowel involvement.
- Involvement of digital arteries, present as Raynaud's phenomenon.
- Calcinosis, Raynaud's, esophageal hypomotility, sclerodactyly, and telangiectasia are the presentation of CREST syndrome.
- *Investigations:* Anemia, raised ESR, elevated IgG, presence of antinuclear antibodies and anticentromere antibodies (in CREST)—are different laboratory findings. Skin and peripheral arterial biopsy is confirmative.
- *Treatment*—is difficult. Drugs like D pencillamine, colchicines, p aminobenzoic acid, vitamin E, dimethyl sulfoxide, ranitidine are tried at various levels. Vasodilators, warming and massaging skin, avoiding detergent soaps, oil and hydrophilic ointment application are used.
- Steroids, oxygen therapy for irreversible pulmonary fibrosis; hemodialysis for renal failure; digitalis and other drugs for cardiac failure are needed later.
- Death is due to cardiac/pulmonary/renal failure.

THAKAYASU'S PULSELESS ARTERITIS

- *It is progressive, initially symptomless panarteritis involving aortic arch and branches of aorta of unknown cause* but probably immunological.
- It is common in young females (85%); common in Japan; subclavian artery is commonly involved (85%).
- It involves all the layers of the arteries in upper limb and neck. It is often bilateral.
- It remains unnoticed for long time.

Features and Management

- Fever, myalgia, arthralgia, hypertension, upper limb claudication, with absence of pulses in neck and upper limb.
- Fainting on turning the neck or change in position; atrophy of face.
- Thrill/bruit along major arteries of upper limb and neck.
- Optic nerve atrophy without papilledema.
- Upper limb weakness and paresthesia.
- Cerebral softening, convulsions, hemiplegia.
- *Complications are*—life-threatening myocardial infarction, embolism and ischemia.
- *Investigations are*—digital subtraction angiography; MR angiography; Doppler study.

Only those who dare to fail greatly, can ever achieve greatly

❖ **Treatment** is—prednisolone 50 mg/day orally and cyclophosphamide; vascular reconstruction whenever needed.

TEMPORAL ARTERITIS

❖ There is localized inflammatory giant cell infiltration of arterial wall (*giant cell arteritis*) involving superficial temporal, facial, retinal, upper limb, coronary and vertebral arteries.
❖ It is common after 50 years. Common in females (2:1).
❖ Claudication of facial muscles, ischemic severe headache, tender, thrombosed superficial temporal artery and its branches are the features.
❖ Retinal ischemia leading into irreversible blindness is dangerous feature. Involvement of coronary artery may cause myocardial infarction.
❖ *Temporal artery biopsy is diagnostic*—shows giant cell granuloma with CD4+ T lymphocytes.
❖ High dose long-term *prednisolone 80 mg/day* is needed. In involvement of retinal artery IV hydrocortisone/*methylprednisolone* may be needed initially.

ERYTHROMELALGIA/ERYTHRALGIA

❖ It is severe burning pain and redness in the feet. Sensation of heat is so severe that patient keeps the feet in cold water to reduce it.
❖ It presents as episodic attack.
❖ There will be flushing in feet; prominent veins; warmness in the skin; severe hyperesthesia is typical; even touching can be painful.
❖ It can be primary or secondary. *Secondary* is which is not uncommon is observed in arterial obliterative conditions, erythrocyanosis frigida, polycythemia, gout and frostbite. *Primary* is due to unknown etiology; it is very rare.

❖ Vasodilators and sympathectomy may be beneficial.

LIVEDO RETICULARIS

It is a condition often associated with systemic lupus erythematosus presenting as features of *arteriolar spasm and dilatation of venules* which is worsened by cold.

SUBCLAVIAN STEAL SYNDROME

❖ Following obstruction of the first part of subclavian artery, vertebral artery provides collateral circulation to the arm by reversing its blood flow. This causes *cerebral ischemia with syncopal attacks, visual disturbances, diminished blood pressure in the affected limb* (Fig. 11.7).
❖ Symptoms will be aggravated by arm exercise.

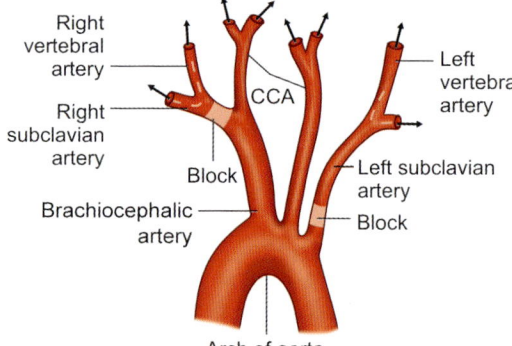

Fig. 11.7: Subclavian steal syndrome.

❖ **Investigations:** Duplex scan and angiogram. Digital subtraction angiography (DSA) is useful.
❖ **Treatment**
 – Transluminal balloon angioplasty.
 – Endarterectomy or bypass graft.

ARTERIES OF LOWER LIMB

Abdominal aorta bifurcates at the level of fourth lumbar vertebra (corresponds to the level of the umbilicus in anterior abdominal wall), into two common iliac arteries.

*The smallest act of kindness is worth more than the greatest intention—**Kahlil Gibran***

- *Common iliac artery* is about 5 cm in length passes downward and laterally, and at the level of lumbosacral intervertebral disc, anterior to sacroiliac joint, it divides into external and internal iliac arteries. Internal iliac artery supplies pelvic organs.
- *External iliac artery* continues as *common femoral artery* at the level of inguinal ligament.
- About 5 cm below the inguinal ligament common femoral divides into *superficial femoral and deep femoral* (Profunda femoris) arteries.
- *Deep femoral* provides collateral circulation around the knee joint and also communicates above with gluteal vessels to maintain collateral circulation around the gluteal region.
- *Superficial femoral artery* at the hiatus in the adductor magnus, continues as popliteal artery up to the inferior angle of the popliteal fossa where it divides into anterior and posterior tibial arteries.
    - *Anterior tibial artery* supplies anterior compartment of leg and ankle, continues as dorsalis pedis artery, which forms dorsal arterial arch of the foot.
    - *Posterior tibial artery* supplies posterior compartment of leg and ends as medial and lateral plantar arteries, which forms plantar arterial arch of the foot. Posterior tibial artery gives *peroneal artery*, which runs close to fibula supplying calf muscles.

ARTERIAL DISEASES

1. **Stenosis** due to trauma, atherosclerosis, emboli.
   It may be:
   - In the brain causing transient ischemic attacks,
   - In the limbs causing claudication and rest pain,
   - In the abdomen causing pain, bloody stool,
   - In the kidney causing hematuria.
2. **Dilatations are aneurysms**.
3. **Arteritis**.
4. **Small vessel abnormalities**.

INTERMITTENT CLAUDICATION

Claudio means *'to limp'* a Latin word. It is a crampy pain in the muscle seen in the limbs. Due to arterial occlusion, metabolites like lactic acid and substance P accumulate in the muscle and cause pain. The site of pain depends on site of arterial occlusion.
- Commonest site is calf muscles.
- Pain in foot is due to block in lower tibial and plantar vessels.
- Pain in the calf is due to block in femoro-popliteal site.
- Pain in the thigh is due to block in the superficial femoral artery.
- Pain in the buttock is due to block in the common iliac or aortoiliac segment, often associated with impotence and is called as **Leriche's syndrome**.

Note:
- Pain commonly develops when the muscles are exercising. Cause for pain is accumulation of substance 'P' and metabolites.
- During exercise increased perfusion and increased opening of collaterals wash the metabolites away.

BOYD'S CLASSIFICATION OF CLAUDICATION

Grade I: Patient complains of pain after walking, and distance at which pain develops is called as *'claudication distance'*. If patient continues to walk pain subsides because the metabolites causing pain are washed away in the circulation due to increased blood flow in the muscle and also by opening of collaterals.

Grade II: Pain still persists on continuing walk; but can walk with effort.

Grade III: Patient has to take rest to relieve the pain.

Note: *Claudication* is not that common in upper limb but can occur during writing or any upper limb exercise.

Opportunity....Often it comes disguised in the form of misfortune, or temporary defeat

REST PAIN (FIG. 11.8)

- It is continuous ache in calf or feet and toes or in the region depending on site of obstruction.
- It is *'cry of dying nerves'* due to ischemia of the somatic nerves.
- It signifies severe decompensated ischemia.
- Pain aggravates by elevation and is relieved in dependant position of the limb.
- Pain is more in the distal part like toes and feet.
- It aggravates with movements and pressure.
- Hyperesthesia is common association with rest pain.

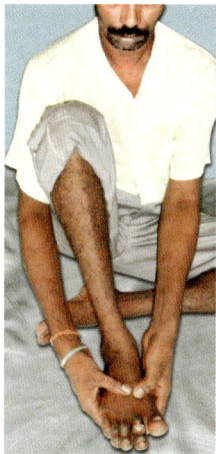

Fig. 11.8: Rest pain due to ischemia. Patient holds the limb to relieve pain. Touch and pressure sensation masks the transmission pathway.

CRITICAL LIMB ISCHEMIA

It is persistently recurring ischemic rest pain or ulceration or gangrene of the foot or toes with an ankle systolic pressure <50 mm Hg or toe systolic pressure <30 mm Hg.

DEFINITIONS

- **Pregangrene:** It is the changes in tissues, which indicates that blood supply is inadequate to keep the tissues alive and presents with rest pain, color changes, edema, *hyperesthesia* with or without ischemic ulceration.
- **Gangrene:** It is macroscopic death of tissue in situ putrefaction.
- **Dry gangrene:** It is dry, desiccated, mummified tissue caused by gradual slowing of bloodstream. There is a line of demarcation and is localized.
- **Wet gangrene:** It is due to both arterial and venous block with superadded putrefaction and infection. It spreads proximally and there is no line of demarcation. It spreads faster. Organs where wet gangrene can develop—appendix, bowel, gallbladder, testis, and pancreas.
- **Necrosis:** It is microscopic cell death.
- **Sequestrum:** It is dead bone in situ.
- **Slough:** It is dead soft tissue.
- **Line of demarcation (Fig. 11.9):** It is a line between viable and dying tissue indicated by a band of hyperemia. It also indicates that disease is well-localized. *Final separation* between healthy and gangrenous tissues occurs by development of a layer of granulation tissue in between. It is hyperesthetic due to *exposed nerve endings*.

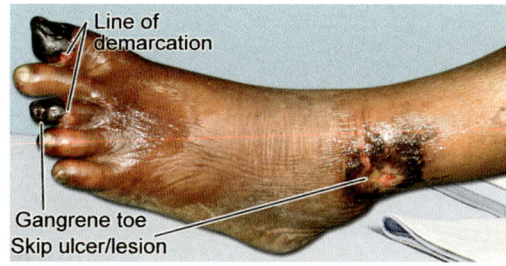

Fig. 11.9: Gangrene toes. Note clear line of demarcation of gangrenous area.

Type of separation
• Separation by aseptic ulceration, seen in dry gangrene.
• Separation by septic ulceration. Seen in infected cases and wet gangrene.

Beauty is eternity gazing at itself in a mirror; But you are eternity and you are the mirror—**Kahlil Gibran**

Features of Ischemia

Features of ischemia (Fig. 11.10)
- Marked pallor, purple-blue cyanosed appearance.
- Thinning of skin.
- Diminished hair.
- Loss of subcutaneous fat.
- Brittle nails, with transverse ridges.
- Ulceration in digits.
- Wasting of muscles.
- Tenderness and reduced temperature (cold).

Levels of block
- *Aortoiliac block* causes claudication in buttocks, thighs, and calves; absence of femoral and distal pulses, bruit over aortoiliac region. *Impotence occurs due to defective perfusion through internal iliac arteries and so into the penis causing erectile dysfunction (Leriche's syndrome).*
- *Iliac artery obstruction* causes claudication in thigh and calf; bruit over iliacs with absence of femoral and distal pulses.
- *Femoropopliteal obstruction* causes claudication in calf muscles with absence of distal pulses but with palpable femoral.
- *Distal obstruction* shows absence of ankle pulses with palpable femoral and popliteal pulses.

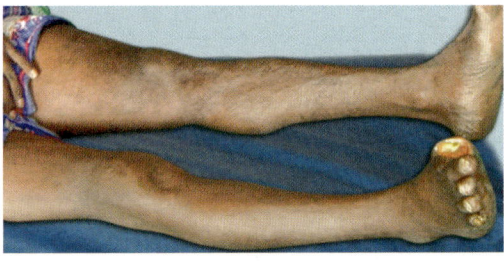

Fig. 11.10: Leg showing muscle wasting and other features of early ischemia such as loss of hair, loss of normal luster of skin, etc.

❖ **Delayed capillary filling:**
Blanched nails or pulp of fingers on pressure, shows delay in refilling (to turn pink) after release of pressure.

❖ **Delayed venous refilling:**
Two fingers are placed over the vein. Finger nearer to heart is moved away so as to empty the vein. Distal finger is released to observe the venous refilling. Delay in filling is called as *Harvey's sign*, signifies ischemia (venous filling will be increased in AV fistulas).

❖ **Paresthesia:**
Over the skin of the foot is due to shunting of blood from the skin to muscles in deeper plane.

❖ **Sensation** in gangrenous area is absent, but the skin is hyperesthetic at the line of demarcation.

❖ **Disappearing pulse syndrome:**
After feeling the pulse the limb is exercised. Pulse disappears once patient develops claudication. Vasodilatation and increased vascular space occurs due to exercise wherein arterial tension cannot be kept adequately and so pulse disappears (unmasking the arterial obstruction).

❖ **Buerger's postural test:**
Patient lying down on his back is asked to raise the leg. In normal individuals limb (plantar aspect of foot) remains pink even after raising above 90°. Ischemic limb, when elevated shows marked pallor and empty veins. The angle at which pallor develops is called as *Buerger's angle of vascular insufficiency*. If it is less than 30° it indicates severe ischemia.

❖ **Systolic bruit:**
It may be heard over stenosed artery like subclavian artery, femoral artery, carotid artery, iliacs, renal artery.

❖ **Adson's test (Scalene maneuver)**
The radial pulse is felt in a patient sitting on a stool. The patient is then asked to take a deep breath (to allow the rib cage to move upwards so as to narrow the cervicoaxillary channel) and turn the face to same side (to contract scalenus anterior muscle so as to narrow the scalene triangle). If the radial pulse disappears or become feeble it signifies cervical rib or *scalenus anticus syndrome*.

❖ **Elevated arm stress test (EAST; modified Roos test)**
With both arms kept in position of 90° abduction and external rotation, patient is

Paralyze resistance with persistence

asked to make a fist and release repeatedly for 5 minutes. Patient continues to do the maneuver in normal side, whereas in diseased (thoracic outlet syndrome) side patient complains of pain and paresthesia with difficulty in continuing the maneuver. Patient drops the arm down to get relieved from the symptoms.
- **Costoclavicular compression maneuver**
Radial pulse becomes absent when patient draws his shoulders backwards and downwards in excessive military position. This is because at this position, subclavian artery is compressed between first rib and clavicle, leading to feeble or absent radial pulse.
- **Hyperabduction maneuver (Halsted test)**
When affected arm is hyperabducted, radial pulse becomes absent or feeble due to compression of artery by pectoralis minor tendon.
- **Allen's test**
It is done to find out the patency of radial and ulnar arteries. Both the arteries are compressed near the wrist and allowed to blanch completely in one minute (in the mean time patient closes and opens the fist several times for further venous outflow). Palm appears pale and white. One of the arteries is released and color of hand is noted. Normally hand becomes pink and flushed in no time; where as in obstruction, the area still remains pale. Other artery is also released and looked for changes in hand. Often test has to be repeated to get proper information.

Note: Abdomen should be examined for the presence of abdominal *aortic aneurysms.* It presents as pulsatile mass above the umbilicus, vertically placed, smooth, soft, nonmobile, not moving with respiration, resonant on percussion. Expansile pulsation is confirmed by placing the patient in knee-elbow position.

Palpation of Blood Vessels

- *Dorsalis pedis artery* is felt against the navicular and middle cuneiform bones, just lateral to the extensor hallucis longus tendon at the proximal end of first web space. It is absent in 10% cases.
- *Posterior tibial artery* is felt against the calcaneus just behind the medial malleolus, midway between it and tendo-Achilles.
- *Anterior tibial artery* is felt in the midway anteriorly between the two malleoli against the lower end of tibia just above the ankle joint lateral to extensor hallucis longus tendon.
- *Popliteal artery* is difficult to feel. It is palpated better in prone position with knee flexed about 40–90° to relax popliteal fascia. It is felt in the lower part of the fossa over the flat posterior surface of upper end of tibia. In upper end of the fossa, artery is not felt, as there is no bony area in intercondylar region.
- *Femoral artery* in the groin is felt just below the inguinal ligament midway between anterosuperior iliac spine and pubic symphysis. Often hip has to be flexed for about 10–15° to feel it properly.
- *Radial artery* is felt at the wrist on the lateral aspect against lower end of the front of radius.
- *Ulnar artery* is felt at the wrist on the medial end against lower end of the front of ulna.
- *Brachial artery* is felt in front of the elbow just medial to biceps brachii tendon.
- *Axillary artery* is felt in apex of the axilla against head of the humerus.
- *Subclavian artery* is felt against first rib just above the middle of the clavicle.
- *Facial artery* is felt against body of mandible at the insertion of masseter.
- *Common carotid artery* is felt medial to sternomastoid muscle at the level of

*When you part from your friend, you grieve not; for that which you love most in him may be clearer in his absence, as the mountain to the climber is clearer from the plain—**Khalil Gibran***

thyroid cartilage against carotid tubercle (*Chassaignac tubercle*) of 6th cervical vertebra (in carotid triangle).
* *Superficial temporal artery* is felt just in front of the tragus of the ear against temporal bone.

INVESTIGATIONS FOR ARTERIAL DISEASES

* Blood tests: Hb%, blood sugar, lipid profile, peripheral smear, platelet count.
* Doppler to find out the site of block (Fig. 11.11).
* Duplex scan:
  - To study the site, extent, severity of block, and also about collaterals.
  - Plethysmography.

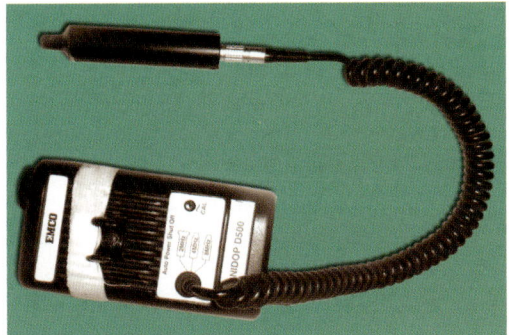

Fig. 11.11: Hand held Doppler.

Ankle-brachial pressure index:
Normally it is 1. If it is less than 0.9, it means ischemia is present. If it reaches 0.3 or less, then it signifies severe ischemia with gangrene.

Angiography

* *Retrograde transfemoral Seldinger angiography (Fig. 11.12)*
  - It is the commonly done procedure. It is done only when femorals are felt. If femoral pulsation is not felt then angiogram is done either *transbrachially (left brachial artery), or transaortic.*
  - Other angiograms are carotid angiogram, celiac angiogram, superior mesenteric angiogram, and coronary angiogram.

  - Femoral artery is cannulated with a guidewire. Through that Seldinger arterial catheter is passed proximally in retrograde direction and water-soluble iodine dye (Sodium diatrizoate) is injected. X-rays are taken to see the block, and its extent in the affected limb.
  - In TAO, *corkscrew* appearance is characteristic. *Distal run off through* collaterals is also important.
  - If catheter is passed still proximally angiogram of opposite side is possible.
  - Seldinger technique can also be used (to study) to do renal angiogram, to detect renal artery stenosis, renal carcinomas, and renal anomalies (vascular).

Indications for angiogram

* TAO; atherosclerosis.
* Raynaud's phenomenon.
* AV fistulas; hemangiomas.
* Thoracic outlet syndrome (e.g. cervical rib).
* Aneurysms; neoplastic conditions.

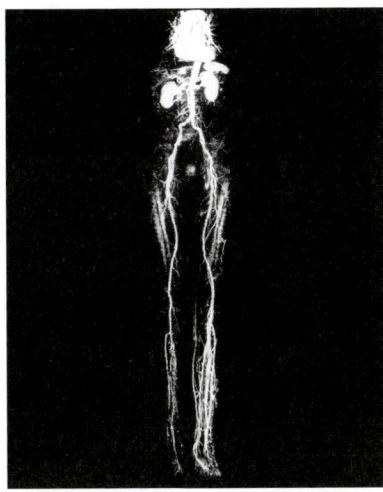

Fig. 11.12: Lower limb angiogram.

Complications of retrograde angiogram

* Bleeding.
* Dissection of vessel wall.
* Hematoma formation.
* Thrombosis.
* Infection.
* Anaphylaxis.

Our greatest glory is not in never falling, but in rising every time we fall

- *Direct aortic angiogram*
  - Practiced earlier, is discouraged at present because of the risk of aortic dissection and paraplegia due to blockage of anterior spinal artery.
- *Digital substraction angiography (DSA)*
  - Here vessel (artery) is delineated in a better way by eliminating other tissues through computer system. AV fistulas, hemangiomas, lesion in circle of Willis, vascular tumors, and other vascular anomalies are well made out.
  - Dye is injected either to an artery or vein. Injecting into a vein is technically easier but larger dose of dye is required. Injecting into an artery is technically difficult but small dose of dye is sufficient.
  - *Advantages*: Only vascular system is visualized; other systems are eliminated by computer substraction. Small lesion, its location and details are better observed with greater clarity.
  - *Disadvantages*: Cost factor and availability.
  - *Complications*: Anaphylaxis, bleeding, thrombosis.
- CT angiogram/CT aortogram (Fig. 11.13).

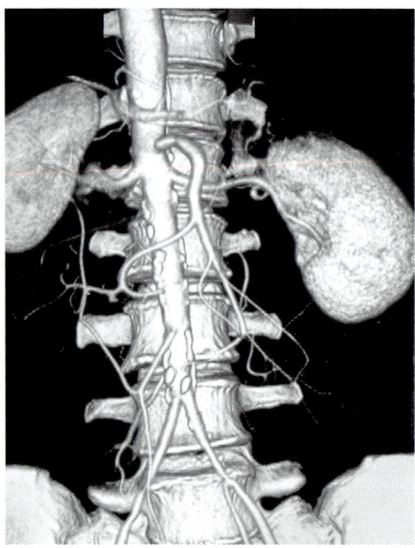

Fig. 11.13: Aortic angiogram.

Ultrasound Abdomen

To see abdominal aneurysm or nature of aorta and other vessels.

DISEASES OF THE ARTERIES

- Atherosclerosis:

Risk factors
• Hypercholesterolemia, hypertriglyceridemia and hyperlipidemia, cigarette smoking.
• Hypertension, diabetes mellitus.
• Age—elderly, common in males.
• Sedentary life, family history.

- Thromboangiitis obliterans (TAO; Buerger's disease).
- Raynaud's disease.
- Conditions causing Raynaud's phenomenon: Like scleroderma, rheumatoid arthritis, SLE, granulomatosis, vasculitis of other causes.
- Embolus.
- Aneurysms.

ATHEROSCLEROSIS

It is a chronic, complex inflammatory condition of elastic and muscular arteries, involving as systemic and segmental. It begins in childhood as fatty streaks.

Risk factors
Definitive
• Hypercholesterolemia, and hyperlipidemia (cholesterol >200 mg%; high LDL (>100 mg%); low HDL (<35 mg%).
• Cigarette smoking.
• Hypertension.
• Diabetes mellitus.
Relative
• Age—elderly.
• Common in males.
• Hypertriglyceridemia.
• Sedentary life, obesity.
• Family history.

*Solitude has soft, silky hands, but with strong fingers it grasps the heart and makes it ache with sorrow—***Kahlil Gibran**

Pathogenesis

- All risk factors cause initial endothelial injury, both mechanical as well as toxic. This reduces significantly *normal atheroprotective features* of endothelium (*barrier function; antiadhesive effect; antiproliferative effect* on smooth muscles of arterial wall). Progressive atheromatous plaque formation, thrombosis, migration and proliferation of vascular smooth muscle cell occur. *Smooth muscle cells migrated* into intima act as neointima and this migration is stimulated by PDGF (platelet derived growth factor released by endothelium smooth muscles, platelets); which (this migrated smooth muscle) newly becomes secretory to produce large quantity of matrix of the plaque. Lipid (LDL) gets oxidized to release factors which promote inflammation and coagulation and factors which prevent production of *protective nitric oxide*. Macrophages stabilize the plaque.
- *Pathology* constitutes of atherosclerotic plaque which contains smooth muscle cells, connective tissue matrix, macrophages and lipid (the feature of atherosclerosis). Ulceration and calcification occurs in these plaques. *Ulcerated plaque* is highly thrombogenic causing thrombosis and further critical block of the vessel leading to tissue ischemia and infarction distally.
- Plaques are more at the *dividing junctions* of the artery where stress and shear force of the blood flow is more. Plaques are dynamic in nature with progression and regression phases.
- Plaque progression has got a unique ability of *adaptation* so that as the plaque progresses, lumen caliber is been tried to be preserved until critical stage occurs. Stenosis more *than 40%* is said to be *critical*. Beyond this, compensatory mechanism fails causing rapid progression and further stenosis of lumina. Stenosis more than 40% causes *atrophy of tunica media* making arterial wall mechanically unstable leading into dilatation and aneurysm.
- *Common arteries involved are*—infrarenal part of abdominal aorta, coronary arteries, iliofemoral vessels, carotid bifurcation, popliteal arteries. It is less common in upper limb arteries, common carotid, renal and mesenteric arteries.

Features and Evaluation

- It is common after 50 years, but can occur at earlier age group.
- It occurs in males and females. Family history is common.
- Smoking, hypertension, diabetes, raised cholesterol are common causes.
- Veins are not diseased. Arterial wall is thickened on palpation.
- Thrill and bruit over femoral, renal, carotid arteries may be felt/heard. It suggests localized stenosis with turbulence of blood flow.
- Features of ischemia in the affected limb. Absence/feeble pulses including of main arteries of the limb—femorals. Abdomen should be examined for aortic aneurysm.
- Transient ischemic attacks, chest pain, eye problems, mesenteric ischemia, altered renal function may be associated.
- Blood sugar, fasting lipid profile, Doppler, angiogram (CT/DSA), US abdomen, ECG, echocardiography are essential investigations. Angiogram shows typical narrowed artery, site, extent, percentage of stenosis, collaterals.

Management

- *Risk factor modification*: Avoid smoking; control of hypertension, diabetes, hypercholesterolemia; weight reduction by diet and exercise.
- *Drugs*: Antiplatelet (aspirin 75 mg, clopidogrel 75 mg); cilostazol 50 mg

Our chief want in life is somebody who will make us do what we can.

bd; atorvastatin to reduce cholesterol; pentoxiphylline.
- *Percutaneous transluminal angioplasty (PTA)* is very useful for iliac blocks and lower limb blocks.
- *Surgeries:*
  - Thrombectomy, endarterectomy, profundaplasty.
  - Reverse/in situ saphenous vein graft.
  - Bypass grafts—iliofemoral, aortofemoral, iliopopliteal, femorofemoral grafts.

Amputations if limb is gangrenous—toe/below knee, above knee. Forefoot and Syme's amputations are not feasible in vascular conditions.

THROMBOANGIITIS OBLITERANS

Thromboangiitis obliterans (TAO) (Syn. Buerger's disease) is a disease exclusively seen in males of young age group (Not seen in females due to genetic reason). Seen only in smokers and tobacco users. Always starts in lower limb, may start on one side and later on the other side. Upper limb involvement occurs only after lower limb is diseased (Fig. 11.14).

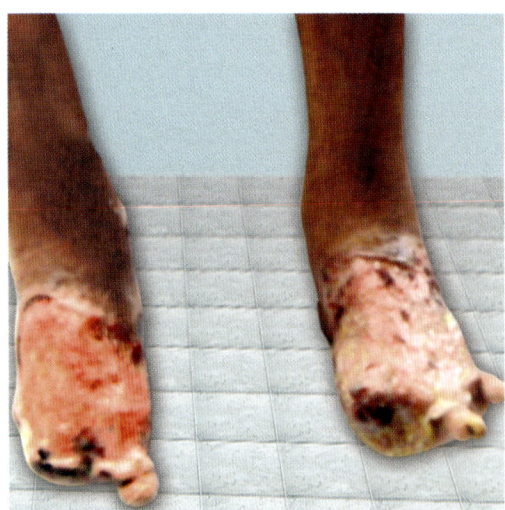

Fig. 11.14: Bilateral TAO in a young male with large ischemic ulcers. Patient underwent amputation of both limbs (below knee).

Investigations

- Hb%. Blood sugar.
- Arterial Doppler and Duplex scan (Doppler + B mode ultrasound).

Pathogenesis

Smoke contains *carbon monoxide* and acid
↓
Causes initially vasospasm and hyperplasia of intima
↓
Thrombosis and so obliteration of vessels occurs. Commonly medium sized vessels are involved
↓
Panarteritis is common. Usually involvement is segmental
↓
Eventually artery, vein and nerve are together involved
↓
Nerve involvement causes rest pain
↓
Patient presents with features of ischemia in the limb
↓
Once blockage occurs, plenty of collaterals open up depending on the site of blockage either around knee joint or around buttock
↓
Once collaterals open up, through these collaterals, blood supply is maintained to the ischemic area
↓
It is called as compensatory peripheral vascular disease
↓
If patient continues to smoke, disease progresses into the collaterals, blocking them eventually, leading to severe ischemia and is called as decompensatory peripheral vascular disease
↓
It is presently called as critical limb ischemia. It causes rest pain, ulceration, and gangrene

Smoking index (SI) =

Number of years of smoking × Number of cigarettes smoked per day

SI > 300 is a risk factor.

Pack years index (PYI) =

Number of years of smoking × Number of packets of cigarettes per day

PYI > 40 is a risk factor

*Trees are poems that the earth writes upon the sky—**Khalil Gibran***

- **Transfemoral retrograde angiogram through Seldinger technique**:
  - Shows blockage.
  - *Corkscrew* appearance of the vessel—collaterals.
  - *Distal run off* is amount of dye filling in the main vessel distal to the obstruction through collaterals. If distal run off is good then ischemia is compensated. If distal run off is poor then ischemia is decompensated.
- **Transbrachial angiogram:** If femorals are not felt, then transbrachial angiogram (through left side brachial artery—left subclavian artery—and so to descending aorta) should be done.
- Ultrasound abdomen.
- Arterial biopsy usually of dorsalis pedis artery.

Treatment

*Stop smoking. Opt for either cigarette or limb but not both (**Stop smoking; start walking**).*

Drugs:
- Vasodilators, e.g. nifedipine.
- Pentoxiphylline increases the flexibility of RBC's and helps them reach the microcirculation in a better way so as to increase the oxygenation.
- Small dose of Aspirin.
- Prostacyclins, Ticlopidine, Praxilene.
  All drugs act at the collateral level than at the diseased vessel.

Buerger's exercise, Buerger's position, heel raise, analgesics, care of feet (Chiropady), *proper footwear are advised.*

Surgery:
- *Lumbar sympathectomy* to increase the cutaneous perfusion so as to promote the ulcer healing.
- *Omentoplasty* to revascularize the affected limb.
- *Profundaplasty* is done for blockage in profunda femoris so as to open more collaterals across the knee joint (It often makes better perfusion to the knee joint and flap of below knee amputation).
- *Amputations are done* at different levels depending on site, severity and extent of vessel occlusion. Usually either below-knee or above-knee amputations are done.

TREATMENT OF ARTERIAL DISEASES

Stop smoking; start walking.
- **Medical:**
  - General measures.
  - Stop smoking.
  - Reduction of weight.
  - Change in lifestyle.
  - Exercise.
  - Care of feet.
  - Control of diabetes and hypertension.
  - Buerger's position and exercise.

  Drugs:
  Nifedipine, Praxilene, Pentoxiphylline, small dose of Aspirin, Prostacyclin, Dipyridamole, Ticlopidine.
- **Surgery:**
  1. **Transluminal balloon angioplasty**:
     Through transfemoral Seldinger approach, initially angiogram is done. Then under guidance (fluoroscopic) stenosed area is approached. Balloon of the angioplasty catheter is inflated at stenosed area *for one minute* and repeated if required. Catheter is withdrawn. It is useful in cases of localized stenosed areas.

     Complications: Thrombosis, bleeding, sepsis.
  2. **Atherectomy**:
     It is removal of atheroma from the wall of medium sized vessels either through open surgery or by percutaneous route.
  3. **Thrombectomy**:
     It is removal of thrombus from larger vessels through an arteriotomy. Done in aortoiliac, femoropopliteal region.
  4. **Endarterectomy**:
     It is removal of thrombus along with diseased intima through an arteriotomy.

Our aim should be service, not success

5. *Intraluminal stent* placement.
6. *Profundaplasty*:
   It is done when there is localized block in opening of profunda femoris (deep femoral). Profunda femoris is opened, thrombus if present, is removed. Opening is widened using either venous or synthetic (Dacron or PTFE) grafts. This procedure allows collaterals across the knee joint to open through profunda femoris and so gives good blood supply to below knee level and may prevent patient going in for above knee amputation (Fig. 11.15). (May be able to save knee joint with below knee amputation and better prosthesis).

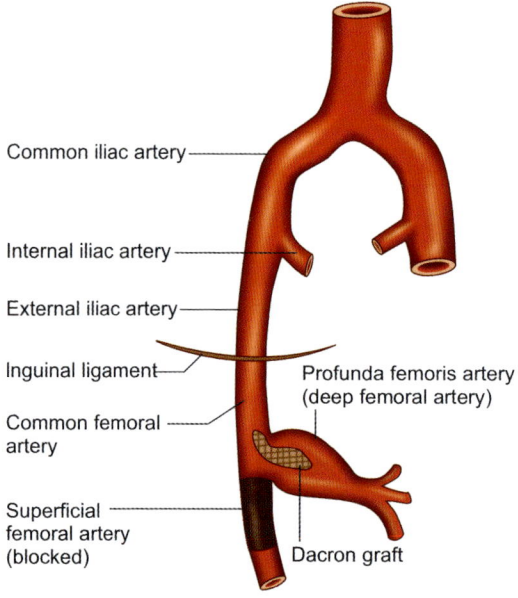

Fig. 11.15: Profundaplasty for deep femoral block.

7. *Reverse saphenous vein graft*:
   In case of femoropopliteal block, saphenous vein is dissected out, reversed and sutured above to the femoral artery and below to popliteal segment so as to bypass the blood through reverse saphenous vein graft. Saphenous vein is reversed to nullify the action of valves so as to allow easy flow of blood.

8. *In situ saphenous vein graft*:
   It is arterialization of saphenous vein. Saphenous vein intact in same position is sutured above and below the blocked femoropopliteal region to bypass the blood across. Venous valves are removed through valvulotomy instrument so as to allow the blood to pass.

9. *Arterial/venous grafts (Fig. 11.16)*:
   Synthetic:
   – Dacron woven graft.
   – Dacron knitted graft.
   – PTFE—polytetrafluoroethylene graft.
   Natural:
   – Internal mammary artery.
   – Long saphenous vein either reverse or in situ.
   Grafts of different length and size are available.

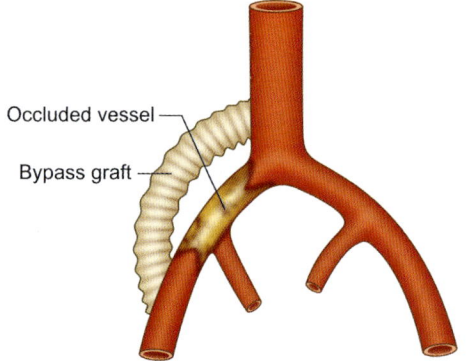

Fig. 11.16: Bypass graft.

Different procedures

- Aortofemoral bypass graft (Figs. 11.17 and 11.18).
- Ileofemoral bypass graft.
- Femorofemoral bypass graft.
- Femoropopliteal graft (Fig. 11.19).
- Femorodistal graft.

Problems with grafts:
Leak, infection, thrombosis, cost factor, availability, re-block.

10. *Lumbar sympathectomy*:
    Indications:
    – Peripheral vascular disease like TAO.

Faith is an oasis in the heart which will never be reached by the caravan of thinking—**Kahlil Gibran**

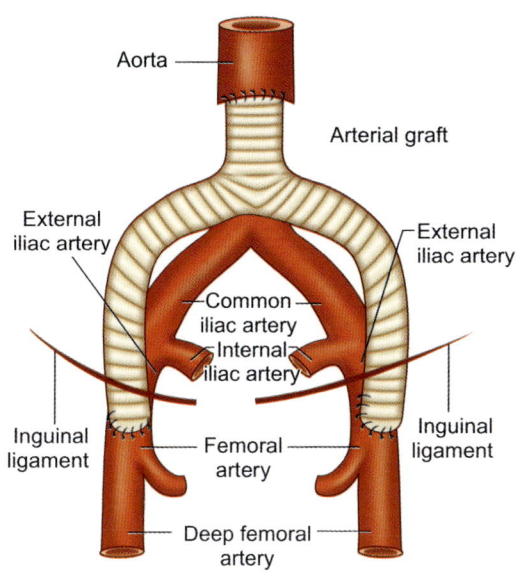

Fig. 11.17: Aortofemoral bypass graft (end to side).

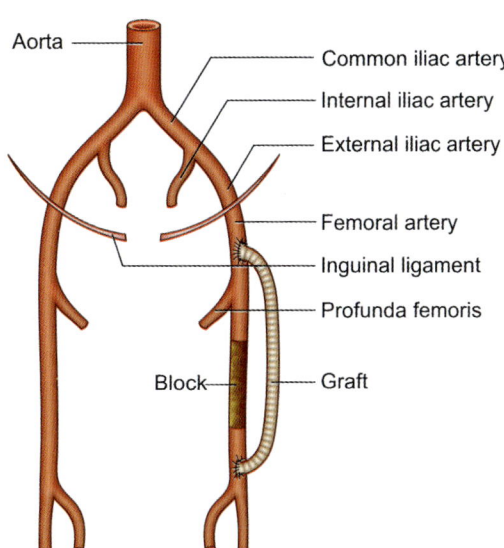

Fig. 11.19: Femoropopliteal bypass graft.

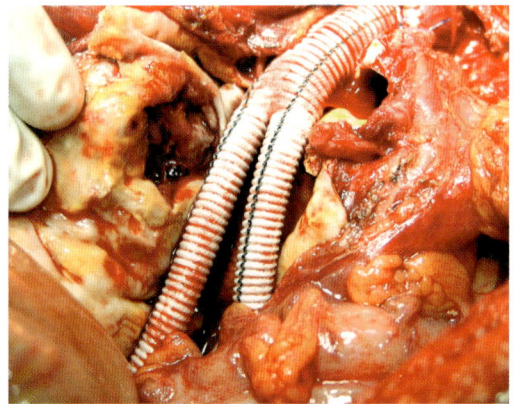

Fig. 11.18: Aortofemoral bypass graft.

- To promote healing of cutaneous ulcers.
- To change the level of amputation and make flaps to heal better after amputation.
- Causalgia of lower limb (it is common in upper limb).
- Hyperhidrosis.

Principle:
It increases the cutaneous blood supply and so healing of ulcer and skin flaps in amputations is better.

Procedure:
Under general or spinal anesthesia, ganglia are approached through a transverse incision in the loin at the level of umbilicus. Through extraperitoneal approach, by dividing external oblique, splitting internal oblique and transverse abdominis muscles, inferior vena cava on right side, aorta on left side are identified. Sympathetic chain is identified by its rami L_2-L_5 ganglia are removed. L_2 is identified by its size (*larger*) and more number of rami. L_1 is retained on one side in bilateral cases. If it is removed it leads to failure of ejaculation and so sterility.

Complications:
- Injury to IVC or aorta.
- Bleeding lumbar veins.
- Spinal vessel spasm and so ischemia of spinal cord and paraplegia.
- Injury to bowel and ureter.
- Wound infection and abscess formation.
- Its effects are only temporary (3–4 weeks). Long-term results are doubtful. It can be combined with omentoplasty.

- It can also be done along with below-knee amputation to increase the blood supply of skin flap so as to have better healing.
- Limb will become warmer immediately after sympathectomy.

11. **Chemical sympathectomy**:
    It is done in lateral position using a long spinal needle under local anesthesia. Position is confirmed by injecting dye under fluoroscopy. Later 5 mL of *phenol* in water or absolute alcohol is injected lateral to the vertebral bodies of fourth and second lumbar vertebrae. Care should be taken to see that the needle does not enter IVC or aorta.
    Procedure is contraindicated in patients with *bleeding disorders* and in patients who are on *anticoagulants*.

12. **Omentoplasty:**
    Indications:
    a. Peripheral vascular disease—to improve circulation.
    b. For lymphedema, it helps by providing lymphatics and so to drain lymph from the limb.
    c. It is also tried for revascularization of pharynx, cranial cavity.
    Omentum is supplied by omental vessels.

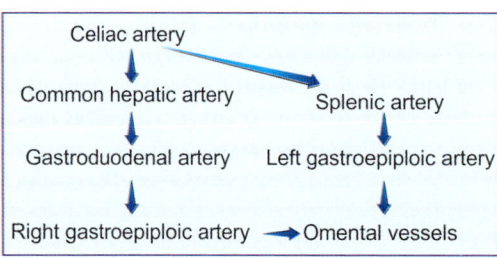

Four layers of omentum have omental arcades of vessels. Omentum is also rich in lymphatics. It has adhesive property. By retaining one of the pedicles, omentum can be mobilized so as to reach the limb to maintain the circulation. It can also be mobilized up to the ankle. It promotes ulcer healing, reduces the pain, and controls the features of ischemia. It can be used in upper limb ischemia. But if patient continues to smoke, disease spreads to these omental vessels also. Often it can be used for both limbs (Fig. 11.20).

Complications of omentoplasty:
- Abdominal sepsis.
- Incisional hernia, where omental pedicle is tunneled into the limb from the abdomen.
- Adhesions and intestinal obstruction.

Procedure:
Under general anesthesia, abdomen is opened with upper midline incision. Omental vessels are identified. Omentum with its blood supply is carefully mobilized to get an adequate length. Lengthened, mobilized omentum is brought into the subcutaneous plane through abdominal wall, lateral to the lower part of rectus muscle. Later this pedicle is mobilized in the subcutaneous tunnel across the leg, burried in the deep fascia.

13. **Other treatment methods:**
    Amputations is done at different levels depending on extent of gangrene, site of block, amount of collaterals.

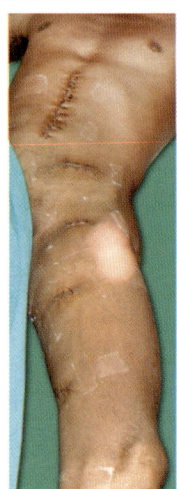

Fig. 11.20: Omentoplasty done for lower limb ischemia. Note the sutured wound in abdomen and limb.

*Your reason and your passion are the rudder and the sails of your seafaring soul—**Kahlil Gibran***

ACUTE ARTERIAL OCCLUSION

Causes
- Trauma.
- Embolism (Figs. 11.21A and B).

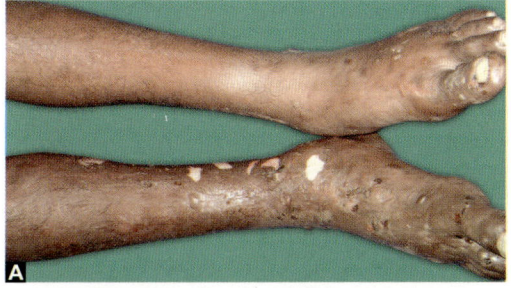

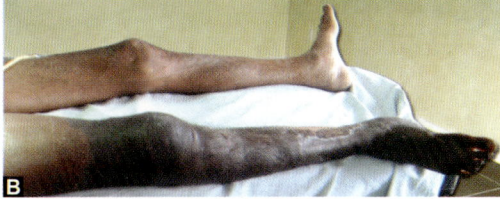

Figs. 11.21A and B: Acute ischemic leg due to acute embolism.

TRAUMATIC ACUTE ARTERIAL OCCLUSION

Causes
- Thrombus due to trauma.
- Subintimal hematoma.
- Acute compartment syndrome.
- During femoral or brachial arterial catheterization, either diagnostic or therapeutic procedures.

Features
- History of trauma, pain, swelling at the site, pallor, pulselessness, cold limb.
- **Investigation:** Duplex scan, angiogram.
- **Treatment:**
  - Wound is explored and tear in the artery is identified. It is sutured by using nonabsorbable monofilament material, polypropylene 6-0. Often venous or dacron graft is required for interposition.
  - Proper antibiotics and heparin are required to prevent thrombosis of the vessel. Later patient is advised to take oral Warfarin for maintenance.

COMPARTMENT SYNDROME

It is common in anterior compartment of leg and in front of forearm. Because of the closed compartment, pressure increases here following fracture and hematoma, which compresses over the vessel. It leads to blockade of vessel causing acute ischemia of the limb presenting with severe pain, pallor, pulselessness.

Treatment
- *Immediate decompression by longitudinal fasciotomy*, is the treatment of choice, where in deep fascia is cut adequately to relieve the compression. Otherwise it may lead to severe limb ischemia, gangrene and may land with amputation.
- Associated fractures, hematoma, vessel tear has to be managed accordingly.

REPERFUSION INJURY

- It occurs after re-establishment of arterial flow to an ischemic tissue bed which further leads to tissue death causing specifically *peripheral muscle infarction*. It is due to sudden release of oxygen-free radicals which blocks the microcirculation, with release of high levels of potassium (hyperkalemia) and myoglobin (myoglobinemia and myoglobinuria). Hemodynamically patient becomes unstable with lactic acidosis, intracellular changes, interstitial edema and cardiac dysfunction. It is often life-threatening.

Participating in pleasures and pressures of life and keeping one's own self, leads to true happiness.

- *Haimovici triad* of revascularization injury (1960)—(1) Muscle infarction; (2) Myoglobinuria; (3) Acute renal failure.
- Severe ischemia causes edema in the muscular compartment with raise in compartment pressure more than the essential capillary perfusion pressure causing *acute compartment syndrome*. It is common in the anterior compartment of the leg. It is basically in the skeletal muscles deep to deep fascia. Compartment pressure when measured using transducer needles will be more than 40 mm Hg or >30 mm Hg for 3 hours or above the mean arterial pressure. Muscle weakness, sensory changes, leg pain which is aggravated by dorsiflexion of toes.
- *No reflow phenomenon* due to tissue edema causing to capillary perfusion block. Even though compartment syndrome and 'no reflow' phenomemenon are separate entities they are always seen together along with reperfusion injury.
- Metabolic acidosis, acute tubular necrosis causing acute renal failure and cardiac arrhythmias may set in and become life-threatening.
- **Features are**—toxemia; oliguria; persistent pain and edema in the leg with muscular tenderness; raised blood urea and serum creatinine with features of acute ischemia in the limb. Raised creatinine level (renal failure), creatine kinase (muscle lysis) are typical.
- **Treatment:**
  - Mannitol to prevent renal failure; fluid therapy.
  - Fasciotomy to reduce raised compartment pressure. All four compartments of lower limb should be decompressed surgically. Long vertical lateral deep fasciotomy incision in the calf behind the fibula along the deep fascia and its fibular attachments is a must. Bleeding is common after fasciotomy as patient is heparinized. Infection of the wound can occur. Later, once the patient is stabilized and edema subsides with healthy wound, secondary suturing or skin grafting is done. If fasciotomy is not done and if patient survives then eventually it leads to Volkmann's ischemic contracture.
  - Antibiotics and supportive therapy.

EMBOLISM

It is due to a solid material which is floating and traveling in the bloodstream, eventually blocking the vessel on its pathway.
- **Arterial emboli:**
  Source—due to mural thrombus following:
  - Myocardial infarction.
  - Mitral stenosis.
  - Atrial fibrillation.
  - Aortic aneurysms.
  - Cervical rib causing poststenotic dilatation of subclavian artery.
- **Venous emboli** are due to DVT causing pulmonary embolism.
- **Fat embolism**.
- **Air embolism**.

Effects of Arterial Embolism

- Brain: Blockage at middle cerebral artery causes hemiplegia, transient ischemic attacks (TIA), visual disturbances.
- Blockage at central retinal artery causes amaurosis fugax, or permanent blindness.
- Blockage at mesenteric vessels causes intestinal gangrene.
- Blockage at renal artery leads to hematuria, loin pain.
- Blockage at limb vessels cause pain, pallor, pulseless, paresthesia, paresis, ulceration, gangrene.

Commonest site of arterial emboli is common femoral artery.

Desire is half of life; indifference is half of death—**Kahlil Gibran**

Investigations for Arterial Embolism

- Emergency Doppler, ECG and echocardiography, angiogram.
- Relevant tests for origin of emboli.

Treatment

- **Embolectomy (Fig. 11.22)**:
  - Done as early as possible as an emergency operation. Under fluoroscopic guidance, *Fogarty catheter* (interventional radiology) is passed beyond the embolus and balloon is opened. Catheter is pulled out gently with embolus. Procedure has to be repeated until embolectomy is completed and bleeding occurs. Angiogram is repeated to confirm the free flow.
  - Postoperatively initially heparin and later oral anticoagulant are used. Procedure is done under general anesthesia.
  - *Open arteriotomy and embolectomy* can be done *by direct approach* and later the arteriotomy has to be sutured. Postoperatively, anticoagulants, antibiotics should be given.

- **Intra-arterial thrombolysis using fibrinolysins**:
  After passing arterial catheter, angiogram is done and agents are injected intra-arterially through the arterial catheter. Drugs used are:
  - Streptokinase—lysis occurs in 48 hours.
  - Urokinase.
  - Tissue plasminogen activator (TPA)—lysis occurs in 24 hours.
  - TPA pulse-spray method—lysis occurs in 6 hours.

  Contraindications for thrombolysis:
  - Stroke.
  - Bleeding diathesis.
  - Pregnancy.

  Heparin should not be used concomitantly with fibrinolysins.

SADDLE EMBOLUS

It is an embolus blocking (Fig. 11.23) at the *bifurcation of aorta*.

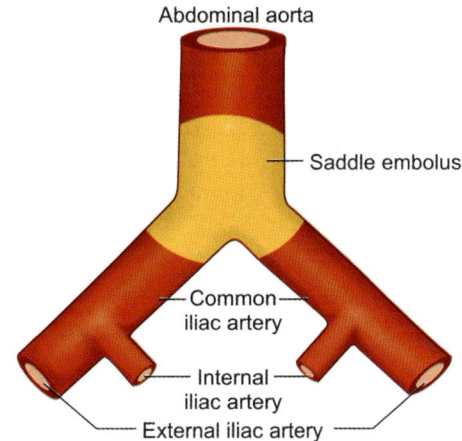

Fig. 11.23: Saddle embolus blocking the bifurcation of abdominal aorta.

Causes

- Mural thrombus after myocardial infarction.
- Mitral stenosis with atrial fibrillation.
- Aortic aneurysm.

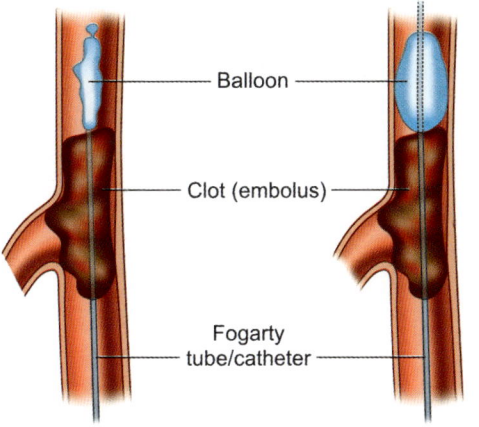

Fig. 11.22: Embolectomy technique.

The embolus, which blocks at aortic bifurcation, is usually large.

Features

- Features of ischemia in both lower limbs.
- Gangrene of both lower limbs.
- Associated infection and its features.
- Investigations
  - Arterial Doppler.
  - Aortic angiogram.
  - Ultrasound abdomen.

Treatment

- Initially, heparin is given intravenously —10,000/units and later 5,000 units/subcutaneously 8th hourly.
- Embolectomy can be done using Fogarty catheter.
- Open arteriotomy and embolectomy can also be tried.
- Antibiotic prophylaxis has to be given to prevent infection.

FAT EMBOLISM

- It is commonly seen after *fracture femur, tibia, or multiple fractures* and occasionally following electroconvulsive therapy.
- Usually occurs in 24–72 hours.
- It is due to aggregation of chylomicrons, derived from bone marrow, causing fat embolism.
- It is often a fatal condition.

Features

1. *Cerebral*: Drowsy, restless, disoriented, constricted pupils, pyrexia, coma.
2. *Pulmonary*: Cyanosis, tachypnea, right heart failure, froth in mouth and nostrils, fat droplets in sputum, eventually respiratory failure.
3. *Cutaneous*: Petechial hemorrhages in the skin.
4. *Retinal artery emboli is the earliest sign to appear, causing striae hemorrhages, fluffy exudates*—confirmed on fundoscopic examination.
5. *Kidney*: Blockage in renal arterioles results in fat droplets in urine.

Treatment

- Oxygen.
- Heparinization.
- Low molecular weight dextran.
- Ventilator support and ICU management.

AIR EMBOLISM

Causes

- Through venous access like IV cannula.
- During artificial pneumothorax.
- During surgeries of neck and axilla.
- Traumatic opening of major veins sucking air inside, causing embolism.
- During fallopian tube insufflation.
- During illegal abortion.

Amount of air required to cause air embolism is *50 mL*.

When the air enters the right atrium, it is churned up into foam, which enters the right ventricle, later blocking the pulmonary artery.

Treatment

Patient has to be placed in Trendelenburg position. By passing a needle, the air has to be aspirated from the right ventricle. Often requires life-saving open thoracotomy to aspirate the excess air causing the block.

THERAPEUTIC EMBOLIZATION

Indications

- Hemangiomas.
- AV fistulas.
- Malignancies like renal cell carcinoma, hepatoma.

Life without liberty is like a body without spirit—**Kahlil Gibran**

- Craniovascular problems.
- To arrest hemorrhage from gastrointestinal tract (GIT), urinary and respiratory tract.

In bleeding duodenal ulcer or gastric ulcer, embolization is used to occlude gastroduodenal artery or left gastric artery respectively.

It is also useful in bleeding esophageal varices, liver secondaries (mainly due to carcinoids), hepatoma.

Materials used	
• Blood clot.	• Human dura.
• Gel foam.	• Plastic microspheres.
• Balloons.	• Ethyl alcohol.
• Quick setting plastics.	• Wool.
• Stainless coils.	

CAISSON'S DISEASE OR DECOMPRESSION DISEASE

It occurs due to rapid decompression from high altitude, aircraft, compressed air chambers causing bubbling of nitrogen which blocks the small vessels, resulting in:
- Excruciating pain *(bends)* in joints and muscles.
- Spinal cord ischemia causing neurological deficits.
- Choking with chest pain, tightness and dry cough when lungs are affected.
- Treatment
  - Oxygen therapy.
  - Recompression and gradual decompression.

ANEURYSMS

It is dilatations of localized segment of arterial system.
- *True* aneurysm contains all three layers of artery (Fig. 11.24).
- *False* aneurysm contains single layer of fibrous tissue as wall of the sac and it usually occurs after trauma.

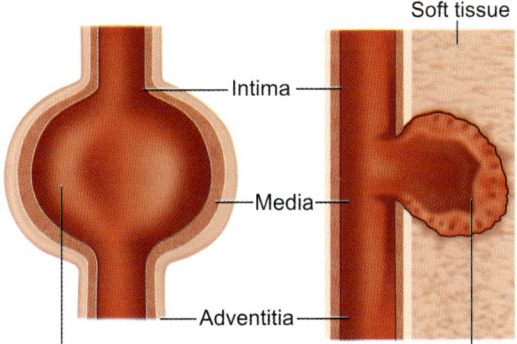

Fig. 11.24: True and false aneurysms. In true type all layers are intact. In false type all layers breached with hematoma having a false capsule.

Types (Fig. 11.25)		
• Fusiform	• Saccular	• Dissecting.

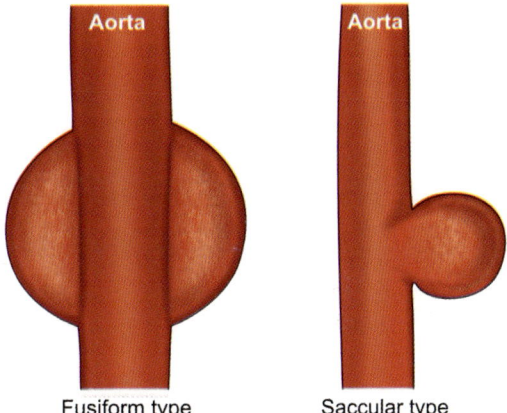

Fig. 11.25: Fusiform and saccular types of aneurysms.

Causes

- Atherosclerosis.
- Syphilis.
- Traumatic.
- Collagen diseases like Marfan's syndrome.

Sites

- Aorta.
- Femoral.

Pay attention to the small things, the kite flies because of its tail

- Popliteal.
- Subclavian.
- Cerebral, mesenteric, renal, splenic arteries.
  Commonest type is true, fusiform, atherosclerotic, aortic aneurysms.
  Berry's aneurysms are multiple aneurysms occurring in circle of Willis.

Clinical Features of Aneurysms

- Swelling at the site which is *pulsatile (expansile)*, smooth, soft, warm, compressible, with thrill on palpation and bruit on auscultation. Swelling reduces in size when pressed proximally.
- Distal edema due to venous compression.
- Altered sensation due to compression of nerves.
- Erosion into bones, joints, trachea or esophagus.
- Aneurysm with thrombosis can throw an embolus causing gangrene of toes, digits, often extending proximally.

Differential Diagnosis

- Pyogenic abscess: Abscess has to be always confirmed by aspiration; especially in axilla, popliteal region, groin.
- Vascular tumors.
- Pulsating tumors—sarcomas, pulsating secondaries.
- Pseudocyst of pancreas mimics aortic aneurysm.
- AV fistula.

Investigations

- Doppler study, duplex scan, angiogram, DSA.
- Tests relevant for the cause, like blood sugar, lipid profile, echocardiography.

Treatment

- Reconstruction of artery using arterial grafts.

- Arterial endoaneurysmorrhaphy—MATA's.
- Therapeutic embolization.
- Clipping the vessel under guidance (e.g. cranial aneurysms).

ABDOMINAL ANEURYSMS

Abdominal aortic aneurysm is the commonest aortic aneurysm. 2% incidence.

Causes

- Atherosclerosis: 95%.
- Others: Syphilis, dissecting, traumatic, collagen diseases.

Classification I

- Infrarenal—commonest. 95%.
- Suprarenal 5%.

Classification II

1. *Asymptomatic*: Found incidentally either on clinical examination or on angiography or on ultrasound. Repair is required if diameter is over 5.5 cm on ultrasound.
2. *Symptomatic without rupture*: Present as *back pain, abdominal pain, mass abdomen* which is smooth, soft, nonmobile, not moving with respiration, vertically placed above the umbilical level, pulsatile both in supine as well as knee-elbow position with same intensity, resonant on percussion. GIT, urinary, venous symptoms can also occur. Hypertension, diabetes, cardiac problems should be looked for and dealt with.
   Investigations
   - Blood urea, serum creatinine.
   - Ultrasound, aortogram.
   - DSA, CT scan, MRI.
   Treatment
   If aneurysm is *more than 5.5 cm then surgery is the choice*.
   Options are:
   Open surgical aneurysm repair using PTFE or dacron graft (Fig. 11.26).

But man is not made for defeat. A man can be destroyed but not defeated—**Ernest Hemingway**

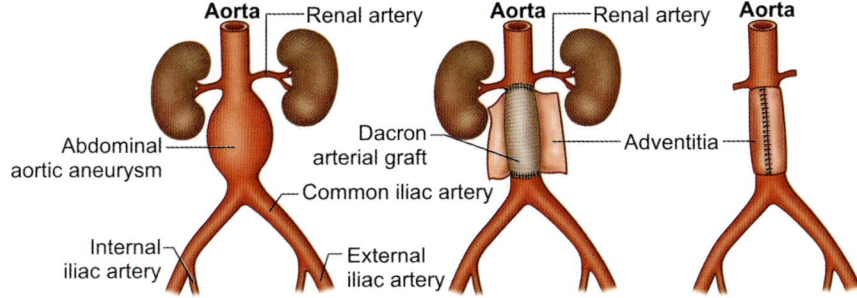

Fig. 11.26: Infrarenal aortic aneurysm repair. It is the commonest site of aortic aneurysm.

Endoluminal stent graft procedure using interventional radiology with Seldinger technique.

Adequate amount of blood is required for surgery.

3. **Symptomatic ruptured aortic aneurysm**: Risk of rupture is 1%, if diameter is within 5.5 cm in size. Risk increases to 20% once the diameter = 7 cm.

It may be *anterior rupture (20%)* into the free peritoneal cavity causing severe shock and very early *death*; or *posterior rupture (80%)* forming a *retroperitoneal hematoma* of large size causing severe back pain, hypotension, shock, absence of femoral pulses and with palpable mass in the abdomen.

Management

- Immediate diagnosis by ultrasound.
- Resuscitation.
- Massive blood transfusions (10–15 bottles).
- *Emergency surgery is the only life-saving procedure in these cases.*

Patient has to be shifted to the operation theater. Abdomen is opened. *Vascular clamps or bulldog* clamps are applied to the aorta above and below the aneurysm. Adventitia is opened and the clot is removed. Aneurysm is excised and the *arterial graft* either *PTFE (Polytetrafluoroethylene), knitted dacron graft, or woven dacron graft* is placed. The graft is sutured to the vessel above and below using monofilament, nonabsorbable suture material, polypropylene 5-zero.

Complications

- Hemorrhage, colonic ischemia.
- Renal failure, sexual dysfunction.
- Aortoduodenal fistula, aortovenacaval fistula.
- Graft leak, graft thrombosis, graft failure.
- Spinal cord ischemia.

PERIPHERAL ANEURYSMS (FIG. 11.27)

- *Peripheral aneurysms* are less common compared to aneurysms in the cavity. Such surface aneurysms are easily visible and amenable for clinical examination better. But same time it may be mistaken for abscess and inadvertent wrong attempt of incision and drainage can occur leading to disastrous consequences.
- Popliteal type is the *commonest* one. Brachial, radial, femoral and axillary are

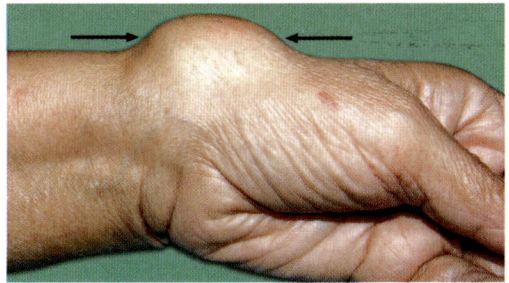

Fig. 11.27: Radial artery aneurysm.

People forget how fast you did the job, but they remember how well you did it.

other rarer sites. Expansile pulsation which is confirmed using two finger placement with thrill and bruit is typical. Infection, thrombosis make is less pulsatile mimicking an abscess.

- Erosion into adjacent bone and skin, rupture are known to occur. Distal emboli may lead into digital gangrene.
- Pressure on the affected artery proximally reduces the size, and eliminates the thrill/bruit; pressure distal to aneurysm causing prominence of the aneurysm swelling with bounding pulsation.
- X-ray, arterial Doppler, angiogram, echocardiogram are needed.
- *Treatment* is open repair using arterial graft or endovascular stenting.

Popliteal Aneurysm

- It is commonest (70%).
- 65% are bilateral.
- 25% cases are associated with abdominal aortic aneurysm.
- 75% causes complications in 5 years.

Presentations

1. *Swelling in popliteal region*, which is smooth, soft, pulsatile, well-localized, warm, compressible, often with thrill and bruit. *It may mimic a pyogenic abscess.*
2. *Thrombosis and emboli* from popliteal aneurysm can cause distal gangrene which may be spreading proximally and may lead to amputation.
3. *Rupture* may cause torrential hemorrhage.

Investigations

- Duplex scan; angiogram
- CT scan; MRI.

Treatment

- Aneurysmorrhaphy.
- Repair with arterial graft using PTFE, dacron.
- Endoluminal stenting.

DISSECTING ANEURYSM

It is the dissection of media of the aorta after splitting through intima creating a channel in the *media of* the vessel wall (Fig. 11.28).

Causes

- Hypertension (it is associated in 80% of dissecting aneurysms).
- Cystic medial necrosis.
- Trauma.
- Weakening of the elastic layers of the media due to shear forces.

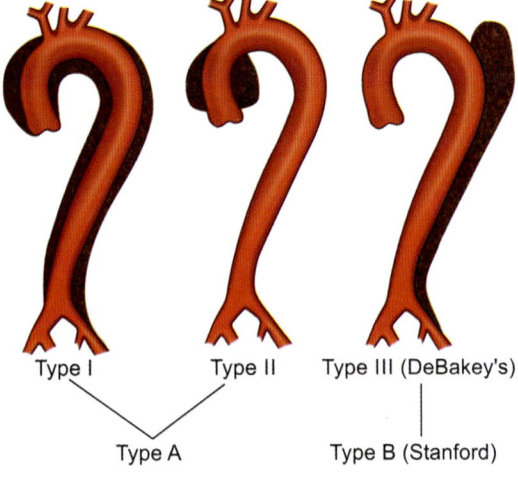

Fig. 11.28: Dissecting aneurysm.

Features

- It is always seen in thoracic aorta, common in ascending aorta (70%).
- It is uncommon in other parts of aorta or other vessels.
- It can occur in aortic arch or thoracic descending aorta.
- This dissected aortic channel gets lined by endothelium, often reopens distally into the aorta causing *double-barrelled aorta*, which in fact prevents complications.
- It is commonly associated with aortic insufficiency.
- Dissecting aneurysm is a misnomer. It is only aortic dissection.

Education is the passport to the future, for tomorrow belongs to those who prepare for it today—**Malcolm X**

- Atherosclerosis is not an usual cause for dissecting aneurysm.

Classification (DeBakey's)

Type I: Dissection begins in ascending aorta extends into descending thoracic aorta (70%).

Type II: Dissection origins and extends only up to the origin of the major vessels. It is safer type with less complications.

Type III: Dissection begins in the descending thoracic aorta beyond the origin of the left subclavian artery.

Dissecting aneurysm can be:
- Acute.
- Chronic.
- Healed dissecting aneurysm which communicates distally again to lumen of aorta forming a *double-barrelled aorta*.

Complications

- *Acute:* Rupture into the pericardium or pleura. Dangerous type.
- *Chronic:* Blockage of coronary vessels, major vessels like carotid, subclavian arteries. Aortic insufficiency.

Features

- Pain in the chest, and back, which is of excruciating type.
- Features of ischemia due to blockage of different vessels.
- **Investigations**
  - Chest X-ray shows mediastinal widening.
  - Arterial Doppler; angiogram.
- **Treatment**
  - Antihypertensives.
  - *Surgery*: Using dacron graft, reconstruction of aorta has to be done with cardiopulmonary bypass.

Indications for surgery
- Progressive disease.
- Significant ischemia.
- Impending rupture.

CAROTID ARTERY ANEURYSM (FIG. 11.29)

- It is common in carotid artery bulb; often extends into the internal carotid artery.
- It is 4% of peripheral aneurysms.

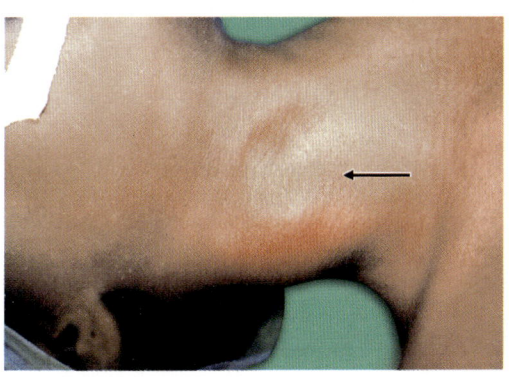

Fig. 11.29: Carotid artery aneurysm.

Causes

Atherosclerosis, trauma, syphilis, Marfan's syndrome, Ehler-Danos syndrome, congenital.

Features

- It is 10% bilateral.
- Presents as swelling in the neck at the level of thyroid cartilage below the angle of mandible which is—(expansile) pulsatile; smooth, soft, nontender, horizontally mobile with thrill on palpation and bruit on auscultation.
- In 50% of cases embolism with neurological features can develop.
- Hoarseness of voice, Horner's syndrome, dysphagia can present.

People seldom improve when they have no other model but themselves to copy after

Differential Diagnosis

- Abscess in the neck.
- Carotid body tumor.
- Neurofibroma arising from vagus.

Complications

Rupture, thrombosis, embolism, hemiplegia.

Investigations

Doppler neck; carotid angiogram, DSA, CT angiogram.

Treatment

- Removal of aneurysm with reconstruction of the artery with graft.
- Ligation of carotid artery as only as life-saving procedure but may lead into hemiplegia.
- Intravascular carotid stent placement.

GANGRENE

It is *macroscopic death* of tissue in situ (in continuity with adjacent viable tissue) with or without putrefaction.

It can occur in:
- Limbs (Fig. 11.30)
- Appendix
- Bowel
- Testes
- Gallbladder.

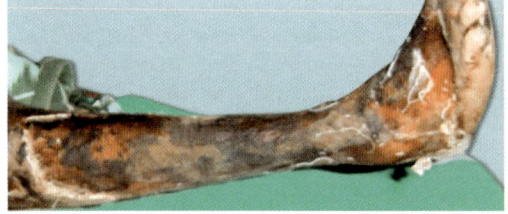

Fig. 11.30: Gangrene leg and foot.

Causes

- Secondary to arterial obstruction like atherosclerosis, emboli, diabetes, TAO, Raynaud's disease, ergots, etc.
- *Infective*: Boil, carbuncle, gas gangrene, Fournier's gangrene, cancrum oris.
- *Traumatic*: Direct, indirect.
- *Physical*: Burns, scalds, frostbite, chemicals, irradiation, electrical.
- Venous gangrene.

Clinical Features

- *Color changes*:
  Pallor, grayish, purple, brownish-black discoloration due to disintegration of hemoglobin to sulfide.
- *Absence of pulse*, loss of sensation, loss of function.
- *Line of demarcation* is visible between viable and dead tissue by a band of hyperemia and hyperesthesia with development of a layer of granulation tissue.
  - In dry gangrene separation occurs by aseptic ulceration with minimum infection. Gangrene is dry, and mummified.
  - In moist gangrene separation occurs by septic ulceration. Often demarcation is vague with *skip lesions* more proximally and so ending with higher level of amputations. Even after amputation skin flap may show *die back* process, leading to failure of take up of amputation flap and so requires still higher level of amputation.
- *Proximal ischemic features may be present* with rest pain, color changes, hyperesthesia—pregangrene.

Types of Gangrene

1. *Dry gangrene* is due to slow and gradual loss of blood supply to the part causing dry, desiccated, wrinkled, mummified part with proper line of demarcation (Fig. 11.31).
2. *Wet gangrene* is due to infection with putrefaction, causing proximally spreading, edematous, swollen, discoloration, with vague line of demarcation.

*An investment in knowledge pays the best interest—**Benjamin Franklin***

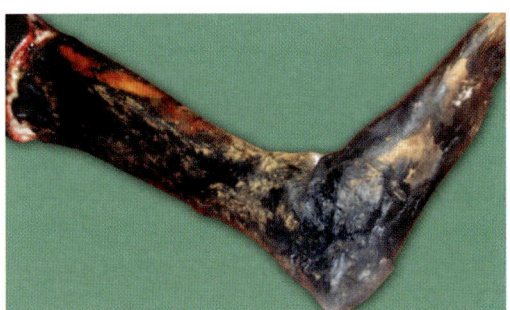

Fig. 11.31: Dry gangrene leg. Patient needed above knee amputation.

Investigations

- HB%, blood sugar.
- Arterial Doppler, angiogram (Seldinger technique).
- Ultrasound abdomen to find out the status of aorta.

Treatment

Limb-saving methods:
- Drugs: Antibiotics, vasodilators, Pentoxiphylline, Praxilene, Dipyridamole, small dose of Aspirin, Ticlopidine.
- Care of feet and toes:
  - The part has to be kept dry.
  - Any injury has to be avoided.
  - Proper footwear is advised [Microcellular rubber (MCR) footwear].
  - Measures for pain relief is taken.
  - Nutrition supplementation is done.
  - The limb should not be heated.
  - Pressure areas has to be protected.
  - Localized pus has to be removed.
- Cause has to be treated.
- Diabetes has to be controlled.
- Surgeries to improve the limb perfusion: Lumbar sympathectomy, omentoplasty, profundaplasty, femoropopliteal thrombectomy or endarterectomy, arterial graft bypass are done according to the need.

Life-saving procedures:
- Amputations may have to be done occasionally.
- *Level of amputation* is decided based on skin changes, temperature, line of demarcation, Doppler study.
1. *Below knee amputation* is a better option as BK prosthesis can be fitted better and also the movements of knee joint are retained. There is no need of external support and limp is absent.
2. In *above knee amputation* ranges of movements are less, limp is present, and often requires third (stick) support to walk.

Different amputations done are *Ray amputation*, below knee amputation (*Burgess amputation*), *Gritti-Stokes transcondylar amputation*, above knee amputation.

DIABETIC FOOT AND DIABETIC GANGRENE (FIG. 11.32)

Foot is a complex structure with many layers of muscles, ligaments, joints, arches, fat, thick plantar fascia, vascular arches, neurological system which maintains weight-bearing, gravity, normal walk (swing and stance phases).

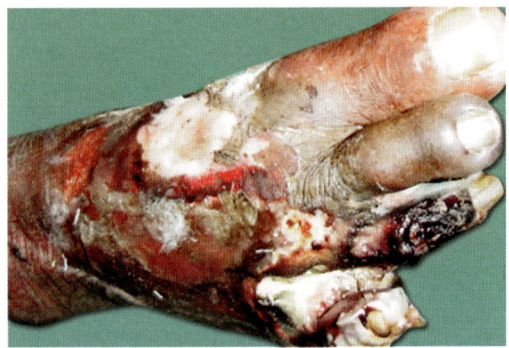

Fig. 11.32: Gangrene 3rd and 5th toes in a diabetic patient already underwent amputation of 4th toe earlier for gangrene.

Success is the ability to go from one failure to another with no loss of enthusiasm

Problems in Diabetic Foot

- Callosities, ulceration.
- Abscess and cellulitis of foot.
- Osteomyelitis of different bones of foot like metatarsals, cuneiforms, calcaneum.
- Diabetic gangrene.
- Arthritis of the joints.

Meggitt's classification of diabetic foot
Grade 0: Foot symptoms like pain only.
Grade 1: Superficial ulcers.
Grade 2: Deep ulcers.
Grade 3: Ulcer with bone involvement.
Grade 4: Forefoot gangrene.
Grade 5: Full foot gangrene.

Pathogenesis of Diabetic Foot/Gangrene (Fig. 11.33)

- High glucose level in tissues is a good culture media for bacteria. So infection is common.
- *Diabetic microangiopathy* causes blockade of microcirculation leading to hypoxia.
- *Diabetic neuropathy*: Due to sensory neuropathy, minor injuries are not noticed and so infection occurs. Due to motor neuropathy, dysfunction of muscles, arches of foot and joints, and loss of reflexes of foot occurs causing more prone for trauma, abscess, etc. Due to autonomic neuropathy, skin will be dry, causing defective skin barrier and so more prone for infection.
- *Diabetic atherosclerosis* itself reduces the blood supply and causes gangrene. Thrombosis can be precipitated by infection causing infective gangrene. Blockage occurs at plantar, tibial, and dorsalis pedis vessels.
- *Increased glycosylated hemoglobin* in blood causes defective oxygen dissociation leading to more hypoxia. At tissue level there will be increased glycosylated tissue protein, which prevents proper oxygen utilization and so aggravates hypoxia.

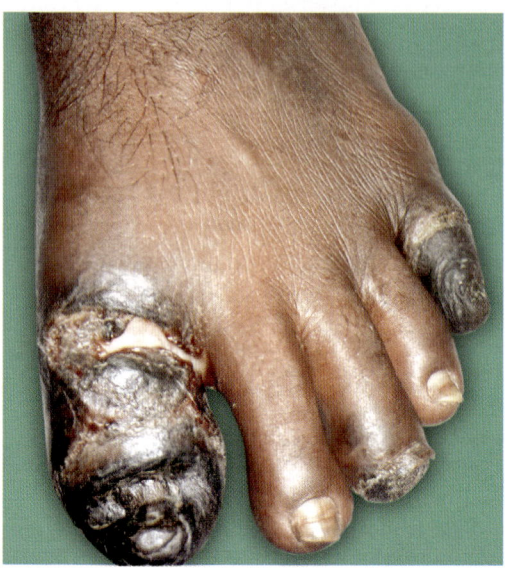

Fig. 11.33: Diabetic foot showing gangrene.

Clinical Features

- Pain in the foot.
- Ulceration.
- Absence of sensation.
- Absence of pulsations in the foot (posterior tibial and dorsalis pedis arteries).
- Loss of joint movements.
- Abscess formation.
- Change in temperature and color when gangrene sets in.

Investigations

- Blood sugar, urine ketone bodies.
- Blood urea and serum creatinine.
- X-ray of part to see osteomyelitis.
- Pus for culture and sensitivity.
- Doppler study of lower limb to assess arterial patency.
- Angiogram to see proximal blockage.
- Ultrasound abdomen to see status of abdominal aorta.

*Develop a passion for learning. If you do, you will never cease to grow—**Anthony J D'Angelo***

Treatment

Foot can be saved only if there is good blood supply.
* Antibiotics—decided by *pus C/S*.
* Regular dressing.
* Drugs: Vasodilators, Pentoxiphylline, Dipyridamole, small dose of Aspirin.
* Diabetes has to be controlled *by insulin only*.
* Diet control, control of obesity.
* Surgical debridement of wound.
* Amputations of the gangrenous area. If blood supply is not present, then below-knee or above-knee amputation may be required. Level of amputation is decided by skin and temperature changes or Doppler study.
* Care of feet in diabetic:
  - Any injury to feet has to be avoided.
  - MCR footwears must be used.
  - Feet have to be kept clean and dry, especially the toes and clefts.
  - Hyperkeratosis has to be avoided.

AINHUM (FIG. 11.34)

* Commonly affects males (can also occur in females).
* Common in blacks, in Negroes.
* History of running barefoot in childhood is common.
* *Fifth toe* is commonly affected.

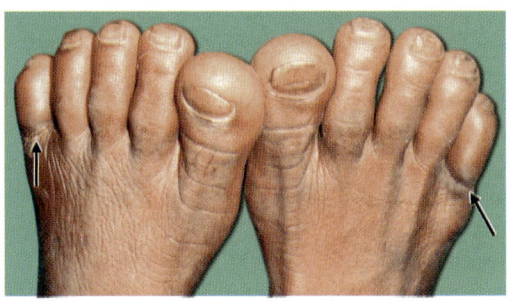

Fig. 11.34: Bilateral ainhum.

* A fissure develops in interphalangeal joint, which becomes a fibrous band, that encircles the digit causing necrosis (Gangrene of little toe).
* Often it can be bilateral.
* **Treatment**
  - If early 'Z' Plasty.
  - Amputation is often required later; Most often autoamputation occurs.

VASCULAR ANOMALIES

* It is a *collective term* used for hemangioma and vascular malformations.
* It can cause gigantism, bleeding, thrombosis, ulceration, thrombocytopenia, bone erosions, sepsis, and disfigurement.
* Doppler and CT or MR angiogram is very useful to identify type, extent, complication, feeding vessels.
* Many show self-involution.
* **Treatment:** Therapeutic embolization, laser therapy, ligation of feeding vessels. Cosmesis is important while treating. Excision and reconstruction is also done occasionally.

Hemangioma (Fig. 11.35)

* *Hemangioma* is a benign tumor containing hyperplastic endothelium with cellular proliferation with increased mast cells.
* It usually shows biphasic growth.
* It is the most common tumor in children (10% of deliveries). It is common in girls (3:1).
* It can be *capillary* or *cavernous* hemangiomas.
* It is common in skin and subcutaneous tissues but can occur anywhere in the body. It is common in head and neck region.
* It may be associated with ocular/visceral/intracranial anomalies, spinal dysraphism, hemangiomas in liver.
* It can cause ulceration, bleeding, thrombosis, sepsis, platelet trapping and thrombocytopenia.
* Bone erosions and skeletal changes can occur. Growth in tissue culture is observed.

Don't wait for your ship to come; swim out to it

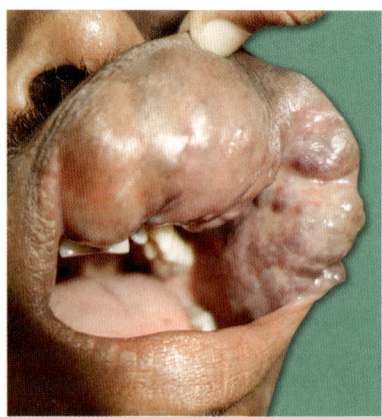

Fig. 11.35: Hemangioma lip—cavernous type. Note the bluish discoloration; it is compressible.

Vascular Malformations

* *Vascular malformations* are single layer endothelium lined spaces derived from arterial, capillary, venous or lymphatic system.
* There is no growth in tissue culture. Raise in mast cells is not seen.
* 90% cases are seen at birth; only few at later period. It is equal in both sexes (1:1).
* Quiescent endothelium with vessels showing progressive ectasia is the feature. Intravascular coagulation and mild thrombocytopenia can develop. Skeletal changes and over growth are common. Spontaneous involution is not common.
* Salmon patch and port wine stains are vascular malformations.
* Disfigurement, tissue destruction, deformity, dysfunction, telangiectasia, skin scarring—are common.

Note:
Hamartomata: Hamartano/hamartia means 'I miss' (Greek) or 'fault' or 'misfire'. Presently this term is not in use. It is benign lesion with aberrant differentiation producing a mass of disorganized but mature specialized cells or tissue indigenous to the particular site. It is tumor like overgrowth of tissue proper to the particular site.

CAPILLARY VASCULAR MALFORMATIONS

Types

* *Salmon patch (Fig. 11.36):*
  Present at birth. Usually on face, scalp, limb. Often involves wide area of skin. With age it goes for spontaneous regression and disappears completely. Hence, *masterly inactivity* is adviced. It is also called as stork bite or naevus simplex.
* *Port-wine stain (Nevus flammeus):*
  Present at birth and persists throughout life without any changes. No spontaneous regression. It presents as reddish-blue, warm area commonly on face. Often it is nodular. *It requires cosmetic coverage, excision and grafting or laser ablation.*

CAPILLARY HEMANGIOMA (Strawberry Hemangioma) (FIG. 11.37)

* Child is normal at birth. Between 1 and 3 weeks it appears as red mark which rapidly increases in 3 months to form strawberry or raspberry hemangioma which *contains immature vasoformative tissues.*

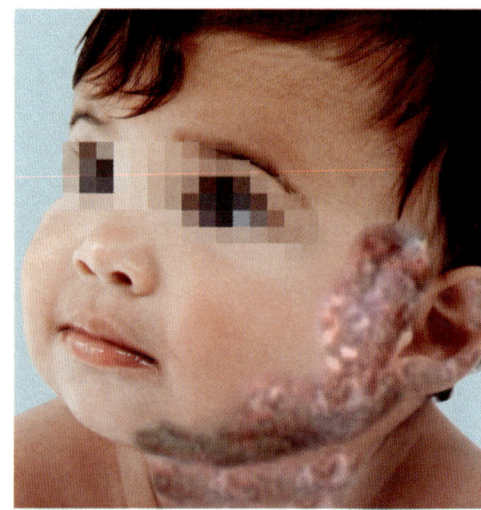

Fig. 11.36: Capillary hemangioma—Salmon patch in an infant.

CAVERNOUS HEMANGIOMA

- It is present at birth and consists of a multiple venous channels.
- Its size increases gradually and may cause problems.
- It often contains feeding vessels which is of surgical importance.
- **Sites:** Face, limbs, liver and other internal organs (Figs. 11.38 and 11.39).

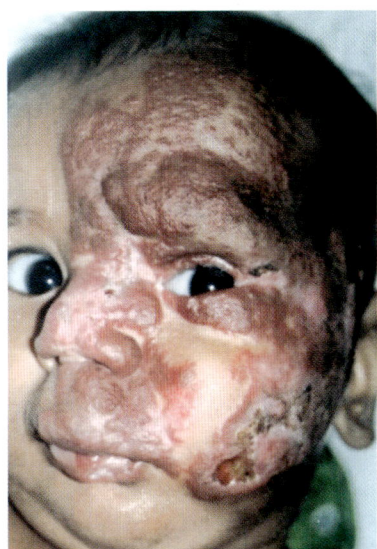

Fig. 11.37: Hemangioma in a child involving face extensively.

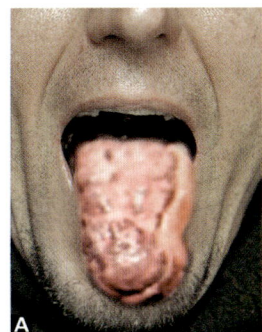 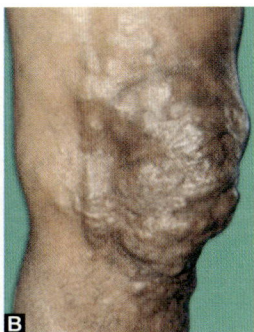

Figs. 11.38A and B: Cavernous hemangioma over (A) Tongue; (B) Knee.

- It is clinically warm, compressible, and bluish in color.
- History of bleeding after minor trauma.
- It involves skin, subcutaneous tissue and often muscle also.
- After one year of age, it slowly involutes and by 7–8 years it disappears completely (commonly).

Treatment
- Allow for spontaneous regression.
- Otherwise by **laser therapy**.
- CO_2 snow therapy.
- Sclerosant therapy.

Associated syndromes

- **Klippel-Trenauny-Weber syndrome:** Nevus flammeus + osteohypertrophy of extremities + AV fistula.
- **Kasabach-Merritt syndrome:** Capillary hemangioma + DIC (Disseminated intravascular coagulation).
- **Sturge-Weber syndrome:** Hemangiomas + hemiplegia and epilepsy (Calcified vascular cerebral and meningeal deposits) + glaucoma.
- **Maffucci syndrome:** Cavernous hemangioma + dyschondroplasia.

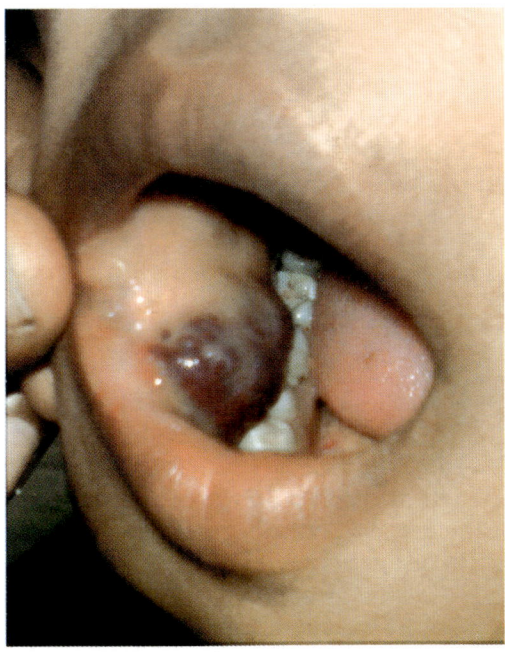

Fig. 4.39: Hemangioma cheek.

Today well lived makes every yesterday, a dream of happiness and tomorrow, a vision of hope

- **Features:** Smooth, bluish, well-localized, soft, compressible, warm swelling from skin and subcutaneous tissue.
- **Complications**
  - Hemorrhage.
  - DIC.
  - Thrombosis.
  - Infection and septicemia.
  - Erosion into the adjacent bone.
- **Investigations**
  - Ultrasound; Doppler.
  - Angiogram to find out feeding vessel.
  - Platelet count.
- **Treatment**
  - Ligation of feeding artery.
  - Therapeutic embolization.
  - If small in accessible area then excision.
  - Sclerosant therapy.
  - Laser ablation.

CIRSOID ANEURYSM

- It is a rare variant of capillary hemangioma occurring in skin, beneath which abnormal artery communicates with the distended veins.
- Commonly seen in superficial *temporal artery* and its branches.
- Often the underlying bone gets thinned out due to pressure.
- Sometimes extends into the cranial cavity.
- Ulceration is the eventual problem which will lead on to uncontrollable hemorrhage.

Features

- Pulsatile swelling in relation to superficial temporal artery, which is warm, compressible, with arterialization of adjacent veins and with bone thickening (due to erosion).
- **Investigations**
  - Doppler study.
  - CT scan; angiogram.
  - X-ray of the part.

Treatment

- Ligation of feeding artery and excision of lesion, often requires preliminary ligation of external carotid artery.
- Intracranial extension requires formal neurosurgical approach.

ARTERIOVENOUS FISTULA

Arteriovenous Fistula (AVF) is a type of **arteriovenous malformations.**

Types	
• Congenital.	• Traumatic.

CONGENITAL AVF (FIGS. 11.40A AND B)

During developmental period AV communications occur.

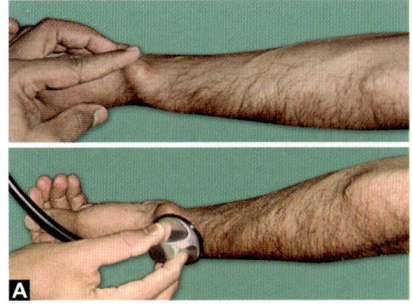

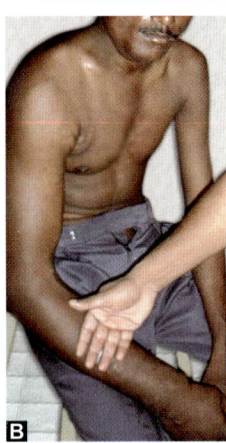

Figs. 11.40A and B: Acquired and congenital arteriovenous fistula.

Health is the greatest gift, contentment the greatest wealth, faithfulness the best relationship—Buddha

Sites

- Limbs either part or whole of the limb. Part may be in toes or fingers.
- Lungs.
- Brain in circle of Willis.
- Other organs like bowel, liver.

Clinical Features

Structural changes in the limb:
- Limb is *lengthened* due to increase blood flow since developmental period (Fig. 11.41).
- Limb *girth* also increased.
- Limb is *warm*.
- *Continuous thrill and continuous machinery murmur* all over the lesion.
- *Dilated arterialized varicose veins* are seen due to increased blood flow and due to valvular incompetence.

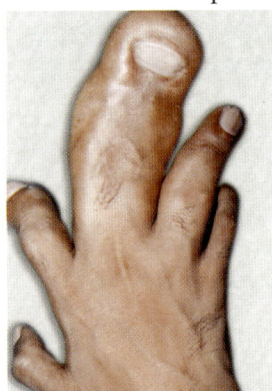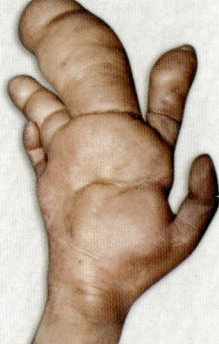

Fig. 11.41: Hypertrophic changes due to AV malformation.

- Often there will be *bone erosion* or extension of AVF into the bone as such.

Physiological changes: Because of the hyperdynamic circulation, there will be *increased cardiac output* and so often *congestive cardiac failure*.

Complications

Hemorrhage; thrombosis; cardiac failure.

Investigations

Angiogram (Fig. 11.42); Doppler study; X-ray of the part.

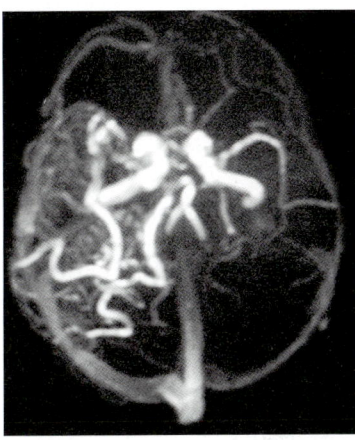

Fig. 11.42: MR angiogram of AV malformation in cranial cavity.

Treatment

- Avoid injury.
- Ligation of feeding artery.
- Sclerosant therapy.
- Therapeutic embolization.
- Amputation when required (only) as life-saving procedure.

ACQUIRED AVF (FIG. 11.43)

Causes

1. Trauma in:
   a. Femoral region.
   b. Popliteal region.
   c. Brachial region.
   d. Wrist.
   e. Aorta venacaval.
   f. Abdomen: It may be following road traffic accidents, penetrating wounds, cock-fight injury ! (common in South India).
2. After vascular surgical intervention for major vessels.

He who attempts the absurd can achieve the impossible

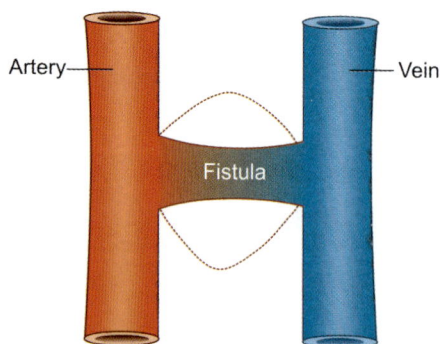

Fig. 11.43: AV fistula.

3. Therapeutic: For renal dialysis, AVF is created (**cimino fistula**) to achieve arterialization of veins and also to have hyperdynamic circulation. So as to have easy adequate venous access for long time *hemodialysis*.

Common sites are *wrist, brachial, and femoral* region.

Pathophysiology

❖ **Physiological changes:** *Cardiac failure due to hyperdynamic circulation.*
❖ **Structural changes**:
  – **Changes at the level of fistula:** Blood flows from high pressure artery to low pressure vein causing diversion of most of the blood. Between the artery and vein, at the site of fistula, dilatation develops along with fibrous sac formation called as *aneurysmal sac*. This presents as warm, pulsatile, smooth, soft, compressible swelling at the site with *continuous thrill and continuous machinery murmur*. It is warm at the site.
  – **Changes below the level of the fistula**: Because of diversion of arterial blood *distal part becomes ischemic*. Because of high pressure *veins become arterialized*, with valvular incompetence causing *varicose veins*.
  – **Changes proximal to the fistula:** *Hyperdynamic circulation* causing cardiac failure.
    If pressure is applied to the artery proximal to the fistula, swelling will reduce in size, thrill and bruit will disappear, pulse rate and pulse pressure becomes normal. This is called as *Nicoladoni's sign or Branhan's sign*.
    Cardiac failure may be very severe in traumatic AVF (often resistant to drug therapy).

Investigations

❖ Doppler; angiogram.
❖ Electrocardiogram; echocardiography.

Treatment

❖ **Excision** of fistula and **reconstruction** of artery and vein with graft (Fig. 11.44).
❖ In emergency situation, **quadruple ligation**, i.e. both artery and vein above and below should be ligated without touching the fistula and sac. Patient recovers well from cardiac failure (Fig. 11.45).
❖ Therapeutic embolization may be tried.

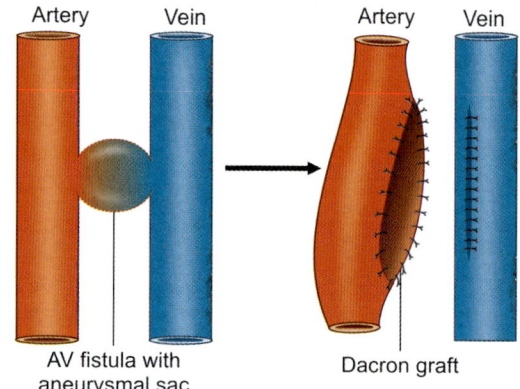

Fig. 11.44: Reconstruction of AV fistula using graft.

*The mind is everything. What you think you become—**Buddha***

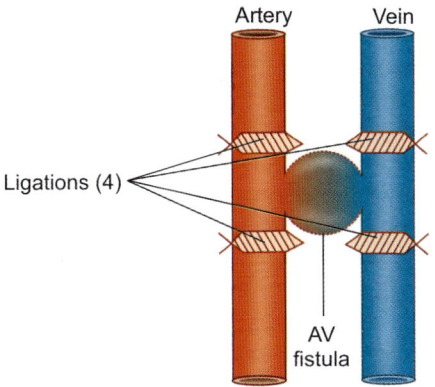

Fig. 11.45: Quadruple ligation of AV fistula.

Note:
Hunter's ligation should be avoided: It is used as life-saving measure because it invariably causes limb ischemia and gangrene even though patient recovers from cardiac failure. It is ligation of only artery proximally so as to make cardiac function normal. But it invariably steals the blood from the limb leading to gangrene.

CHAPTER 12

Venous Diseases

Chapter Outline

- Anatomy of Veins of Lower Limb
- Physiology of Venous Blood Flow in Lower Limb
- Deep Vein Thrombosis
- Varicose Veins
- Venous Ulcer
- Thrombophlebitis
- Anticoagulants

ANATOMY OF VEINS OF LOWER LIMB

DEEP VEINS

1. Tibial, popliteal, femoral veins are called as *'veins of conduits'* which drain blood into iliac veins and then to inferior vena cava (IVC).
2. **Pumping veins**: They are venous sinuses existing in the calf muscles, which pump blood towards major veins. They are better termed as *musculovenous pumps*. They are also called as the *peripheral heart*.

SUPERFICIAL VEINS (FIG. 12.1)

- ❖ *Great (Long) saphenous vein (GSV/LSV)*: The GSV originates from dorsal venous arch of the first toe (great toe), after passing anterior to the medial malleolus, it runs up the medial side of the leg. At the knee, it runs over the posterior border of the medial epicondyle of the femur, coursing laterally to lie on the anterior surface of the

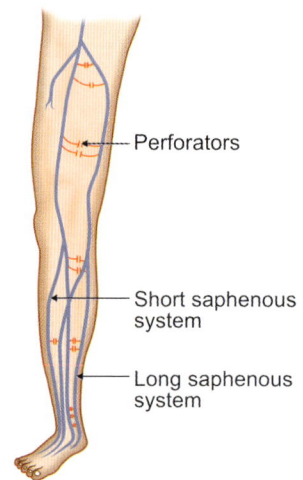

Fig. 12.1: Anatomy—veins of lower limb.

thigh before entering an opening in the fascia lata called the saphenous opening. It joins with the femoral vein at femoral triangle as saphenofemoral junction (SFJ). Tributaries of GSV are posterior arch vein, anterolateral vein, posteromedial vein

*Life lived for others is a life worthwhile—**Albert Einstein***

and accessory vein. It is accompanied by saphenous nerve in the leg. It has got 3–13 valves (Fig. 12.2A).

- **Small (short/lesser) saphenous vein (SSV):** It originates from lateral aspect of the foot along the 5th toe from dorsal venous arch, runs upwards along the posterior and lateral aspect of the leg, in between two heads of gastrocnemius muscle joining the popliteal vein at or above the knee joint level. It may join the popliteal vein at different levels as variation or join great saphenous vein or Giacomini vein. It is superficial vein located in subcutaneous plane in saphenous fascia. Vein accompanies the sural nerve. Number of valves in SSV is 1–8 (Fig. 12.2B).

Superficial veins have got multiple valves, which facilitates blood flow towards heart. Superficial veins usually drain about 10% of lower limb blood, i.e. from skin and subcutaneous tissues.

PERFORATOR VEINS (FIG. 12.2C)

They are the veins, which connect superficial to deep veins at various levels. They travel from superficial fascia through an opening in the deep fascia before entering the deep veins. The direction of flow of blood here is from superficial to deep veins. These perforators are also guarded by valves so that the blood flow is unidirectional, i.e. towards deep veins. Reversal of flow occurs due to incompetence of perforator, which will lead to *varicose veins*.

Types

1. Ankle perforators.
2. Lower leg perforators.
3. Gastrocnemius perforators (of Boyd).
4. Mid-thigh perforators.
5. Hunter's perforator in the thigh.

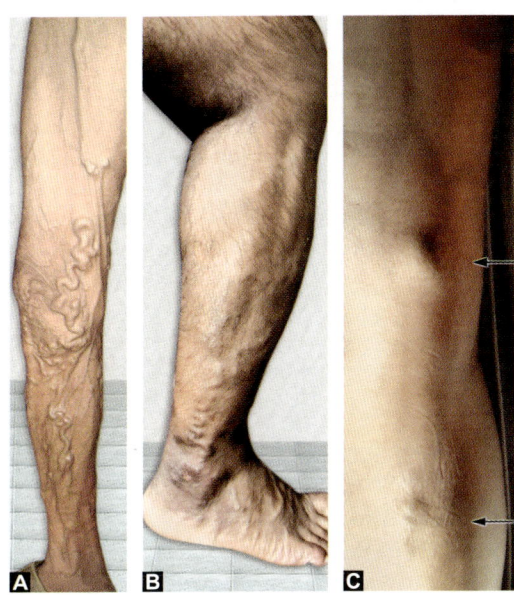

Figs. 12.2A to C: (A) Great saphenous vein varicosity; (B) Small saphenous vein varicosity; (C) Perforator incompetence (blow-outs).

PHYSIOLOGY OF VENOUS BLOOD FLOW IN LOWER LIMB

- Veins are thin-walled vessels with collapsible walls that assume an elliptical configuration in collapsed state and circular configuration in the filled state.
- Venous valves are abundant in the distal lower extremity and the number of valves decreases proximally, with no valves in superior and inferior vena cava.

Factors Affecting the Venous Return

- Arterial pressure across the capillary increases the pumping action of vein.
- **Calf musculovenous pump:** During contraction phase of walking, pressure in the calf muscles increases to 200–300 mm Hg. This pumps the blood towards the heart. During relaxation phase of walking, pressure in the calf falls and so it allows blood to flow from superficial to deep

Take time to read; it is the foundation to wisdom

veins through perforators. Normally while walking, pressure in the superficial system at the level of ankle is 20 mm Hg.
- During walking, foot pump mechanism propels blood from plantar veins into the leg.
- Gravity.

Factors responsible for venous return

- Negative pressure in thorax.
- Peripheral pump—calf muscle.
- Vis-a-tergo of adjoining muscle.
- Non-refluxing valves in course of veins.

DEEP VEIN THROMBOSIS

Deep vein thrombosis (DVT) is formation of *blood clot* in the deep venous system due to varied causes; it is common in iliofemoral/femoropopliteal and soleal (leg) veins. But venous thrombosis can also occur in pelvic veins and upper limb (axillary vein).

Etiology

Factors:

Virchow's triad

1. Stasis.   3. Vein wall injury.
2. Hypercoagulability.

Causes

- Following childbirth.
- Trauma.
- Muscular violence.
- Immobility.
- Debilitating illness, obesity, immobility, bed rest, pregnancy, puerperium, oral contraceptives, and estrogens.
- Postoperative thrombosis: Common after the age of 40 years. Incidence following surgeries is 30%. In 30% of cases both legs are affected. Usually seen after prostate surgery, hip surgery, major abdominal surgeries, gynecological surgeries, and cancer surgeries. Bedridden for more than 3 days in the postoperative period increases the risk of DVT.
- *Spontaneous thrombosis* is common in visceral neoplasm like carcinoma pancreas or carcinoma stomach. It is often migrating type.
- Thrombus may start in a venous tributary, which eventually may extend into the main vein causing DVT.
- *Axillary vein thrombosis* can occur spontaneously, following compression by cervical rib, by various causes of thoracic inlet syndrome, or arm being in the hyperabducted state for prolonged period (e.g. painting the ceiling), after axillary lymph node block dissection, after radiotherapy to axilla, occasionally as a complication of venous cannulation.
- Polycythemia vera, thrombocytosis.
- Deficiencies of antithrombin III, protein C, protein S.

Sites

- Pelvic veins—common.
- Leg veins—common in femoral and popliteal veins (common on left side) (Fig. 12.3).
- Upper limb veins—not uncommon (axillary vein thrombosis).

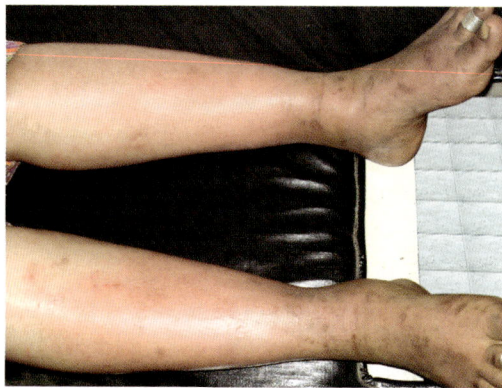

Fig. 12.3: Deep vein thrombosis (DVT) both legs.

*Old words are reborn with new faces—**Crissjami***

Phlegmasia alba dolens: It is DVT of *femoral vein* (deep femoral vein commonly) causing painful congestion and edema of leg, with lymphangitis, which further increases the edema and worsens the situation (*White leg*).

Phlegmasia cerulea dolens: It is extensive DVT of *iliac and pelvic veins* causing *blue leg* with either venous gangrene or areas of infarction.

Clinical Features

- Pain and swelling in the calf and thigh (often). Commonly associated with fever. Pain is often so severe that the patient finds difficult to flex (or move) the leg.
- Leg is tense, tender, warm, pale or bluish with stretched and shiny skin.
- **Positive Homan's sign**: Passive forceful dorsiflexion of the foot with extended knee causes tenderness in the calf.
- **Mose's sign**: Gentle squeezing of lower part of the calf from side to side is painful. Gentleness is very important otherwise it may dislodge a thrombus to form an embolus.
- Most often, DVT is *asymptomatic* and presents suddenly with *features of pulmonary embolism like chest pain, breathlessness and hemoptysis*.

Investigations

- Venous Doppler.
- Duplex scanning.
- Venogram.
- Radioactive I^{125} fibrinogen study.
- Hemogram with platelet count.

Treatment

- Rest, elevation of limb, bandaging the whole limb with crepe bandages.
- Anticoagulants: Heparin, warfarin, phenindione.
- For *fixed thrombus:* Initially high dose of heparin of 25,000 units/day for 7 days has to be given. Then later patient is advised to continue with warfarin for 6 months. Low molecular weight heparin (LMWH) can also be used. Dose is controlled by assessment of *activated partial thromboplastin time (APTT)*. Duration of heparin treatment is usually for 5 days.
- For *free thrombus: Fibrinolysins*—streptokinase or urokinase or tissue plasminogen activator are used to dissolve thrombus (it should not be given when patient is on heparin).
- Venous thrombectomy is done using Fogarty venous balloon catheter.
- Thrombotic emboli is prevented from reaching the heart by filtering it at inferior vena cava (IVC) level using Kim ray Greenfield filter, suture sieve plication, stapler plication, vena caval ligation, Mobin Uddin umbrella filter.

Note: Streptokinase is derived from streptococci. Urokinase is derived from human urine.

Prevention of DVT

- Care to be taken to see for proper positioning of legs with no pressure on the calf muscles.
- Pressure bandage to the legs has to be applied during major surgeries, and laparoscopic surgeries. During postoperative period, elevation, massaging, pressure bandage, early ambulation, maintaining hydration are essential measures.
- Low dose heparin/low molecular weight heparin is given in suspected cases, in major surgeries and continued during postoperative period till the patient is ambulated. 5000 units is given subcutaneous 2 hours before surgery.
- Various measures like graduated static compression, elastic stockings, electrical stimulation of calf muscles, pneumatic compression are used to prevent sluggish flow of blood.

Observation is the best teacher

❖ Dextran 70, intravenously 500 mL during surgery and another 500 mL postoperatively in 24 hours can also be used to prevent DVT.

Effects and sequelae of DVT

- Pulmonary embolism—15%.
- Infection; Venous gangrene.
- Partial recanalization, chronic venous hypertension around the ankle region causing venous ulcers.
- Recurrent DVT—30%.

VARICOSE VEINS

They are *dilated, tortuous, elongated veins in the leg* (Fig. 12.4). There is reversal of blood flow through its faulty valves.

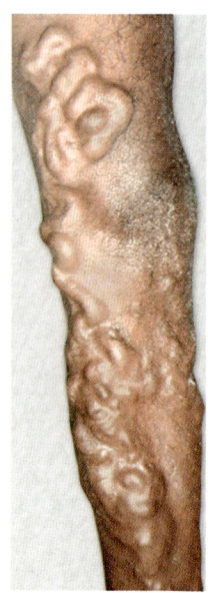

Fig. 12.5: Long saphenous vein varicosity.

Types

❖ *Long saphenous vein varicosity* (Fig. 12.5).
❖ *Short saphenous vein varicosity* (Fig. 12.6).
❖ Varicose veins due to *perforator incompetence*.

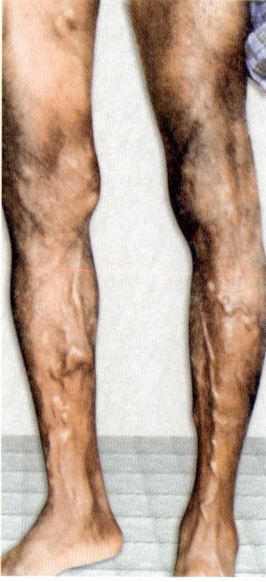

Fig. 12.4: Varicose veins in lower limbs. Note the bilateral long saphenous vein varicosity.

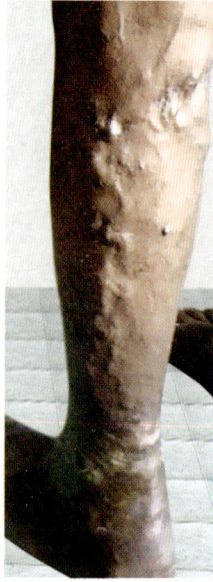

Fig. 12.6: Short saphenous vein varicosity.

❖ *Thread veins (or dermal flares)*: These are small varices in the skin usually around ankle, which look like dilated, red or purple network of veins.

Out of suffering have emerged the strongest souls; the most massive characters are searched with scars— **Kalil Gibran**

❖ *Reticular varices*: These are slightly larger varices than thread veins located in subcutaneous region.
❖ Combinations of any of above.

Pathogenesis

Theories
1. Fibrin cuff theory.
2. White cell trapping theory.

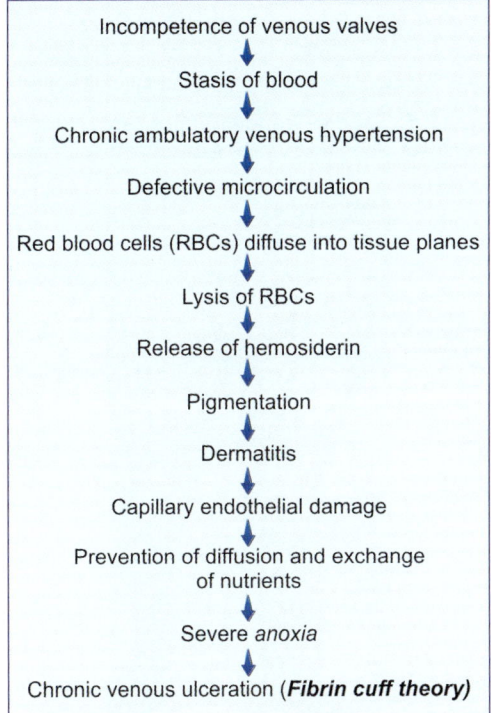

Inappropriate activation of trapped leukocytes release proteolytic enzymes, which causes cell destruction and ulceration—**White cell trapping theory**. Fibrin deposition, tissue death, scarring occurs together, called as *lipodermatosclerosis*.

Etiology of Varicose Veins

Varicosities are more common in lower limb because of erect posture and long column of blood has to be supported which can lead to weakness and incompetence of valves.

Primary Varicosities

Due to:
❖ Congenital incompetence or absence of valves.
❖ Weakness or wasting of muscles.
❖ Stretching of deep fascia.

Secondary Varicosities

❖ Recurrent thrombophlebitis.
❖ Occupational—standing for long hours.
❖ Obstruction to venous return like abdominal tumor, retroperitoneal fibrosis, lymphadenopathy.
❖ Pregnancy (due to progesterone hormone).
❖ Atriovenous (AV) malformations—congenital or acquired.
❖ Iliac vein thrombosis.

Sites where varicosities can occur
• Lower limb.
• Pampiniform plexus of veins in scrotum.
• Vulva.
• Sites of portosystemic anastomosis.

CEAP classification of lower limb varicose veins (2004)
CEAP Classification
C – *Clinical* signs (grade 0–6); (A) for asymptomatic or (S) for symptomatic presentation
E – *Etiological* classification—congenital (Ec), primary (Ep), secondary (Es), no venous etiology (En)
A – *Anatomic* distribution—superficial (As), deep (Ad) or perforator (Ap), no venous location identified (An)
P – *Pathophysiologic* dysfunction—reflux (Pr), obstructive (Po), both, or no pathophysiology identified (Pn)
Grading of clinical signs (C)
0 – No visible or palpable signs of venous diseases
1 – Telangiectases, reticular veins or malleolar flare
2 – Varicose veins
3 – Edema without skin changes
Contd...

A good head and an industrious hand are worth gold in any land.

Contd...

4 – Skin changes due to venous diseases like pigmentation, eczema or lipodermatosclerosis
4a – pigmentation; 4b – lipodermatosis, atrophia blanche
5 – Skin changes as above with healed ulceration
6 – Skin changes as above with active ulceration
Anatomical distribution (A)
As – superficial system:
1 – Telangiectasis, reticular veins
2 – Great saphenous vein above the knee – ostial and preterminal
3 – Great saphenous vein below the knee
4 – Small saphenous vein
5 – Nonsaphenous – 43%
Ad – deep system:
   From 6 to 16
Ap – perforator system
   17 – Perforator vein (PV) of the thigh
   18 – Perforator (PV) of the calf and leg
An – no anatomical lesion identified

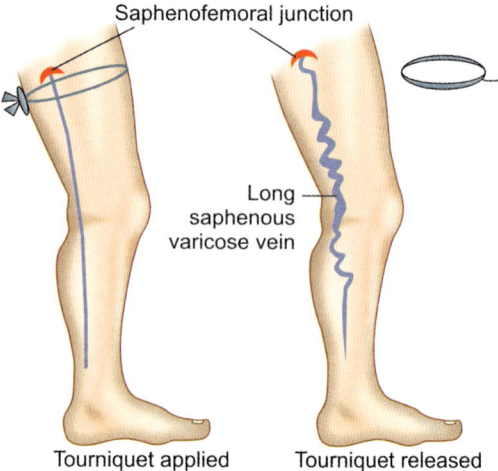

Fig. 12.7: Brodie-Trendelenburg test. Note the reversal of blood flow while releasing the tourniquet.

Clinical Features

It is more common in females (10:1). It is much more common in females with a family history. Often it is familial. *Familial varicose veins* begins in younger age group, seen bilaterally, involves all veins including deep veins.

- Visible dilated veins in the leg with pain, distress, nocturnal cramps, feeling of heaviness, pruritus.
- Pedal edema, pigmentation, dermatitis, ulceration, tenderness, and restricted ankle joint movement.
- Bleeding, thickening of tibia occurs due to periostitis.
- Positive cough impulse at the saphenofemoral junction.
- ***Brodie-Trendelenburg test (Figs. 12.7 and 12.8)***
  - Vein is emptied by elevating the limb and a tourniquet is tied just below the saphenofemoral junction (or using thumb, saphenofemoral junction is occluded). Patient is asked to stand quickly. When tourniquet or thumb is released, rapid filling from above

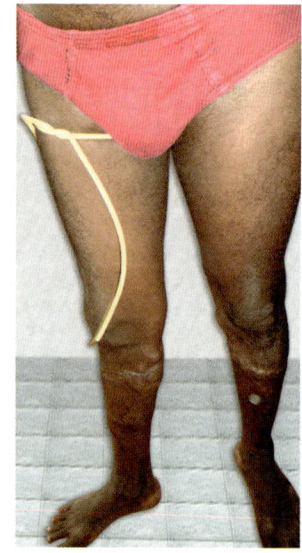

Fig. 12.8: Tourniquet test for varicose vein.

signifies saphenofemoral incompetence. *This is Trendelenburg test I.*
  - In *Trendelenburg test II*, after standing tourniquet is not released. Filling of blood from below upwards rapidly can be observed within 30–60 seconds. It signifies perforator incompetence.

Beauty is not in the face, beauty is a light in the heart— **Kalil Gibran**

- **Perthe's test**:
 The affected lower limb is wrapped with elastic bandage and the patient is asked to walk around and exercise. Development of severe cramp like pain in the calf signifies DVT.
- **Modified Perthe's test**:
  - Tourniquet is tied just below the saphenofemoral junction without emptying the vein. Patient is allowed to have a *brisk* walk, which precipitates *bursting pain* in the calf and also makes superficial veins more prominent. It signifies DVT.
  - DVT is contraindicated for any surgical intervention of superficial varicose veins. It is also contraindicated for sclerosant therapy.
- **Three-tourniquet test**:
 To find out the site of incompetent perforator, three tourniquets are tied after emptying the vein.
  - At saphenofemoral junction.
  - Above-knee level.
  - Another below knee level.

  Patient is asked to stand and looked for filling of veins and site of filling. Then tourniquets are released from below upwards to again see for incompetent perforators.
- **Schwartz test**:
 In standing position, when lower part of the vein in leg is tapped, impulse is felt at the saphenous junction or at the upper end of the visible part of the vein. It signifies continuous column of blood due to valvular incompetence.
- **Pratt's test**:
 Esmarch bandage is applied to the leg from below upwards with a tourniquet at saphenofemoral junction. After that the bandage is released to see the '*blow outs*' as perforators.
- **Morrissey's cough impulse test**:
 The varicose veins are emptied. The leg is elevated and then the patient is asked to cough. If there is saphenofemoral incompetence, expansile impulse is felt at saphenous opening.
- **Fegan's test**:
 On standing, the site where the perforators enter the deep fascia bulges and this is marked. Then on lying down, button like depression in the deep fascia is felt at the marked out points, which confirms the site of perforator.
- Examination of the abdomen is done to look for pelvic tumors, lymph nodes, etc. which may compress over the veins to cause varicosity.

Clinical tests for varicose veins

- Cough impulse test.
- Brodie-Trendelenburg test.
- Modified Perthe's test.
- Three-tourniquet test.
- Fegan's test.

Investigations

- ***Venous Doppler***
 It is done with the patient standing; the Doppler probe is placed at saphenofemoral junction and later wherever required (Fig. 12.9). Basically by hearing

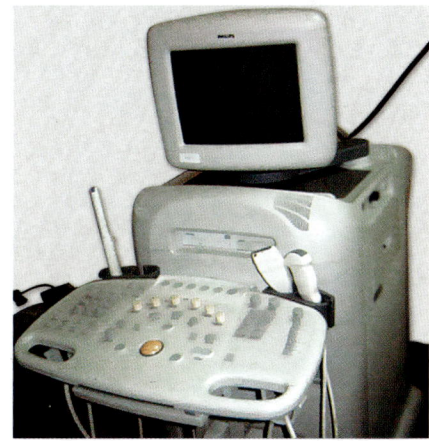

Fig. 12.9: Doppler machine. Doppler is good investigation for venous diseases.

A man who is proud of this money rarely has anything else to be proud of the changes in sound venous flow, venous patency, and venous reflux can be very well-identified.

* **Duplex scan (Figs. 12.10A and B)**
It is a highly reliable ultrasound Doppler imaging technique (here high resolution B mode ultrasound imaging and Doppler ultrasound is used) which along with direct visualization of veins, gives the functional and anatomical information, and also color map. Examination is done in standing and lying down position and also with Valsalva maneuver. Hand held Doppler probe is placed over the site and visualized for any block and reversal of flow. DVT is very well-identified by this method.

* **Venography**:
Ascending venography was very common investigation done before Doppler period. A tourniquet is applied above the malleoli and the vein of dorsal venous arch of foot is cannulated. Water-soluble dye injected, flows into the deep veins (because of the applied tourniquet). X-rays are taken below and above knee level.

Any block in deep veins, its extent, perforator status can be made out by this.

It is a good reliable investigation for DVT.

If DVT is present, surgery or sclerotherapy are contraindicated.

Descending venogram is done when ascending venogram is not possible and also to visualize incompetent veins. Here contrast material is injected into the femoral vein through a cannula in standing position. X-ray pictures are taken to visualize deep veins and incompetent veins.

* **Plethysmography.**
* **Ambulatory venous pressure**.
* **Arm-foot venous pressure** (foot pressure is not more than 4 mm Hg above the arm pressure).
* **Other investigations: Ultrasound abdomen**, peripheral smear, platelet count, and other relevant investigations are done depending on the cause of the varicose veins. If venous ulcer is present, then the discharge is collected for culture and sensitivity, biopsy from ulcer edge is taken to rule out Marjolin's ulcer, plain X-ray of the part is done to find out periostitis.

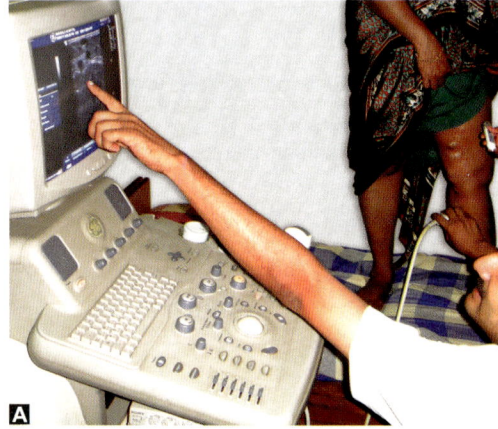
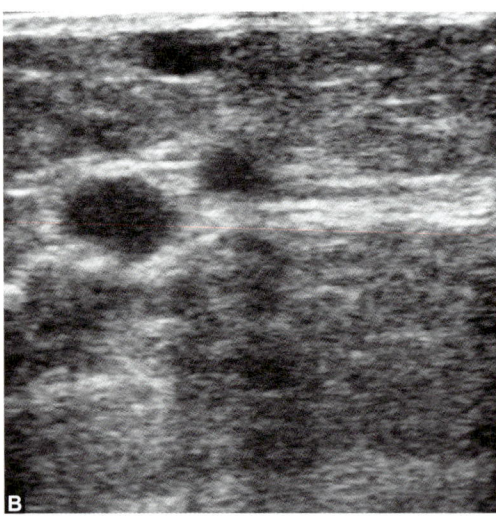

Figs. 12.10A and B: Duplex scan for venous diseases of lower limb should also be done in standing position.

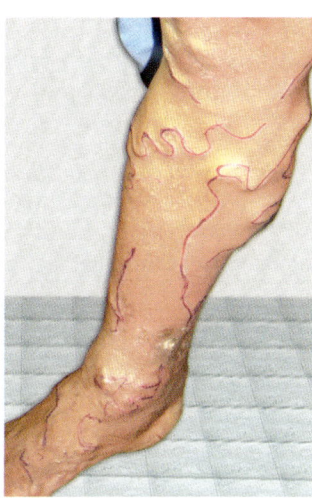

Fig. 12.11: Veins should be marked just prior to surgery using marking ink.

Note: Venous hemodynamic mapping (VHM) should be done; all veins and perforators should be marked prior to surgery (Fig. 12.11).

Treatment

Indications for intervention
• Cosmesis.
• Severe recurrent leg pain.
• Complications.

1. **Conservative treatment**
   - Elastic crepe bandage application from below upwards or use of pressure stockings to the limb (Fig. 12.12).
   - Diosmin therapy, which increases the venous tone.
   - Elevation of the limb.

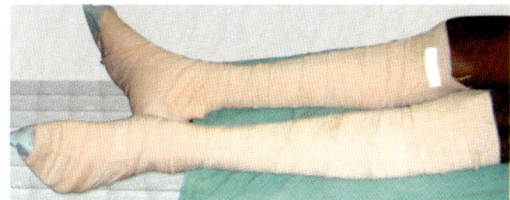

Fig. 12.12: Crepe bandages applied to both legs in bilateral varicose veins.

2. ***Injection—sclerotherapy*** (Fegan's technique).

By injecting sclerosants into the vein, complete sclerosis of the venous walls can be achieved.

Indications
- Uncomplicated perforator incompetence.
- In the management smaller varices.
- Recurrent varices.

Sclerosants used are
• Sodium tetradecyl sulphate 3% (STDS).
• Sodium morrhuate.
• Ethanolamine oleate.
• Polidocanal.

Mechanisms of action
- Causes aseptic inflammation leading to thrombosis.
- Causes perivenous fibrosis leading to block.
- Causes approximation of intima leading to obliteration.

After emptying, with the patient sitting down and the leg horizontal, a 23-gauge needle is inserted into the vein. 0.5 mL of sclerosant is injected into the vein and immediately compression is applied on the vein (to prevent the entry of blood which may cause thrombosis, which in turn gets recanalized later, thereby further worsening the condition), so as to allow the development of sclerosis and proper endothelial apposition.

Usually injection is started at the ankle region and then proceeded upwards along the length of veins at different points. Later pressure bandage is applied for 3 weeks. Often injection may have to be repeated after a week.

Microsclerotherapy
Very dilute solution of sclerosing agent like STDS, polidocanal is injected into the thread veins and reticular veins followed by application of compression bandage (30-G needle). Dermal flare disappears well by this method.

Many people worry a lot today about tomorrow because they didn't worry a little yesterday about today

> **Foam sclerotherapy by Tessari (Figs. 12.13A and B)**
>
> - 1 mL of STDS is taken in a 5/10 cc syringe which is rapidly passed into a syringe containing air (4 mL) repeatedly through a 3 way system to form 5 mL of foam. This foam is injected into the superficial vein. Maximum total of 6 mL of STDS, i.e. 30 mL of foam can be injected. Air gets absorbed eventually. Foam minimizes thrombosis of vein and foam is less likely to pass distally along the venous flow to cause serious side effects like DVT.
> - *Advantages:* Technique is cheap, easier, done on OPD basis.
> - *Complications:* Headache, transient blindness, stroke, air embolism, thrombophlebitis, pain and pigmentation.
> - *Contraindications:* Peripheral arterial disease, DVT.

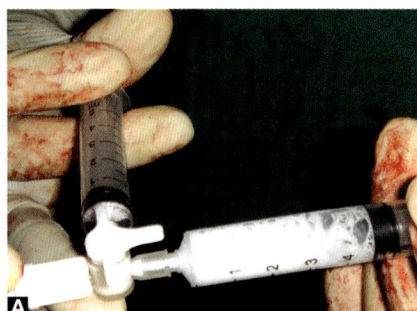

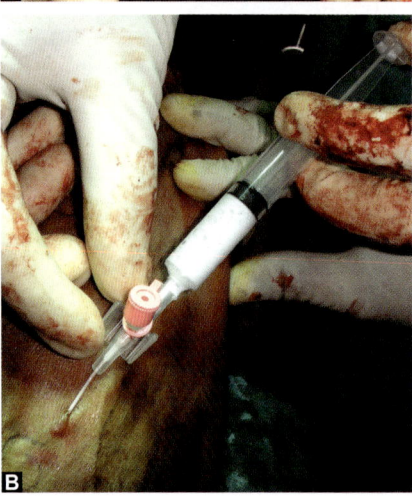

Figs. 12.13A and B: Technique making foam and injecting into the vein. 4 mL air with 1 mL STD is mixed vigorously using 3 way stopcock and two 5 mL syringes. Created foam is injected into the vein immediately. Total of 6 mL STD (30 mL foam) can be injected.

Advantages
- It can be done as an outpatient procedure.
- It does not require anesthesia.

Disadvantage
Inadvertent subcutaneous injection can cause skin necrosis or abscess formation.

> **Contraindications for sclerotherapy**
>
> - Saphenofemoral incompetence.
> - Varicose veins with venous ulcer.
> - Deep vein thrombosis.

3. **Surgery**
   - *Trendelenburg operation:* It is juxtafemoral flush ligation of long saphenous vein (i.e. flush with femoral vein), after ligating named (superficial circumflex, superficial external pudendal, superficial epigastric veins) and unnamed tributaries. All tributaries should be ligated, otherwise recurrence will occur *(saphena varix)* (Fig. 12.14).

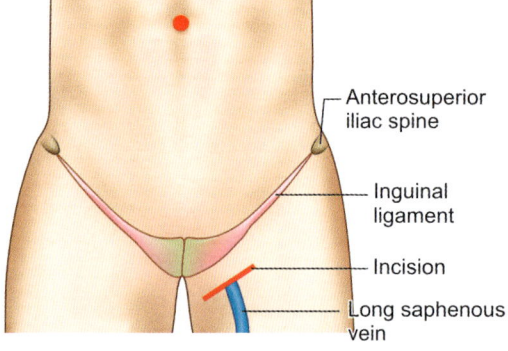

Fig. 12.14: Incision for juxtafemoral flush ligation of long saphenous vein (Trendelenburg operation).

   - *Stripping of vein*: Using *Myer's stripper* vein is stripped off. Stripping from below upwards is technically easier. Immediate application of crepe bandage reduces the chance of bleeding and hematoma formation (Figs. 12.15 and 12.16A). Complication is injury to saphenous nerve causing *saphenous neuralgia*.
   Stripping is not usually done for the veins in the lower part of the leg.

*Let there be spaces in your togetherness—**Kalil Gibran***

A special telescope is introduced deep to deep fascia through a single small vertical incision at proximal leg selecting healthy skin. Potential space between muscle and deep fascia with loose areolar tissue is easy to dissect using endoscope. Technique is done under tourniquet 300 mm Hg pressure. Endoscope is advanced down along the medial border of the tibia. Perforators travelling in subfascial plane are identified and fulgurated using bipolar cautery or clips can be applied into the perforators. It is recommended in chronic venous insufficiency (CVI). But its limitation is difficulty in getting 'lift off' of the skin in cases with severe lipodermatosclerosis making it difficult to identify the perforators.

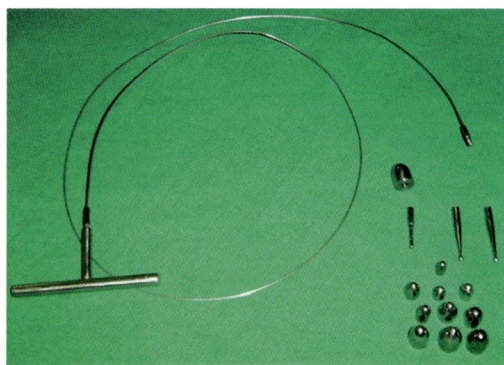

Fig. 12.15: Myer's stripper with olive tips.

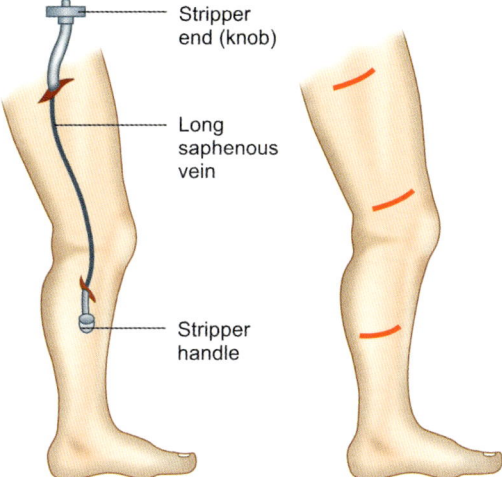

Figs. 12.16A and B: (A) Picture showing stripping of the vein using a stripper; (B) Cockett and Dodd subfascial ligation of perforators using multiple small horizontal incisions.

- *Subfascial ligation of Cockett and Dodd:* Perforators are marked out by Fegan's method. Perforators are ligated deep to the deep fascia through incisions in anteromedial side of the leg (Fig. 12.16B).
- *Ligation of short saphenous vein* at saphenopopliteal junction.
- *Removal of superficial varicose veins by hook phlebectomy.*
- *Subfascial endoscopic perforator ligation surgery (SEPS) (Hauer, 1985) (Fig. 12.17)*

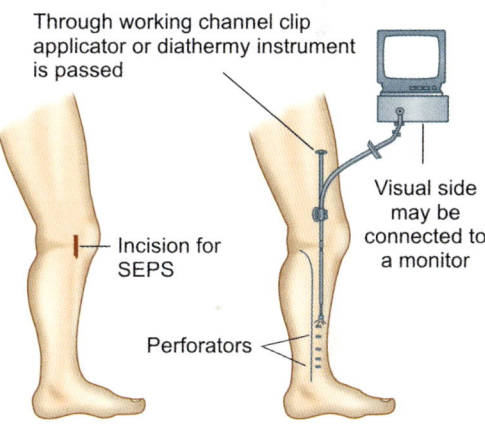

Fig. 12.17: Subfascial endoscopic perforator ligation surgery (SEPS).

Contraindication for surgery

- Deep vein thrombosis.

---

4. **Thermoablation of varicose veins**
   - **Radiofrequency ablation (RFA) method (VNUS closure):** A RFA catheter is passed into long saphenous vein near saphenofemoral junction under guidance to create 85°C temperature which causes

One cannot love what he cannot respect, whether it be himself or another endothelial damage, denaturation and venous occlusion.

❖ **Endovenous laser ablation (EVLA)(Fig. 12.18):** Long saphenous vein (LSV) is cannulated; guidewire is passed; 5 French catheter is passed over guidewire; tip is placed 1 cm distal to the junction. Laser fiber is inserted through the catheter; laser fiber should protrude 2 cm beyond the catheter tip. Fiber is fired at every 3 mm gap for 3 seconds. It creates a temperature of up to 1000°C at the tip which causes thermal endothelial damage and sealing of the vein completely. *Problems are*—pain, ecchymosis, hematoma, burn injury, infection.

Complications of varicose vein surgery

- Infection.
- Hematoma formation.
- DVT.
- Saphenous neuralgia.
- Recurrence.

Complications of varicose veins

- Hemorrhage: Venous hemorrhage can occur from the ruptured varicose veins or sloughed varicose veins, often torrential, but can be controlled very well by elevation and pressure bandage.
- Pigmentation, eczema and dermatitis.
- Periostitis causing thickening of periosteum. It delays healing of ulcer due to poor perfusion of ulcer bed.
- Venous ulcer.
- *Marjolin's ulcer*—due to *unstable scar of long duration*—very well-differentiated squamous cell carcinoma.
- Lipodermatosclerosis.
- Ankylosis of the ankle joint is due to fibrosis of soft tissues around ankle joint—fibrous ankylosis.
- Talipes equinovarus, wherein patient walks on the tip of toes like horse.
- Deep venous thrombosis per se due to varicose vein is rare but can occur if there is associated deep vein disease or recurrent thrombophlebitis.
- Calcification of the wall of varicose veins or of sclerosed soft tissue.
- Recurrent thrombophlebitis, clot formation on the superficial system often at perforator level which often get infected causing fever and tenderness over the spot.

VENOUS ULCER

It is the complication of varicose veins or deep vein thrombosis.

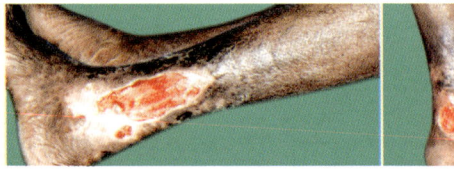

Fig. 12.19: Venous ulcers in the lower limb.

Area where venous ulcer commonly develops is around and above the medial malleoli (Fig. 12.19) because of presence of large number of perforators, which transmit pressure changes directly into superficial system. This area is called as *Gaiter's zone*. It can also be on both malleoli.

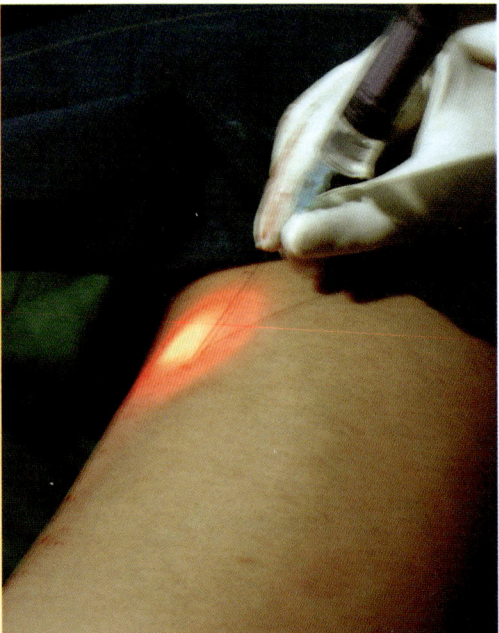

Fig. 12.18: Laser diode fiber tip in the LSV close to SAFJ which is glowing red.

Forget not that the earth delights to feel your bare feet and the winds long to play with your hair—**Kalil Gibran**

Ulcer is often large, nonhealing, tender, recurrent with secondary infection. Vertical group of inguinal lymph nodes are usually enlarged and tender.

Often it leads to scarring, ankylosis, Marjolin's ulcer formation. Slough from the ulcer bed may give way causing venous hemorrhage.

Periostitis is common which also prevents ulcer from healing.

Due to regular walking on toes so as to relieve the pain causes contracture and extra-articular fibrosis of Achilles tendon. Proper exercise is the remedy—*talipes equinovarus*.

Pathogenesis

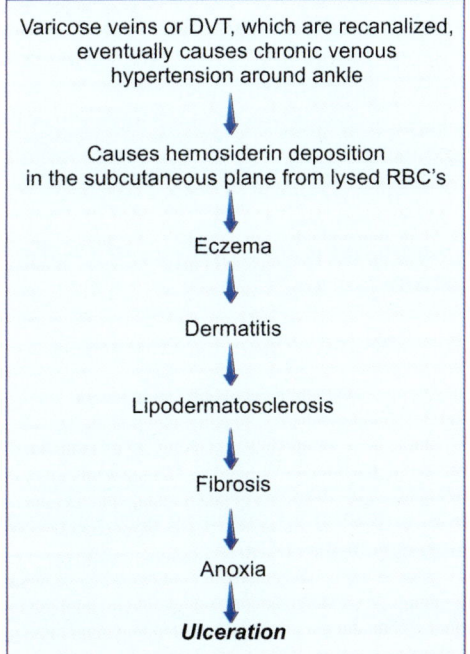

Investigations

* Discharge from the ulcer for culture/sensitivity.
* X-ray of the area to look for periostitis.
* Biopsy from the ulcer edge to rule out Marjolin's ulcer.

Treatment

Bisgaard Method

* Foot elevation.
* Massage of the indurated area and whole calf.
* Passive and active exercise.
* Pressure bandage (crepe bandage).
* Care of ulcer by regular cleaning with povidone iodine, H_2O_2.
* Dressing with EUSOL.
* Antibiotics depending on culture and sensitivity of the discharge.

Once ulcer bed granulates well, split skin grafting (SSG) is placed (*Thiersch graft*).

Note: Specific treatment for varicose veins should be undertaken—Trendelenburg operation, stripping of veins, perforator ligation.

50% of venous ulcer occur as a result of recanalization of DVT, and the leg is commonly called as *postphlebitic limb (leg)*. It presents with all complications of venous diseases like eczema, ulceration, lipodermatosclerosis, and venous ulcers. Here surgery for superficial varicose veins is contraindicated. Venous valve repair (*valvuloplasty*) or drugs like *Stanazolol* that reduce the fibrous tissue, which in turn, increases the oxygenation are beneficial.

Complications of venous ulcers	
• Hemorrhage.	• Periostitis is common over the tibia.
• Marjolin's ulcer.	
• Infection.	• Disability.
• Talipes equinovarus.	• Calcification.
• Calcification.	

(*EUSOL* is Edinburgh University solution of lime containing *boric acid, hypochlorite, calcium hydroxide*).

We always have time enough, if we will use it in a right way

THROMBOPHLEBITIS

It is the inflammation of veins, usually superficial veins due to different causes.

Types

- *Acute*: Due to IV cannulation, trauma, minor infections, hypercoagulability.
- *Recurrent*:
- *Spontaneous:* Polycythemia vera, polyarteritis, Buerger's disease.
- *Thrombophlebitis migrans (Trousseau's sign)*: It is spontaneous migrating thrombophlebitis seen in visceral malignancy like pancreas, stomach of affected veins.

Features

- Pain, redness, tenderness, cord-like thickening of veins, fever.
- It can be seen either in upper limb or lower limb.
- **Complications**
  - Destruction of venous valves resulting in varicose veins.
  - DVT, embolism, infection.
- **Treatment**
  - Elevation.
  - Anti-inflammatory drugs, antibiotics.
  - Application of crepe bandage.

ANTICOAGULANTS

HEPARIN

- It is a natural anticoagulant, a mucopolysaccharide.
- It prevents clotting of blood both in vivo and in vitro by acting on all three stages of coagulation. It *prolongs clotting time and activated thromboplastin time* in specific (by 1.5–2.0 times the control).
- Heparin also causes hyperkalemia.
- Commercial heparin is derived from lung and intestinal mucosa of pigs and cattle.
- The onset of action is immediate after administration lasting for 4 hours.
- It is metabolized in the liver by heparinase.
- It does not cross placental barrier and not secreted in breast milk.

Indications

- As prophylaxis in major surgeries, postoperative period, puerperium.
- As therapy in DVT.

Dose

- For prophylaxis: 5,000 units/SC 8th hourly.
- For therapy: 10,000 units/IV 6th or 8th hourly. Later change to subcutaneous dose.
- In severe cases, 5000 units to 20,000 units is given daily through IV infusion at a rate of 1000 units per hour. Daily dose should not exceed 25,000 units.

Heparin should not be given intramuscularly and should not be combined with streptokinase or urokinase. Heparin is not given orally.

Heparin administration should always be monitored with activated partial thromboplastin time (APTT).

Complications

Allergy, bleeding, thrombocytopenia.

LOW MOLECULAR WEIGHT HEPARIN

It is a commercially prepared with a molecular weight of 4000 to 6500.

Advantages

- They are absorbed more completely.
- Have a longer duration of action.
- Have a better anticoagulant effect.
- Less interaction with platelets.
- Less antigenic.
- Usage is easier and acceptable.
- Dosage is once daily; blood monitoring is not needed.

Your children are not your children. They are the sons and daughters of Life's longing for itself—**Kalil Gibran**

Disadvantages

They are expensive. Presently LMWH are becoming very popular. Enoxaparin, Dalteparin, Parnaparin, Reviparin.

Heparin Antagonist

50 mg of 1% Protamine sulfate solution is given slow intravenous.

ORAL ANTICOAGULANTS

They are given orally and are slow acting.

Types

1. **Coumarin derivatives**
   - Bishydroxycoumarin (Dicoumarol)—first coumarin drug derived from sweet clover.
   - Warfarin sodium—commonest oral anticoagulant used.
2. **Indandione derivative**
   - Phenindione.
   - Anisindione.

Modes of action of oral anticoagulant therapy
- By suppressing synthesis of prothrombin, factors VII, IX, and X.
- By inhibiting carboxylation of glutamic acid through vitamin K.
- Oral anticoagulant does not have in vitro action.
- They are slow acting and long acting.
- Control of oral anticoagulant therapy is by *monitoring prothrombin time*.
- PT becomes normal only 7 days after cessation of the drug.

- They cross placental barrier and known to cause teratogenicity when given in 1st trimester.
- They are secreted in breast milk.

Indication

In DVT, after cessation of heparin for maintenance therapy.
After valve replacement surgery.

Side Effects

- Bleeding—it may require blood transfusion to control.
- Cutaneous gangrene.
- Fetal hemorrhage and teratogenicity.
- Alopecia, urticaria, dermatitis.
- Drug interactions: With NSAIDs, Cimetidine, Omeprazole, Metronidazole, Cotrimoxazole, Erythromycins, Barbiturates, Rifampicin, Griseofulvin.

WARFARIN SODIUM (**W**iskonsin **A**lumini **R**esearch **F**oundation + coum**ARIN** derivative) is the commonest drug used. It has got lesser side effects. It has got cumulative action and so given in tapering dose.
- Dose is 5 mg per day.
- It should be discontinued 7 days before any surgery like tooth extraction and prothrombin time should return to normal level. During surgery if excess bleeding occurs blood transfusion may be given.
- Its dosage is monitored by measuring international normalized ratio (INR) which should be more than 2-2½ times control value.

> **In vitro anticoagulants:** Oxalates, citrates ethylenediaminetetraacetic acid (EDTA).

Differences between oral anticoagulants and heparin

	Oral anticoagulant	Heparin
	Slow acting.	Immediate.
	Long acting.	Short acting.
	Only in vivo action.	Both in vitro and in vivo action.
	Crosses the placental barrier.	Does not cross the placenta.
	Secreted in milk.	Not secreted in milk.
Monitored by:	Prothrombin time.	Partial thromboplastin time.
Administration:	Orally.	Intravenously.

We always have time enough, if we will use it in a right way

CHAPTER 13

Lymphatics

Chapter Outline

- Lymphangiography
- Isotope Lymphoscintigraphy
- Lymphangitis
- Lymphedema
- Differential Diagnosis for (Cervical) Lymphadenopathy
- Lymphomas
- Hodgkin's Lymphoma
- Non-Hodgkin's Lymphoma
- Burkitt's Lymphoma (Malignant Lymphoma of Africa)
- Tuberculous Lymphadenitis

LYMPHANGIOGRAPHY

Indications

- Congenital lymphedema like aplasia, hypoplasia, hyperplasia.
- Lymphomas, it shows reticular pattern. It is also useful to assess the response to treatment.
- Secondaries in lymph nodes, especially iliac and para-aortic lymph nodes as irregular filling defects.

Technique

Patent blue dye or 1 mL Isosulphan blue is injected subcutaneously between toes. Dye will be taken up by lymphatics, which will be visualized clearly. After making incision, one of the lymphatic vessels is dissected and 30-G needle is passed. Ultrafluid lipiodol, which is an oily contrast medium, is injected slowly using pressure pump at a rate of 1 mL in 8 minutes (total quantity is 7 mL). Slowly in 24 hours, it passes through the lymphatics and reaches the iliac and para-aortic lymph nodes. Radiographs taken, helps to visualize both lymphatic vessels as well as lymph nodes.

- Secondaries in lymph nodes cause filling defects.
- Lymphomas show enlarged nodes, which have foamy or reticular appearance.

Disadvantages

- Technically difficult.
- Extravasation of dye can occur.
- Dye might not have reached the required area.
- Time-consuming and invasive procedure.

Lymphangiographic Classification of Lymphedema

- *Congenital hyperplasia (10%).*
- *Distal obliteration (80%).*
- *Proximal obliteration (10%).*

Do not dwell in the past; do not dream of the future, concentrate the mind on the present moment—**Buddha**

ISOTOPE LYMPHOSCINTIGRAPHY

Radioactive technetium labeled antimony sulfide colloid particles are injected into the web space using fine needle. These particles are specifically taken up by lymphatics. Using gamma camera, limb and inguinal region are exposed to visualize the lymphatics and inguinal lymph nodes. In 3 hours it reaches para-aortic lymph nodes, other abdominal lymph nodes and liver. Later thoracic duct also can be visualized. It can be compared to the take up on the other limb.

Advantages

- It is more sensitive (94%) and specific (100%).
- Technically easier and faster compared to lymphangiography.
- Thoracic duct, other lymph nodes and liver can be visualized.

LYMPHANGITIS (FIG. 13.1)

- It is inflammation of the lymphatics usually acute due to staphylococcal or streptococcal bacterial infection.
- It causes acute pain, fever, redness along the line of lymphatics vessels.
- Streaks of redness which blanches on pressure and reappears after release is typical.
- Tender regional lymph nodes are commonly present.
- Treatment is limb elevation, antibiotics like amoxycillin, analgesics. diethyl carbamazine citrate (DEC) is also used often.
- Recurrent lymphangitis can occur in many; often also in filarial/malignant patients.

LYMPHEDEMA

It is accumulation of fluid (lymph) in extra-cellular and extravascular fluid compartment, commonly in subcutaneous tissues. It is primarily due to defective lymphatic drainage. It is protein rich interstitial fluid.

Classification

Kinmoth classified lymphedema as:
- *Primary* without any identifiable lymphatic disease.
- *Secondary* is acquired due to definitive cause. *Most common form.*

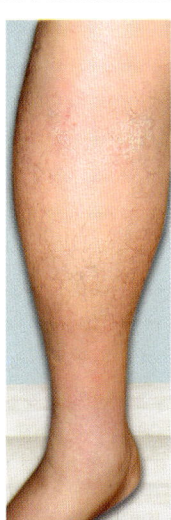

Fig. 13.1: Lymphangitis leg. Redness and blanching on pressure is typical feature.

Primary type
It affects commonly females.
It is common in lower limb and left side.
It can be:
• Familial.
• Syndromic.
It can be:

• Lymphedema congenita
  – Present at birth.
  – Familial type is called as **Milroy's disease**.

• Lymphedema praecox
  – Present at puberty—up to 35 years.
  – Familial type is called as **Meige's disease**.

• Lymphedema tarda—present in adult life—after 35 years.

Contd...

Contd...

It can be radiologically (lymphangiography):
- Hypoplasia 70%
- Aplasia 15%
- Hyperplasia (varicose lymphatics) 15%

It can be lymphangiographically and clinically:
- Distal obliteration
  - Here proximal part is normal. It is common in young females.
- Proximal obliteration
  - Common type 85%. Common in both sexes.
  - With distal *hyperplasia*.
  - With distal *obliteration*.
- Congenital hyperplasia—it shows dilated incompetent *megalymphatics*.

Causes of secondary lymphedema

- Trauma.
- Surgery—inguinal block or axillary block dissection.
- Filarial lymphedema due to *Buchereria Bancrofti*. Common cause in coastal region.
- Tuberculosis.
- Syphilis.
- Fungal infection.
- Advanced malignancy—hard, fixed lymph nodes in axilla or in inguinal region.
- Postradiotherapy lymphedema.
- Bacterial infection.
- Rare causes: Rheumatoid arthritis, snake and insect bites, deep vein thrombosis (DVT), chronic venous insufficiency.

Pathology *(Commonly in Filarial Lymphedema)*

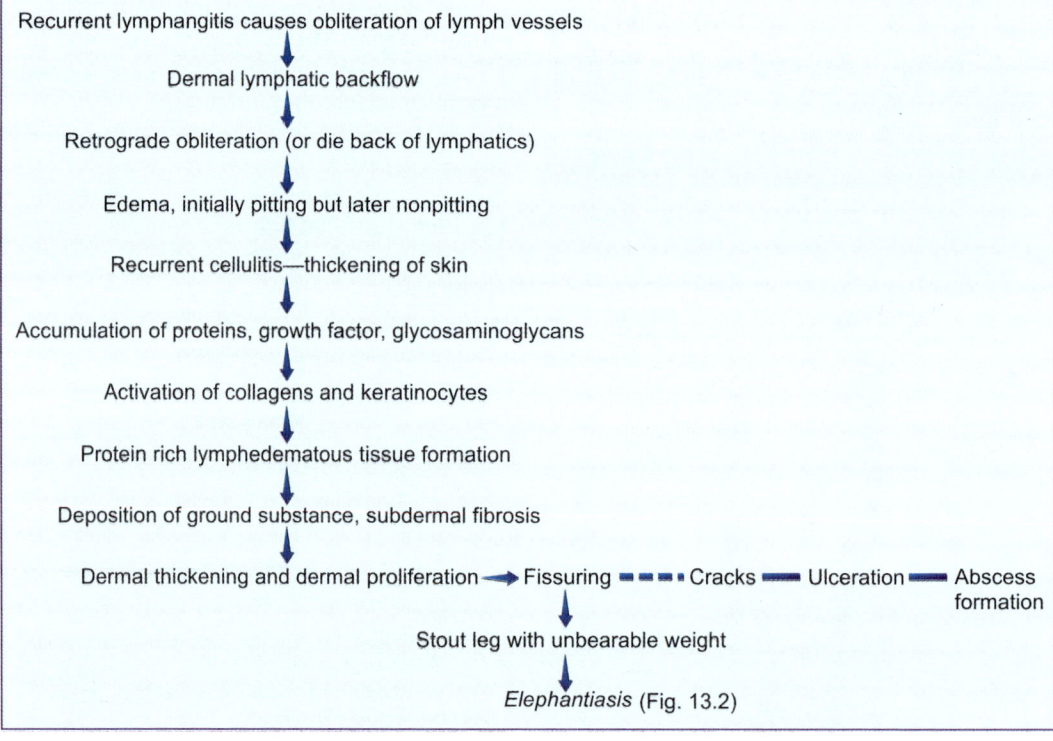

Rarely, it causes protein losing diarrhea, chylous ascites, chylothorax, chyluria, lymphorrhea. Recurrent lymphadenitis occurs in the region, which aggravate the condition.

Disease in the limb is confined to skin and subcutaneous tissue, i.e. only superficial lymphatics are involved by the disease, deep lymphatics are not. Superficial and

*Just as a candle cannot burn without fire, men cannot live without a spiritual life—**Buddha***

Chapter 13 : Lymphatics

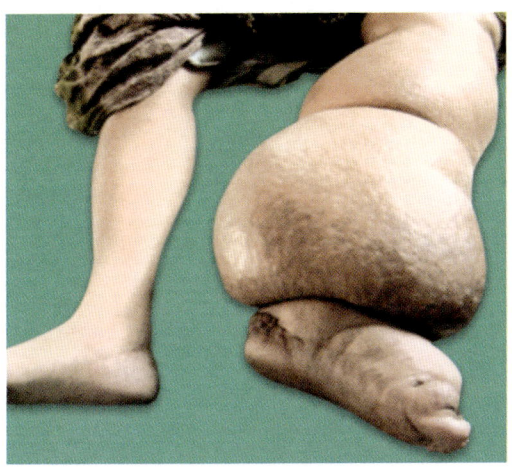

Fig. 13.2: Showing elephantiasis left leg with skin thickening and fissuring.

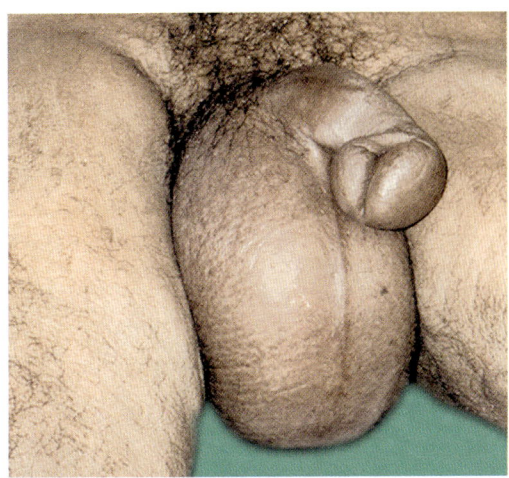

Fig. 13.3: Ram's horn penis.

deep lymphatics are not communicating with each other (unlike the veins in the limb where superficial and deep veins are freely communicating with each other).

Sites of lymphedema
1. Lower limb—commonest.
2. Upper limb.
3. Scrotum, penis (*Ram's horn penis*) (Fig. 13.3).
4. Breast—requires reduction mammoplasty.
5. Labia.
6. Eyelid.
7. Localized lymphedema.

Clinical Features

- Swelling in the foot, extending progressively into the leg (Fig. 13.4).
- *Buffalo hump* in the dorsum of the foot.
- Squaring of toes.
- Skin over the dorsum of foot cannot be pinched because of subcutaneous fibrosis—*Stemmer's sign*.
- Initially pitting edema, which later becomes nonpitting.

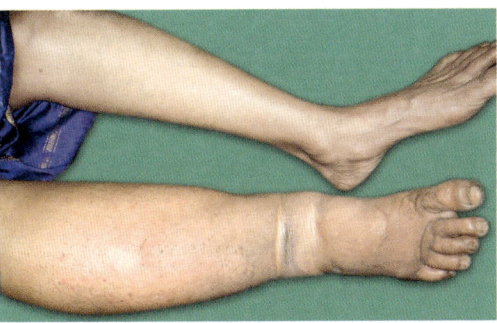

Fig. 13.4: Lymphedema right leg.

- Eczema, fissuring, papillae formation, ulceration, lymph ooze, elephantiasis are other features.

Brunner's grading of lymphedema
Latent subclinical: No clinically apparent lymphedema.
Grade I: Pitting edema which more or less disappears on elevation of the limb is due to excess deposition of interstitial fluid.
Grade II: Nonpitting edema which does not reduce on elevation.
Grade III: Edema with irreversible skin changes like fibrosis, papillae, fissuring (Figs. 13.5A and B).

Our worst misfortunes never happen, and most miseries lie in anticipation

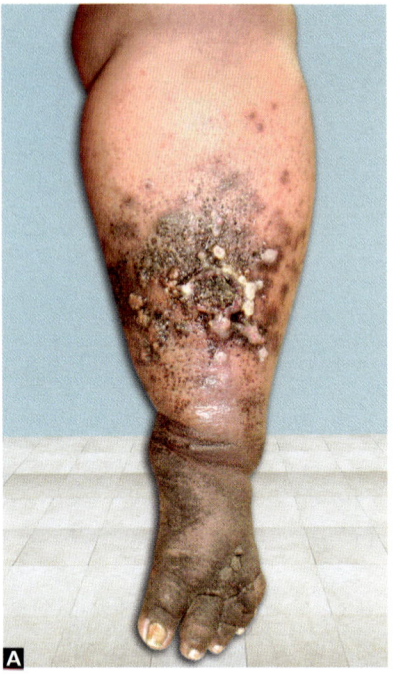
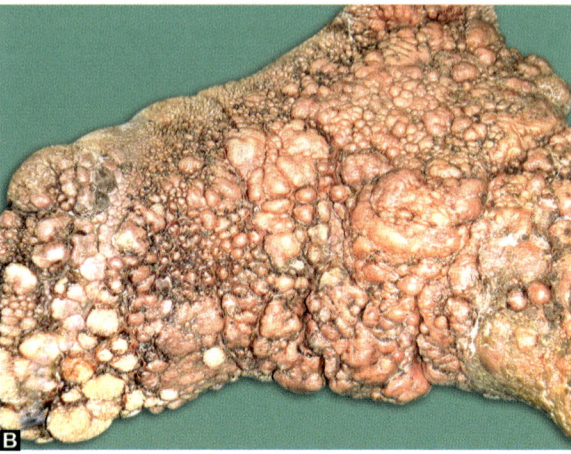

Figs. 13.5A and B: Elephantiasis leg. In another patient is obvious changes in the foot with nodules formation.

Differential diagnosis

- Cardiac causes, hypoproteinemias, malnutrition, nephrotic syndrome.
- Myxedema.
- Trauma.
- Venous diseases like DVT.
- Lipodystrophy and lipoidosis.
- Arterial diseases including AV malformations.
- Gigantism.
- Drug induced—steroids, estrogens, nifedipine.
- Elephantiatic neurofibromatosis and lipomatosis.
- *Lipedema* is bilateral symmetrical enlargement of legs exclusively seen in women at the age of puberty due to deposition of abnormal fat.

Investigations

- For the cause.
- Erythrocyte sedimentation rate (ESR), peripheral smear.
- Lymphangiography.
- Isotope—lymphoscintigraphy.

Complication

- Skin thickening.
- Recurrent cellulitis with nonhealing ulcers, morbidity and disability.
- Lymphangiosarcoma.

Treatment

Conservative

- Elevate the limb, weight reduction; exercise.
- Massaging and avoiding prolonged standing.
- Diuretics to reduce the edema are controversial. It more often causes electrolyte imbalance than being beneficial.
- Benzopyrones are proteinolytic agents *(Lympedin)*.
- Daily wearing of below knee stockings.

*Holding on to anger is like grasping a hot coal with the intent of throwing it at someone else; you are the one who gets burned —**Buddha***

- Avoid trauma and infection.
- Intermittent pneumatic compression devices.
- Antibiotics—Flucloxacillin, Erythromycins, long acting Penicillins.
- Topical antifungal 1% Clotrimazole and systemic Griseofulvin 250–1,000 mg.
- Regular washing and keeping the limb clean is very important.
- Diethyl carbamazine citrate 100 mg tid for 3 weeks.
- **Complex decongestive therapy** with elevation, exercise, massaging and compression wraps.
- **Manual lymphatic drainage** using gentle superficial massaging of the skin, initially on the opposite side then on the same side.

Surgery

Surgeries for lymphedema has been classified as:
- **Excisional**
  - Charle's operation.
  - Homan's operation.
- **Physiological**
  - Omentoplasty.
  - Nodovenous shunt (Fig. 13.6).
  - Lymphovenous shunt.
  - Ileal mucosal patch.

  Here either communication between superficial and deep lymphatics is created or new lymphatic channels are mobilized to the site.

  Omentoplasty (omental pedicle): As omentum contains plenty of lymphatics, omental transfer with pedicle will facilitate lymph drainage.
- **Combined**

  Both excision + creation of communication between superficial and deep lymphatics.
  - Sistrunk operation.
  - Thompson's operation.
  - Kondolean's operation.

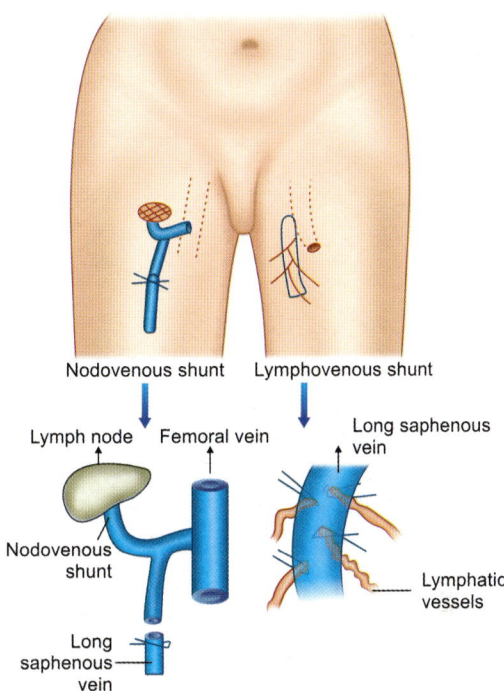

Fig. 13.6: Nodovenous (right sided) and lymphovenous shunt (left sided) surgeries for lymphedema.

- **Bypass procedure**
  Skin bridge across the thigh and abdomen.
  - Nodovenous shunt.
  - Lymphovenous shunt using microscope.
  - Ileal mucosal patch.
- **Limb reduction surgeries**
  - *Sistrunk operation*: Along with excision of lymphedematous tissue, window cuts in deep fascia is done, so as to allow communication into normal deep lymphatics.
  - *Homan's operation*: Excision of lymphedematous tissue after raising skin flaps. Later skin flaps are trimmed to required size and sutured primarily.
  - *Thompson's operation*: Lymphedematous tissue is excised under the skin flaps. Epidermis and part of the dermis of one of the skin flaps is shaved off using Humby's knife. It is buried under oppo-

Pleasure in the job puts perfection in the work

site flap, deep to the deep fascia like a *swiss roll (Swiss roll operation or buried dermal flap operation) (Fig. 13.7)*.

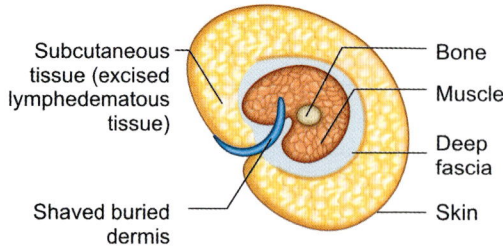

Fig. 13.7: Thompson's swiss roll operation. After removal of lymphedematous tissue deep fascia is opened to bury the abraded epidermis to achieve the communication.

Problems here are epidermal cysts and sinus formation.

- **Kondolean's operation**: Along with excision of lymphedematous tissue, vertical strips of deep fascia are removed so as to open the deep lymphatics, which creates communication between superficial and deep lymphatics.
- **Charle's operation**: Done in severe lymphedema with elephantiasis. Along with excision of lymphedematous tissues, skin grafting is done. It reduces the size and weight of the limb. Patient becomes ambulatory (Figs 13.8A and B).

In severe type, amputation may be required occasionally.

DIFFERENTIAL DIAGNOSIS FOR (CERVICAL) LYMPHADENOPATHY

Cervical lymphadenopathy is the common condition which clinicians come across and various causes attribute for the same. It is often difficult to find out the cause unless relevant investigations are made (Figs. 13.9A and B).

Differential diagnosis for cervical lymphadenopathy

Infective causes
- Acute lymphadenitis.
- Chronic nonspecific lymphadenitis.
- Tuberculous lymphadenitis.
- Infectious mononucleosis.
- Toxoplasmosis.
- Cat scratch fever.

Neoplastic causes
- Metastatic lymph node enlargement (secondaries)
- Lymphomas—HL/NHL/Burkitt's.
- Chronic lymphatic leukemia (CLL).

Other causes
- Autoimmune diseases like systemic lupus erythematosus, rheumatoid arthritis (juvenile), etc.
- HIV infection, immunosuppression.

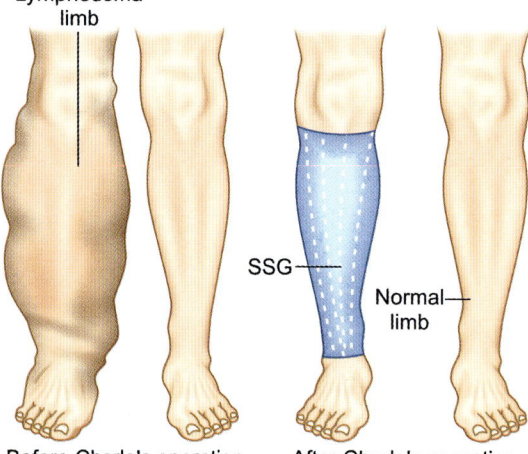

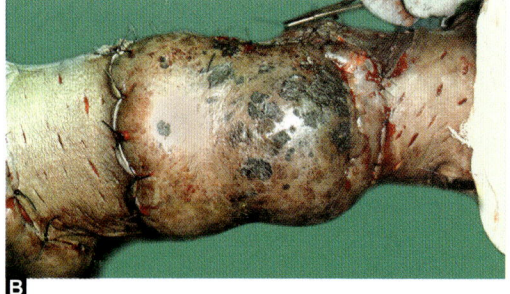

Figs. 13.8A and B: Charle's operation. Here lymphadematous tissue is excised and split skin graft is used to cover the defect. Often graft is taken from the same area prior to excision.

Whatever words we utter should be chosen with care for people will hear them and be influenced by them for good or ill —Buddha

Chronic Nonspecific Lymphadenitis

Infections like chronic/recurrent tonsillitis, scalp infection; recurrent dental infection can cause nonspecific lymphadenitis. Patient presents with firm nontender, usually multiple bilateral lymph node enlargement in the neck. It may mimic lymphoma or tuberculosis of lymph nodes. Fine needle aspiration cytology (FNAC)/open biopsy of lymph node confirms the diagnosis. Histology shows reactive hyperplasia or sinus histiocytosis.

Tuberculous Lymphadenitis

It is caused by *Mycobacterium tuberculosis* infection. It causes matted lymph node enlargement, cold abscess or sinus formation. FNAC, biopsy confirms the diagnosis. It is treated by antituberculous drugs.

Infectious Mononucleosis

It is due to Epstein-Barr virus infection (glandular fever). It affects young individuals causing sore throat, fever, generalized lymphadenopathy, skin rashes, hepatosplenomegaly. Monospot test is positive. Symptomatic treatment is sufficient.

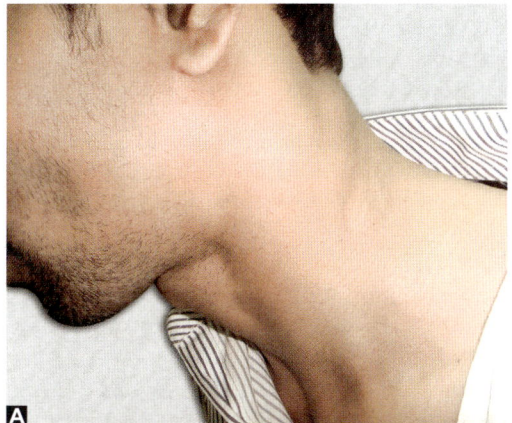
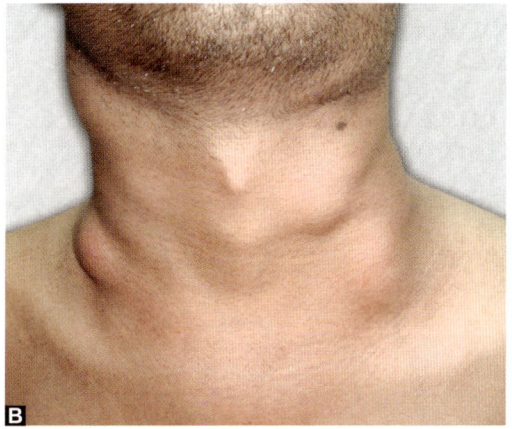

Figs. 13.9A and B: Lymphadenopathy in the neck. It could be lymphoma or tuberculosis or secondaries in the neck. HIV infection also commonly causes cervical lymphadenopathy.

Acute Suppurative Lymphadenitis

It is bacterial infection causing acute inflammation and suppuration of the lymph node caused by group A streptococci or staphylococci, usually focus is from tonsils or throat. Fever, chills, tender enlarged firm or soft palpable neck lymph nodes are the usual features. Total count will be raised. Antibiotics like amoxicillin or cloxacillin controls the infection. Often pus requires needle aspiration or incision and drainage. It may cause septicemia and local complications like internal jugular vein thrombosis, laryngeal edema.

Toxoplasmosis

It is caused by *Toxoplasma Gondii*, protozoa through meat. It causes fever, myalgia, lymphadenopathy. It is crescent shaped protozoa. Cats are the definitive host. During its enteric cycle in cat, it forms oocyst which is excreted in feces. Intermediate hosts are birds or other animals where oocysts get ingested to form sporozoites and tachyzoites and trophozites infecting cells in different organs. *Toxoplasma* transmits from mother to fetus through placenta. In adults, with acquired infection can be asymptomatic or cervical lymphadenopathy (commonest); chorioretinitis; or rarely contral nervous system (CNS) involvement. It is diagnosed by serological test (Sabin-Feldman dye test).

The remedy for injuries is not to remember them.

Cat Scratch Disease

Cat scratch fever is caused by *Bartonella henselae*, transmitted through cat. It causes fever and lymphadenopathy. It is diagnosed by lymph node biopsy with '*Warthin Starry*' staining. It is self-limiting disease.

Secondaries in Neck Lymph Nodes

It is usually from proximal aerodigestive tract—oral cavity, laryngopharynx, trachea and esophagus. It can also be from lungs, breast, thyroid, gastrointestinal tract (GIT), testes, etc. nodes are hard, well defined often fixed. It can later on fungate. Primary is diagnosed by endoscopies, blind biopsies, CT of the area or direct incision biopsy. FNAC is done for secondaries. Primary is treated independently. Secondaries are treated by radical neck dissection. If nodes are fixed, then chemotherapy is given.

Lymphomas

It is primary malignant lymphoproliferative disease involving lymph nodes, liver, spleen and/or bone marrow; occasionally viscera or other organs. Any organ can be involved by lymphoma. It can be Hodgkin's (HL) or non-Hodgkin's (NHL) lymphoma.

LYMPHOMAS

They are progressive neoplastic condition of lymphoreticular system arising from stem cells.

WHO modified **REAL** (**R**evised **E**uropean **A**merican **L**ymphoma) classification of lymphoma:
1. B-cell neoplasms
   I. Precursor B-cell neoplasm—ALL, LBL.
   II. Peripheral B-cell neoplasm—it includes all B-cell related non-Hodgkin's lymphomas.
2. T-cell and putative NK cell neoplasms
   I. Precursor T-cell neoplasms—ALL and LBL T-cell related.
   II. Peripheral T-cell and NK cell neoplasm—It includes all T-cell related non-Hodgkin's lymphomas.

Contd...

Contd...

3. Hodgkin's lymphoma
   I. Predominant HL—nodular lymphocyte type.
   II. Classical HL.
      – Nodular sclerosis.
      – Lymphocyte rich.
      – Mixed cellularity.
      – Lymphocyte depletion.

Types

- Hodgkin's lymphoma (HL).
- Non-Hodgkin's lymphoma (NHL).

HODGKIN'S LYMPHOMA

- It is the commonest type of lymphoma.
- Grossly lymph nodes are fleshy, pinkish gray, and rubbery in consistency (Fig. 13.10).

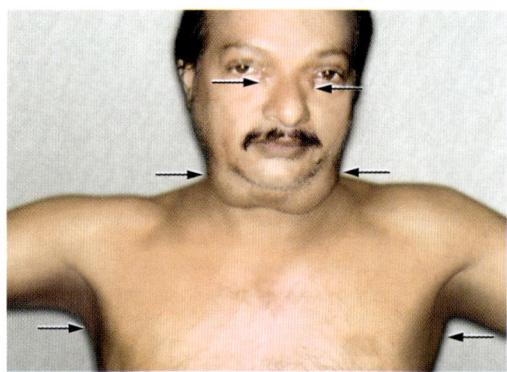

Fig. 13.10: Enlarged, bilateral rubbery neck nodes—lymphoma.

- Microscopically contains cellular infiltration with lymphocytes, reticulum cells, histiocytes, fibrous tissue and **Reed-Sternberg** cells (Reed-Sternberg cells are giant cells with two large mirror image nuclei).

Rye's classification

1. Lymphocytic predominance. Has got *good prognosis*.
2. Mixed cellularity.
3. Nodular sclerosis.
4. Lymphocytic depletion. Has got *bad prognosis*.

---

*We are what we think. All that we are arises with our thoughts. With our thoughts, we make the world—**Buddha***

Reed-Sternberg cells are also seen occasionally in certain other conditions like glandular fever.

Clinical Features

- It is more common in males.
- It has got bimodal presentation. It is seen in young and adolescents (20–30 years) as well as in elderly (> 50 years) (Fig. 13.11).
- Painless progressive enlargement of lymph nodes. They are smooth, firm, nontender, typical with *India rubber* consistency.

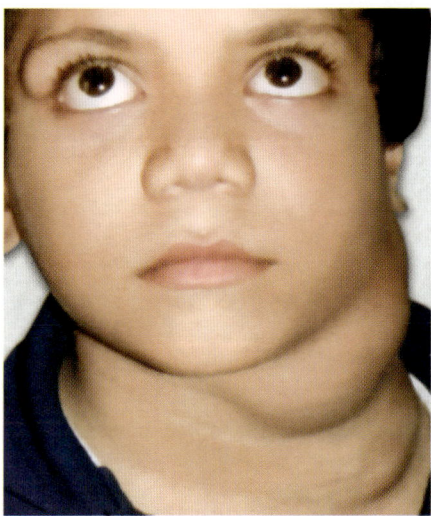

Fig. 13.11: Hodgkin's lymphoma in young boy with typical look of neck nodal involvement. HL is common in young and elderly patients with bimodal representation.

Site

- Cervical lymph nodes, commonest. 82% (lower deep cervical group in posterior triangle).
- Others include axillary, mediastinal, inguinal, abdominal.

Specific Features

- Nodular sclerosis is most common type.

- Consecutive group of lymph nodes are involved.
- *Splenomegaly* is very common (45%).
- Hepatomegaly with jaundice—jaundice is due to hemolysis or due to diffuse liver involvement.
- Constitutional symptoms like *fever, night sweats, weight loss* may be present, which signifies stage 'B', and has got poor prognosis. Stage 'A' is absence of these symptoms, which signifies better prognosis.
- Mediastinal lymph node involvement may cause compression features like superior vena cava (SVC) obstruction.
- Occasionally bone may get involved, like vertebrae. But it is not common in HL.
- Anemia, pancytopenia.

Differential Diagnosis

- Tuberculosis.
- NHL.
- HIV.
- Chronic lymphatic leukemia.
- Nonspecific lymphadenitis.
- Sarcoidosis.
- Secondaries in lymph nodes (Fig. 13.12).

Ann-Arbor clinical staging

Stage 1: Confined to one group of lymph node.
Stage 2: More than one group of lymph nodes on one side of the diaphragm.
Stage 3: Nodes involved on both sides of the diaphragm.
Stage 4: Extranodal involvements like liver, bone marrow.
Suffix 'S'—Spleen involved,
Suffix 'B'—Presence of constitutional symptoms,
Suffix 'A'—Absence of constitutional symptoms.

Investigations

- Blood: Hb%, ESR, peripheral smear, blood urea, serum creatinine.
- FNAC of lymph nodes.

Following the happiness is like chasing the wind or clutching the shadow

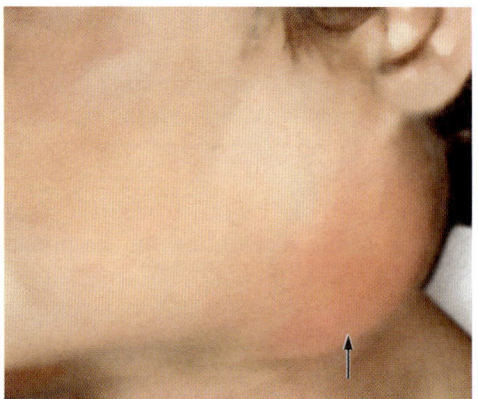

Fig. 13.12: Secondaries in neck is hard, often fixed mass. It is a differential diagnosis for lymphoma.

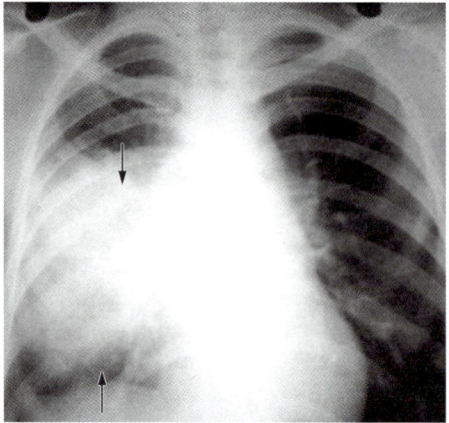

Fig. 13.13: Chest X-ray showing mediastinal lymphoma.

- Excision biopsy of lymph nodes. Full lymph node has to be excised to retain the architecture of the lymph node. It is important to grade the tumor.
- Chest X-ray to see mediastinal lymph nodes, pleural effusion (Fig. 13.13).
- Ultrasound abdomen—to look for the involvement of liver, spleen, and abdominal lymph nodes.
- CT scans of mediastinum and abdomen (Fig. 13.14).
- Lower limb lymphangiography to see the pelvic and retroperitoneal lymph nodes.
- Bone marrow biopsy to stage and also to see the response to treatment.
- *Staging laparotomy*:
  - After opening the abdomen, splenectomy is done mainly to remove the tumor bulk, as spleen is commonly involved and also to avoid irradiation to splenic area, which often causes unpleasant pulmonary fibrosis (due to damage to lower lobe of left lung). Biopsies are taken from both lobes of the liver (needle biopsy) from para-aortic, mesenteric, iliac nodes. In females ovaries are fixed behind the uterus to prevent radiation oophoritis (oophoropexy). It is done in suspected stage I and II cases. Presently it is not commonly done due to availability

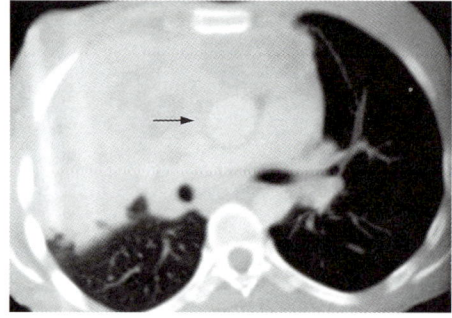

Fig. 13.14: CT scan showing mediastinal tumor suggestive of mediastinal lymphoma.

of better modalities of staging like ultrasound, CT scan, MRI, etc. Advanced radiotherapy technique makes it safer to irradiate splenic area without causing much damage to left sided lung.

Treatment for HL

- Stage I and II:
  1. Mainly **radiotherapy**—external high cobalt RT.
     - Above the diaphragm—'Y' field therapy, covering cervical, axillary, mediastinal lymph nodes.
     - Below the diaphragm, *mantle or inverted 'Y' field therapy*, covering para-aortic and iliac nodes.
  2. Chemotherapy.

You will not be punished for your anger; you will be punished by your anger—Buddha

- Stage III and IV: Mainly *chemotherapy*. Drugs used includes:
  - Mustine. **M**. (Mechloroethamine) 6 mg/sq m
  - Oncovine. **O**. (Vinca alkaloids) 1.4 mg/sq m
  - Procarbazine. **P**. 100 mg orally for 10 days of the cycle.
  - Prednisolone. **P**. 15–45 mg for first 10 days.
  - Other regimens available—MVPP, ABVD. *A (Adriamycin) B (Bleomycin) V (Vinblastin) D (Dacarbazine) is commonly used* and more popular now.

Prognosis: 5-year-survival rate is 80%.

Prognostic factors

1. Stage I and II has got better prognosis.
2. Lymphocytic predominance has got better prognosis.
3. Stage 'A' without constitutional symptoms has got better prognosis.

Causes of death in lymphoma

- Disseminated diseases like liver involvement (liver failure).
- Stage IV lymphoma with bone marrow involvement.
- Recurrent severe opportunistic respiratory tract infection.
- Spine involvement with paraplegia and pathological fracture.
- Immunosuppression—septicemia.

NON-HODGKIN'S LYMPHOMA (FIGS. 13.15A TO C)

- It occurs in middle-aged and elderly. It is more aggressive than HL.
- It involves asymmetrical group of lymph nodes.
- General condition is poor.
- Inner Waldeyer ring, epitrochlear lymph nodes, peripheral lymph nodes are commonly involved.
- Spleen is not commonly involved.
- Hepatomegaly is common.
- Vertebral involvement is common; paraplegia can occur.
- Secondary infection, cachexia and immunosuppression is more common.
- Open biopsy, chest CT scan, USG abdomen, liver function tests, MRI spine, immunohistochemistry are needed investigations.

Types

- Nodular (follicular).
- Diffuse lymphocytic.
- Undifferentiated.
- Histiocytic type.

Rappaport classification	Working classification
1. Nodular	a. Low grade
2. Diffuse	b. Intermediate grade
	c. High grade

Differences between Hodgkin's lymphoma (HL) and non-Hodgkin's lymphoma (NHL)

	Hodgkin's lymphoma	*Non-Hodgkin's lymphoma*
Age:	Young and elderly.	Middle age and elderly.
Pattern of involvement:	Symmetrical and consecutive.	Asymmetrical.
Cervical lymph node:	Commonly involved.	Any group can be involved.
Splenomegaly:	Common.	Not common.
Peripheral lymph node involvement (e.g. epitrochlear nodes).	Not common.	Common.
Treatment:	Mainly radiotherapy. Chemotherapy.	Mainly chemotherapy.
Prognosis:	Better.	Poor.

A long life may not be good enough but a good life is long enough.

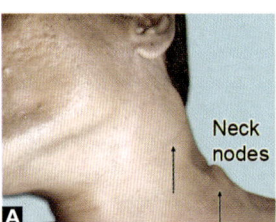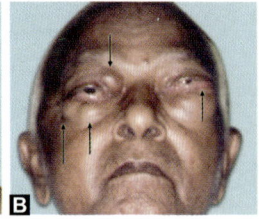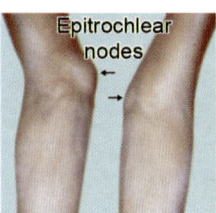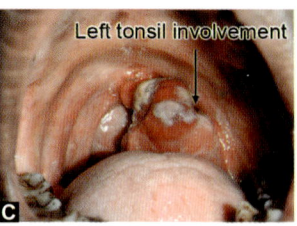

Figs. 13.15A to C: Non-Hodgkin's lymphoma showing involvement of neck lymph nodes, eyelids, epitrochlear lymph nodes and left tonsils.

Treatment

Mainly **chemotherapy**.
Various regimens are available which include:
- **CHOP regime is used**— Cyclophosphamide; Hydroxydaunorubicin; Oncovin; Prednisolone. This is the standard regime commonly used.
- *R CHOP regime* is adding Rituximab when lymphoma is B cell type.
- *R-CHOEP regime* is when Etoposide is added.
- *Side effects are*—hemorrhagic cystitis (Mesna is given); alopecia; nausea and vomiting; neutropenia; severe sepsis.
- ABVD—Adriamycin, Bleomycin, Vincristine, Dacarbazine.
- ABVP—Adriamycin, Bleomycin, Vincristine, Prednisolone.
- Combinations of above.
- *Rituximab* may be used with chemotherapy regimes.

Role of radiotherapy in NHL: When vertebra is involved.
Prognosis is poor in NHL compared to HL.

BURKITT'S LYMPHOMA (Malignant Lymphoma of Africa)

- It is common in South Africa and New Guinea.
- *Epstein-Barr virus* may be the etiological agent. It is common in children.
- It is associated with infectious mononucleosis.
- It is common in malaria endemic area.
- The tumor is multifocal, rapidly growing, painless.
- Different groups of lymph nodes can also be affected.

Microscopy

Primitive lymphoid cells with large clear histiocytes—*starry night (starry sky)* pattern.

Site

It is common in jaw—either lower or upper.
Abdominal presentation and renal involvement is common (75%).
Renal involvement often may be bilateral.
In females ovaries are commonly affected.

Investigation

- FNAC and biopsy confirms the diagnosis.
- X-ray jaw shows osteolytic lesions.
- Ultrasound abdomen to see involvement of kidneys.
- Blood urea and serum creatinine estimation is done.

Work out your own salvation. Do not depend on others —**Buddha**

Treatment

Radiotherapy

Chemotherapy: Cyclophosphamide, Methotrexate, Orthomelphalan.

Surgery is usually not indicated unless it is localized or in case of involvement of ovaries.

Prognosis is good.

TUBERCULOUS LYMPHADENITIS

Causative organism:
Mycobacterium tuberculosis (not *M. bovis*).

Site

- Common in neck lymph nodes.
- Common in *upper deep cervical (jugulo-digastric—54%)* lymph nodes.
- Next common is posterior triangle lymph nodes (22%).

Mode of Infection

- Usually through *the tonsils,* occasionally through blood from lungs.
- It may be associated with pulmonary tuberculosis or renal tuberculosis.

> **Stages of tuberculous lymphadenitis (Fig. 13.16)**
> 1. Stage *of infection and lymphadenitis.*
> 2. Stage of *periadenitis with matting.*
> 3. Stage of *caseating necrosis and cold abscess formation* (Fig. 13.17).
> 4. Stage of formation of *collar stud abscess.*
> 5. Stage of *formation of sinus* which discharges yellowish caseating material.

- Often fibrosis and calcification can occur with or without treatment.

Gross pathology:
Firm, matted, lymph node, with cut section showing yellowish caseating material.

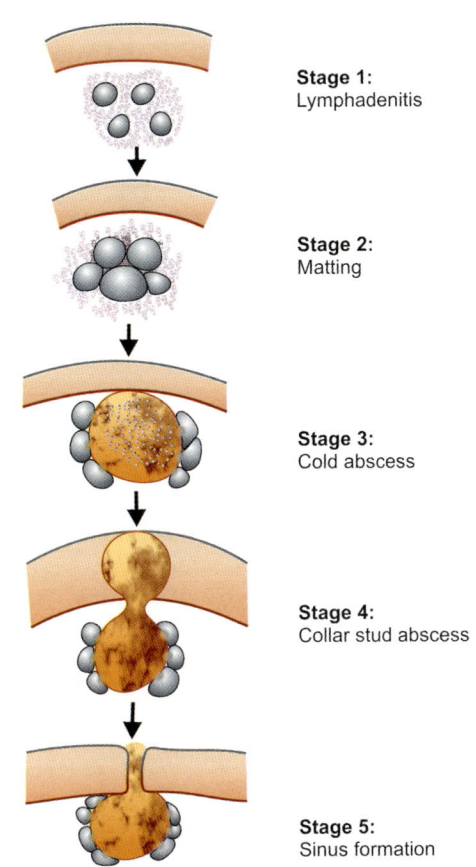

Fig. 13.16: Stages of tuberculous lymphadenitis.

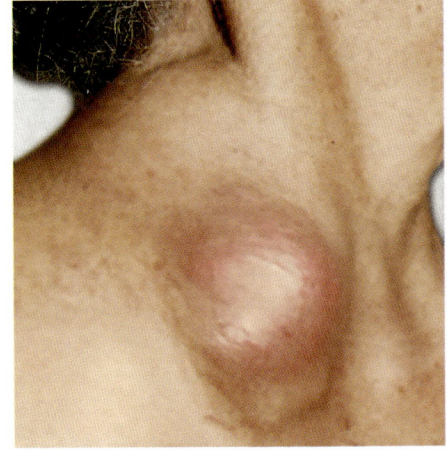

Fig. 13.17: Cold abscess in the neck which has formed collar stud abscess. It eventually leads to sinus formation.

You my say you KNOW, but by your actions it is KNOWN.

Tuberculous lymphadenitis—types	
Hyperplastic	**Caseating**
a. 20% common.	80% common.
b. Discrete, firm or hard.	*Matted* due to periadenitis.
c. Occurs in the cortex of lymph node.	Involves medulla with periadenitis.
d. Host immunity is good.	Body resistance is not adequate.
e. Drugs act better.	Drugs do not reach in proper concentration and may not be effective.
f. Drug resistance is uncommon.	Drug resistance is common.
g. No cold abscess or sinus formation.	Cold abscess or sinus are common.
h. Blood spread.	From tonsils.

Microscopic appearance:
- *Epithelioid cells with caseating material* are seen along with *Langhan's type* of giant cells.
    - Disease can also occur in other lymph nodes like, axillary lymph nodes, para-aortic lymph nodes, mesenteric lymph nodes, and inguinal lymph nodes.
    - Disease may be associated with HIV infection, and lymphomas.

Clinical Features

- Swelling in the neck, which is *firm, matted*.
- *Cold abscess* is soft, smooth, nontender, fluctuant, without involvement of the skin.
- As a result of increased pressure, cold abscess ruptures out of the deep fascia to form *collar stud abscess* which is adherent to the overlying skin.
- Once collar stud abscess bursts open, discharging sinus is formed.
- *Tonsils may be studded with tubercles* and so clinically should always be examined.
- Associated pulmonary tuberculosis should also be looked for.

Differential Diagnosis

- Nonspecific lymphadenitis.
- Lymphomas.
- Secondaries in the neck.
- Branchial cyst mimics cold abscess.
- Lymph cyst mimics cold abscess.
- HIV with lymph node involvement.
- When there is discharging sinus—actinomycosis.

Investigations

- Hematocrit, ESR.
- FNAC of lymph node.
- HIV test.
- Open biopsy when FNAC is inconclusive.
- Chest X-ray to look for pulmonary tuberculosis.

Treatment

- ***Antituberculous drugs*** has to be started—
    - Rifampicin 450 mg OD in empty stomach. It is bactericidal. It discolors urine red. It is also hepatotoxic.
    - INH—300 mg OD. It is bactericidal. It causes intolerance, neuritis, hepatitis (INH).
    - Ethambutol 800 mg OD. It is bacteriostatic. It causes GIT intolerance, retrobulbar neuritis (green color blindness).
    - Pyrazinamide 1500 mg OD or 750 mg BD. It is bactericidal. It is hepatotoxic, also causes hyperuricemia and increases psychosis.

Better than a thousand hollow words, is one word that brings peace—**Buddha**

Duration of treatment is usually 6–9 months.

- ❖ **Aspiration**
  - When there is cold abscess, initially it has to be aspirated [Needle is introduced into the cold abscess in a nondependent site along a *'Z' track* (in zigzag pathway) so as to prevent sinus formation].
- ❖ **Drainage**
  - But if it recurs, then it should be drained. Drainage is done through *a nondependent incision*. After draining the caseating material, *wound is closed without placing a drain*.
- ❖ **Surgery**
  Surgical removal of tubercular lymph nodes are indicated when:
  - There is no local response to chemotherapy
  - When sinus persists.

  It is done by raising skin flaps and removing all caseating material and lymph nodes. Care should be taken not to injure major structures.

Peace comes from within. Do not seek it without—**Buddha**

14

Nerves and Tendon

Chapter Outline

- Peripheral Nerve Injuries
- Brachial Plexus Injuries
- Causalgia
- Median Nerve Injuries
- Carpal Tunnel Syndrome
- Ulnar Nerve Injuries
- Claw Hand
- Radial Nerve Lesions
- Common Peroneal Nerve
- Axillary Nerve Injury
- Long Thoracic Nerve (Nerve of Bell)
- Trigeminal Neuralgia
- Tendon
- Tendon Repair
- Tendon Transfer
- Tendon Graft

PERIPHERAL NERVE INJURIES

Seddon's Classification

- *Neuropraxia:*
  It is a *temporary physiological paralysis* of nerve conduction. Here recovery is complete. There is no reaction of degeneration. Cross-section of an intact nerve is shown in Figure 14.1.
- *Axonotmesis*:
  It is *division of nerve fibers or axons* with intact nerve sheath. There is reaction of degeneration distally with near complete recovery. Patient can present with sensory loss, paralysis of muscles or causalgia.
- *Neurotmesis*:
  Here *complete division of nerve fibers* with sheath occurs. Degeneration occurs proximally up to the first node of Ranvier as well as distal to the injury. Recovery is incomplete even after nerve suturing.

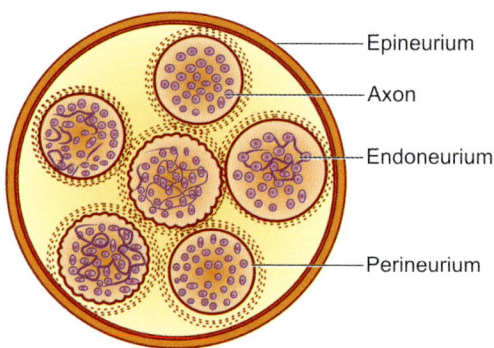

Fig. 14.1: Cross-section of a nerve.

There is complete loss of motor and sensory functions with loss of reflexes. If the nerve is mixed type rather than pure motor or sensory recovery is still poorer.

Injuries may be:
- Incised or lacerated or crushed one.
- Cut end of the nerve forms *neuroma* proximally and *glioma* distally.

The best antiques are old friends

Neuromas may be:
* True neuroma or false neuroma.
* End neuroma or Side neuroma.

Sunderland's classification
I. Conduction block—temporary neuronal block.
II. Axonotmesis but endoneurium is preserved.
III. Axonotmesis with disruption of endoneurium but perineurium is preserved.
IV. Here there is disruption of endo and perineurium but epineurium is intact.
V. Neurotmesis with disruption of endo, peri and epineurium.

Clinical Features
* Loss of sensory, motor, autonomous and reflex functions.
* Secondary changes in the skin and joint.

Management
* Associated injuries like fracture, vessel injury, injuries in other systems should be looked for.
* Regular checking of sensation, muscle power, and reflexes assesses nerve injury.
* Nerve conduction studies.
* Investigations relevant to associated injuries.
* Exploration of the wound.
  Debridement of the area is done. If injury is incised type, then nerve is sutured with 8-0 or 10-0 nonabsorbable interrupted sutures (polypropylene).

Types of Nerve Suturing
* **Primary nerve suturing** is done if it is a clean incised wound (Fig. 14.2).
* **Secondary nerve suturing** is done after 3 weeks if it is a crushed wound (Fig. 14.3).

Usually operative microscope or loup is used for nerve suturing.
i. *Epineurorrhaphy*: Only epineurium is sutured using interrupted sutures.
ii. *Epiperineurorrhaphy*: Initially perineural sheath and then epineurium is sutured.
* If nerve is lacerated, *marker stitches (using silk)* are placed at the cut end site to identify the nerve for suturing at a later period.
* If nerve suturing fails or if could not be done, then tendon transfer is done at a later period after 4–6 months.
* *Incomplete injury* usually does not require any suturing.
* **6-0 polypropylene is usually used**.

Easier suturing is achieved by following methods:
* Relaxing incisions.
* Transpositioning of the nerve.
* Shortening of the bone.

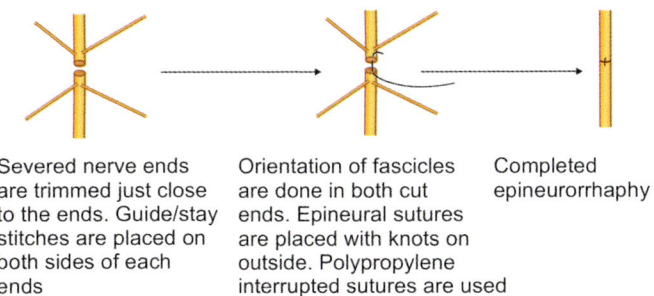

Severed nerve ends are trimmed just close to the ends. Guide/stay stitches are placed on both sides of each ends

Orientation of fascicles are done in both cut ends. Epineural sutures are placed with knots on outside. Polypropylene interrupted sutures are used

Completed epineurorrhaphy

Fig. 14.2: Primary nerve repair.

*Ever has it been that love knows not its own depth until the hour of separation—**Kalil Gibran***

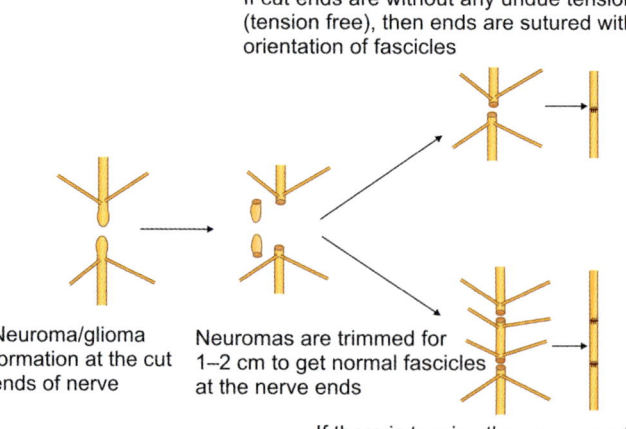

Fig. 14.3: Secondary nerve repair.

- Nerve graft—usually sural nerve is used for nerve graft.
- Positioning of the limb.
- Initially *neurolysis* (release of the scar tissue adjacent to injury) is done in case of secondary suturing.

Prognostic factors in healing of the nerve injury

- Higher the lesion worse the prognosis.
- More the gap between the cut ends worse the prognosis.
- Associated injuries alter the prognosis.
- Children do better with nerve injury.
- Type of the injury also decides the prognosis.

Tinel's Sign

It is the clinical sign (prognostic indicator) used to assess the level of regeneration. It is elicited 3 weeks after the nerve injury (regeneration begins after the completion of nerve degeneration).

Tapping is done over the course of the nerve *from distal to proximal* end to elicit a sensation of *'pins and needles' or hyperesthesia*. If sensation is felt at the site as well as distally along the distribution of the nerve that means good recovery can be expected. If sensation is felt only at the site of tapping, then result is equivocal. If no sensation is felt it means no recovery can be expected.

Causes of peripheral nerve lesions

- Traumatic: Either closed or open injury.
- Inflammatory: Leprosy, Herpes zoster, diphtheria.
- Compression neuropathies.
- Lead poisoning.
- Arsenical poisoning.
- Alcoholism.
- Diabetes mellitus.
- Vitamin B_1 deficiency.
- Porphyria.
- Neurofibroma and other neural tumors.
- Idiopathic.

BRACHIAL PLEXUS INJURIES

Types

It can be:
- Supraclavicular injury : 65%.
- Infraclavicular injury : 25%.
- Combined : 10%.

It can be:

Preganglionic injury.	Postganglionic injury.
Avulsion injury.	Usually less severe.
More dangerous.	Better recovery.
Extends into the spinal cord.	

Difficulties come not to obstruct, but to instruct

It can be:

Upper plexus injury (Erb-Duchenne paralysis)	Lower plexus injury (Klumpke's paralysis)
It is due to depression of shoulder by trauma.	Forcible hyperabduction causes this injury.
In newborn after difficult labor.	In newborn due to difficult breech delivery.
Here C_5 and C_6 roots are injured.	Here C_8 and T_1 roots are injured.
Muscles affected are deltoid, biceps, brachioradialis and supinator.	Intrinsic muscles of the hand are involved.
Effects are:	
Elbow will be extended, pronated and upper limb is internally rotated. (Policeman receiving tip).	1. Combined median and ulnar claw hand. 2. Horner's syndrome.

Investigations

- Nerve conduction studies.
- CT/MRI.
- Electromyogram.
- X-ray cervical spine and part.

Treatment

- Conservative.
- Nerve repair.
- Tendon transfer.
- Physiotherapy.

CAUSALGIA

It is severe burning pain in the distribution of a peripheral nerve due to *incomplete injury* to the peripheral nerve.

Sites

- Common in upper limb, seen in brachial plexus or median nerve injuries.
- In the lower limb, it can be seen in distribution of sciatic nerve or tibial nerve.
- *Clinically*, there will be hyperesthesia and severe, *disabling burning pain* along the distribution of the nerve.

Management

- Nerve conduction studies.
- Sympathectomy—cervical for upper limb, lumbar for lower limb.

MEDIAN NERVE INJURIES

- Median nerve arises from lateral ($C_{5,6,7}$) and medial cord (C_8 and T_1) of the brachial plexus. It lies initially lateral to the axillary artery and becomes medial in the lower part of the arm and in the cubital fossa. It passes through the pronator teres, descends in relation to flexor muscles and enters the palm through the carpal tunnel at the wrist.
- It supplies pronator teres, flexor carpi radialis, palmaris longus and flexor digitorum superficialis. Anterior interosseous branch of the median nerve supplies pronator teres, lateral half of the flexor digitorum profundus, flexor pollicis longus and pronator quadratus.
- In the wrist, it supplies abductor pollicis brevis, flexor pollicis, opponens pollicis of thenar eminence and lateral two lumbricals. It gives sensory supply to lateral three and half fingers of the hand.

Median nerve is affected in

1. Injuries
   a. Supracondylar fracture of the elbow.
   b. Fracture-dislocation of the elbow.
   c. Direct cut injuries.
2. Leprosy.
3. Carpal tunnel syndrome.
4. As a part of brachial plexus injury.

In the sweetness of friendship let there be laughter and sharing of pleasures

Clinical Features of Median Nerve Palsy

In high median nerve palsy
- Wasting of the thenar eminence. Loss of sensation in lateral three and half fingers.
- *Ochsner's clasping test* shows pointing index because of the inactivity of lateral two divisions of the profundus.
- *'Ape or Simian thumb deformity'* is due to over action of the adductor pollicis, which is supplied by the deep branch of ulnar nerve. As all other thenar muscles are paralyzed, thumb lies in the same plane of the metacarpals.
- *'Pen test'*: In median nerve injury, pen held in front of the hand cannot be touched by thumb, as abduction is not possible due to paralysis of the abductor pollicis brevis.

In low median nerve palsy
Profundus is not paralyzed and so *pointing index* is *not seen*.

Investigations
- Nerve conduction studies.
- X-ray of the part in case of fracture.
- Electromyogram.

Treatment
- Nerve suturing or nerve graft.
- Tendon transfer.
- The condition is treated like carpal tunnel syndrome.

CARPAL TUNNEL SYNDROME

- It is the *compression neuropathy of median nerve* in the carpus, deep to flexor retinaculum.
- Flexor retinaculum (transverse carpal ligament) maintains the concavity of wrist and extends laterally from trapezium and scaphoid to pisiform and hook of the hamate medially.

Carpal tunnel is formed by carpal bones behind and flexor retinaculum in front. It contains median nerve and long flexor tendons of fingers and thumb. Ulnar nerve lies superficially, not within the carpal tunnel. Median nerve gets compressed if space of the carpal tunnel gets reduced.

Causes
- Lunate dislocation.
- Mal united Colles' fracture.
- Radiocarpal arthritis.
- Flexor tendon tenosynovitis.
- Myxedema; acromegaly; pregnancy.

Features
- Common in *females*.
- Tingling, numbness, paresthesia and burning sensation in the lateral three and half fingers supplied by median nerve. Burning sensation gets aggravated at night.
- Ape thumb deformity, wasting of thenar muscles, weakness of opponens pollicis and abductor pollicis brevis, i.e. features of low median nerve palsy.
- When BP cuff is inflated patient feels the typical pain in the fingers.
- Tapping the median nerve at the distal end of forearm with the wrist held in extension aggravates the symptoms.
- Condition is often bilateral.
- **Differential diagnosis**
  - Cervical spondylosis.
  - Cervical rib syndrome.
- **Diagnosis:** Nerve conduction studies; MRI cervical spine.
- **Treatment**
  - Surgical decompression of median nerve by cutting both superficial and deep part of flexor retinaculum completely, by 'S' shaped incision.
  - Postoperatively *good physiotherapy* is required.
  - Condition is permanently curable.

Circumstance do not make man, they reveal him

ULNAR NERVE INJURIES

- After arising from the medial cord of the brachial plexus (C_8 and T_1), it runs on the medial aspect of the axillary artery up to middle of the arm. Then it enters the posterior compartment in relation to triceps muscle. After passing behind the medial epicondyle and through two heads of flexor carpi ulnaris, it runs in front of the flexor digitorum profundus (FDP) in the forearm. It reaches the hand in front of the flexor retinaculum through *Guyon's canal*. Here it divides into superficial and deep branches.
- Ulnar nerve supplies flexor carpi ulnaris, medial half of flexor digitorum profundus, all muscles of the hypothenar eminence (palmaris brevis, abductor digiti minimi, opponens digiti minimi, flexor digiti minimi), adductor pollicis of the thenar eminence and all interossei of the hand. It also gives sensory supply to medial part of the hand, medial one and half fingers.

Ulnar nerve is affected in

- Supracondylar fracture; Tardy ulnar palsy.
- Injury to the medial epicondyle.
- Leprosy; cubitus valgus deformity.

Features

- *Claw hand* deformity.
- Weakness of all the muscles supplied by the ulnar nerve.
- '*Card test*':
  A card is placed between the two fingers of the patient to grasp. In weak palmar interossei, patient cannot grasp [palmar interossei are adductors of the fingers (*PAD*)].
- Abduction of fingers is checked [(dorsal interossei are abductors (*DAB*)].
- *Froment's sign*: A book is placed to grasp between fingers and thumb of the patient. Normally thumb will be straight because of the action of adductor pollicis muscle. As it is paralyzed in ulnar palsy, grasp is achieved by the action of flexor pollicis longus and there will be flexed thumb.
- Loss of sensation over medial one and half fingers and hand.
- **Investigations:** Nerve conduction studies; electromyogram.
- **Treatment:** Nerve suturing or nerve grafting; tendon transfer.

> **Intrinsic minus deformity:** It is due to loss of intrinsic muscle power, i.e claw hand.
> **Intrinsic plus deformity:** It is due to muscle contracture and fibrosis.
> **Ulnar paradox:** In ulnar palsy, higher the lesion, lesser the deformity, lower the lesion more the deformity. In higher lesion, FDP is also paralyzed. In lower lesion, FDP is intact and so FDP causes more flexion (overaction) and so the claw hand is aggravated.

CLAW HAND

- It is the *hyperextension of the metacarpophalangeal (MCP) joint with flexion of the interphalangeal (IP) joints of the hand.*
- Extension of MCP joint is due to action of extensor digitorum.
- Flexion of MCP joint and extension of interphalangeal joints are by extensor hood of interossei and lumbricals. So, extensor hood is functioned mainly by ulnar nerve and also by median nerve. In ulnar or median nerve palsies, these actions are paralyzed and so patient develops claw hand (Fig. 14.4).
- It is actually *intrinsic minus deformity*.

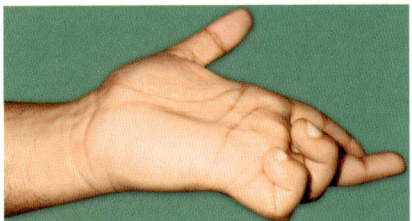

Fig. 14.4: Ulnar claw hand.

*Work is love made visible—***Kalil Gibran**

Causes
- Leprosy • Trauma
- Entrapment neuropathies • Tardy ulnar palsy
- Klumpke's palsy.

Clinical Features

- Typical claw hand.
- Loss of sensation along the distribution of the nerve.
- Inability to grasp card between the fingers.
- While holding the book between the thumb and fingers, thumb will be flexed in ulnar claw hand (*positive Froment's test*).

Types

1. *Ulnar claw hand*: Only medial two fingers are involved.
   - *Low ulnar palsy*: Here lesion is in the wrist (at Guyon's canal). Here deformity is more because of the overaction of the FDP.
   - *High ulnar palsy*: Here as FDP is also paralyzed, there is no overaction. Deformity is less.
     » Ulnar paradox: Higher the lesion lesser the deformity, lower the lesion more the deformity.
2. *Median claw hand*: Only lateral two fingers are involved. It is less common.
3. *Combined median and ulnar claw hand*: Here all four fingers of the hand are involved.

Investigations

- Electromyogram.
- Nerve conduction studies.

Treatment

- *Paul Braund's operation*: Extensor carpi radialis longus or brevis (ECRB) is transferred with a graft to the extensor hood through the lumbrical canal. Graft is taken from palmaris longus or plantaris muscle.
- *Stye-Bunnell's operation*: Flexor digitorum superficialis of index finger is used (only in ulnar claw hand) to transfer to extensor hood.
- *Anterior transpositioning* of the ulnar nerve in case of tardy ulnar palsy.

RADIAL NERVE LESIONS

- Radial nerve is derived from the posterior cord of the brachial plexus ($C_{5,6,7,8}$ and T_1). It descends behind the axillary artery in front of the subscapularis, latissimus dorsi and teres major. It passes through the medial and lateral heads of the triceps muscle, winds round the humerus through the radial groove and enters the forearm in front of the lateral epicondyle in relation to brachioradialis, brachialis and extensor carpi radialis longus muscles.
- In the arm, it supplies triceps, anconeus, brachioradialis, extensor carpi radialis longus and part of the brachialis. It gives posterior and lower lateral cutaneous nerves of the arm and posterior cutaneous nerve of the forearm.
- *Superficial branch* of the radial nerve from the elbow runs in the forearm in relation to supinator and brachioradialis and ends by forming 5 digital nerves, which gives sensory supply to lateral three and half fingers on the dorsal aspect.
- *Deep branch* also called as posterior interosseous nerve winds round the radius supplying supinator and extensor carpi radialis brevis. It gives 3 short branches to extensor digitorum, extensor digiti minimi and extensor carpi ulnaris. It also gives two long branches—one to abductor pollicis longus and extensor pollicis brevis; another to extensor digitorum, extensor carpi ulnaris and extensor digiti minimi.

Tolerance is another word for indifference

Conditions where radial nerve is affected

In the axilla
- *Crutch palsy*—it is neuropraxia.
- Fracture upper end of the humerus.
- Bony or soft tissue growth.

In the radial groove
- Pressure on the arm from the edge of the operating table.
- *Saturday night palsy*—an individual with excessive alcohol consumption compresses his arm over the chair or by fall. It is neuropraxia.
- Prolonged tourniquet application—*Tourniquet palsy*.
- Fracture of the shaft of the humerus.
- *Rarely* intramuscular injection of drugs can cause radial nerve palsy.

In the elbow
- Dislocation or fracture neck of the radius.

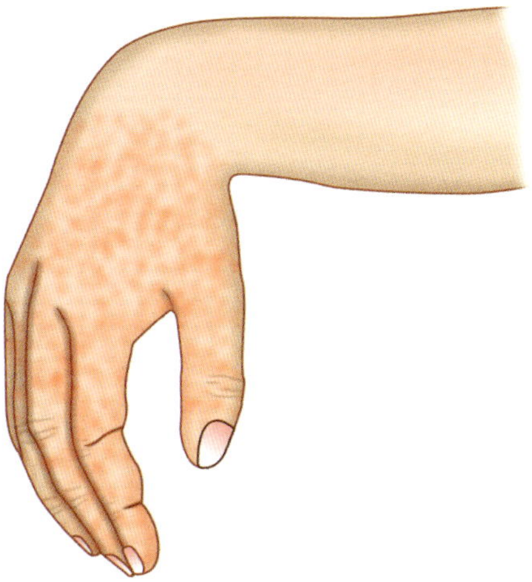

Fig. 14.5: Wrist drop.

Features

- *Wrist drop* because of inability to extend the wrist (Fig. 14.5).
- Inability to extend MCP joint, but extensions of the IP joints is normal.
- Inability to extend the forearm.
- Inability to extend the thumb.
- Flexion of the elbow against resistance with forearm in mid-prone position is difficult because of the weakness of the brachioradialis muscle.
- Loss of sensation in back of the arm, forearm, hand and lateral three and half fingers. Posterior interosseous nerve is purely motor and so sensation is intact when it gets injured.
- **Investigations:** X-ray of the part; nerve conduction studies.
- **Treatment:** Nerve suturing or nerve graft; tendon transfer.

COMMON PERONEAL NERVE

This nerve supplies the extensor and peroneal group of muscles; and sensory supply to the skin over the front and lateral aspect of the leg and dorsum of the foot (Fig. 14.6).

Common peroneal nerve is affected in
- Fracture neck of the fibula.
- Leprosy.
- Lead poisoning.
- Iatrogenic.

Clinical Features
- Foot drop with high stepping gait.
- Talipes equinovarus deformity.
- Loss of sensation in the lateral side of the leg and dorsum of the foot.

Management
- Treating the foot drop.
- Micro cellular rubber (MCR) chappals.
- Tendon transfer using tibialis posterior muscle. Tendon of the muscle is detached from the navicular insertion and with a tendon graft (from plantaris) it is transferred to cuboid and cuneiform bones to get dorsiflexion and eversion.

AXILLARY NERVE INJURY

Axillary nerve supplies the deltoid and teres minor muscle and also sensory supply to the skin over the upper lateral aspect of the arm.

The teacher who is indeed wise does not bid you to enter the house of his wisdom but rather leads you to the threshold of your mind—**Kalil Gibran**

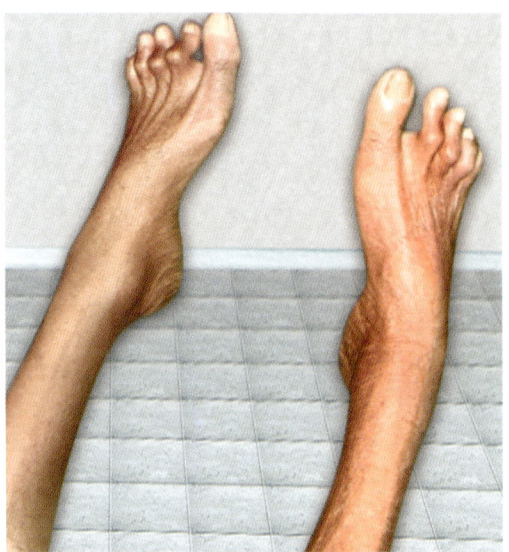

Fig. 14.6: Foot drop with claw toes.

Axillary nerve is affected in:
- Fracture neck of the humerus.
- Dislocation of humeral head.
- Following IM injection into the deltoid.
  Clinically, there will be loss of abduction of the shoulder and anesthesia of the skin over the lateral part of the arm.

LONG THORACIC NERVE (NERVE OF BELL)

- It supplies serratus anterior muscle. It arises from $C_{5,6,7}$ cervical roots. The nerve is injured commonly in malignancy, during breast, axillary or chest wall surgeries.
- *Clinically,* when outstretched (elbow extended) arm is pushed against the wall, the inferior angle of the scapula becomes prominent (*Winging of the scapula*).

TRIGEMINAL NEURALGIA

- It is the excruciating pain and hyperesthesia along the distribution of the trigeminal nerve.
- **Causes:** Postherpetic (zoster); malignancy.

Features
- Paroxysmal, shooting, sharp, sudden, short pain.
- It is usually unilateral.
- Second and third division of 5th cranial nerve is affected.
- Sensory or motor loss will not be present.
- Touching/washing/shaving face or brushing are triggering factors.
- It begins behind the ear and spreads towards orbit, ear/chin.
- Often it begins below the orbit and spreads to nose, upper lip or to cheek.
- **Treatment**
  - Carbazepine tablets 100mg three times a day.
  - Peripheral neurectomy.
  - Injection into gasserian/trigeminal ganglion using alcohol/lignocaine.
  - Intracranial decompression of trigeminal ganglion pathway or intramedullary trigeminal tractotomy is done only in severe intolerable intractable cases (rarely).

TENDON

- Tendon is the continuity of the muscle to have its action at the site especially in hand, foot and digits.
- It is covered by synovial sheath with a thin layer of fluid in between which allows smooth gliding of the tendon.
- Tendon injuries may be cut wound, lacerations, injury associated with nerve or vessel injury.

After injury tendon heals by:
1. **Intrinsic healing method**—occurs through synovial fluid when tendon is not under stress.
2. **Extrinsic healing method**—occurs through proliferation of fibroblasts across epitenon. It occurs when tendon is under

Determination is the wake-up call to the human will

stress. It forms a mass of fibrous tissue at the site called as '*tenoma*'. It may interfere with the proper gliding of the tendon.

Stages of Tendon Healing

1. By 21 days weak healing occurs and contraction of muscle possible.
2. At 6 weeks, mild traction can be applied to the tendon.
3. At 3 months, moderate stress may be used.
4. By 8 months, full tensile strength is recovered.

TENDON REPAIR

1. *Primary repair* is done within 24 hours.
2. *Delayed repair* within a week after 24 hours.
3. *Secondary repair* anytime after one week.

Types of Suturing the Tendon (Figs. 14.7A and B)

1. **Goldner method**: Here knot comes away from the cut ends of the tendon.
2. **Kessler method**: Here knot comes in the cut part of the tendon.

Suture material used is monofilament non-absorbable suture material (polypropylene, 3 or 4 zero).
- Continuous sutures are used for suturing.
- Epitenon can be later apposed with interrupted sutures.
- Postoperative immobilization is required for 3–4 weeks.
- Later passive and active exercise is required with the help of a physiotherapist.

Complications of tendon suturing are infection, adhesion, stiffness and failure.

TENDON TRANSFER

- It is the transfer of one tendon from its existing site to another site to have a function required at the newer site.

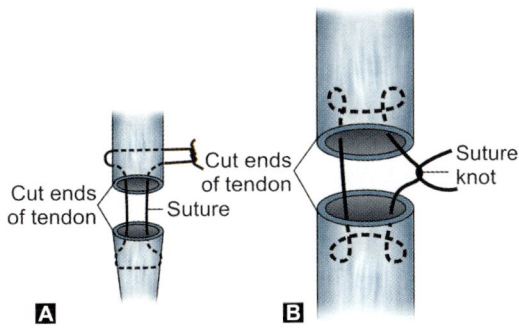

Figs. 14.7A and B: Types of tendon suturing (A) Goldner method; (B) Kessler method.

- Other tendons should maintain function of the transferred tendon.
- Tendon should able to acquire the function at the newer site properly.
- For example, flexor digitorum superficialis (FDS) (of index finger) tendon transfer in ulnar claw hand to lumbrical canal of the digits to have flexion at MCP joint and extension of proximal IP joint.

TENDON GRAFT

When tendon suturing or transfer is not possible because of inadequate length, tendon of a muscle, which is not much helpful functionally, is taken as a graft to obtain required length.

Common grafts used are:
- Palmaris tendon in forearm.
- Plantaris tendon in leg.

For example, ECRB is lengthened using tendon graft to transfer to lumbrical canals in claw hand.

Problems in tendon graft: Infection, adhesions, graft failure, and stiffness of the part.

There is no service than doing something for someone who will never find it out!

CHAPTER 15

Neoplasm and Soft Tissue Tumors

Chapter Outline

- Neoplasm
- Spread of Malignant Tumors
- Paraneoplastic Syndromes
- Investigations for Neoplasm
- Soft Tissue Tumors (Sarcomas)
- Kaposi's Sarcoma

NEOPLASM

Definition

Willis defined neoplasm as '*it is an abnormal mass of tissue, the growth of which exceeds and is uncoordinated with that of the normal tissues and persists in the same excessive manner even after cessation of the stimuli*.'

Neoplasia is:
Progressive.   **P**ervasive.
Persistent.   **P**erverted.
Purposeless.   **P**roliferative mass of tissue.

Components

Parenchyma:
It contains proliferating neoplastic cells.
Stroma:
It contains supporting connective tissues and blood vessels.

Features of anaplasia
• Lack of differentiation.
• Pleomorphism—variation in size and shape.
• Hyperchromatism—dark staining nuclei.
• Anisocytosis.
• Anisonucleosis.
• Abnormal mitotic activity.

Classification

Benign	Malignant
Well-differentiated.	Lack of differentiation.
Structures are typical of tissue/cell of origin.	Atypical structure with anaplasia.
Smooth, slow, progressive rate of growth.	Erratic, rapid growth.
Normal mitotic figures.	Abnormal mitotic activity.
Well-localized and capsulated.	Not localized. Not capsulated.
Do not infiltrate surrounding normal tissues.	Infiltrate the surrounding tissues.
No metastasis.	Metastasize to lymph node or blood.
Curable.	May not be completely curable.
Few benign tumors after long time may turn into malignancy:	
Treatment is simple.	Treatment is complex and complicated.

A friend is your second identity

Sarcoma	Carcinoma
Arising from mesenchymal tissues.	Arising from epithelial cells derived from any of the three germ layers.
'Sar' means flesh-[Greek]. 'Oma' means tumor.	'Carc' means crab-like.
Smooth, firm or hard swelling.	Hard, proliferative, with everted edge.
Warm and vascular with dilated veins over the surface.	Spreads through lymphatics as well as blood.
Spreads mainly through blood commonly to lungs, e.g. liposarcoma, fibrosarcoma, etc.	Squamous cell carcinoma, renal cell carcinoma, adenocarcinoma.

Neoplasms which are only locally malignant: No blood spread. No lymph node spread—Marjolin's ulcer, rodent ulcer, verrucous carcinoma, adamantinoma.

Neoplasms which are locoregionally malignant: Regional lymph node spread is observed—squamous cell carcinoma, papillary carcinoma thyroid.

Neoplasms which are systemic and spread through blood and often also to lymph node—melanoma, carcinoma breast (Figs. 15.1 to 15.3).

Features of malignant tissues

- Altered differentiation, anaplasia.
- Rapid rate of growth.
- Local invasion.
- Metastasis.
- Not capsulated.

Dysplasia:

It means 'disordered growth'. It is loss in the uniformity of the cells with pleomorphism and hyperchromatism as well as loss in their architectural orientation.

Etiological factors

Age
It is more common in elderly. But it is variable.

Heredity
- Familial: Familial polyposis of colon.
- Multiple endocrine neoplasia (MEN) syndrome.
- Neurofibromatosis.
- von Hippel-Lindau syndrome.
- Familial breast and ovarian cancers.

Genetic
- Xeroderma pigmentosa.
- Ataxia telangiectasia.
- Fanconi anemia, bloom syndrome.

Acquired causes
- Chronic atrophic gastritis.
- Solar keratosis.
- Leukoplakia of oral cavity.
- Ulcerative colitis.

Chemical carcinogens
- Alkylating agents.
- Hydrocarbons.
- Amides, azo dyes.
- Aflatoxin B1.
- Arecoline, collagenases and tannins (present in betel nuts).
- Nitrosamines, vinyl chloride, insecticides.

Radiation carcinogens
- UV rays, ionizing radiation.

Microbial carcinogens
- Human papilloma virus—carcinoma cervix.
- Epstein-Barr virus—Burkitt's lymphoma, nasopharyngeal carcinoma.
- Hepatitis 'B' virus.
- Human T-cell leukemia virus type I.
- *Helicobacter pylori* can cause carcinoma of stomach and is associated with lymphomas. [Mucosa associated with lymphoid tissue (MALT)].

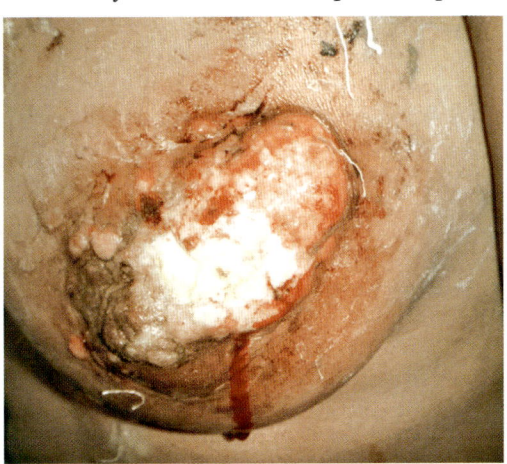

Fig. 15.1: Fungating carcinoma of breast.

Beware of the little expenses; a small leak can sink a great ship

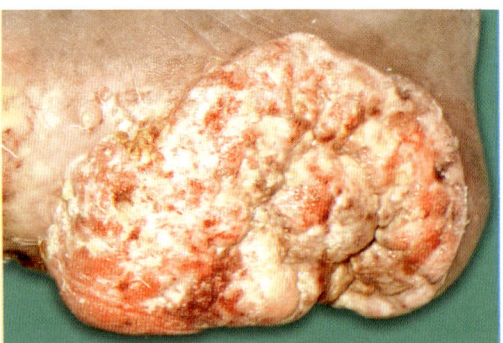

Fig. 15.2: Squamous cell carcinoma heel showing proliferative lesion.

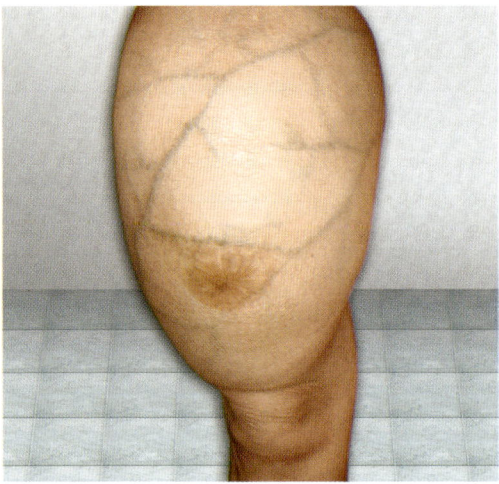

Fig. 15.3: Soft tissue sarcoma of thigh showing swelling with dilated vessels on the surface.

Carcinoma in situ:
When dysplasia involves entire thickness of the epithelium, which is preinvasive, it is called as carcinoma in situ. Basement membrane is intact in carcinoma in situ.

SPREAD OF MALIGNANT TUMORS

1. **Local spread:**
   It spreads into adjacent structures like soft tissues, vessels, bone, etc.
2. **Lymphatic spread:**
   - *By permeation*: Here malignant cells proliferate through lymphatic vessels up to lymph node level, e.g. in carcinoma breast, malignant cells permeate into axillary lymph nodes.
   - *By embolization:* Here cells get dislodged from lymphatic vessels and freely travel to spread into further level of lymph nodes. In carcinoma breast, spread occurs from axillary lymph node to supraclavicular lymph node by embolization.
   - *Retrograde lymphatic spread:* It occurs once malignant infiltration blocks lymph vessel. In carcinoma breast, retrograde spread occurs to opposite breast, opposite axilla, or to mediastinum. In melanoma through dermal lymphatics and retrograde spread '*in transit nodules*' occur in the skin.
3. **Blood spread:**
   - Occurs through veins, as veins are thin and infiltration is easier (arteries contain elastic fibers which resist malignant infiltration).
   - Both by **permeation** (e.g. permeation through renal vein is common in renal cell carcinoma) and by **embolization** (in other malignancies).
   - Blood spread is commonly to **lungs, bone** (upper end of femur and humerus, ribs, skull), liver, brain, adrenals, and other organs.
   - In carcinoma prostate, due to increased pressure and venous block, retrograde venous spread occurs through vertebral venous plexus, which causes **osteoblastic secondaries** in pelvic bones and vertebrae.
4. **Seedling:**
   - From lower lip cancer to upper lip as *kiss cancer*.

*Only when you drink from the river of silence shall you indeed sing—**Kalil Gibran***

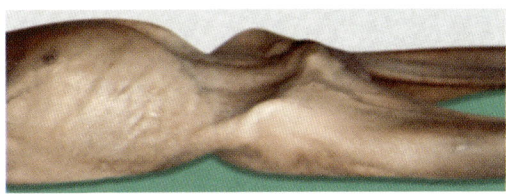

Fig. 15.4: Typical malignant cachexia in an advanced GI malignancy.

- Recurrence in the scar after surgery for malignancy, e.g. deposition of malignancy in the scar of suprapubic catheter (SPC) from bladder tumor.
- Seedling in the peritoneal cavity from abdominal malignancy is common causing intractable ascites.
5. **Transcoelomic spread**:
Due to spillage or dislodge of malignant cells from primary site causing seedling in other organ, e.g. in carcinoma stomach, secondaries in ovary is caused by transcoelomic spread (***Krukenberg tumor***). Here cells get deposited onto the raw surface of ovary during ovulation (So it occurs in menstruating age group only). Advanced malignancy can be associated with severe cachexia (Fig. 15.4).

PARANEOPLASTIC SYNDROMES

Certain symptom complexes, which are not specifically explained by the tumor, but are relevant, often problematic and life-threatening are called as *paraneoplastic syndromes* (Table 15.1).

Incidence:
Seen in 10% of patients.

Grading of tumor
- it signifies aggressiveness of tumor.
- It is based on differentiation of tumor cells and mitotic activity.

Staging of the tumor
- it is based on the size of the primary tumor, nodal spread and blood spread.
- It is called as 'TNM' staging.
- 'TNM' staging is more relevant than grading in managing and predicting prognosis.

Table 15.1: Paraneoplastic syndromes

Syndrome	Cause	Types of tumor
Cushing's syndrome.	ACTH or ACTH-like substance.	Small cell carcinoma lung. Neural tumor. Pancreatic tumor.
Syndrome of inappropriate ADH.	ADH	Small cell carcinoma lung. Brain tumor.
Carcinoid syndrome.	Serotonin, bradykinin.	Bronchial adenoma. Gastric and pancreatic cancer.
Hypoglycemia.	Insulin. Insulin-like substance.	Fibrosarcoma. Hepatoma.
Hypercalcemia.	PTH related peptide.	Renal cell carcinoma. Carcinoma breast, SCC lung. Ovarian cancer, leukemia.
Polycythemia.	Erythropoietin.	Renal cell carcinoma, hepatoma. Cerebellar hemangioma.
Myasthenia.	Immunologic.	Carcinoma lung.
Acanthosis nigricans.	Epidermal growth factor.	Lung cancer, uterine cancer, gastric cancer.
Dermatomyositis.	Immunologic.	Lung cancer, breast carcinoma.
Clubbing and hypertrophic osteoarthropathy of fingers.		Carcinoma lung.
Migrating thrombophlebitis. (Trousseau phenomenon).	Tumor product mucin, It activates clotting.	Carcinoma pancreas, lung.

*Trust in dreams, for in them is hidden the gate of eternity—**Kalil Gibran***

Broder's grading of squamous cell carcinoma— based on keratin/epithelial pearls

- *Grade I:* Well-differentiated—>75% epithelial pearls.
- *Grade II:* Moderately differentiated—50–75% epithelial pearls.
- *Grade III:* Poorly differentiated—25–50% epithelial pearls.
- *Grade IV:* <25% epithelial pearls.

INVESTIGATIONS FOR NEOPLASM

I. BIOPSY

- '*Bio*' means life or tissue. '*Opsis*' means vision or microscopy.
- Biopsy means study of tissues using microscopy.
  - Or *life by vision*.
  - Or *vision for life* (to save life).

Incision Biopsy

- It is done from the edge of the lesion like an ulcer. It is not taken from the center, as there will be central necrosis.
- Incision biopsy is contraindicated in melanoma where excision biopsy is preferred.

Excision Biopsy

In small lesions, excision biopsy is done. Lymph node biopsy is done in case of lymphoma.

Fine Needle Aspiration Cytology

Fine needle aspiration cytology (FNAC) is a cytological study of tumor cell to find out the disease and also to confirm whether it is malignant or not.

Procedure:
It is done using 23 or 24 gauge needle with specialized syringe (Fig. 15.5), which create negative pressure by aspiration and contents are smeared in the slides. Dry slides as well as 100% methanol are used for study.

- It is done in parotid, thyroid, lymph node, breast and all other surface lesions.
- In follicular carcinoma of thyroid, it is not very useful as angioinvasion and capsular invasion which are specific cannot be detected.
- In lymph node, it is useful for secondaries and tuberculosis.
- Ultrasound guided or CT guided FNAC are popular at present.

It is absolutely contraindicated in testicular tumor. Because the tough tunica albuginea usually prevents tumor spread and once FNAC disrupts it, spread can occur.

Advantages

- Very sensitive.
- Done on OP basis.
- Least invasive. Safer.
- Anesthesia is not required.

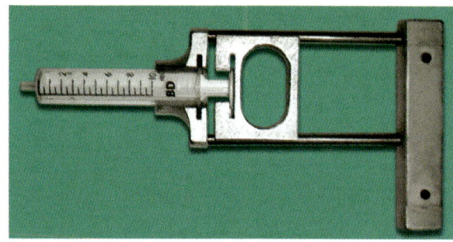

Fig. 15.5: Instrument used for FNAC. It creates suction during aspiration to get more cells.

Types of biopsies			
• Incision biopsy.	• FNAC.	• Excision biopsy.	• Frozen section biopsy.
• Trucut biopsy (Fig. 15.6).	• Punch biopsy.	• Pap smear.	• Ultrasound guided biopsy.
• CT guided biopsy.	• Laparoscopic biopsy.		• Thoracoscopic biopsy.
• Endoscopic biopsy (gastroscopic or colonoscopic or through ERCP or through cystoscopy).			
• Proctoscopic biopsy.			
• Open biopsy either laparotomy or thoracotomy or craniotomy using Dandy's brain cannula.			

To strengthen your heart, forgive yourself and others

❖ Tumor dissemination through the track is not there (except in testicular tumor where it is not done).

Disadvantage

Negative result cannot rule out malignancy.

Trucut Biopsy (Fig. 15.6)

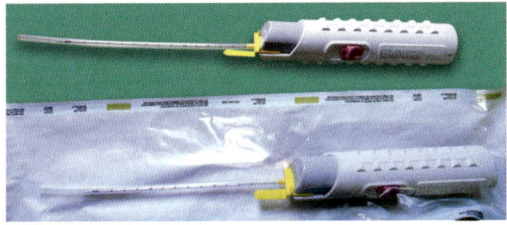

Fig. 15.6: Instrument used for trucut biopsy. Incision biopsy is ideal for soft tissue sarcoma. Trucut biopsy also can be done. FNAC is of very least significant in STS

❖ The *'Trucut' biopsy needle* consists of an inner solid needle, the obturator and an outer hollow needle and the cannula. The obturator has a pointed end for tissue penetration and behind this is a notch for the biopsy specimen. The cannula serves as a cutting sheath. Outer cannula is usually of 14 or 18 Gage sized. Technique is by push, slide and withdraw method.
❖ It is mainly used in breast lump (standard and ideal). Sample insufficiency is rare compared to FNAC; histological and tumor receptor status can be assessed so the treatment plan can be properly planned. Technically, it is safer (as breast is a surface organ). Tissue architecture is revealed in trucut biopsy unlike as in FNAC.
❖ It is also used now for many other organs under image guidance like liver, prostate, other solid organs.

Frozen Section Biopsy

It is done in carcinoma breast or in follicular carcinoma of thyroid when FNAC fails.

II. IMMUNOHISTOCHEMISTRY

❖ *To categorize leukemias or lymphomas.* Either 'T' cell or 'B' cell.
❖ *To find out site of origin of metastatic tumors,* e.g. by assessing levels of prostate specific antigen in prostate cancer or levels of thyroglobulin in thyroid carcinomas.
❖ *Detection of receptors or molecules*: For example, estrogen receptors in breast cancer. ER +ve has got better prognosis. Presence of oncoprotein product c–erbB2 in breast cancer signifies poor prognosis.

III. TUMOR MARKERS

❖ Tumor markers are biochemical indicators for presence of a tumor. They are not used for primary pathological diagnosis. They are of prognostic value.
❖ Presence of tumor marker signifies recurrence or residual tumor.

Malignancies which are curable
• Basal cell carcinoma. • Adamantinoma. • Verrucous carcinoma. • Marjolin's ulcer. • Papillary carcinoma of thyroid. • Carcinoma colon.

Sarcomas which spread to lymph nodes also	
• Synovial sarcoma. • Lymphosarcoma. • Rhabdomyosarcoma.	• Ewing's sarcoma. • Kaposi's sarcoma.

SOFT TISSUE TUMORS (SARCOMAS)

Features

❖ Sarcomas are much lesser in incidence compared to carcinomas.
❖ It occurs in younger age group compared to carcinomas.
❖ They can arise from bone (osteosarcoma) or from any soft tissues (soft tissue sarcomas) (Fig. 15.7) (Mesenchymal tissue).

*Friendship is always a sweet responsibility, never an opportunity—**Kalil Gibran***

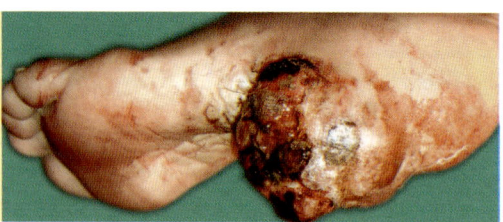

Fig. 15.7: Soft tissue sarcoma foot. Note the vascularity.

- They are much more aggressive compared to carcinomas.
- They are rapidly growing tumors with fleshy appearance.
- They are not encapsulated but are having pseudocapsule.
- They spread through blood, especially to lungs often also to other organs.
- Lymphatic spread is not common with certain exceptions.
- Main method of treatment is surgery, i.e. wide excision, amputation.
- In inoperable cases, debulking is the accepted method of treatment.
- Radiotherapy and chemotherapy are adjuvant therapies used.
- Commonest sarcoma of bone is **osteosarcoma (Fig. 15.8)**.
- Commonest soft tissue sarcoma is **liposarcoma**.
- *Usual clinical features* are: Diffuse swelling which is smooth, hard, warm and very vascular.

Important features of sarcoma

- More aggressive.
- Rapidly spreading.
- Not very much radiosensitive.
- Blood spread.
- Painless soft tissue mass is the presentation.
- Very vascular.

Soft tissue sarcoma—incidences

- 1% of adult malignancies.
- 15% of pediatric malignancies.
- Incidence:
  - 35% occur in lower limb (commonest site).
  - 15% upper limb, 15% retroperitoneum.
  - 10% trunk, 10% viscera, 10% other areas.
- Soft tissue tumor >5 cm size should be biopsied to rule out sarcoma.

Etiology of sarcoma

- *Genetic*:
  - von Recklinghausen disease.
  - Gardner's syndrome.
  - Tuberous sclerosis.
  - Basal cell nevus syndrome.
  - Li-Fraumeni syndrome.
- *Chemicals*—PVC, tetrachlorodibenzodioxin, arsenic.
- *Viral*—HIV in Kaposi's sarcoma.
- *Ionizing radiation*—malignant fibrous histiocytoma (p53).

Clinical Features of Soft Tissue Sarcoma (Figs. 15.9 and 15.10)

- Painless swelling of short duration with progressive increase in size—*soft tissue mass*.
- Compression of adjacent structures.
- Smooth, hard/firm/soft, warm and vascular.
- Features of secondaries in lung—cough, hemoptysis and chest pain.

Investigations

- *Incision biopsy* is the main method of diagnosis.

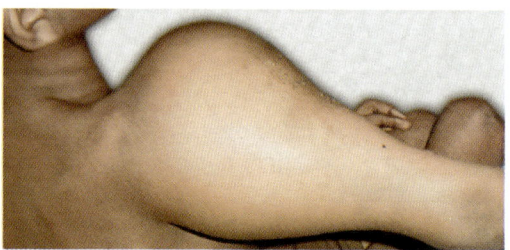

Fig. 15.8: Osteosarcoma of the upper end of humerus in an adolescent boy.

*Conflict is the primary engine of creativity and innovation—**Ranold Heifetz***

Remember about soft tissue sarcoma

- **Soft tissue sarcoma (STS)** arises from pluripotent mesenchymal stem cell without in situ changes. Transformation from benign lesion to sarcoma is not observed/disproved now except MPNST (Malignant peripheral nerve sheath tumor).
- Ratio of soft tissue sarcoma to bone sarcoma is 3:1.
- Soft tissue sarcoma is more common in males (4:1).
- Ratio of benign soft tissue tumor to malignant soft tissue tumor is 100:1. Most of the sarcomas arise as de novo. Per se benign will not turn into malignancy, as it is now found that cell of origin to begin with multiples with anisocytosis in soft tissue sarcoma. In olden days, it was accepted to consider benign (precursor tumor) turning into malignancy like lipoma turning into liposarcoma which is disproved now. But this argument does not hold good for nerve sheath tumor and probably lymphedema turning into lymphangiosarcoma (postmastectomy).
- 50% of STS occurs in extremities called as extremity STS; 35% lower and 15% upper limb.
- 3% of sarcoma spreads to lymph nodes.
- Soft tissue tumor >5 cm should be biopsied in suspicious of sarcoma.
- Commonest sarcoma of bone is *osteosarcoma*. (*Note:* Commonest malignancy of bone is secondaries).
- Commonest soft tissue sarcoma is *liposarcoma / malignant fibrous histiocytoma* (MFH—25%) overall; in the extremities both *MFH and liposarcoma*; in the retroperitoneum, it is *liposarcoma*.
- Commonest visceral (GIT) sarcoma is leiomyosarcoma.
- In genitourinary system, leiomyosarcoma is commonest in adults and rhabdomyosarcoma in *pediatric age group*; in uterus leiomyosarcoma; in myocardium angiosarcoma; in hand and foot synovial sarcoma; in skin Kaposi's sarcoma; in head and neck region angiosarcoma.
- *Lung* is the commonest site of secondary. Secondaries in *liver* especially in visceral STS as a principal site.
- Incision biopsy is the best method for tissue diagnosis.
- CT chest and abdomen to find out spread as—metastatic work up.
- Immunohistochemistry is a must to identify type, to plan adjuvant therapy and predict prognosis.

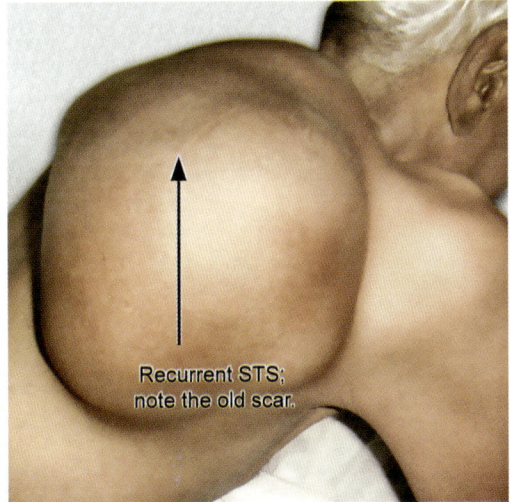

Fig. 15.9: Recurrent soft tissue sarcoma back. Note the scar on the surface. It could be synovial sarcoma.

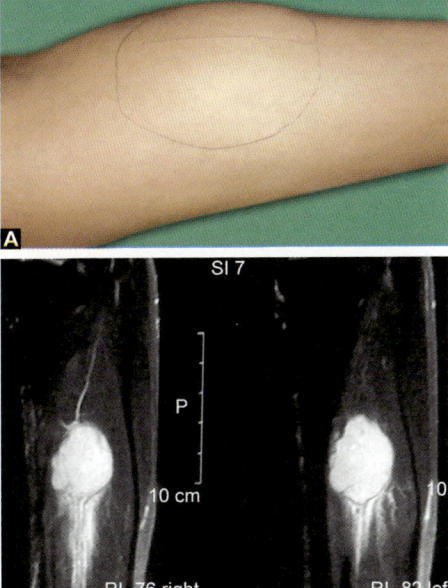

Figs. 15.10A and B: Soft tissue sarcoma leg. MRI pictures of the same patient showing the lesion. MRI is the ideal investigation to assess the local extension of soft tissue tumor.

❖ Excision biopsy is done if the tumor size is <3 cm.
❖ CT scan or MRI of the part to see the extent and invasion.

*Conflict is the primary engine of creativity and innovation—**Ranold Heifetz***

- MRI is the investigation of choice as it determines the vascularity, relation to vessel and fascial planes (Fig. 15.11).
- Chest X-ray is done to look for secondaries.
- CT chest is ideal to see early lung secondaries. It is done in all deep-seated, high grade and tumor more than 5 cm in size.
- Angiogram may be required to find out the tumor vascularity.
- Radionuclide scintigraphy (Gallium-67).
- P-MRS (P-Magnetic Resonance Spectroscopy and FDG (Fluor-2-Deoxy Glucose) PET are done to assess the metabolic activity of tumor.

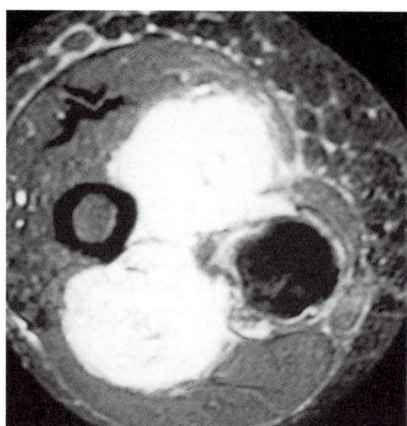

Fig. 15.11: MRI picture of the soft tissue tumor thigh encasing vessels partially and eroding the bone. Patient needed high level above knee amputation.

FNAC is less useful for sarcomas. Core/trucut biopsy can be done but is not equal to incision biopsy.

Incision biopsy for soft tissue sarcoma

- It is the ideal tool to conclude sarcoma histologically.
- Incision should be placed in such a way that it can be included in wide tumor excision at later period.
- Incision should be longitudinal in limbs.
- Injury to vessels and nerves should be avoided.
- Flaps should not be undermined.
- Adequate hemostasis is needed, as tumors are vascular.
- Immunohistochemistry and cytogenetics are possible and often essential.

Staging STS

It is done based on grading, tumor size, nodal status, metastases (GTNM staging). Grade is the single most important factor in staging STS. Nodal spread (3%) is rare but carries poor prognosis.

(G) TNM Staging of soft tissue sarcoma (of trunk and extremities)

T – Tumor (T)
TX – Primary tumor cannot be assessed
T0 – No evidence of primary tumor
T1 – Tumor 5 cm or less in greatest dimension
T2 – Tumor more than 5 cm and less than or equal to 10 cm in greatest dimension
T3 – Tumor more than 10 cm and less than or equal to 15 cm in greatest dimension
T4 – Tumor more than 15 cm in greatest dimension
T Suffix (m) Select if synchronous primary tumors are found in single organ

N – Nodes (N)
N0 – No regional lymph node metastases or unknown lymph node status
N1 – Regional lymph node metastasis
N Suffix (sn) if regional lymph node metastasis identified by SLN biopsy only
(f) if regional lymph node metastasis identified by FNA or core needle biopsy only

M – Distant Metastasis (M)
M0 – No distant metastases
M1 – Presence of distant metastases
The terms pM0 and MX are not valid categories in the TNM system.
Assignment of the M category for clinical classification may be cM0, cM1, or pM1
cM0 – No distant metastasis

Contd...

*Generosity is giving more than you can, and pride is taking less than you need—**Kalil Gibran***

Contd...

cM1 – Distant metastasis
pM1 – Distant metastasis, microscopically confirmed
Definition of FNCLCC (Fédération Nationale des Centres de Lutte Contre le Cancer)

Histologic Grade (G)
The FNCLCC grade is determined by three parameters: Differentiation, mitotic activity, and extent of necrosis. Each parameter is scored as follows differentiation (1–3), mitotic activity (1–3), and necrosis (0 –2)
The scores are added to determine the grade
GX – Grade cannot be assessed
G 1 – Total differentiation, mitotic count and necrosis score of 2 or 3
G 2 – Total differentiation, mitotic count and necrosis score of 4 or 5
G 3 – Total differentiation, mitotic count and necrosis score of 6, 7, or 8

Tumor differentiation score:
1. Sarcomas closely resembling normal adult mesenchymal tissue (e.g. low grade leiomyosarcoma)
2. Sarcomas for which histologic typing is certain (e.g., myxoid/round cell liposarcoma)
3. Embryonal and undifferentiated sarcomas, sarcomas of doubtful type, synovial sarcomas, soft tissue osteosarcoma, Ewing sarcoma/primitive neuroectodermal tumor (PNET) of soft tissue

Mitotic count (score):
In the most mitotically active area of the sarcoma, 10 successive high-power fields (HPF; one HPF at 400 × magnification = 0.1734 mm^2) are assessed using a 40 × objective.
Mitotic count score: 1: 0 – 9 mitoses per 10 HPF. 2: 10 – 19 mitoses per 10 HPF. 3: ≥20 mitoses per 10 HPF.

Tumor necrosis score:
0–No necrosis. 1–<50% tumor necrosis. 2–≥ 50% tumor necrosis.

Staging
IA: T0, N0, M0, GX/G1.
IB: T1,2,3; N0, M0, GX/G1.
II: T1, N0, M0, G2/G3.
IIIA: T2, N0, M0, G2/G3.
IIIB: T3,4; N0, M0, G2/G3.
IV: Any T, Any N, M0, Any G; Any T, Any N, M1, Any G.

Note: Staging of STS differs in thorax, abdomen and heads and neck.

Differential diagnosis for soft tissue sarcoma
- Hematoma.
- Abscess.
- Aneurysm.
- Myositis.
- Recurrence of sarcoma (Fig. 15.12).

Treatment

- **Wide excision** is the treatment of choice with 3–5 cm clearance with adequate depth.
- **Compartment resection** is a radical limb saving procedure. Here muscle group of one compartment (anterior, posterior or medial) is resected entirely from its origin to insertion with the tumor. It is done only when tumor is intracompartmental. It is not suitable when tumor is extracompartmental or many compartments are involved or encased to major neurovascular bundle.
- Amputation is done in large tumors of upper or lower limbs.
- Preoperative radiotherapy or chemotherapy followed by wide excision.

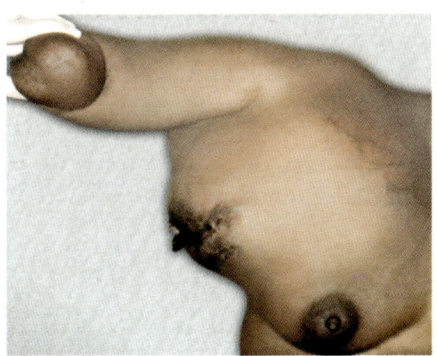

Fig. 15.12: Recurrent chest wall tumor, could be secondary as patient was earlier amputated for soft tissue tumor hand (forearm amputation).

*One cannot make a slave of a free person, for a free person is free even in a prison—***Pluto**

Principles of treatment

- Surgery is the *main treatment* modality. Amputation rate for STS has come down drastically from 50% in 1960 to 5% at present. It is also because of proper adjuvant radiotherapy following function/limb sparing complete excision, application of microvascular surgeries. Neoadjuvant chemotherapy, perioperative/post operative RT also play a major role.
- In low grade tumor without any spread—functional/limb sparing complete wide excision is sufficient without any adjuvant therapy. If microscopic margin is positive for tumor then postoperative external beam RT (EBRT) is given.
- In high grade tumor <5 cm size, function sparing wide excision with more than 1 cm clearance margin is sufficient. If clearance margin is less than 1 cm or shows microscopic positive margin, then perioperative brachytherapy OR postoperative EBRT is given.
- In high grade tumor which is between 5–10 cm size, function limb sparing complete wide excision with perioperative brachytherapy OR postoperative EBRT is given.
- In high grade tumor more than 10 cm in size, initial neoadjuvant chemotherapy; then functional/limb sparing complete wide excision with postoperative brachytherapy and EBRT should be given.

❖ **Postoperative radiotherapy** is commonly used because of less tumor burden and less wound problems. During surgery, titanium clips are placed at high-risk areas to identify the sites to concentrate proper RT.
  - *Brachytherapy* is very effective in local control of the tumor. Initially precise mapping of the area is done in the operation theater. *After loading, catheters* are placed in surgical field peroperatively. Later these catheters are loaded with iridium 192.
  - Permanent radioactive sources also can be placed to the area.
  - Palliative external radiotherapy can be given to prevent bleeding, fungation and to reduce pain in advanced cases. It is also used in secondaries in brain and bone.
❖ Primary radiotherapy alone (radical) is less beneficial in soft tissue sarcoma.

❖ Chemotherapy drugs *VAC* are *(Vincristine, Adriamycin, Cyclophosphamide)* commonly used. Other drugs used are Ifosfamide, Dacarbazine in combination with above drugs. *Mesna* is used as a protection for hemorrhagic cystitis. Chemotherapy is used when tumor is more than 5 cm or high grade. Usually postoperative chemotherapy is given.

Indications for amputations in soft tissue sarcoma

- Major neurovascular encasement.
- Bone involvement (Fig. 15.13).
- Multiple compartment involvement.
- Limb itself is diseased like lymphedema.
- Recurrence with multicentricity.
- Debulking surgery is useful in large advanced tumors like retroperitoneal sarcomas.

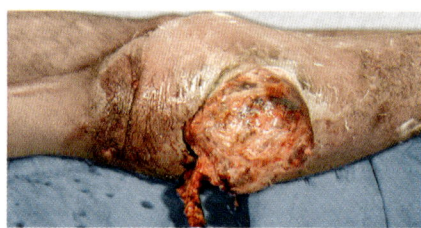

Fig. 15.13: Osteosarcoma upper tibia with tumor fungation.

❖ *Neoadjuvant chemotherapy* is used to make the primary tumor better operable.
❖ *Isolated limb perfusion using cytotoxic drugs and tumor necrosis factor* with hyperthermia is also often used.
❖ *Pulmonary metastasis* can be treated with wedge resection, segmentectomy, lobectomy, pneumonectomy. Surgery is done only when primary is well-controlled. Radiotherapy and chemotherapy are also tried. Metastases in lung more than 3 in number signifies poor prognosis.

Prognostic factors

- Size >5 cm.
- High grade.
- More than one compartment involvement.
- Deep tumors and multicentric.
- Neurovascular invasion.
- Lung secondaries.

*Progress lies not in enhancing what is, but in advancing toward what will be—***Kalil Gibran**

LIPOSARCOMA

- It is the **commonest type** of soft tissue sarcoma arising from the fat cells (of primitive mesenchymal cells).
- Common sites: Retroperitoneum; thigh; back; shoulder.
- *Types:*
  - Well-differentiated.
  - Myxoid.
  - Round cell.
  - Pleomorphic has got poor prognosis.
- Microscopically, it contains lipoblasts with '*signet ring*' malignant cells. It is low grade type.
- *Spread is to lungs.*
- Treatment is wide excision or radiotherapy with surgical debulking in places where complete removal of tumor is not possible like in retroperitoneal liposarcoma.

FIBROSARCOMA

- It can arise from **the bone** or from **soft tissues** (Fig. 15.14).
- It is the next common soft tissue malignancy after liposarcoma.
- It arises from fibroblasts.
- Commonest site is thigh.
- Spindle fibroblasts with '*herring bone*' pattern is typical feature on microscopy.

Types

- Well-differentiated.

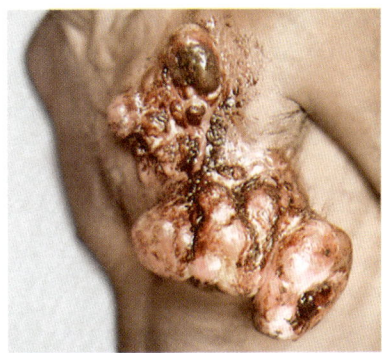

Fig. 15.14: Dermatofibrosarcoma protuberance over left chest wall.

- Poorly differentiated.
- Dermatofibrosarcoma protuberance. It is common in trunk.
- Aggressive fibromatoses are variant of fibrosarcoma, which are locally malignant in which desmoid tumor is also included.
  - Fibrosarcoma is slow growing tumor, which attains large size.
  - Clinically it is smooth, hard, warm, localized tumor.
  - It compresses or infiltrates the adjacent structures like neurovascular bundle.

LEIOMYOSARCOMA

- It arises from smooth muscle. Cut section shows whorled appearance.
- It is of undetermined grade.
- It is common in retroperitoneum and viscera, but can occur in limbs and skin.
- Recurrence is common. It has got poor prognosis.

RHABDOMYOSARCOMA

It arises from striated muscle. It is common in *head and neck*, upper thigh and arm.

Types

- Pleomorphic—commonest type of rhabdomyosarcoma.
- Embryonal—common in infants and children.
- Botryoidal.
- Alveolar.
  It is more aggressive tumor with poorer prognosis (*High grade*). It also metastasizes to lymph nodes.

SYNOVIAL SARCOMA

- It originates from synovial cells.
- It is common in thigh, leg, shoulder, hand and foot.
- Occasionally, it can occur in the abdominal wall and retroperitoneum.
- It is common in young individuals.

You will never win if you never begin—Helen Rovelandlin Powel

> **Chondrosarcoma**
> - It arises from chondroblasts.
> - It attains large size with slow growing nature.
> - Common sites are ribs and flat bones.
>
> **Hemangiosarcoma**
> - It originates from blood vessel endothelium.
> - *Types*
>   - Malignant hemangioendothelioma.
>   - Malignant hemangiopericytoma.
>
> **Lymphangiosarcoma**
> - It arises from lymph vessel endothelium.
> - It commonly occurs after radical lymph node dissection.

- It occurs adjacent to joint but uncommon to involve the synovial sheath of the joint.
- It spreads both through blood as well as to **lymph nodes (20%)**.
- It is very aggressive soft tissue sarcoma (high grade).

MALIGNANT NEURILEMMOMA

- It is commonly associated with multiple neurofibromatosis of von Recklinghausen's disease.
- It produces pain, tenderness and paresthesia.

KAPOSI'S SARCOMA

- It is malignant blood vessel tumor of multicentric origin arising from vascular smooth muscle or pericytes.
- It is seen commonly in HIV patients due to immunosuppression.
- Primary tumor commonly occurs in skin, mucous membrane, lymph nodes or viscera.
- It is linked with Human Herpes Virus 8 (HHV8) as causative agent.

Types

- *European Kaposi's sarcoma:* It is common in old age. Kaposi first described it in 1862. It mainly involves skin especially of lower extremity. Visceral involvement is rare.
- *African Kaposi's sarcoma:* It occurs commonly in children and young individual. It commonly involves skin and lymph nodes. It resembles lymphoma.
- *Transplant associated Kaposi's sarcoma:* It is due to drug-induced immunosuppression. It involves mainly skin and often regresses once immunosuppression is discontinued.
- *AIDS-associated Kaposi's sarcoma:* It occurs in 30–40% of AIDS patients. It is common in homosexuals. It has got wide, disseminated involvement with metastases. It is very aggressive. It is often associated with lymphoma and other malignancies.

Features

- Multiple reddish-blue nodules in the skin with ulceration over the nodule.
- Lymph node enlargement.
- Koebner phenomenon is common in areas of trauma.
- **Differential diagnosis:** Lymphomas; Cutaneous angiomatoses; mycobacterial infection of skin.
- **Investigations:** Biopsy of the skin lesion; Tests for HIV infection.
- **Treatment**
  - Irradiation.
  - Chemotherapy: Drugs used are Adriamycin, Bleomycin and Vinblastine.
  - Antiretroviral therapy; Interferons.

> **Sarcomas, which also spread through lymph nodes**
> - Synovial sarcoma.
> - Lymphangiosarcoma.
> - Rhabdomyosarcoma—alveolar type.
> - Ewing's sarcoma.
> - Angiosarcoma.
> - Epitheloid sarcoma.
> - Carcinosarcoma of uterus.

Modern man lives increasingly in the future and neglects the present

CHAPTER 16

Skin Tumors

Chapter Outline

- Classification of Skin Tumors
- Skin Adnexal Tumors
- Merkel Cell Carcinoma
- Dermatofibroma
- Dermatofibrosarcoma Protuberance
- Keratoacanthoma (Molluscum Sebaceum)
- Rhinophyma (Potato Nose)
- Premalignant Conditions of the Skin
- Squamous Cell Carcinoma (Epithelioma)
- Marjolin's Ulcer
- Basal Cell Carcinoma (Rodent Ulcer)
- Nevi/Naevi
- Melanoma

CLASSIFICATION OF SKIN TUMORS

Epidermal
- *Benign*—papilloma, seborrheic keratosis
- *Malignant*—basal cell carcinoma (BCC), squamous cell carcinoma (SCC)

Melanocytic
- *Benign*—all types of nevi
- *Malignant melanoma*

Skin adnexal tumor
- *Benign*—syringoma, hidradenoma, sebaceous adenoma, trichofolliculoma, trichilemmoma
- *Malignant*—hidradenocarcinoma, sebaceous carcinoma

Dermal tumors
- Neurofibroma, dermatofibroma, dermatofibrosarcoma protuberans

Note:
- Skin cancer is the most common of all cancers.
- Skin cancers (SC) are also classified as **melanotic (MSC) or nonmelanotic (NMSC).** NMSC are commonest (95%). BCC is 80%; SCC is 18%.

Contd...

Contd...

Patient who had BCC/SCC has higher risk to develop 2nd new skin cancer (35% in 3 years; 50% in 5 years). NMSC can be low-risk or high-risk groups. Lesion more than 2 cm in trunk and limbs; more than 1 cm in forehead and neck; more than 6 mm in central face; poorly defined margin; recurrent type; moderate or poor differentiation; perineural/vascular invasion; presence of immunosuppression; previous RT (radiotherapy)— are high-risk lesions.

SKIN ADNEXAL TUMORS (FIG. 16.1)

- They are tumors arising from accessory skin structures like sebaceous glands, sweat glands, hair follicles, etc.
- It is not uncommon. It may be **benign or malignant**.

To understand the heart and mind of person, look not at what he has already achieved, but what at he aspires to be—**Kalil Gibran**

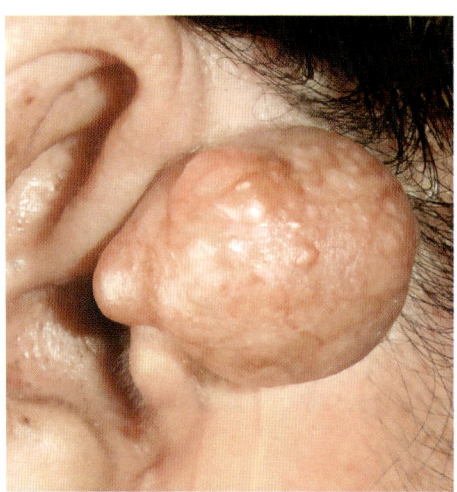

Fig. 16.1: Skin adnexal tumor.

- It presents as protruding well-localized swelling in the skin.
- Malignant skin adnexal tumor forms a nodular, hard, indurated swelling in the skin, often with involvement of hard, nodular regional **lymph glands**.
- It mimics **squamous cell carcinoma of skin**.

Differential Diagnosis

- Squamous cell carcinoma of skin.
- Dermatofibrosarcoma protuberans.
- **Diagnosis**
  - Biopsy.
  - Fine needle aspiration cytology (FNAC) of lymph node.
- **Treatment**
  - *Excision* of benign tumor.
  - **Wide excision and regional lymph node block** dissection when required.

MERKEL CELL CARCINOMA

- It is an aggressive malignant condition arising from *neuroendocrine receptor cells of the skin* (dermis) which mimics histologically oat cell carcinoma.
- It is common in white elderly females (4:1); may be due to UV rays.
- *Treatment* is wide excision and radiotherapy.

DERMATOFIBROMA (FIG. 16.2)

(Sclerosing angioma or subepithelial benign nodular fibrosis).
- It is a benign tumor arising from skin.
- It is the formation of firm, single or multiple nodules commonly occurring in extremities (limbs).
- It can be red, brownish yellow (due to lipid), or bluish black (due to hemosiderin).

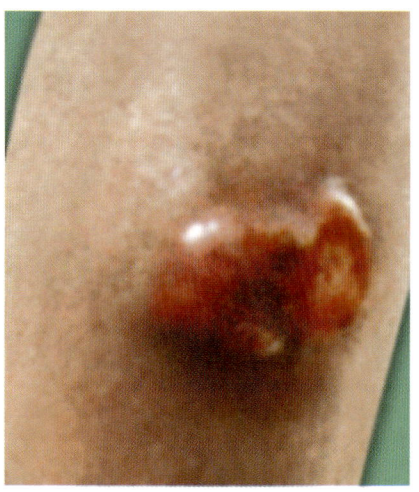

Fig. 16.2: Dermatofibroma.

- **Differential diagnosis**
  - Squamous cell carcinoma of skin.
  - Melanoma; basal cell carcinoma.
  - Skin adnexal tumor.
- **Treatment:** Excision.

DERMATOFIBROSARCOMA PROTUBERANCE

- It is a low-grade fibrosarcoma, which grows slowly but persistently.
- Occurs in the limb, abdominal wall, and back (Fig. 16.3).

Optimism is the faith that leads to achievement. Nothing can be done without hope and confidence—**Hellen Keller**

- It is not a rare entity, often attains a large size with multiple, nodular, hard, swelling with often involvement of lymph nodes.
- Rarely it spreads into lungs through blood.
- It mimics squamous cell carcinoma of skin, and skin adnexal tumor.

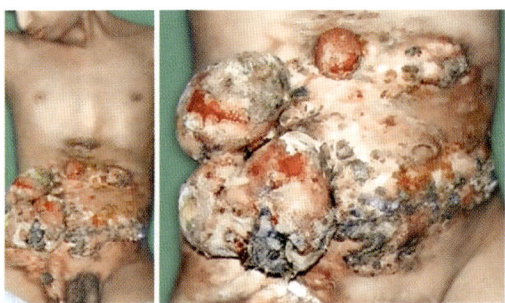

Fig. 16.3: Dermatofibrosarcoma.

Diagnosis

- Biopsy of the lesion.
- Chest X-ray, CT scan chest.
- FNAC of the lymph node.

Treatment

- Wide excision and follow-up.
- Recurrence is common.
- Prognosis is good.

KERATOACANTHOMA (MOLLUSCUM SEBACEUM)

- It is an overgrowth and subsequent spontaneous regression of *pilosebaceous glands* commonly seen in adults.
- Cause is unknown. It may be self-limiting benign neoplasm of viral origin.
- It presents as a rapidly growing, painless, single swelling in the skin with central brown area (Fig. 16.4).
- It grows usually for 4 weeks and later shows spontaneous regression in 4 months.
- During regression phase, central area separates from the lesion leaving a deeply seated scar.

- Mobile, hard, painless, nontender, lump with a central brownish area.
- No lymph nodes are enlarged.
- It is a benign condition. It mimics squamous cell carcinoma.
- Treatment is excision. Always specimen should be sent for histopathological study after excision.

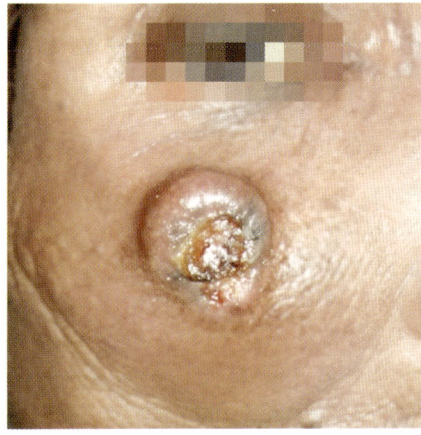

Fig. 16.4: Keratoacanthoma.

RHINOPHYMA (POTATO NOSE)

- It is a ***glandular form of acne rosacea*** causing immense thickening of ***distal part of skin of nose*** with visible openings of sebaceous follicles. Nose is bluish red in color with dilated capillaries (Fig. 16.5).

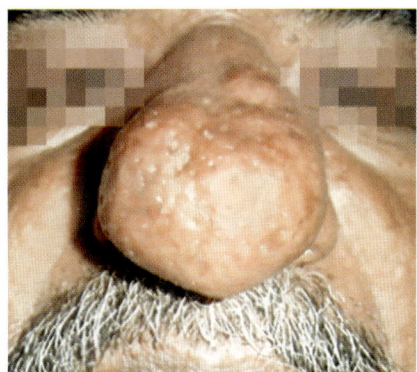

Fig. 16.5: Typical rhinophyma.

*A man with one watch knows what time it is; a man with two watches is never sure—**Unknown***

PREMALIGNANT CONDITIONS OF THE SKIN

- **Bowen's disease** of skin: It is an intradermal precancerous condition. It presents as brownish induration with a well-defined edge. Microscopically, it contains large clear cells. Eventually it turns into carcinoma.
- **Paget's disease** of nipple.
- Leukoplakia.
- Senile or solar keratosis: It is multiple, dry, hard, scaly, lesions in face and back of hands due to exposure to sunlight, occurs after middle age. Squamous cell carcinoma occurs later.
- Radiodermatitis: **Squamous cell carcinoma** can occur due to radiodermatitis. It is more observed in X-ray machine/X-ray room workers. Protective coverage while taking/using X-rays may prevent it.
- Chronic scars develop into *Marjolin's ulcer*.
- *Xeroderma pigmentosa* wherein there is defective DNA excision repair mechanism. It turns into malignant melanoma.
- Chronic lupus vulgaris.
- Prolonged irritation of skin by various chemicals like dyes, tar, soot, etc.

SQUAMOUS CELL CARCINOMA (EPITHELIOMA) (FIGS. 16.6 AND 16.7)

- It occurs in premalignant conditions like Bowen's disease, chronic scars, chemically induced chronic irritation, radiodermatitis, senile keratosis.
  For example, Khangri cancer in Kashmir, chimney scrotal cancer, Kang cancer in Tibetans.
- It arises from squamous layer of the skin.
- It *spreads* **locally** slowly into deeper tissues like fascia, muscle, tendons and later gets fixed to the bone underneath.
- *Regional lymph node (Fig. 16.8)* spread occurs *presenting* as—stony hard, nontender single or multiple, discrete or adherent to each other, mobile or fixed to deeper structures. Fungation or ulceration in lymph node metastases can occur at a later stage. It may erode into the vessels underneath to case torrential hemorrhage. Often lymph nodes may get enlarged by *secondary infection* making it firm tender and palpable. A course of proper antibiotics may reduce the lymph node size.

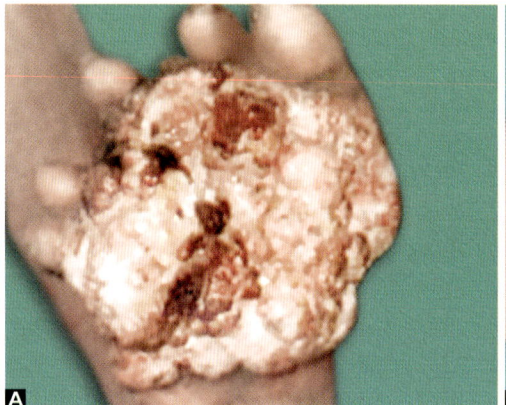
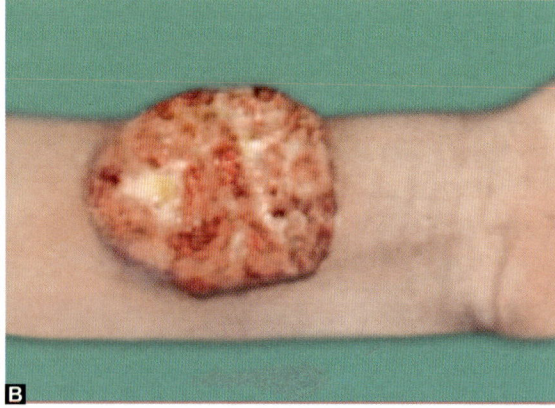

Figs. 16.6A and B: Squamous cell carcinoma in (A) Foot; (B) Hand.

Time does not heal, it merely tucks the pain away into the recesses of memory—**Maureen Murari**

Chapter 16 : Skin Tumors

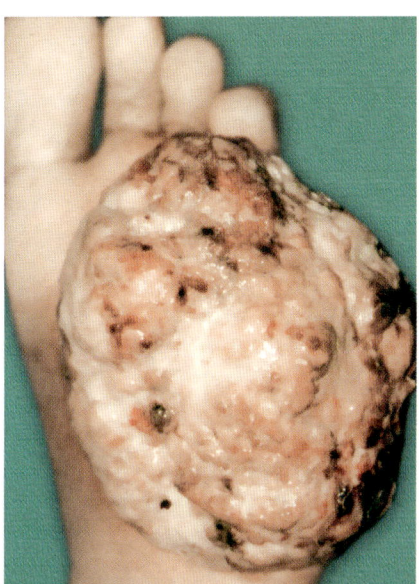

Fig. 16.7: Squamous cell carcinoma in the plantar aspect of the foot. Note the proliferative cauliflower-like lesion.

Etiology of squamous cell carcinoma
• Bowen's disease. • Chronic scars and sinuses. • Lupus vulgaris. • Solar keratosis. • Chemically induced chronic irritation. • Radiodermatitis. • **Kangri cancer** is due to constant placing of the hot charcoal pot(kangri) over the abdominal wall to control cold. Seen in Kashmir. • **Kang cancer** is seen in buttocks and heel of Tibetians due to sleeping over oven bed to control cold. • **Chimney sweep cancer** is observed in scrotum due to constant irritation by tar. *SCC is more common in immunosuppressed individuals.*

❖ **Indurated** base and surrounding tissue.
❖ Bloody discharge is seen in the floor of the lesion.
❖ Restricted mobility when ulcer infiltrates deeper structure (bone).
❖ Regional lymph nodes are commonly involved with hard, nodular features, initially mobile but eventually fixed to underlying structures.
❖ Usually no blood spread.

Variants

❖ *Marjolin's ulcer,* which occurs in chronic scar, is a type of squamous cell carcinoma without lymph node spread.
❖ *Verrucous carcinoma* is a squamous cell carcinoma, that commonly occurs in mucous membrane or mucocutaneous junction without lymph node spread. It is dry exophytic, warty, indurated growth. It has got good prognosis. It is curable malignancy.

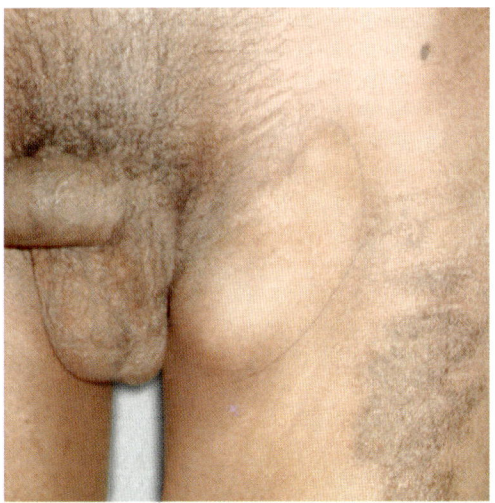

Fig. 16.8: Squamous cell carcinoma (SCC) causing secondaries in regional lymph nodes.

Clinical Features

❖ An ulcerative or ulceroproliferative lesion.
❖ **Raised and everted edge**.

Histology

Whorls of malignant squamous cells with epithelial or *keratin pearls* are characteristics.

*With a new day come a new strength and a new thought—**Eleanor Roosevelt***

Broder's grading of squamous cell carcinoma—based on epithelial/keratin pearls
• Grade I: Well-differentiated—>75% epithelial pearls. • Grade II: Moderately differentiated—50–75% epithelial pearls. • Grade III: Poorly differentiated—25–50% epithelial pearls. • Grade IV: Dedifferentiated—<25% epithelial pearls.

Differential Diagnosis

- Basal cell carcinoma (BCC).
- Melanoma.
- Keratoacanthoma.
- Skin adnexal tumors.

Investigations

- Wedge biopsy.
- FNAC from lymph node.

Treatment

- **Radiotherapy**
  - It is given using radiation, needles, moulds, etc. 6000 cGy units/6 weeks with 200 units/day.
- **Surgery**
  - *Wide excision* is better with a margin of 1 cm clearance. If defect is small, it is closed with primary suture. If defect is wide then split skin graft is needed to cover the defect.
  - *Amputation* at one joint above level.
  - When lymph nodes are involved, *block dissection* of the regional lymph nodes (like of ilioinguinal dissection, axillary dissection or neck node dissection depending on the location of primary tumor and site of secondaries) is done.
- **In advanced disease**
  With fixed lymph nodes, *palliative external radiotherapy* is given to palliate pain, fungation and bleeding.

- **Chemotherapy**
  It is given using Methotrexate, Vincristine, Bleomycin, Cisplatin or 5-fluorouracil. Postoperative adjuvant as well as palliative chemotherapy is used.

Problems with block dissection
• Lymphorrhea. • Infection, seroma formation. • Flap necrosis. • Bleeding due to blowout of the vessel underneath (like femoral/carotid). • Lymphedema.

MARJOLIN'S ULCER (FIG. 16.9)

- It is a well-differentiated squamous cell carcinoma, which occurs in chronic scars like burn scar, scar of venous ulcer.
- As it develops in a scar due to chronic irritation and as there are **no lymphatics** in scar tissue, *it will not spread to lymph nodes*.
- Because scar is relatively avascular, it grows slowly. As scar does not contain nerves, it is painless.
- Once it reaches the normal skin, it may behave like any other squamous cell carcinoma, i.e. it will spread to lymph nodes.

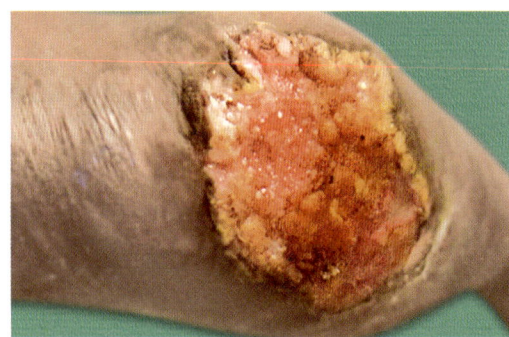

Fig. 16.9: Marjolin's ulcer in a long standing ulcer over elbow.

Clinical Features

- History of pre-existing venous ulcer or burns.
- Indurated, painless, nontender, ulcer with raised and everted edge.

Biopsy from the edge: Confirms the diagnosis.

Treatment

- **Wide excision**.
- If ulcer is large, **amputation** is required.
- **Radiotherapy should not be given** as it may turn into poorly differentiated squamous cell carcinoma.
- It is a curable malignancy.

BASAL CELL CARCINOMA (RODENT ULCER) (FIG. 16.10)

- It is a low grade, locally invasive, carcinoma arising from basal layer of skin or mucocutaneous junction. **It does not arise from mucosa**.
- It is more common in white skinned people than blacks. Common in places where exposure to UV light is more (**Australia**).
- It is common in males, in middle-aged and elderly.

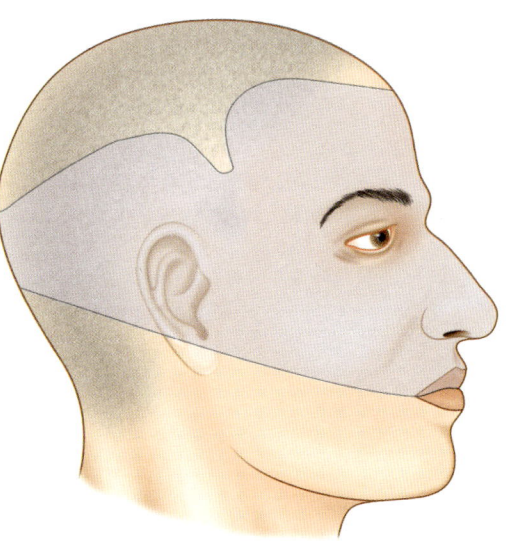

Fig. 16.11: Note the common site of BCC—in the face above between angle of mouth and ear lobule.

- Common site of occurrence is **face** (Fig. 16.11)—above the line drawn between angle of mouth and ear lobule. It is called as *tear cancer* because it is commonly seen in area where tears roll down. Often can occur in mucocutaneous junctions.
- **It is only locally malignant**. It does not spread through lymphatics or through the blood. But it erodes deeply into local tissues including cartilages, bones causing extensive local destruction (Fig. 16.12). Hence the name '*rodent ulcer*'.

Types

- *Nodular.*
- *Cystic.*
- *Ulcerative.*
- *Multiple,* often associated with syndromes and other malignancies.
- *Pigmented BCC (Fig. 16.13)*—mimics melanoma.
- *Geographical or field fire or forest fire BCC* is wide area involvement with

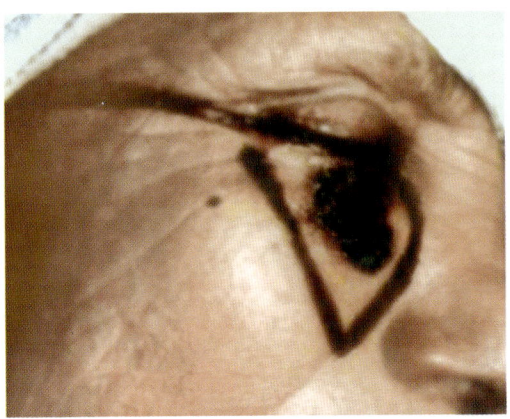

Fig. 16.10: Basal cell carcinoma.

I'd rather attempt to do something great and fail than to attempt to do nothing and succeed—Robert H Schuller

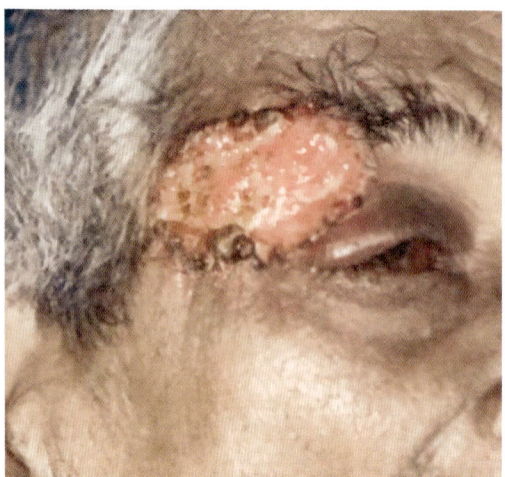

Fig. 16.12: Rodent ulcer lateral aspect of the eyebrow. Note the typical beaded edge.

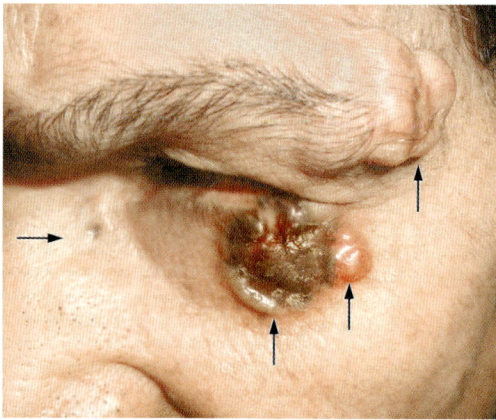

Fig. 16.13: Basal cell carcinoma. It is often multiple.

It contains malignant cells arranged as outer palisading columnar cells with central polyhedral cells *without prickle cells or keratinization*.

Clinical Features

* *Slowly growing, locally invasive ulcer on the face in a middle-aged man, which is nontender, dry, and nonmobile, with raised, beaded edge and central scab.*
* Erodes into the underlying deeper tissue like muscle, bone, cartilage producing *severe disfigurement* of face.
* Site of beading signifies the area of active proliferating cells. In between beaded areas, dormant nonactive cells are present.
* No lymph node or blood spread.

Differential Diagnosis

* Squamous cell carcinoma.
* Melanoma.
* Keratoacanthoma.

Investigations

Wedge biopsy, X-ray of the part.

Treatment

* **Radiotherapy**
  – BCC is ***radiosensitive***.
  – If lesion is away from vital structure (like away from eyes), then curative radiotherapy can be given.
  – Radiotherapy is not given once it erodes cartilage or bone.
* **Surgery**

Indications for surgery
• Rodent ulcer eroding into cartilage or bone.
• BCC close to the eye.
• Recurrent BCC.

central scabbing and peripheral active proliferating edge.
* *Basisquamous BCC*—behaves like squamous cell carcinoma with spread into lymph nodes. BCC, which has not been treated for long time can turn into basisquamous carcinoma.

Microscopic Types

* Superficial type.
* Morphia type.

The most beautiful things in the world cannot be seen or even touched, they must be felt with the heart—**Helen Keller**

– *Wide excision* with 1 cm clearance with primary closure if defect is small; split skin grafting or flap if defect is wider. Rhomboid/Z local flaps or forehead/pectoralis major myocutaneous flap can be used.
– Laser surgery.
– Cryosurgery.
– **Microscopically oriented histographic surgery** (MOHS).

NEVI/NAEVI

It is a *hamartomata* of melanocytes due to excessive stimulation.

It may present during birth or appear later in life.

Types (Figs. 16.14 and 16.15)

- Hairy mole is a mole with a hair growing on its surface.
- Nonhairy mole.
- **Blue nevus:** It is seen in children. It is located deep in the dermis, hence appears blue. It is common over buttock (Mongolian spot), hand, feet.
- **Junctional nevus:** It is centered in the junctional layer (basal layer) of the epidermis as clusters. It is immature, unstable and premalignant. Microscopically there is proliferation of melanocytes at the epidermal junction. Features of malignant transformation are—change in the size, color, bleeding, ulceration, crusting, satellite spots.
- **Compound nevus:** It is combination of intradermal and junctional nevus. Intradermal part is inactive but junctional part is potentially malignant.
- **Juvenile melanoma:** It is appearance of junctional like mole before puberty. It is seen in children over the face.
- **Hutchinson's freckle:** It is seen in elderly with large area of dark pigmentation. In the macular stage, it is smooth and brown. In the tumor stage, it is dark and irregular. It commonly turns into melanoma.

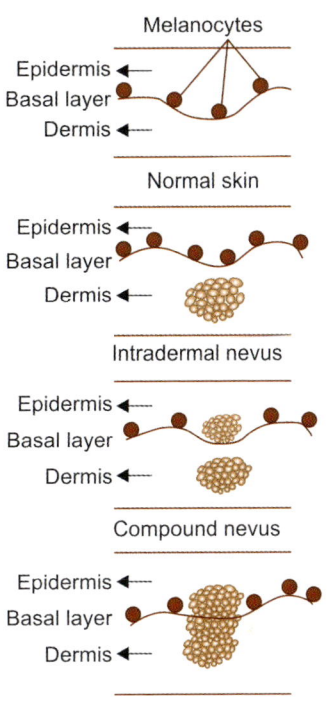

Fig. 16.14: Different types of nevi.

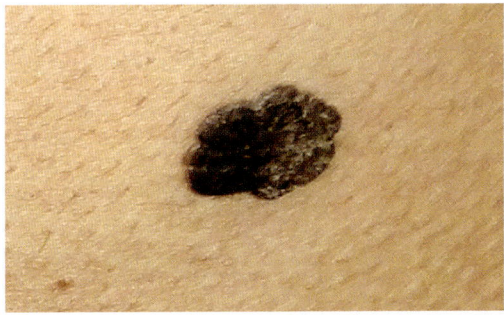

Fig. 16.15: Junctional nevus.

Treatment

- Excision.
- The tissue always should be sent for histopathology.

A = x+y+z; A = success, x = work, y = play, z = keep your mouth shut—**Albert Einstein**

MELANOMA

- It is a malignant tumor arising from the *epidermal melanocytes*.
- Its incidence is equal in both sexes. Its incidence is increasing over the years.
- It is the most aggressive malignant cutaneous tumor.

Sites (Figs. 16.16 to 16.18)

- In females, leg is the commonest site.
- In males, it is front or back of the trunk.
- In the Bantu tribe, sole is the commonest site.
- **Other sites:** Eyes, mucocutaneous junction, meninges, anus and mouth.

Risk Factors

- Exposure to sunlight.
- Ethnic factors, socioeconomic status, life style, climate.
- Albinism, family history.
- Xeroderma pigmentosa (Fig. 16.19).
- Junctional nevus.

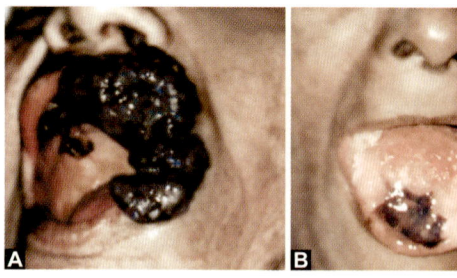

Figs. 16.16A and B: Oral melanoma in: (A) Lip; (B) Tongue.

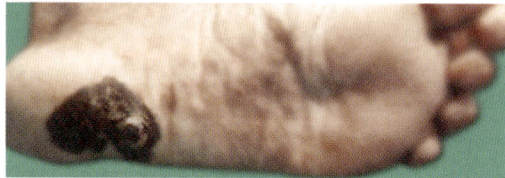

Fig. 16.17: Large melanoma in the sole. Note the pigmentation.

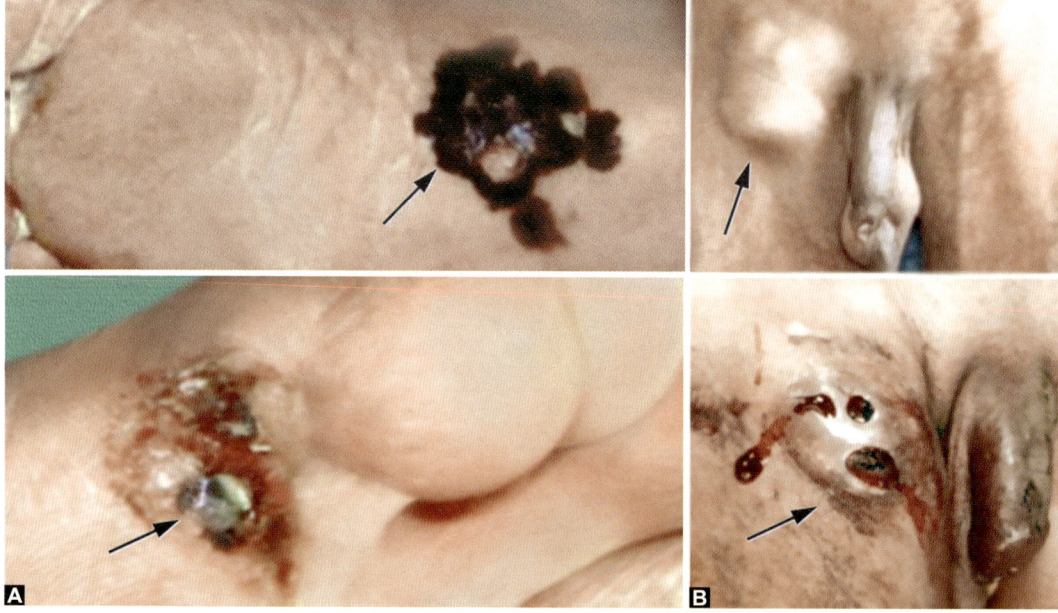

Figs. 16.18A and B: (A) Melanoma foot; (B) Lymph node secondaries.

*Never bend your head, always hold it high. Look the world straight in the eye—***Helen Keller**

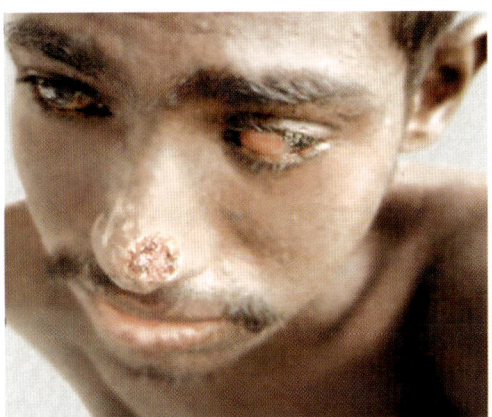

Fig. 16.19: Xeroderma pigmentosa with BCC in the nose. Such patients are prone for other malignancies of skin like melanoma also. There is defective DNA excision repair.

Classifications

Breslow's classification: Based on thickness of invasion measured by optical micrometer.
I: Less than 0.75 mm.
II: Between 0.76 to 1.5 mm.
III: 1.51 mm to 4 mm.
IV: More than 4 mm.

Clark's levels (Fig. 16.20)
Level 1: Only in epidermis.
Level 2: Extension into papillary dermis.
Level 3: Filling of papillary dermis completely.
Level 4: Extension into reticular dermis.
Level 5: Extension into subcutaneous tissue.

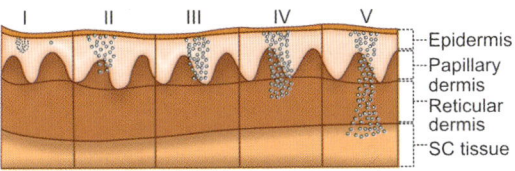

Fig. 16.20: Clark's level.

Clinical Types

1. **Lentigo maligna melanoma**:
   About 7–15%. *Least common, least malignant.* Occurs in old age and common in face *(Hutchinson's melanotic freckle)*.

2. **Superficial spreading**:
   Most common. Occurrence is 64%. Occurs in any part of the body with variegated irregular look.

3. **Nodular melanoma**:
   About 12–25%. *More malignant* than the above two. It is common in younger age group, occurring in any part of the body. Common in genitals/anal canal; causes early metastases.

4. **Acral lentiginous melanoma**:
   Occurs in palms, soles and subungual region. Common in *Japan*. It has got a *poor prognosis*.

5. **Amelanotic melanoma**:
   This is the *worst form*. Because of the undifferentiation, tumor cells loose their capacity to synthesize melanin. It presents as pinkish fleshy growth which is rapidly progressive. It may mimic soft tissue sarcoma.

Clark's concept:
Initial radial growth phase that occurs horizontally and later vertical growth phase with invasion.

Clinical Features

- It can start in a pre-existing **nevus** (commonly junctional nevus)—90% or as **de novo** in a normal skin—10%.
- Melanoma is **unknown before puberty**.
- Pigmentation with irregular surface and margin with rapid growth.
- Ulceration, bleeding, itching, changes in the color.
- When a mole becomes malignant, following changes should be observed:
  - *Major signs*: Change in size, shape and color.
  - *Minor signs*: Inflammation, crusting, bleeding, itching, diameter more than 5 mm, halo around a mole.
- **No induration occur in melanoma**.

Smart people speak from experience. Smarter people, from experience do not speak

Five most important features of melanoma (ABCDE)	
1. **A**symmetry.	4. **D**iameter > 6 mm.
2. **B**order irregularity.	5. **E**levation.
3. **C**olor variation.	

Spread

- *Through lymphatics (Fig. 16.21)*
  - It spreads to regional lymph nodes either by permeation or by embolization.
  - *Intransit nodules (beyond 2 cm up to nodal level) or satellite nodules (within 2 cm)* in the skin between primary and regional lymph node area are often seen due to retrograde spread to dermal lymphatics.
- *Through blood*:
  - To lungs (cough with hemoptysis), liver (massive enlargement of liver), brain (convulsions, raised intracranial pressure), skin, bones (paraplegia if spine is involved, pathological fracture, bone pain). Secondaries are typically black in color.
  - Extensive visceral involvement causes *melanuria*.
  - Sometimes primary is very small and so unnoticed (in anus, subungual region). They present with features of secondaries only.

Melanoma

- Incidence—5% of all skin cancers.
- 20 times more common in whites than blacks.
- Mucosal melanoma has got poor prognosis.
- Can spread from mother to fetus.
- Multiple melanomas are 1% common.
- Melanoma in retina will not cause lymph node involvement, as retina has no lymphatic drainage.
- 10% of melanomas are familial.
- *Satellite nodules* are secondary skin nodules within 2 cm of primary.
- *Intransit nodules* are secondary skin nodules beyond 2 cm of primary anywhere up to lymph node region.

TNM staging (8th edition, 2018, AJCC)

T (Tumor)
T0 – No evidence of primary tumor; Primary site of tumor is unknown
Tis – in situ carcinoma (thickness, ulceration not applicable)
T1: < 1 mm; T1a – < 0.8 mm without ulceration; T1b – < 0.8 mm with ulceration or > 0.8 to 1 mm with or without ulceration.
T2: 1–2 mm; T2a without ulceration; T2b is with ulceration.
T3: 2–4 mm; T3a is without ulceration; T3b is with ulceration.
T4 > 4 mm; T4a is without ulceration; T4b is with ulceration.

N – Nodes
N0: No regional nodes involved.
N1: N1a – Clinically occult. One node detected by SLNB: N1b – Clinically detected one node; N1c – No nodes but presence of in transit, satellite or microsatellite metastasis.
N2: N2a – 2 or 3 clinically occult node; N2b – 2 or 3 nodes with at least one clinically detectable node; N2c – One clinically occult or detectable node with in transit, satellite or microsatellite metastasis.
N3: N3a – 4 or more clinically occult nodes; N3b – 4 or more nodes with at least one clinically detectable nodes; N3c – 2 or more clinically occult or detectable nodes with in transit, satellite or microsatellite metastasis.

M – Metastases
M 0 – No distant spread
M1: M1a – Skin, soft tissue, non-regional node spread without [M1a (0)] or with LDH elevation [(M1a (1)]. M1b – Distant spread to Lungs with or without M1a without raise in LDH [M1b (0)] or with raised LDH [M1b (1)]. M1c – Distant spread to non-CNS viscera with or without M1a or M1b without raise in LDH [M1c (0)] or with raise in LDH [M1c (1)]. M1d – Distant spread to CNS with or without M1a,b,c without raise in LDH [M1c (0)] or with raise in LDH [M1c (1)].

Staging
Stage 0: Tis, N0, M0.
Stage IA: T1a, T1b, N0 M0. **Stage IB**: T2a, N0 M0.
Stage IIA: T2b, T3a, N0, M0. **Stage IIB**: T3b, T4a, N0, M0.
Stage IIC: T4b, N0, M0.
Stage IIIA: T1a/b, T2a; N1a or N2a; M0. **Stage IIIB**: T1a/b, T2a; N1 b/c, N2b; M0. T2b, T3a, N1a, N2b, M0; T0, N1b/c, M0. **Stage IIIC**: T1a to T3a, N2c or N3a/b/c, M0; T3b/T4a, any N ≥ N1, M0; T4b, N1a to N2c, M0; T0, N2b, N2c, N3b/N3c, M0. **Stage IIID**: T4b, N3a/b/c, M0.
Stage IV: Any T, Any N, M1.

Faith is the strength by which a shattered world shall emerge into light—**Helen Keller**

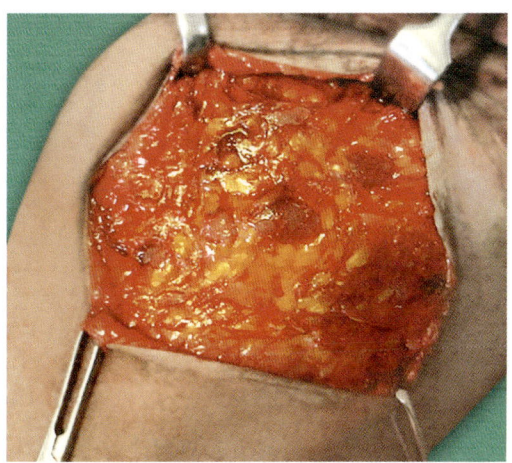

Fig. 16.21: Secondaries in inguinal lymph nodes from a primary in the leg.

Investigations

- **No incision biopsy:** Incision biopsy may accelerate the blood spread.
- Excision biopsy of the primary.
- FNAC of lymph node.
- Ultrasound abdomen to see liver secondaries (usually huge hepatomegaly occurs).
- Chest X-ray to see secondaries.
- Other relevant methods depending on site and spread.
- Urine for melanuria.
- Sentinel lymph node biopsy (SLNB).

Treatment

Surgery: It is the main treatment.

For primary

- *Wide excision,* with a clearance margin of 3–5 cm (presently extent of margin of clearance is controversial).
- Handley's **wide local excision (WLE)** is wide excision with clearance margin as well as depth (clearance margin used in olden days was 3–5 cm).
- *Present recommendation* is in situ melanoma needs 0.5 cm clearance; melanoma <1 mm thickness needs 1.0 cm clearance; 1–2 mm thickness needs 1–2 (1.5) cm clearance; 2 cm/3 cm clearance is sufficient for >2.0 mm thickness. Procedure can be done under regional or local anesthesia. Evidence says that more than 2 cm clearance will not show any additional advantage in treating primary tumor.
- Primary closure or split-thickness skin graft (SSG) or local flaps are used to cover the defect.
- If wider area is involved, then *amputation* with one joint above.
- In fingers and toes, *disarticulation* is required.
- Melanoma in anal canal may require *abdominoperineal resection.*
- *Enucleation* of eye in case of melanoma in eye.

For lymph node secondaries

- In a clinically palpable lymph node, FNAC of lymph node is done, the spread is confirmed and then regional block dissection is done, i.e. ilioinguinal or axillary or neck.
- In a fixed lymph node, only chemotherapy is the treatment because it is inoperable.
- *Lymphatic mapping and sentinel node biopsy*: Radioactive colloid is injected around primary site and lymphoscintigraphy is done using hand held gamma camera to visualize the micrometastasis in the nodal field. If there is micrometastasis then regional block dissection is done.
- Prophylactic regional block dissection, which was previously advocated is now controversial. But still used in many centers.

For locoregional recurrent melanoma:

- *Isolated limb perfusion* using cytotoxic agents like Dacarbazine (DTIC/Dimethyl triethyl imidazole carboxamide), Melphalan.
  - *Melphalan* is injected at high temperature of 41°C with a pump and oxygenator

*Make sure you have finished speaking before your audience has finished listening—**Dorothy Sarnoff***

through cannulas into femoral vein and artery with a proximal tourniquet in situ. Hyperthermia and oxygenation increase the metabolic activity of tumor cells to make it more vulnerable to melphalan.
  - *Complications* of isolated limb perfusion are—deep venous thrombosis (DVT), sepsis, bleeding.
* Laser ablation of multiple small cutaneous lesions.

Chemotherapy

Indications

* In secondaries in lungs, liver and bones.
* Postoperatively after surgery for melanoma. Usually it is given intravenously.
  Drugs are:
  DTIC: Diethyl Trimethyl Imino Carbazine.
  Melphalan (Phenyl alanine mustard). (Melphalan for melanoma).

Immunotherapy

* BCG and specific tumor antibodies through melanoma antigens are beneficial.
* Radiotherapy has no role, as melanoma is radioresistant.

Prognosis

* As it is aggressive tumor, prognosis is not good.
* Females have got better prognosis.
* Extremity melanoma has got better prognosis.
* Old people carry poor prognosis.
* *Poor prognostic factors are*—tumor thickness, nodal spread, ulceration, vascular invasion, vertical growth, in transit nodule, distant spread, stage III/IV, high mitotic activity.

CHAPTER 17

Neck

Chapter Outline

- Anatomy of Lymphatics of Head and Neck
- Branchial Cyst
- Branchial Fistula
- Pharyngeal Pouch
- Laryngocele
- Cystic Hygroma (Cavernous Lymphangioma)
- Ludwig's Angina
- Parapharyngeal Abscess
- Retropharyngeal Abscess
- Carotid Body Tumor (Potato Tumor, Chemodectoma, Non-chromaffin Paraganglioma)
- Torticollis (Wry Neck)
- Sternomastoid Tumor
- Subhyoid Bursitis
- Secondaries in Neck Lymph Nodes
- Pancoast Tumor (Superior Sulcus Tumor)

ANATOMY OF LYMPHATICS OF HEAD AND NECK

Inner Lymphatic Ring (Inner Waldeyer's Ring)

It consists of adenoids above, lingual tonsils below and two palatine tonsils laterally, one on each side (Fig. 17.1).

Outer Circular Chain of Nodes (Outer Waldeyer's Ring) (Fig. 17.2)

It consists of occipital, postauricular, preauricular, parotid, facial, submandibular, submental, superficial cervical and anterior cervical nodes.

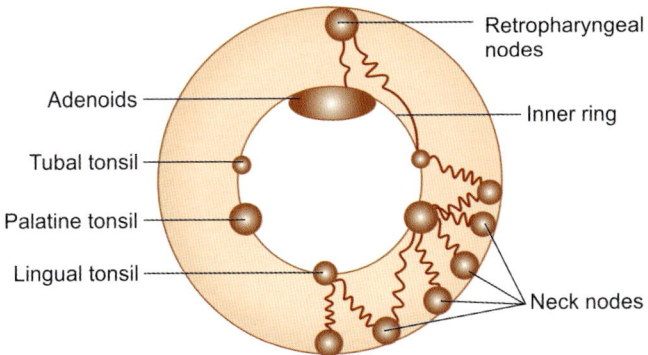

Fig. 17.1: Inner and outer Waldeyer's ring.

There's only one way you can fail, and that's to quit

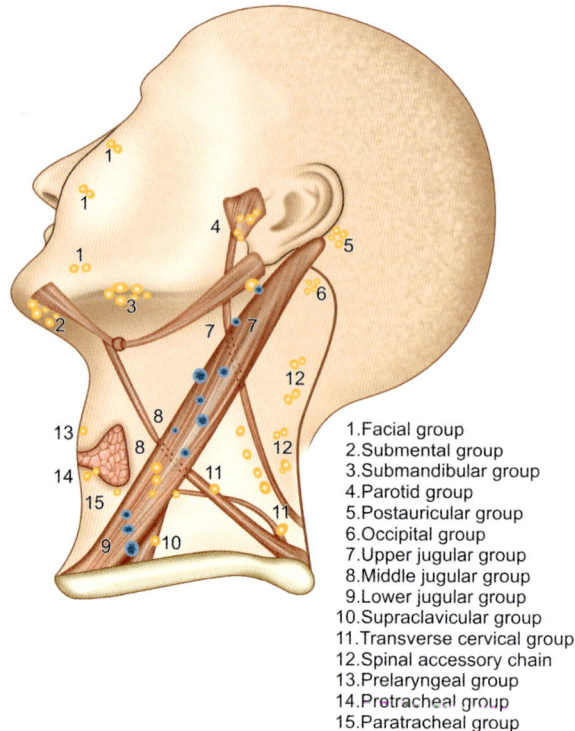

Fig. 17.2: Lymphatic drainage in the neck.

1. Facial group
2. Submental group
3. Submandibular group
4. Parotid group
5. Postauricular group
6. Occipital group
7. Upper jugular group
8. Middle jugular group
9. Lower jugular group
10. Supraclavicular group
11. Transverse cervical group
12. Spinal accessory chain
13. Prelaryngeal group
14. Pretracheal group
15. Paratracheal group

Facial nodes are:
- Superficial:
  - Upper-infraorbital.
  - Middle-buccinator.
  - Lower-supramandibular.
- Deep groups—in relation to pterygoids.

Submandibular lymph nodes drain
- The side of the nose.
- The cheek.
- Angle of the mouth.
- Entire upper lip.
- Outer part of the lower lip.
- The gums.
- Side of the tongue.

Submental lymph nodes drain from the central part of the lower lip, floor of the mouth and apex of the tongue.

Superficial cervical nodes. They lie on outer surface of the sternomastoid around the external jugular vein. They drain the parotid region and lower part of the ear.

Deep cervical lymph nodes
- Upper deep cervical lymph nodes—jugulodigastric nodes.
- Lower deep cervical lymph nodes—juguloomohyoid nodes.

They drain ipsilateral half of head and neck; finally form a *jugular lymph trunk* from lower deep cervical to join thoracic duct on the left side; junction of right subclavian and right jugular vein on right side.

Other lymph node groups
- Parotid—from nose, eyelids, scalp, auditory meatus and tympanic cavity.
- Preauricular—from ear and side of scalp.
- Postauricular—scalp temporal area, back of ear.

*We could never learn to be brave and patient, if there were only joy in the world—**Helen Keller***

Note:
Nodes are classified as horizontal (circular) and vertical. Circular is classified as outer ring (Waldeyer) and inner ring. Vertical is classified as central and lateral.

Rule of 7 in the neck
• 7 days—inflammation. • 7 months—neoplasm. • 7 years—congenital defect. *Note:* The rule of 7 provides a probable diagnosis of the neck mass based on the average duration of the patient's symptoms.

BRANCHIAL CYST (FIGS. 17.3A AND B)

It arises from the remnants of second branchial cleft. Normally 2nd, 3rd and 4th clefts disappear to form a smooth neck. *Persistent 2nd cleft* is called as *cervical sinus,* which eventually gets sequestered to form *branchial cyst.*

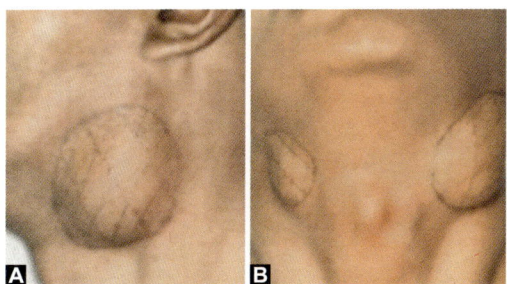

Figs. 17.3A and B: Branchial cyst.

Clinical Features

* Swelling in the neck beneath the anterior border of upper third of the sternomastoid muscle.
* It is smooth, soft, and fluctuant, often transilluminant.
* It contains *cholesterol crystals.*
* Cyst appears at 20–25 years of age, even though it is congenital.

Histology

Histologically, it is lined by *squamous epithelium.*

Differential Diagnosis

* Cold abscess.
* Lymph cyst.
  It may get infected to form an abscess.
  FNAC shows *cholesterol crystals.*

Treatment

* *Excision* under general anesthesia (GA).
* Cyst is in relation to carotids, hypoglossal nerve, glossopharyngeal nerve, spinal accessory nerve, and posterior belly of digastric, and pharyngeal wall. Medially it is close to the posterior pillar of tonsils. During dissection, all these structures should be taken care of.

BRANCHIAL FISTULA

* It is a *persistent second branchial cleft with a communication outside to the exterior.* It is commonly a congenital fistula. Occasionally the condition is secondary to incised, infected branchial cyst. Often it is bilateral.
* *External orifice* of the fistula is situated at *the lower third of the neck* near the anterior border of the sternomastoid muscle.
* Track passes between external and internal carotid arteries.
* *Internal orifice* is located on the anterior aspect of the posterior pillar of the fauces, just behind the tonsils.
* Sometimes fistula ends internally at the posterior pillar of tonsil as blind end, due to *fibrosis.*
* Track is lined by *ciliated columnar epithelium* with patches of lymphoid tissues beneath it, causing recurrent inflammation.
* *Discharge* is mucoid or mucopurulent.

Investigations:
Discharge study, fistulogram, MR fistulogram.
Treatment:
Always surgery.
After passing a probe under general anesthesia, fistula is excised across its full length,

*In order to succeed, your desire for success should be greater than your failure—**Bill Cosby***

up to its internal opening. Care should be taken to safeguard carotids, jugular vein, hypoglossal nerve, glossopharyngeal nerve, and spinal accessory nerve. *Track should be excised fully.*

PHARYNGEAL POUCH

- It is a protrusion of pharyngeal mucosa through *Killian's dehiscence*, a weak area of the posterior pharyngeal wall between *thyropharyngeus (oblique fibers)* and *cricopharyngeus (transverse fibers)* of the *inferior constrictor muscle* of the pharynx.
- Imperfect relaxation of the cricopharyngeus increases the pressure in the pharynx, mainly during swallowing which leads to protrusion of pharyngeal mucosa through the Killian's dehiscence causing pharyngeal pouch (Fig. 17.4).
- *The protrusion is usually toward left.*

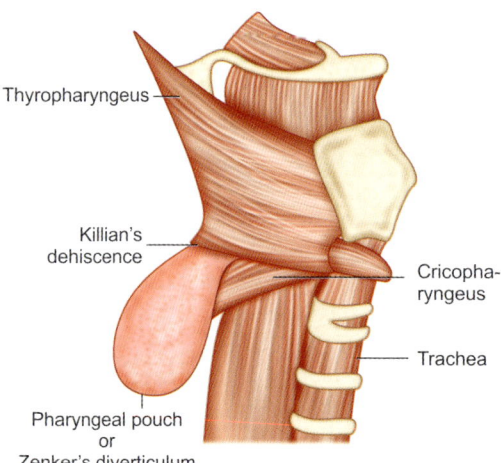

Fig. 17.4: Pharyngeal pouch (Zenker's diverticulum).

Stages

- *Small diverticulum.*
- *Large, globular349*
- *diverticulum* causing regurgitation, cough, dysphagia and respiratory infection.
- *Large pouch*, which is visible in the neck as a globular swelling often tender, smooth and soft. They present with dysphagia, features of respiratory infection like pneumonia and lung abscess, weight loss and cachexia. Pouch may get infected and may form an abscess. Often the pouch descends downward and enters the superior mediastinum.

Clinical Features

Pain, dysphagia, recurrent respiratory infection, swelling in the neck on the left side, which is smooth, soft and tender.

Investigations

- *Barium swallow*—lateral view shows pharyngeal pouch (Fig. 17.5).
- Chest X-ray shows pneumonia.
- Flexible esophagoscopy can show the opening of the pouch.
- *CT scan is ideal.*
- *Indirect laryngoscope* can show pooling of saliva.

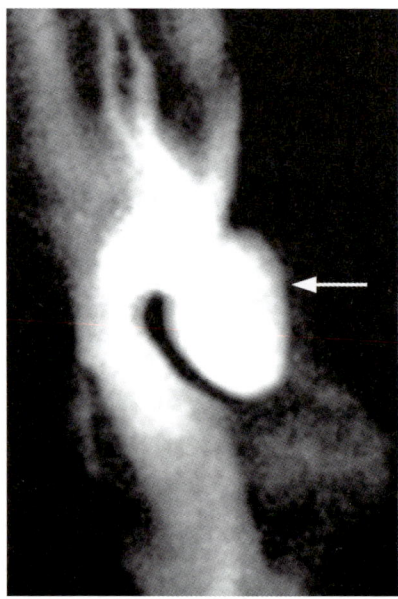

Fig. 17.5: Barium swallow showing pharyngeal pouch.

*Many of life's failures are people who did not realize how close they were to success when they gave up—**Thomas A Edison***

Complications

* Infection either *mediastinitis or lung infection* (Pneumonia or lung abscess).
* Pharyngeal fistula.
* Abscess in the neck.

Treatment

* Antibiotics have to be started.
* *Pharyngeal pouch is excised* by an oblique neck incision (approach from neck). As there is cricopharyngeal spasm, *cricopharyngeal myotomy* (i.e. cutting of cricopharyngeal circular muscle fibers without opening mucosa) is done to prevent the recurrence.
* Conservative in old age with physiotherapy and nutritional support.

LARYNGOCELE

* It is a *unilateral narrow necked, air containing diverticulum resulting from herniation of laryngeal mucosa* (Fig. 17.6).
* It is situated in the anterior third of the laryngeal ventricle, between the false cords and thyroid cartilage and herniates through *the thyrohyoid membrane*.

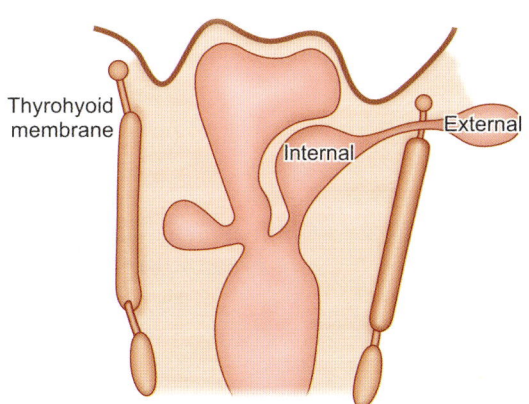

Fig. 17.6: Diagrammatic representation of laryngocele.

* It occurs in professional *trumpet players, glass blowers, and in people with chronic cough*.

Clinical Features

* Swelling seen in the neck in relation to larynx adjacent to thyrohyoid membrane, which is smooth, soft, resonant and becomes more prominent while blowing (Figs. 17.7A to C).
* Infection is quite common in the sac of laryngocele, leading to the blockade of opening of the sac causing an abscess.
* Pus often may be discharged into the pharynx repeatedly.

Diagnosis

Clinical features, X-ray neck, laryngoscopy, CT scan.

Treatment

Excision through neck incision. Neck of the sac should be ligated.

CYSTIC HYGROMA (CAVERNOUS LYMPHANGIOMA) (FIG. 17.8)

* It is a cystic swelling due to sequestration of a portion of jugular lymph sac from the lymphatic system, during the developmental period *in utero*.
* Present during birth and so may cause obstructed labor due to huge size. Occasionally present in early infancy.

Sites

* *Posterior triangle of the neck*—commonest site. Eventually may extend upward in the neck.

More smiling, less worrying. More compassion, less judgment. More blessed, less stressed. More love, less hate—**Roy T Bennett**

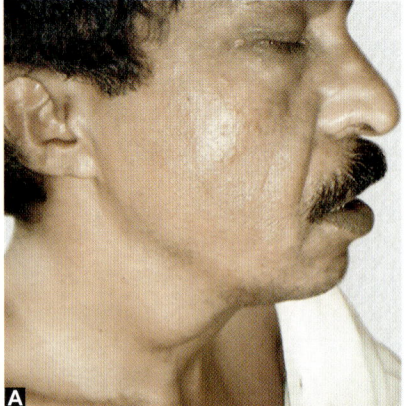

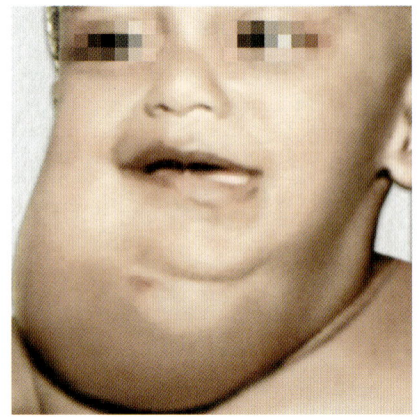

Fig. 17.8: Cystic hygroma.

- Cheek.
- Axilla.
- Tongue—lymphangiogenetic macroglossia.
- Groin.
- Mediastinum.
- Often multiple sites.

Pathology

- It contains aggregation of cysts looking like *soap bubbles*.
- Cysts have *mosaic appearance* with larger cysts lying near the surface and smaller cysts in the deeper planes.
- Each cyst contains clear lymph with endothelial lining.

Clinical Features

- Swelling is *present since birth* in the *posterior triangle of neck* causing obstructed labor.
- Swelling is smooth, soft, fluctuant (cystic), *compressible, and brilliantly transilluminant*.
- Swelling may rapidly increase in size causing *respiratory obstruction—dangerous sign*.
- It may get infected forming an *abscess*, which is a tender, warm, soft swelling.

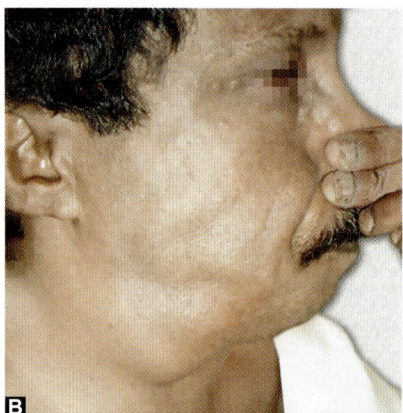

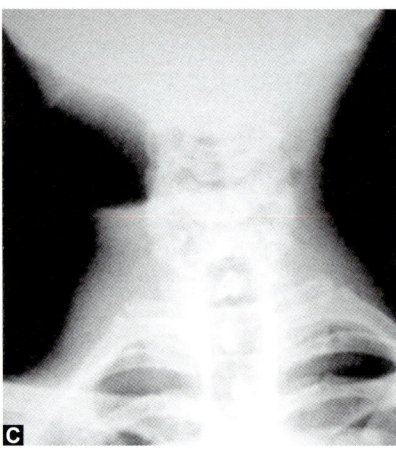

Figs. 17.7A to C: Laryngocele in a patient which increases in size after nasal blowing. X-ray picture of the same patient.

If you want to be happy, do not dwell in the past, do not worry about the future, focus on living fully in the present—**Roy T Bennett**

It may cause septicemia, which may be life- threatening.

Complications

* Respiratory distress due to rapid enlargement.
* Infection → Abscess → Septicemia.
* Surgery itself may cause torrential hemorrhage.

Treatment

* Aspiration of the contents. Later once the sac or capsule gets thickened by fibrous tissue, it is excised.
* When it causes respiratory obstruction, *aspiration and tracheostomy* has to be done.
* Under proper antibiotic coverage, drainage of abscess is done. Later sac is excised.

LUDWIG'S ANGINA

* Ludwig's angina is a serious, potentially life-threatening polymicrobial cellulitis of the submandibular space (neck) and the floor of the mouth with severe diffuse inflammatory edema leading into severe complications (described by Wilhelm Frederick von Ludwig in 1836).
* The organisms commonly isolated are *Streptococcus viridans* and *Staphylococcus aureus*; anaerobes also are frequently involved, including bacteroides, peptostreptococci, and peptococcus, fusiform bacilli, diphtheroids.

Surgical Anatomy

The submandibular space comprises part of the space above the hyoid bone. The total space is divided into the sublingual space superiorly and submandibular space inferiorly. Ludwig's angina begins in the submaxillary space and secondarily involves submental and sublingual space. Typically affected structures are the anterior neck, the pharyngomaxillary space (parapharyngeal), the retropharynx and the superior mediastinum.

Etiology

* It usually originates from an odontogenic infection, especially from the second or third lower molars. These teeth have roots that lie at the level of the mylohyoid muscle and abscesses here can spread to the submandibular space.
* Sialadenitis, peritonsillar abscess.
* Open mandibular fracture, oral lacerations; tongue piercing, trauma to the floor of the mouth.
* Infected thyroglossal cyst, epiglottitis.
* Upper respiratory infections.

Pathology

* Ludwig's angina is a cellulitis of the submandibular space that spreads to the structures of the anterior neck and beyond via connective tissue, muscle, and fascial planes rather than by the lymphatic system. Cellulitis, rather than abscess formation, is the most common presenting finding.
* As the infection progresses, edema of the suprahyoid tissues and supraglottic larynx elevate and posteriorly displace the tongue, resulting in life-threatening airway narrowing. In advanced infection, internal jugular vein thrombosis, cavernous sinus thrombosis and brain abscess, in addition to airway compromise, have been described. Necrotizing mediastinitis usually occur through the retropharyngeal space and the carotid sheath.
* As the infection is deep to deep fascia in a closed fascial plane and rapidly spreading leading to laryngeal edema, acute airway obstruction, sepsis, toxemia.
* *Predisposing factors:* Dental carries; recent dental treatment; diabetes mellitus; malnutrition; alcoholism; compromised

Don't be discouraged; it's often the last key in the bunch that opens the lock

immune status like acquired immunodeficiency syndrome (AIDS); organ transplantation and trauma.

Features

- Poor oral hygeine, tooth pain.
- Tachypnea, tachycardia and fever; toxicity.
- Diffuse swelling and pain in the floor of the mouth.
- Dysphagia, odynophagia, drooling, trismus, and fetid breath.
- Hoarseness, stridor, respiratory distress, cyanosis, dysphonia.
- Board like swelling of floor of mouth; elevation of the tongue.
- Nonfluctuant suprahyoid diffuse swelling with brawny edema with typically a bilateral submandibular edema above the hyoid bone with characteristic "bull's neck" appearance.
- Lymphadenopathy and fluctuation are not usually seen.

Cardinal signs of Ludwig's angina (Fig. 17.9)

- Bilateral involvement of more than a single deep tissue space.
- Gangrene with serosanguinous, putrid infiltration but little or no frank pus.
- Involvement of connective tissue, fasciae, and muscles but not glandular structures.
- Spread via fascial space continuity rather than by the lymphatic system.

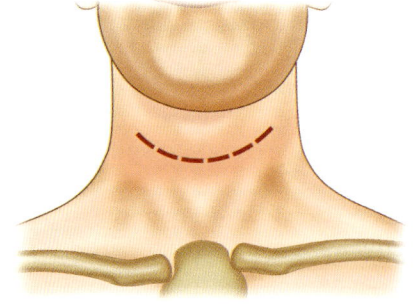

Fig. 17.9: Incision for decompressing the Ludwig's angina.

Management

- Ludwig's angina is a clinical diagnosis.
- Blood count, blood gas analysis, ultrasound neck, blood and fluid/pus culture.
- Airway maintenance is the single most important early management as an emergency basis either by cricothyroidotomy or tracheostomy.
- Proper antibiotics like ampicillin, clindamycin, piperazillin and tazobactum.
- Fluid and electrolyte management.
- Decompression using horizontal submandibular suprahyoid incision by cutting deep fascia often mylohyoid muscles.
- Condition has got high mortality.

PARAPHARYNGEAL ABSCESS

It is an *infection of pharyngo-maxillary/lateral pharyngeal space.*

Surgical Anatomy

This is a cone-shaped space; base is formed by base of the skull, apex is formed by the greater cornu of hyoid bone, medial wall by the superior constrictor with buccopharyngeal fascia, lateral wall is formed by the medial pterygoid, angle of mandible, deep part of the parotid and partly submandibular salivary gland. Space is divided into two compartments by styloid process.

1. *Anterior prestyloid compartment* is bound by tonsillar fossa medially and medial pterygoid laterally.
2. *Posterior poststyloid compartment* is bound by lateral pharyngeal wall medially and parotid laterally. Posterior compartment contains internal carotid artery, internal jugular vein, glossopharyngeal, vagus, spinal accessory and hypoglossal nerves.

Causes

- Usually infection arises from the tonsils (tonsillitis, peritonsilar abscess), after tonsillectomy, from adenoids in children.

- From the submandibular/parotid/retropharyngeal spaces.
- Third molar infection.
- Ear infection.
- Trauma.

Clinical Features

- It causes diffuse swelling in the upper neck behind angle of mandible, trismus, fever, toxicity.
- Medial shift of pharyngeal wall and tonsil with bulging of posterior pillar.
- May present with paralysis of glossopharyngeal, vagus, spinal accessory and hypoglossal nerves and sympathetic chain (Horner's syndrome).
- Dysphagia, odynophagia, laryngeal edema (severe cases) with respiratory distress.

Complications

- Thrombosis of internal jugular vein which may extend above to sigmoid sinus.
- Erosion into the internal carotid artery causing torrential bleeding.
- Spread of infection into other spaces in the neck and into mediastinum.
- Acute laryngeal edema with respiratory distress.
- Septicemia.

Treatment

- Systemic antibiotics, fluid resuscitation.
- Under GA, drainage is done by making lengthy horizontal deep incision between angle of the mandible and hyoid bone. Early drainage is needed. Antibiotics are given.
- Tracheostomy may be needed often.

RETROPHARYNGEAL ABSCESS

Surgical Anatomy

The wall of the pharynx has got 5 layers. Mucosa, submucosa, pharyngobasilar fascia, muscular layer (contains 3 constrictors and stylopharyngeus, salpingopharyngeus, palatopharyngeus muscles), and buccopharyngeal fascia which cover outer part of constrictors and extend over buccinator. Buccopharyngeal fascia is adherent to prevertebral fascia posteriorly in the midline. Retropharyngeal lymph nodes are located between buccopharyngeal fascia and prevertebral fascia in paramedian (eccentric) position (not midline)—*space of Gillette* one on each side.

Types (Fig. 17.10)

- Acute.
- Chronic.

a. *Acute Retropharyngeal Abscess*

- It is infection and suppuration of retropharyngeal lymph nodes due to staphylococci or streptococci organisms.
- Commonly from tonsils or pharynx.
- Common in infants and children.

Clinical features

- It presents as *lateral (paramedian, eccentric) smooth, tender swelling* in the pharynx with dysphagia, dyspnea, cough, toxic features and neck rigidity.
- Diagnosis is obvious on proper clinical examination.

Treatment

- Intravenous antibiotics.
- Drainage is done usually *through per oral incision* under careful anesthesia. Occasionally drainage may be required through a neck incision. Pus should be sent for culture.

b. *Chronic Retropharyngeal Abscess*

- It is invariably due to *tuberculosis of cervical spine.*
- Abscess is in the **midline behind the prevertebral fascia**. There is destruction of the body of the vertebra due to tuberculosis.

*Don't be pushed around by the fears in your mind. Be led by the dreams in your heart—***Roy T Bennett**

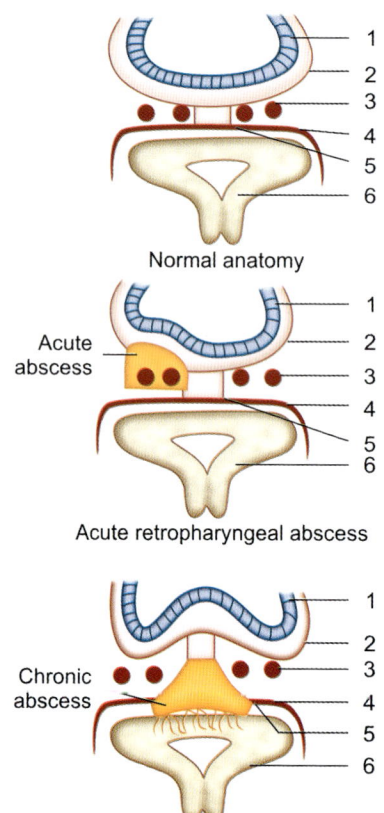

1. Pharyngeal wall, 2. Buccopharyngeal fascia,
3. Retropharyngeal LN, 4. Prevertebral fascia,
5. Median septum, 6. Vertebra

Fig. 17.10: Note acute and chronic retropharyngeal abscess. Normal anatomy is also shown. Acute is eccentric and is due to suppuration of retropharyngeal lymph nodes. Chronic is central, midline and is due to tuberculosis of the cervical vertebra.

Clinical features
- It is *midline swelling in the posterior pharyngeal wall*, which is smooth and nontender.
- Features of tuberculosis of cervical spine will be observed.
- Often abscess may point in the neck in relation to sternomastoid.
- Neurological manifestations may occur in severe disease.

Investigations
X-ray spine, chest X-ray, ESR, MRI of cervical spine are essential investigations.

Treatment
- Antitubercular drugs.
- Drainage of the abscess should be done *through neck approach (never intraoral approach)*.
- Decompression of the vertebra and stabilization is also often required.

CAROTID BODY TUMOR (POTATO TUMOR, CHEMODECTOMA, NON-CHROMAFFIN PARAGANGLIOMA)

- It arises from the carotid body, which is located at the bifurcation of the carotid artery.
- Cells of the carotid body are sensitive to the changes in pH and temperature of the blood.
- Often they are locally malignant tumors, but in 20% cases spread can occur to the regional lymph nodes.
- Blood supply to the tumor is from *external carotid artery*. Tumor does not secrete epinephrine or any endocrine substances.
- They can be *familial*.

Clinical Features (Fig. 17.11)
- Usually unilateral, more common in middle age.
- Swelling in the carotid region of the neck, which is smooth, firm, pulsatile (due to pulsatile vessel overlying its surface) and moves only side to side but not in vertical direction.
- Features of transient ischemic attack due to compression over the carotids.
- Thrill may be felt and bruit may be heard. Often tumor may extend into the cranial cavity along the internal carotid artery as *dumb-bell tumor*.

*Tenderness and kindness are not signs of weakness and despair, but manifestations of strength and resolution—**Kalil Gibran***

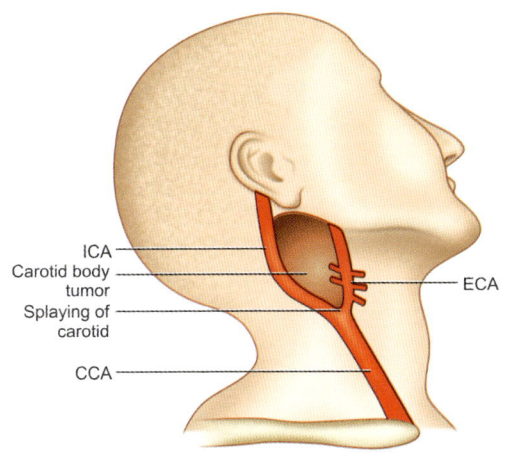

Fig. 17.11: Note the site and location of carotid body tumor. Splaying of the carotid is common.
(CCA: common carotid artery; ECA: external carotid artery; ICA: internal carotid artery)

Investigations

- Doppler.
- Angiogram to see the *'tumor blush'*.
- CT scan.
- *No FNAC: No partial excision.*

Widening/splaying of the carotid artery with tumor blush in an angiogram is called as **Lyre sign**.

Shamblin classification of carotid body tumor
• Type I: Localized easily resectable (26%).
• Type II: Adherent, partially surrounding the carotids (46%).
• Type III: Adherent, encased carotids completely (27%).

Differential Diagnosis

- Carotid aneurysm.
- Soft tissue tumor (sarcoma).
- Lymph node enlargement.
- **Neurofibroma of the vagus nerve** presents as swelling in the carotid triangle in the region of thyroid as vertically placed, oval, hard swelling. On palpation of the swelling, patient often develops bradycardia and dry cough. It does not move with deglutition and has only transverse mobility. As the tumor lies behind the carotid, it can stretch the carotid in front causing transmitted pulsation.

Treatment

- If it is small, it can be excised easily as the tumor is in the adventitia.
- When it is large, as commonly observed, *complete excision has to be done followed by placing a vascular graft.*
- Carotid body tumor is *not radiosensitive.*

TORTICOLLIS (WRY NECK) (FIGS. 17.12A AND B)

It is turning of the neck to one side with chin pointing toward opposite side.

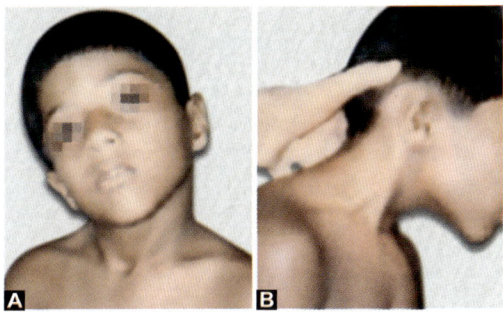

Figs. 17.12A and B: Torticollis neck. Note the side of the neck flexed with chin pointing opposite side.

Causes

- Sternomastoid tumor.
- Traumatic—spinal injury, disk prolapse, spondylosis.
- Inflammatory: Lymphadenitis either tuberculous or suppurative.
- Spasmodic; reflex; rheumatic.
- Burns.
- Ocular causes.

Luck is when opportunity knocks and you answer

Features

- Restricted neck movements.
- Chin pointing toward opposite side.
- Squint.
- Features relevant to the causes.
- **Treatment:** Treat the cause.

STERNOMASTOID TUMOR

- It is due to birth injury to the sternomastoid muscle.
- It is a *misnomer*. It is not a tumor.

Pathogenesis

During childbirth, injury to sternomastoid muscle causes *hematoma* in the muscle, which gets organized to form sternomastoid tumor.

Features

- It is seen in infants of 3–4 weeks age.
- Swelling in the sternomastoid muscle, which is smooth, hard, nontender and adherent to the muscle.
- Chin pointing toward opposite side. Head tilted toward same side (*scoliosis capitis*).
- In later age groups, it causes *hemifacial atrophy* because the external carotid artery is compressed by sternomastoid tumor leading to decreased blood supply.
- Compensatory cervical scoliosis.
- Compensatory squint.
- **Differential diagnosis:** Other causes for torticollis.
- **Treatment:** Division of the lower end of the sternomastoid muscle or excision of the muscle.

SUBHYOID BURSITIS

Subhyoid bursa is space between posterior surface of the body of hyoid bone and thyrohyoid membrane (Fig. 17.13). It lessens friction between these two structures during swallowing.

Due to constant friction, inflammatory fluid collects in the bursa leading to bursitis, which presents as a **horizontally placed** midline swelling between lower part of the hyoid bone and thyrohyoid membrane.

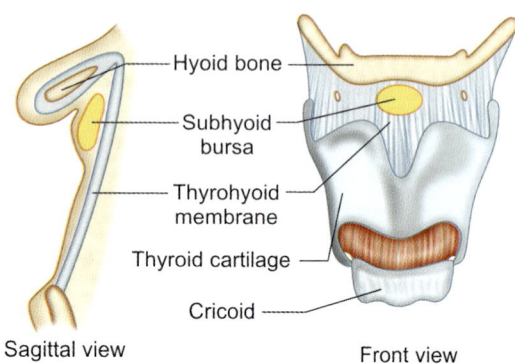

Fig. 17.13: Sagittal and front view showing location and relation of subhyoid bursa.

Features

- Smooth, soft, cystic, fluctuant, non-transilluminating swelling, which moves upward with deglutition but *not while protruding the tongue out*.
- It should be differentiated from thyroglossal cyst and pretracheal lymph nodes.
- It contains turbid fluid, often gets infected to make swelling tender or to form an abscess.
- **Treatment:** Excision under general anesthesia.

Differential diagnosis for neck lymph node enlargement
• Tuberculous lymphadenitis.
• HIV infection.
• Chronic lymphatic leukemia.
• Infectious mononucleosis.
• Secondaries in lymph nodes.
• Lymphomas.
• Nonspecific lymphadenitis.
• Sarcoidosis.

Discussion is an exchange of knowledge; argument is an exchange of ignorance—Unknown

SECONDARIES IN NECK LYMPH NODES

Levels in Neck Nodes (Memorial Sloan–Kettering Cancer Center Leveling of Neck Nodes) (Fig. 17.14)

Level I: Submental lymph nodes (IA) and submandibular lymph nodes (IB).

Level II: Lymph nodes in upper deep cervical region (it extends from base of skull to hyoid bone and from lateral margin of sternothyroid to posterior margin of sternomastoid muscle).

Level III: Lymph nodes in middle cervical region (from hyoid bone to omohyoid muscle or cricothyroid membrane).

Level IV: Lymph nodes in lower cervical region (from omohyoid muscle to clavicle).

Level V: Lymph nodes in posterior triangle including supraclavicular region.

Level VI: Lymph nodes in the midline neck—pretracheal and prelaryngeal.

Level VII: Lymph nodes in the mediastinum.

Common sites of primary	
• Oral cavity, tongue, tonsils.	• Esophagus.
• Salivary glands.	• Lungs.
• Pharynx—nasopharynx.	• Gastrointestinal tract (GIT).
• Larynx.	• Thyroid.

❖ It is *commonly from squamous cell carcinoma*, but can be from adenocarcinoma, or melanoma.

❖ Squamous cell carcinoma is mainly from oral cavity, pharynx. Adenocarcinoma is usually from GIT, commonly involving left supraclavicular lymph nodes.

Features of Secondaries in Neck (Figs. 17.15 to 17.20)

❖ Nodular surface, hard in consistency; often fixed when it is advanced.

❖ But secondaries from *papillary carcinoma of thyroid* can be soft, cystic and contains brownish black fluid.

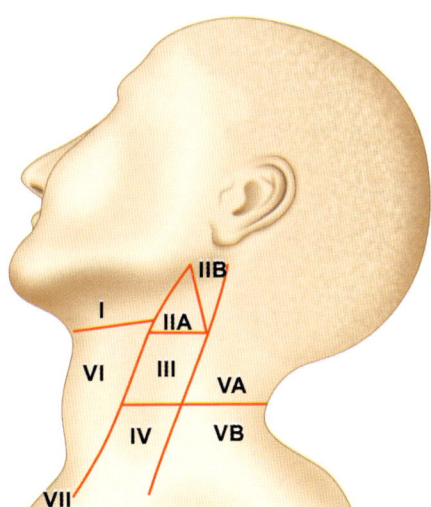

Fig. 17.14: Levels in neck nodes.

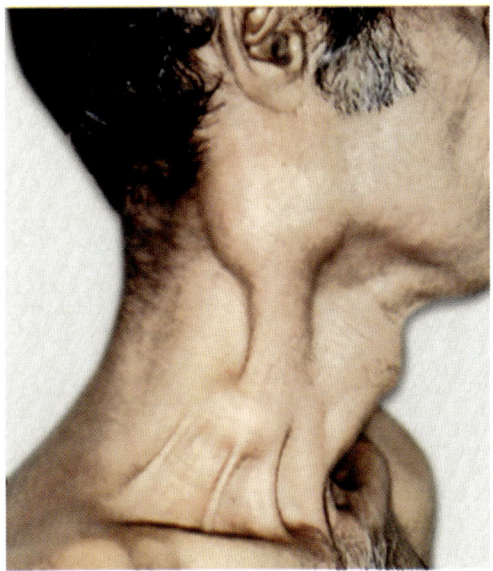

Fig. 17.15: Secondaries in the neck nodes from laryngeal carcinoma.

Accept yourself, love yourself, and keep moving forward. If you want to fly, you have to give up what weighs you down—**Roy T Bennett**

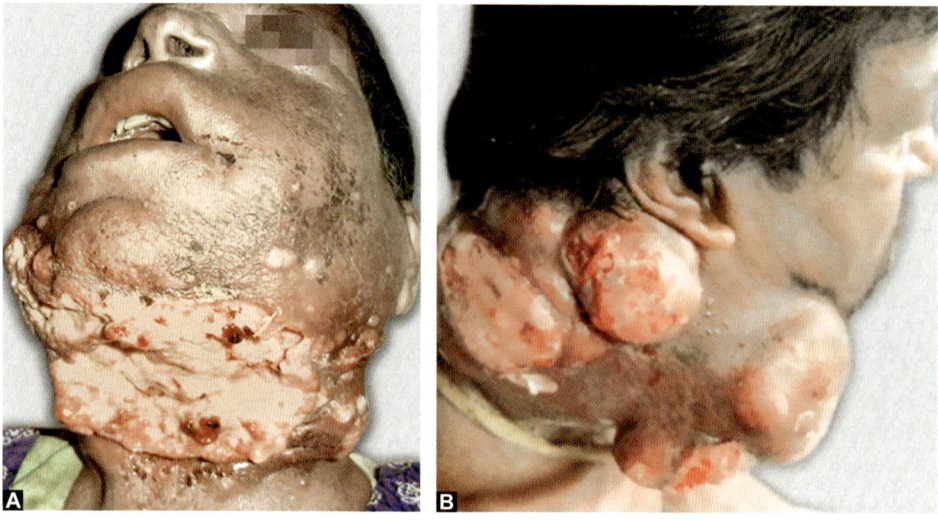

Figs. 17.16A and B: Advanced secondary carcinoma neck with ulceration and fungation.

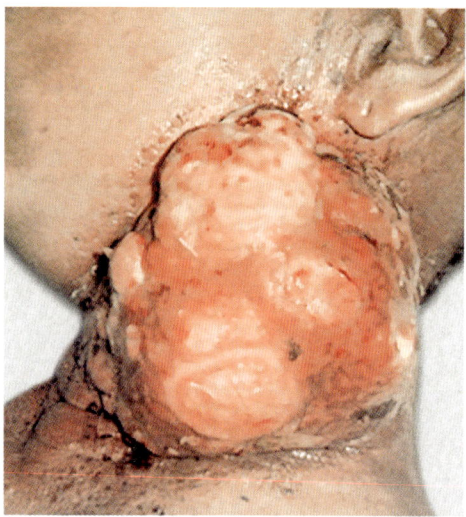

Fig. 17.17: Large secondaries in neck with extensive fungation.

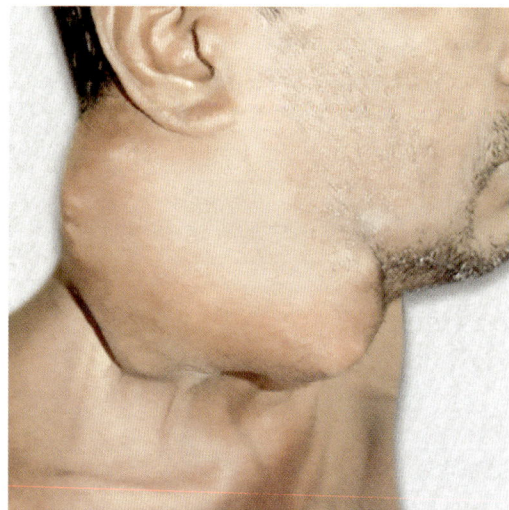

Fig. 17.18: Large secondaries in neck with nodularity with platysma involvement below.

- Secondaries can infiltrate into carotids, sternomastoid, posterior vertebral muscles, spinal accessory nerve (shrugging of shoulder is affected), hypoglossal nerve (tongue deviates toward the same side), cervical sympathetic chain (*Horner's syndrome*).

- Secondaries spread into adjacent soft tissues and also to the skin causing fungation and ulceration. Often because of tumor necrosis, softer area develops in the hard node.
- In advanced cases, tumor may infiltrate into the major vessels like carotids, or

The road to success is lined with many tempting parking places

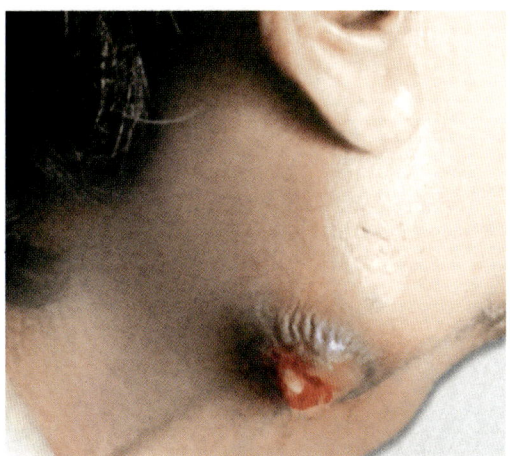

Fig. 17.19: Secondaries in neck with ulcer over the summit.

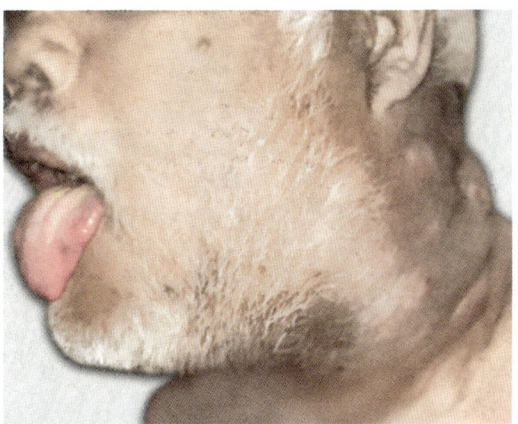

Fig. 17.20: Secondaries in neck with nodules and ulceration. Note the deviation of tongue toward same side due to hypoglossal nerve involvement.

branches of external carotid artery causing torrential hemorrhage.

- *Hoarseness*—carcinoma thyroid, larynx.
- *Dysphagia*—carcinoma posterior 1/3rd of tongue, pharynx, esophagus.
- *Hemoptysis, cough, dyspnea*—carcinoma lung.
- *Ear pain, deafness*—nasopharyngeal carcinoma.
- *Spinal accessory nerve*—shrugging of shoulder is defective.
- *Hypoglossal nerve*—tongue deviates toward same side with wasting.
- *Sympathetic chain*—Horner's syndrome with miosis, anhidrosis, upper eye lid droop (pseudoptosis), enophthalmos, loss of spinociliary reflex.

Types of Secondaries in the Neck

Secondaries in the Neck with Known Primary

- Here secondaries are present and primary has been identified clinically in the oral cavity, pharynx, larynx, thyroid, or other areas.
- Biopsy from the primary and FNAC from the secondaries has to be taken.
- Primary is treated accordingly either by curative radiotherapy or by surgery (wide excision).
- Secondaries when mobile are treated by radical lymph node block dissection in the neck.

Secondaries in the Neck with Clinically Unidentified Primary

- Hard, neck lymph nodes are the secondaries, but primary has not been identified clinically.
- FNAC of the neck node has to be done and secondaries have to be confirmed. Then search for the primary has to be done by various investigations.
  They are:
  - Nasopharyngoscopy.
  - Laryngoscopy.
  - Esophagoscopy.
  - Bronchoscopy.
  - Blind biopsies from the fossa of Rosenmüller, lateral wall of pharynx, pyriform fossa, larynx.
  - FNAC of thyroid and suspected areas.
  - CT scan.
- Once the biopsy confirms the primary, it is treated either by *surgery or by curative radiotherapy*.
- Secondaries in the neck are treated by *radical neck dissection*.

Secondaries in the Neck with an Occult Primary

- Here secondaries in the neck lymph nodes are confirmed by FNAC, *but primary*

We are all different. Don't judge, understand instead—**Roy T Bennett**

has not been revealed by any available investigations.
- Inspite of all the investigations mentioned above are done and if does not show any evidence of primary, only then it is called as *occult primary*.
- Initially the secondaries in the neck are treated by *radical neck dissection*, then *regular follow up* is done (at three monthly intervals) until the primary reveals.
- Once primary is revealed it is *confirmed by biopsy* and treated accordingly, either by *curative radiotherapy or by wide excision* depending on location of revealed primary.
- This type is usually less aggressive and has got better prognosis. *Primary branchiogenic carcinoma may be a differential diagnosis for this.*

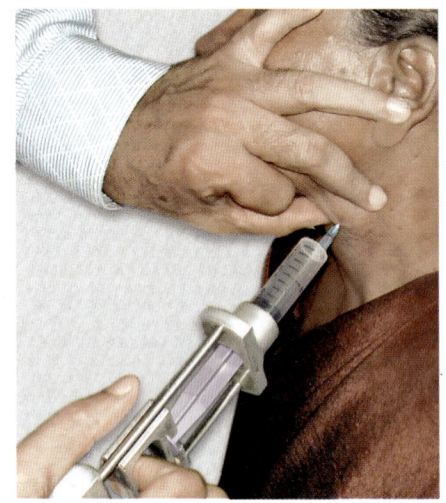

Fig. 17.21: FNAC of neck lymph node. It is very useful method in secondaries in neck node and tuberculosis. Its use is equivocal in lymphoma where open biopsy of the node is preferred method.

Occult primary sites, which can cause secondaries in neck

- Fossa of Rosenmüller.
- Lateral wall of pharynx.
- Posterior third of the tongue.
- Thyroid.
- Paranasal sinuses.
- Bronchus.
- Esophagus.

Investigations for Secondaries in Neck

- FNAC of secondary (Fig. 17.21).
- Biopsy from primary.
- Blind biopsies from suspected areas.
- Nasopharyngoscopy, laryngoscopy, bronchoscopy and esophagoscopy.
- CT scan.

Nodal staging in secondaries (Fig. 17.22)

N_0—nodes not detected
N_1—single node same side <3 cm.
N_{2a}—single node same side 3–6 cm.
N_{2b}—multiple nodes same side <6 cm.
N_{2c}—bilateral/contralateral nodes <6 cm.
N_3—node >6 cm.

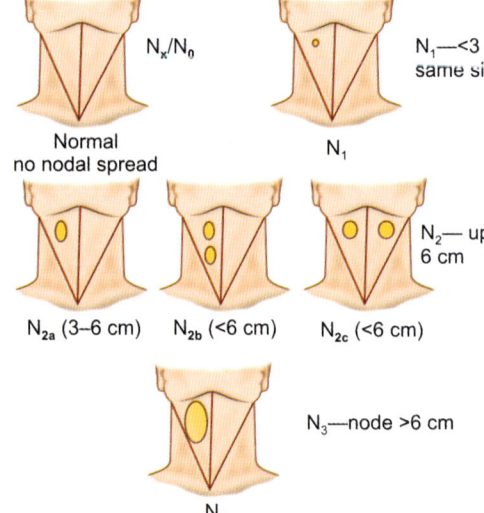

Fig. 17.22: Diagrammatic representation of neck lymph node staging in secondaries.

Differential Diagnosis

- Lymphomas.
- Tuberculous lymphadenitis.
- Nonspecific lymphadenitis.

On the wings of imagination, let your mind explore every realm of life

Treatment

- Primary has to be treated depending on the site, either by *wide excision (surgery)* or by *curative radiotherapy*. Then the secondaries have to be treated.
- Secondaries when are *mobile are* treated *by radical neck dissection*.
- When *fixed* it is *inoperable. Palliative external radiotherapy* has to be given to palliate the pain and to prevent the anticipated bleeding.
- Sometimes *initially, external radiotherapy* has to be given to *downstage* the disease so that it becomes operable and later classical block dissection can be done.

Types of Block Dissection

Classic Radical Neck Dissection

It is resection of lymph nodes, fat, fascia, sternomastoid muscle, strap muscles, internal jugular vein, accessory nerve, submandibular salivary gland, lower part of parotid—enbloc (Criles' operation).

Incision that is commonly made is *McFee* incision, which are two parallel incisions, one at submandibular region, another at supraclavicular region. Blood supply of the flap remains intact and so healing will be better without flap necrosis (Figs. 17.23 and 17.24).

Conservative Functional Block Dissection (Modified Radical Neck Dissection—MRND)

It is done only in selected cases where tumor is very well-differentiated and less aggressive. Structures preserved here are sternomastoid muscle, internal jugular vein and spinal accessory nerve.

- Only spinal accessory nerve is preserved— MRND type I.
- Accessory nerve and internal jugular vein are preserved—MRND type II.
- Accessory nerve, sternomastoid and internal jugular veins are preserved—MRND type III.

Supraomohyoid Block

Only fat, fascia, lymph nodes, muscles, submandibular salivary gland, with dissection

Type of neck dissection	Nodes removed	Structures preserved
Comprehensive:		
Radical neck dissection (RND)	Level I-V	None
MRND type I	Level I-V	Spinal accessory nerve
MRND type II	Level I-V	Spinal accessory nerve; IJV
MRND type III	Level I-V	Spinal accessory nerve; sternomastoid muscle; IJV
Bilateral RND Commando's operation		
Selective node dissection:		
Supraomohyoid neck dissection (N_0)	Level I-III	Spinal accessory nerve; sternomastoid muscle; IJV
Extended supraomohyoid dissection (N_0)	Level I-IV	Spinal accessory nerve; sternomastoid muscle; IJV
Anterolateral neck dissection (N_0)	Level II-IV	Spinal accessory nerve; sternomastoid muscle; IJV
Posterolateral neck dissection (N_0)	Level II-V with suboccipital, retroauricular nodes	Spinal accessory nerve; sternomastoid muscle; IJV
Anterior/central dissection	Level VI	Spinal accessory nerve; sternomastoid muscle; IJV

(IJV: internal jugular vein)

Respect other people's feelings. It might mean nothing to you, but it could mean everything to them—**Roy T Bennett**

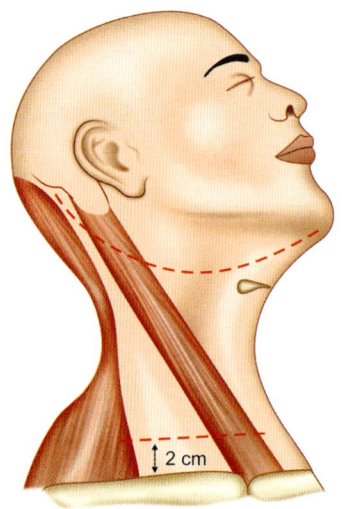

Fig. 17.23: McFee incision for radical neck dissection. Upper incision is from mastoid process along the line of digastric to hyoid bone point then upward to chin. Lower incision is parallel to clavicle 2 cm above from anterior margin of trapezius to midline.

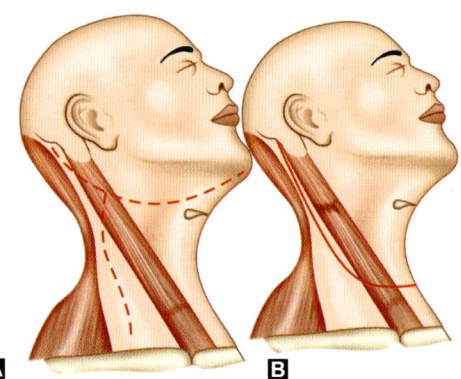

Figs. 17.24A and B: Other incisions used in neck block dissection. (A) Schobinger incision; (B) Hockey stick incision.

above the omohyoid muscle is done. Done only in selected individuals with well-differentiated tumor and involvement of few submandibular lymph nodes (*Levels I, II and III are removed*).

Bilateral Neck Dissection

Internal jugular vein has to be preserved on one side. *Always the side where the vein is preserved is operated first.* (If both the jugulars are ligated, cerebral congestion occurs leading to cerebral edema which is dangerous. If it occurs during surgery, the patient has to be kept in propped position; antibiotics, diuretics, steroids are given, repeated CSF taps are done to control the cerebral edema).

Commando Operation (Combined Mandibular Dissection and Neck Dissection)

It is *enbloc removal*, which includes wide excision of primary tumor with hemimandibulectomy and neck block dissection (*e.g. in tongue*).

Lateral Neck Dissection

It is done in laryngeal and pharyngeal primaries with clinically negative nodes. Levels II, III and IV are removed bilaterally.

Anterior (Central) Dissection

Level VI (pre-, paratracheal) nodes are removed

Posterolateral Dissection

Levels II, III, IV and V are removed for cutaneous malignancies.

Extended Radical Dissection

Additional nodes in the mediastinum are cleared (level VII).

Complications of Block Dissection

- Hemorrhage.
- Infection.
- Lymph ooze.
- Carotid blowout.

Other Treatments

Chemotherapy

- Drugs used are—Methotrexate, Vincristine, Bleomycin, Adriamycin.
- It can be given by *intra-arterial route, through external carotid artery* (never

through internal carotid as it will cause cerebral damage).
* Doppler and angiogram should be done to confirm site of arterial catheter. Drug is usually administered through an arterial pump. Other method is to increase the height of the drip stand to get a pressure above the level of the systolic pressure of the patient (i.e. more than 13 feet).
* Drugs can also be given IV or orally.

Note:
To control hemorrhage in head and neck cancers and during head and neck surgeries (like radical parotidectomy, commandos operation, maxillectomy), often ligation of external carotid artery is required. **Ligation should be done distal to the origin of the superior thyroid artery (Fig. 17.25)**. It should never be ligated below the origin of the superior thyroid artery as this will lead to the formation of Eddy current and thrombus at the carotid artery bifurcation and later to intracranial embolism. Ligation of external carotid artery (ECA) to control bleeding is usually done in continuity.

Carotid blowout:
It is most dangerous complication. It is due to sepsis, wound breakdown, arterial adventitious stripping and necrosis and drying of the artery. Ligation of the carotid is done to save the life of the patient but procedure itself has got 20% mortality and 50% morbidity (hemiplegia).

PANCOAST TUMOR (SUPERIOR SULCUS TUMOR)

It is a type of peripheral lung carcinoma arising from the apex of the lung.

Features

* It invades brachial plexus, sympathetic chain, upper ribs and vertebrae.
* Intractable pain in upper chest and arm.

Pancoast syndrome
• Lower brachial plexus palsy. • Horner's syndrome—miosis (small pupil), enophthalmos (regression of eyeball), anhydrosis (absence of sweating), ptosis (drooping of upper eyelid), loss of spinociliary reflex, nasal congestion. • Rib erosion. • Apical shadow.

Note:
Causes of Horner's syndrome are—posterior inferior cerebellar artery thrombosis, cervical sympathectomy, pancoast tumor, syringomyelia, lower brachial plexus injury (Klumpke's), carotid artery aneurysm, advanced neck malignancies like lymph node secondaries.

* **Investigations:**
  - Chest X-ray.
  - CT scan.
  - Bronchoscopy and biopsy.
  - CT guided biopsy.
  - MRI is better than CT to visualize brachial plexus and sympathetic chain.
* **Treatment**
  - Lobectomy/pneumonectomy.
  - Radiotherapy.
  - Chemotherapy.
* **Prognosis:** Poor prognosis.

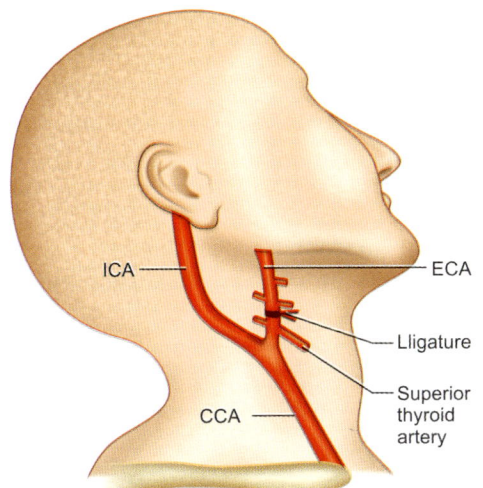

Fig. 17.25: Ligation of external carotid artery should be done when needed distal to the origin of the superior thyroid artery.
(ICA: internal carotid artery; ECA: external carotid artery; CCA: common carotid artery)

*Faith is a knowledge within the heart, beyond the reach of proof—**Khalil Gibran***

CHAPTER 18

Thyroid

CHAPTER OUTLINE

- Development
- Anatomy
- Congenital Anomalies
- Thyroid Function Tests
- Classification of Goiter
- Diffuse Hyperplastic Goiter
- Nodular Goiter
- Solitary Thyroid Nodule
- Retrosternal Goiter
- Thyrotoxicosis
- Thyroid Neoplasm
- Papillary Carcinoma
- Follicular Carcinoma
- Anaplastic Carcinoma
- Medullary Carcinoma of Thyroid
- Malignant Lymphoma
- Hashimoto's Thyroiditis
- De Quervain's Subacute Granulomatous Thyroiditis
- Reidel's Thyroiditis
- Thyroidectomy
- Emil Theodor Kocher
- Hypothyroidism

DEVELOPMENT

- The thyroid gland develops from a median down growth of a column of cells from the pharyngeal floor between the first and second pharyngeal pouches (subsequently marked by the foramen cecum of the tongue).
- The canalized column becomes the *thyroglossal duct,* which is displaced forward by the developing hyoid bone and then lies slightly to one side below the hyoid, more commonly to the left. The duct bifurcates to form the thyroid lobes and a portion of the duct forms the pyramidal lobe.

ANATOMY

- It is located in the anterior triangle of the neck. It weighs about 20 grams (Figs. 18.1 and 18.2).

Parts

- *Right and left lateral lobes* located in a space (thyroid fossa) between trachea and esophagus medially and carotid sheath laterally. Each lobe is 5 × 3 × 1.5 cm in size, extends from the middle of thyroid cartilage to 6th tracheal ring.
- *Isthmus* is the connecting part between two lateral lobes in midline extending from 2nd to 4th tracheal rings.
- *Pyramidal lobe* is upward extension as fibrous strands or muscular strands from the junction of the isthmus and left lateral lobe.
- Gland is invested by *pretracheal fascia.*
- *Berry's ligament* is a strong condensed vascular connective tissue between the lateral lobe and cricoid cartilage on each side.

*A friend is one that knows you as you are, understands where you have been, accepts what you have become, and still, gently allows you to grow—***William Shakespeare**

Chapter 18 : Thyroid

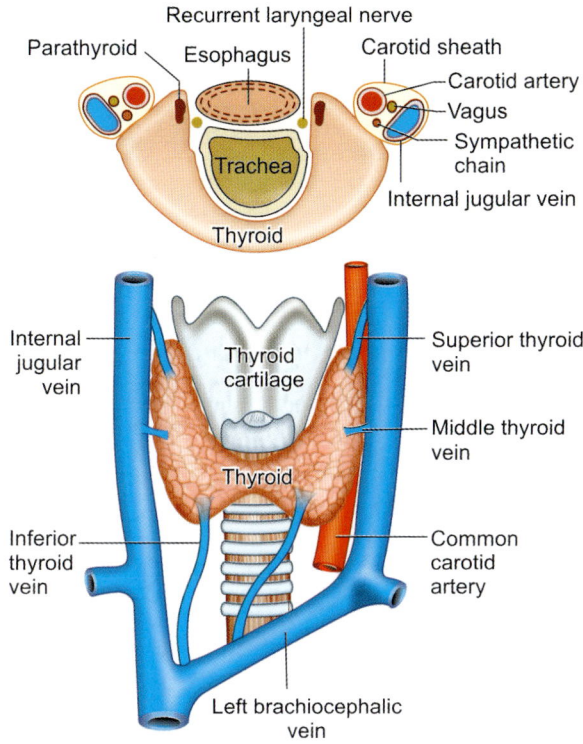

Fig. 18.1: Relations of the thyroid gland.

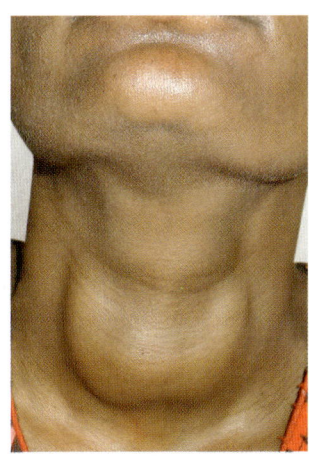

Fig. 18.2: Butterfly-shaped thyroid.

Blood Supply

- *Superior thyroid artery*, a branch of external carotid artery enters the gland near superior pole as a larger anterior superficial branch and a smaller posterior branch.
- *Inferior thyroid artery*, a branch of thyrocervical trunk of subclavian artery passes behind the carotid sheath running medially reaching the posterolateral aspect of the gland.
- *Thyroidea ima artery*, a branch of aorta or brachiocephalic artery enters the isthmus or lower pole of one of the lateral lobes.
- Tracheal and esophageal branches, serve as blood supply to the retained thyroid gland after thyroidectomy.

Venous Drainage

- Superior thyroid vein.
- Middle thyroid vein is short and drains into the internal jugular vein. It is first to be ligated in thyroidectomy.

How a person masters his fate is more important than what his fate is

- Inferior thyroid veins are many in number.
- Kocher's vein may be present which drains lower or middle thyroid.
- *Parathyroid glands*—four in number, two on each side embedded in thyroid.

Lymphatic Drainage (Fig. 18.3)

Primary:
- Tracheoesophageal nodes.
- Prelaryngeal (Delphian) node.
- Pretracheal (Subdelphian) nodes.
- Mediastinal nodes.

Secondary:
- Deep cervical nodes.
- Supraclavicular nodes.
- Occipital nodes.

CONGENITAL ANOMALIES

ECTOPIC THYROID (FIGS. 18.4 AND 18.5)

Ectopic thyroid tissue may lie any where along the line of descent. Whole of the thyroid gland or residual thyroid lies in an abnormal position either in the posterior part of the tongue, or in the upper part of the neck in midline, or intrathoracic region. Radioisotope scan, CT scan for intrathoracic thyroid confirms the diagnosis.

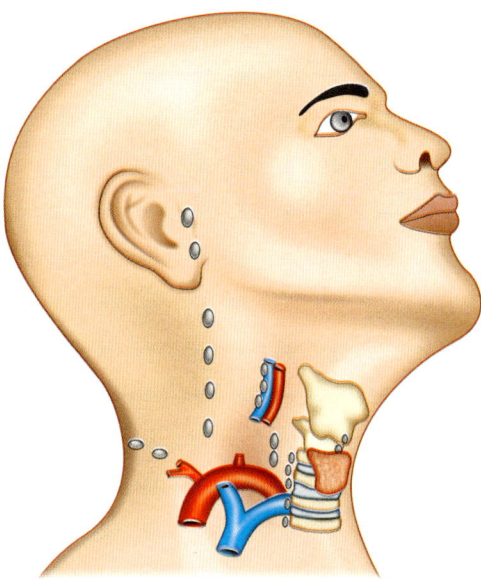

Fig. 18.3: Lymphatic drainage of thyroid.

Important Relations of Thyroid Gland

- *Recurrent laryngeal nerve* lies in the tracheoesophageal groove, in relation to Berry's ligament.
- *Superior laryngeal nerve*, which gives a branch as external laryngeal nerve supplies cricothyroid muscle. It accompanies superior thyroid artery.

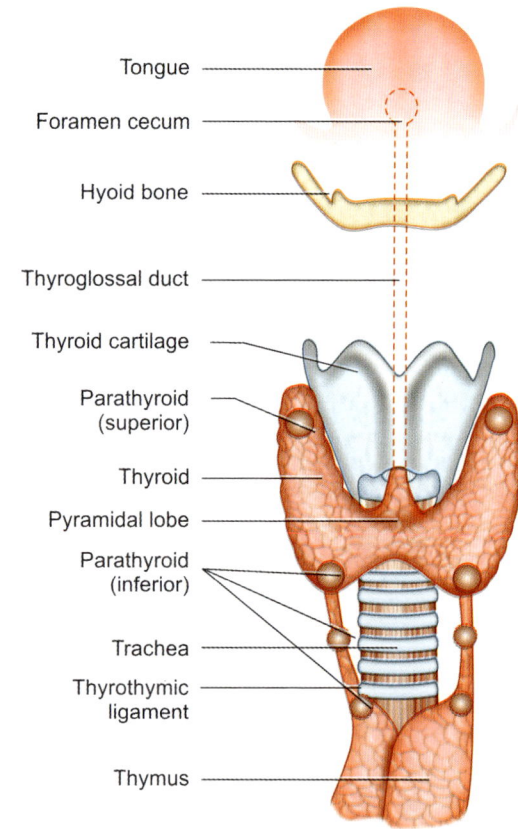

Fig. 18.4: Anatomy of thyroglossal duct showing its pathway.

Always bear in mind that your own resolution to success is more important than any other one thing—**Abraham Lincoln**

Chapter 18 : Thyroid

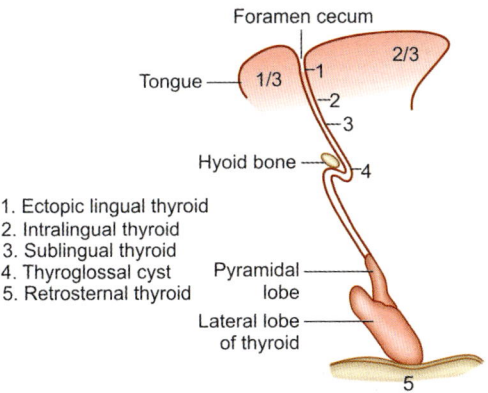

1. Ectopic lingual thyroid
2. Intralingual thyroid
3. Sublingual thyroid
4. Thyroglossal cyst
5. Retrosternal thyroid

Fig. 18.5: Ectopic sites of thyroid.

LINGUAL THYROID

It is a thyroid swelling *in the posterior third of tongue, at the foramen cecum*, presenting as rounded swelling (Fig. 18.6). It may be the only existing thyroid tissue, which may cause:
* Dysphagia.
* Speech impairment.
* Respiratory obstruction.
* Hemorrhage.

Any disease, which can occur in normal thyroid, can also occur in lingual thyroid, i.e. nodularity, toxicity, malignancy.

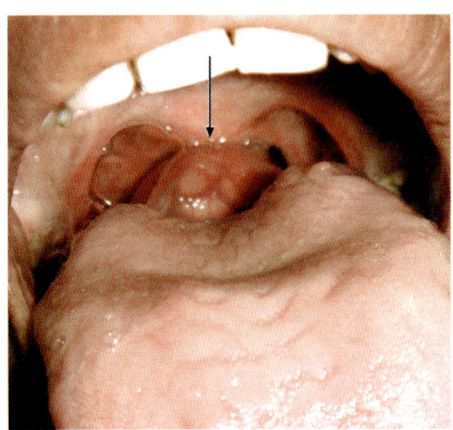

Fig. 18.6: Lingual thyroid visible on the posterior 1/3rd of the tongue. Neck should be palpated for the presence or absence of normal thyroid.

Diagnosis

* *Radioisotope study* shows the uptake of iodine by the lingual thyroid and also says the status of the thyroid in normal fossa.
* Ultrasound neck has to be done to see the absence of thyroid in normal location.

Treatment

* L-thyroxine is given daily orally.
* Often requires surgical excision and is technically easier.
* Radioisotope therapy for ablation is also given.

THYROGLOSSAL CYST (FIG. 18.7)

Thyroglossal cyst is a swelling occurring in the neck in any part along the line of thyroglossal tract.

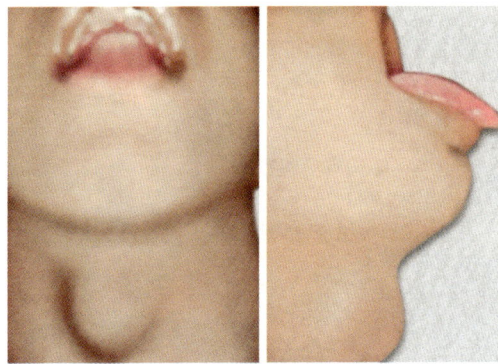

Fig. 18.7: Thyroglossal cyst.

Possible sites for thyroglossal cyst
• Beneath the foramen cecum.
• In the floor of mouth.
• Suprahyoid.
• Subhyoid—commonest site.
• On the thyroid cartilage.

* It is usually congenital wherein there will be degeneration of a part of the tract causing cystic swelling.

A goal is a dream with a deadline

- Normal thyroid may be present in the normal location (fossa).
- Sometimes, thyroid may not be present in the normal site but may be present in the wall of the thyroglossal cyst.

Clinical Features

- Swelling in the *midline, towards the left*.
- Moves with deglutition as well as with the protrusion of tongue. Patient is asked to open the mouth and keep the lower jaw still. Examiner holds the cyst between the thumb and forefinger. When the patient is asked to protrude the tongue, a '*tugging sensation*' can be felt, by the examiner.
- Swelling is smooth, soft, fluctuant (cystic), nontender, mobile, often transilluminant.
- Thyroid fossa is empty, if there is no thyroid in normal location.
- Thyroglossal cyst can get infected and may form an abscess.
- Malignancy can develop in thyroglossal cyst (papillary carcinoma).

Investigations

- Radioisotope study.
- Ultrasound neck.
- Fine needle aspiration cytology (FNAC) from the cyst.

Treatment

- *Sistrunk operation:* Excision of cyst along with entire tract up to the foramen cecum is done along with removal of part of the hyoid bone as the tract passes through it.
- If there is no normal thyroid gland after the surgery, maintenance dose of L-thyroxine 0.1 mg OD is given life long.
- If tract is not completely excised, it results in thyroglossal fistula.

THYROGLOSSAL FISTULA (FIG. 18.8)

- *It is not a congenital condition*.

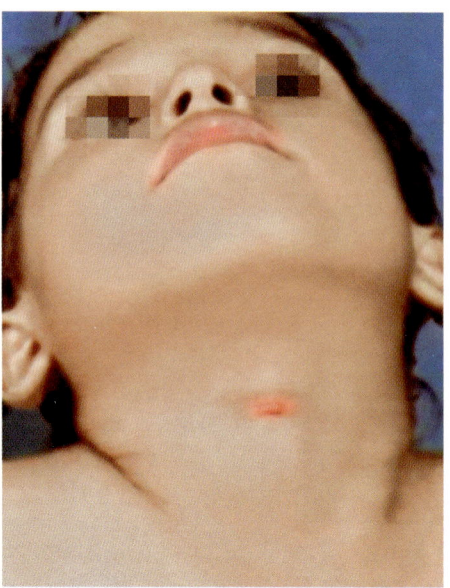

Fig. 18.8: Thyroglossal fistula.

- It either follows infection of thyroglossal cyst, which bursts open or after inadequate removal of the cyst.
- It is lined by columnar epithelium, discharges mucus, and is a seat of recurrent inflammation. '*Hood sign*' is characteristic.
- **Investigations:** Radioisotope study and fistulogram.
- **Treatment:** Sistrunk operation.

(*Note:* One more sistrunk operation is done in case of lymphedema).

LATERAL ABERRANT THYROID

- It is at present considered as a misnomer.
- It is the metastasis into cervical lymph node from a papillary carcinoma of thyroid.
- FNAC has to be done and treated as papillary carcinoma of thyroid.

AGENESIS

Total agenesis of one thyroid lobe may occur. This is rare but can be clinically important.

*A successful man is one who can lay a firm foundation with the bricks others have thrown at him—**David Brinkley***

It leads to confusion in diagnosis, especially in the toxic gland, where it could be diagnosed as a secreting nodule.

DYSHORMONOGENESIS

- It is an *autosomal recessive* condition wherein there is either deficiency of thyroid enzymes (either peroxidase or dehalogenase) or inability to concentrate or to bind or to retain iodine.
- It may be familial and patient presents with large diffuse vascular goiter involving both lobes.
- They respond very well to L-thyroxine and may not require surgery at any time.
- Condition may be associated with congenital deafness which is being called as *Pendred's syndrome*.

THYROID FUNCTION TESTS

- T_3 (Serum triiodothyronine): 1.2–3.1 nmol/liter.
- T_4 (Serum thyroxine): 55–150 nmol/liter.
- TSH 0–5 IU/mL of plasma.
- PBI (Protein bound iodide)—8 µg%.
- Free T_3 is 0.3% (3–9 pmol/liter). It is the best single test in assessing hyperthyroidism.
- Free T_4 is 0.03% (8–26 pmol/liter).
- RA I^{123} scan can show either cold nodule, hot nodule, or warm nodule.
- TRH (Thyrotrophin releasing hormone test): After IV TRH (200 mg), TSH level is estimated.
- TSH level is below 2.5 m units/L in hyperthyroidism and it is exaggerated in hypothyroid patient (more than 20 m units/L).
- Serum creatinine is increased in hyperthyroidism; decreased in hypothyroidism.
- Serum cholesterol is increased in hyperthyroidism and decreased in hyperthyroidism.
- BMR is increased in hyperthyroidism.
- Thyroid autoantibodies are also useful to evaluate the function.
- T_3 suppression test.

FNAC OF THYROID

- It is the investigation of choice in most of the thyroid diseases to conclude the pathological diagnosis.
- It is useful in papillary/medullary (amyloid)/anaplastic carcinomas, lymphomas, colloid nodule, thyroiditis.
- 23-G needle is used. Suspicious solitary/multiple nodules/dominant nodules should be aspirated.
- Karolinska *hospital* (Lowhagen) at Sweden pioneered this method.
- Minimum 6 aspirations should be done. An adequate FNAC smear should have six aspirations with six groups of cells with each group containing 20 cells. USG guided aspiration is better.
- Diagnostic accuracy of FNAC is 95%; sensitivity 85%; specificity 94%.
- Aspiration is *graded* as: Thy 1—nondiagnostic; Thy 2—non-neoplastic; Thy 3—follicular; Thy 4—suspicious of malignancy; Thy 5—malignancy.
- In a cyst of thyroid FNAC may be less reliable; if cyst recurs after 3 aspirations, surgery is needed.
- Malignancy rate in a simple cyst is 5%; in a complex cyst it is 75%.
- FNAC is *not reliable* at present in follicular carcinoma of thyroid as capsular and vascular invasions cannot be detected. But it is possible by newer technique to identify the differences—benign is polyploidy, malignancy is aneuploidy; benign are monoclonal, malignancy are polyclonal; MR spectroscopy and thyroimmunoperoxidase estimation are useful to differentiate.
- FNNAC is fine needle nonaspiration cytology—is said to be more reliable.

Those who wish to sing always finds a song

USG in thyroid

- To identify nodules, number, size, vascularity, echogenicity.
- USG-guided FNAC.
- To identify neck lymph nodes.
- To find out solid or cystic nature.
- Benign lesion is *hyperechoic*, often cystic with well-defined margin; shows peripheral egg *shell calcification* with sonolucent rim (halo) around nodule.
- Malignant lesion is *hypoechoic* with poorly defined margin, with high vascularity, with microcalcification without any halo around.

CLASSIFICATION OF GOITER (FIGS. 18.9 AND 18.10)

1. **Simple nontoxic**
   - Diffuse hyperplastic:
     1. Physiological
        a. Puberty.
        b. Pregnancy.

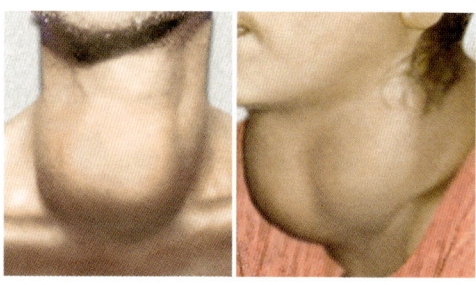

Fig. 18.9: Note the goiters in a male and a female patient.

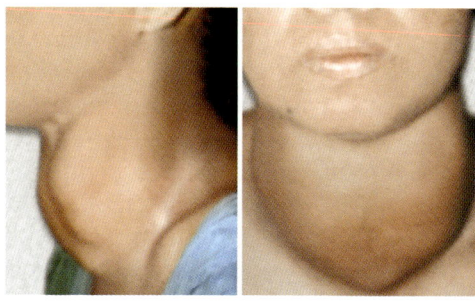

Fig. 18.10: Multinodular goiter.

   2. Primary iodine deficiency (endemic; dietary intake less than 100 ug/day).
   3. Secondary iodine deficiency
      a. Goitrogens of Brassica family, e.g. cabbage, soyabean
      b. Excess dietary fluoride.
      c. Drugs: PAS, Lithium, Phenylbutazone, Thiocyanates.
      d. Dyshormonogenetic goiter.
   - Colloid goiter
   - Nodular goiter (multinodular).
   - Solitary nontoxic nodule.
   - Recurrent nontoxic nodule.
2. **Toxic**
   - Diffuse (*Primary*)—*Graves' disease.*
   - Multinodular (*Secondary*)—*Plummer's disease.*
   - Toxic nodule (solitary) (*Tertiary*).
   - Recurrent toxicosis.
3. **Neoplastic**
   - Benign—adenomas: Papillary, follicular, Hurthle cell, colloid.
   - Malignant—carcinomas: Papillary, follicular, medullary, anaplastic, lymphomas.
4. **Thyroiditis**
   - Hashimoto's autoimmune thyroiditis.
   - de-Quervain's autoimmune thyroiditis.
   - Reidel's thyroiditis.
5. **Rare causes:** Bacterial (suppurative), amyloid.

DIFFUSE HYPERPLASTIC GOITER

- Initial persistent increase in thyroid stimulating hormone (TSH) level causes diffuse active lobules. In late stages of diffuse hyperplasia, TSH stimulation decreases and many follicles become inactive get filled with colloid and it is called *as colloid goiter*.
- As diffuse hyperplastic goiter is a reversible stage, L-thyroxine is beneficial.

When one door of happiness closes, another opens; but often we look so long at the closed door that we do not see the one which has been opened for us—**Helen Keller**

NODULAR GOITER

Pathogenesis

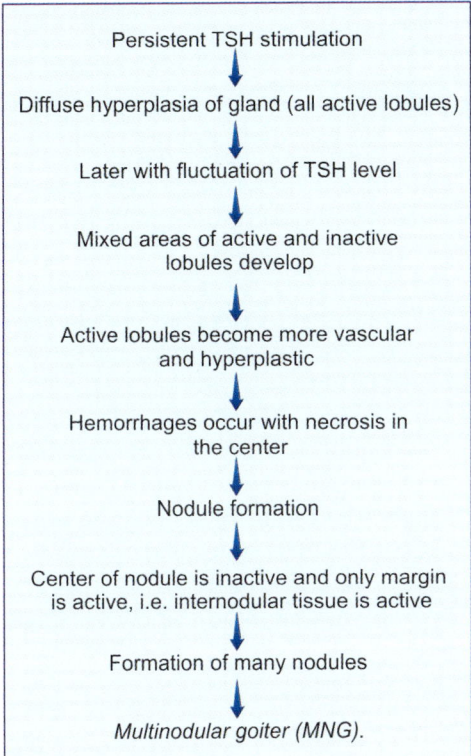

Other factors involved are growth stimulating immunoglobulins and growth prone cell clones.

Clinical Features

- It is a slowly progressive disease with many years of history.
- *Multiple nodules* of different sizes are formed in both lobes, also in isthmus, which is firm, nodular, nontender, moves with deglutition.
- Recent increase in size signifies malignant transformation or hemorrhage.

Complications of multinodular goiter

- Secondary thyrotoxicosis (30%).
- Follicular carcinoma of thyroid.
- Hemorrhage in a nodule.
- Tracheal obstruction.
- Cosmetic problem.

Investigations

T_3, T_4, TSH, ultrasound neck, FNAC, X-ray neck shows ring or rim calcification.

Treatment

- *Nodular goiter is an irreversible stage and so surgery is the treatment.*

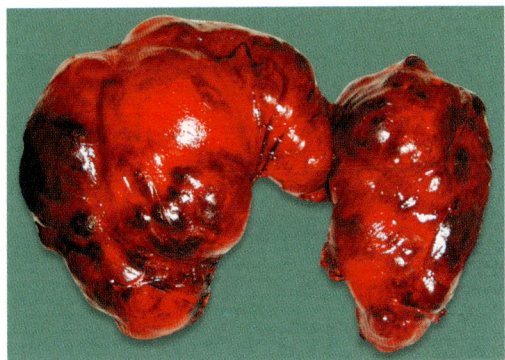

Fig. 18.11: Multinodular goiter surgical specimen—total thyroidectomy was done.

- ***Partial*** or ***subtotal thyroidectomy*** is done depending on the amount of gland involved, amount of normal gland existing, and location of nodules.
- *Total thyroidectomy is the present recommendation* as recurrence is common otherwise. But lifelong L-thyroxine has to be given to the patient (Fig. 18.11).
- Postoperatively L-thyroxine is often given to prevent further fluctuation in TSH level.

Happiness is not a matter of events; it depends upon the tides of the mind

SOLITARY THYROID NODULE

It is a single palpable nodule in thyroid on *clinical or sonological examination*, in an otherwise normal gland.

Causes

- Thyroid adenomas—(a) Colloid, (b) Hürthle cell, (c) Follicular.
- Papillary carcinoma of thyroid.
- Thyroid cysts.
- Thyroiditis.

Types

- Toxic solitary nodule.
- Nontoxic solitary nodule.

Based on radioisotope study:
- *Hot*: Means autonomous toxic nodule.
- *Warm*: Normally functioning nodule.
- *Cold*: Nonfunctioning nodule; may be malignant (need not be always).

Solitary nodule can also be classified as:
- Benign—70%
- Malignant—5%
- Indeterminate—10% (auspicious and follicular carcinoma)
- Nondiagnostic—15%

Clinical Features

- Single nodule palpable in one or other lobes of the thyroid, which is usually smooth and firm.
- *Lahey's test* does not show any other nodules in posterior part of the gland (Fig. 18.12).

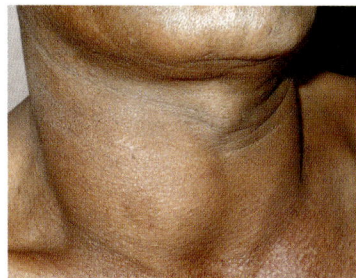

Fig.18.12: Solitary nodule in thyroid in a male patient. Malignancy is more common in male thyroid nodule.

Investigations

- Ultrasound neck (very useful).
- FNAC.
- T_3, T_4, thyroid stimulating hormone.
- Radioisotope study (I^{123}).

Treatment

- If it is a *nontoxic nodule due to any cause*, *hemithyroidectomy* with complete removal of lateral lobe and whole of the isthmus is done.
- If it is *papillary carcinoma thyroid*, then *near total thyroidectomy* is done along with suppressive dose of L-thyroxine given 0.3 mg OD daily.
- *If it is a toxic nodule, radioiodine therapy, I^{131}*—5 milli curie is given orally, if the age of the patient is more than 10 years.

  If age is less than 10 years, then initially toxicity has to be controlled by antithyroid drugs, always followed by surgery—hemithyroidectomy, or radioactive therapy later.

DOMINANT NODULE

It is palpable nodule in an *enlarged thyroid gland*.

RETROSTERNAL GOITER

- Usually arises from the lower pole of a nodular goiter.
- Common in short neck individuals.
- Due to negative intrathoracic pressure, nodule gets drawn into the superior mediastinum. Sometimes it may also be an ectopic thyroid.

Types

1. *Substernal type*: Part of the nodule is palpable in the lower neck.

Life is really simple, but we insist on making it complicated—**Confucius**

2. *Plunging goiter*: An intrathoracic goiter is occasionally forced into the neck by increased intrathoracic pressure.
3. *Intrathoracic goiter* itself.

Features

- Dyspnea at night.
- Cough and *stridor* (stridor is harsh sound on inspiration).
- Dysphagia.
- Engorgement of neck veins and superficial veins on the chest wall.
- *Pembertones' sign* is positive. The patient is asked to raise the arm above the shoulder level. Dilated veins are seen over neck and upper part of chest wall. Stridor and rarely dysphagia may occur. When patient raises the arm above the shoulder level, retrosternal goiter compresses over the easily compressible structures like superior vena cava (SVC) and trachea causing dilated veins and dyspnea respectively.
- Dull note over the sternum on percussion.
- Retrosternal goiter can be either nodular, toxic or malignant.
- **Differential diagnosis:** Mediastinal tumor.
- **Investigations:**
  - Chest X-ray shows soft tissue shadow under the sternum. CT scan is useful
  - I^{123} study is diagnostic.
- **Treatment:**
  - Surgical removal of retrosternal thyroid is done. Commonly it can be removed through an incision in neck (as blood supply of retrosternal goiter is from neck), but in case of large retrosternal extension or malignant type median sternotomy is required.
  - *Radioiodine therapy is not accepted in retrosternal goiter.*

THYROTOXICOSIS (Hyperthyroidism)

It is a symptom complex due to raised levels of thyroid hormones.

Thyrotoxicosis refers to biochemical and physiological manifestations of excessive thyroid hormones. *Hyperthyroidism* is the term used for overproduction of the hormones by thyroid gland. In hyperthyroidism pathology is in thyroid gland itself. Hyperthyroidism is one of the causes of thyrotoxicosis. Thyrotoxicosis can also occur due to other causes other than hyperthyroidism.

Other causes of thyrotoxicosis without hyperthyroidism are—ectopic functioning thyroid, struma ovarii, functioning metastatic follicular carcinoma, trophoblastic tumors, thyrotoxicosis factitia.

Types

1. Diffuse toxic goiter (Graves' disease, **Basedow's disease**, primary thyrotoxicosis) (Fig. 18.13).
2. Toxic multinodular goiter (secondary thyrotoxicosis, **Plummer disease**).
3. Toxic nodule.
4. Hyperthyroidism of rare causes:
   a. *Thyrotoxicosis factitia*—drug induced. Due to intake of L-thyroxine more than normal.

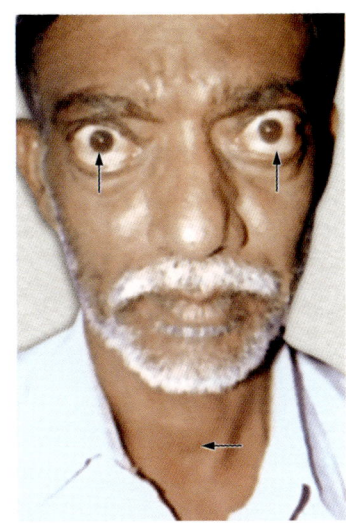

Fig. 18.13: Thyrotoxicosis (primary). Note the exophthalmos.

Success is not final; failure is not fatal: It is the courage to continue that counts—**Winston S Churchill**

b. *Jod Basedow thyrotoxicosis*—because of large doses of iodides given to a hyperplastic endemic goiter.
   c. *Autoimmune thyroiditis or de Quervain's thyroiditis.*
   d. Occasionally *carcinoma thyroid.*
   e. *Neonatal thyrotoxicosis.* It subsides in 3–4 weeks as TsAb titers fall in the baby's serum.

Clinical Features

- It is eight times more common in females.
- Occurs in any age group.
- Primary type is seen commonly in younger age group.
- Secondary is common in older age group.

Symptoms of Hyperthyroidism

Gastrointestinal system
- Weight loss in spite of increased appetite.
- Diarrhea (due to increased activity at ganglionic level).

Cardiovascular system
- Palpitations.
- Shortness of breath at rest or on minimal exertion.
- Angina.
- Cardiac irregularity.
- Cardiac failure in the elderly (CCF).

Neuromuscular system
- Undue fatigue and muscle weakness.
- Tremor.

Skeletal system
- Increase in linear growth in children.

Genitourinary system
- Oligomenorrhea.
- Occasional urinary frequency.

Integument
- Hair loss.
- Pruritus.

Psychiatry
- Irritability.
- Nervousness.
- Insomnia.

Sympathetic overactivity causes dyspnea, palpitation, tiredness, heat intolerance, sweating, nervousness, increased appetite and decrease in weight. Because of the *increased catabolism* they show weight loss in spite of having increased appetite, and so also increased creatinine level, which signifies *myopathy* (due to more muscle catabolism).

Fine tremor is due to diffuse irritability of gray matter.

Thrill is felt in the upper pole of the thyroid and also bruit on auscultation. It is because in upper pole, superior thyroid artery enters the gland superficially, and so thrill and bruit can easily be assessed. In lower pole inferior thyroid artery enters the gland from deeper plane and so thrill cannot be felt.

Signs of Hyperthyroidism

Eye Signs in Toxic Goiter

Eye signs are common in primary thyrotoxicosis. Lid lag, lid spasm can occur in secondary thyrotoxicosis also.

- **Lid retraction:** Here upper eyelid is higher than normal; lower eyelid is in normal position. It is due to *sympathetic overactivity* causing spasm of involuntary smooth muscle part of the levator palpebrae superioris (*Muller's musc*le). It is *a sign of* thyrotoxicosis, *not a sign* of exophthalmos.
- **von Graefe's sign** (Lid Lag's sign): It is inability of the upper eyelid to keep pace with the eyeball when it looks downwards to follow the examiner's finger.
- **Dalrymple's sign:** Upper eyelid retraction, so visibility of upper sclera.
- **Stellwag's sign:** Absence of normal blinking—so *staring look*—first sign to

Happiness is in the taste, not in the thing

Wayne's diagnostic indices (clinical) of thyrotoxicosis

	Symptoms	Present	Absent
1.	Dyspnea on effort	+1	
2.	Palpitation	+2	
3.	Tiredness	+2	
4.	Preference to heat		−5
5.	Preference to cold (Heat intolerance)	+5	
6.	Excessive sweating	+3	
7.	Nervousness	+2	
8.	Appetite increased	+3	
9.	Weight decreased	+3	
	Signs	**Present**	**Absent**
1.	Bruit over thyroid	+2	
2.	Exophthalmos	+2	
3.	Lid retraction	+2	
4.	Lid lag	+1	
5.	Hyperkinetic movements	+4	−2
6.	Fine finger tremors	+1	
7.	Hands hot	+2	−2
	Moist	+1	−1
8.	Atrial fibrillation	+4	−3
9.	Pulse rate 80/minute	0	
	80–90/minute	+3	
	More than 90/minute	+3	
10.	Palpable thyroid		
	<11 points—nontoxic goitre	11–19 equivocal	>19 points—toxic

appear. It is due to widening of palpebral fissure due to lid retraction and also due to contraction of voluntary part of levator palpebrae superioris muscle.

- *Joffroy's sign:* Absence of wrinkling on forehead when patient looks up (frowns) with head is bent down/flexed position.
- *Moebius sign:* It is lack of convergence of eyeball. Defective convergence is due to lymphocytic infiltration of inferior oblique and rectus muscles in case of primary thyrotoxicosis. There will be diplopia. It may be an early sign of eventual ophthalmoplegia.
- *Naffziger's sign:* With patient in sitting position and neck fully extended, protruded eyeball can be visualized when observed from behind.

Note: Other signs (only of academic interest):
- Jellinek's sign: Increased pigmentation of eyelid margins.
- Enroth sign: Edema of eyelids and conjunctiva.
- Rosenbach's sign: Tremor of closed eyelids.
- Gifford's sign: Difficulty in everting upper eyelid in primary toxic thyroid—differentiates from exophthalmos of other causes.
- Loewi's sign: Dilatation of pupil with weak adrenaline solution.
- Knie's sign: Unequal pupillary dilatation.
- Cowen's sign: Jerky pupillary contraction to consensual light.
- Kocher's sign: When clinician places his hands on patient's eyes and lifts it higher, patient's upper lid springs up more quickly than eyebrows.

Order of appearance of signs	
Stellwag's sign	— Mild. First sign to appear.
von Graefe's Sign	— Mild.
Joffroy's sign	— Moderate.
Moebius sign	— Severe.

EXOPHTHALMOS
- It is proptosis of the eye, caused by infiltration of the retrobulbar tissues with fluid and round cells, with *lidspasm* of upper eyelid (lidspasm is spasm of levator palpebrae superioris muscle which is partly innervated by sympathetic fibers).
- Sclera can be seen clearly above the limbus of the eye.
- Proptosis can be measured by *ophthalmometer*.

Life is ours to be spent, not to be saved—DH Lawrence

- Exophthalmos is often self-limiting, but not always. Sleeping in propped up position and lateral tarsorrhaphy will help to protect the eye.

Severe exophthalmos
- Eyelid edema, chemosis, conjunctival injection.
- Diplopia, ophthalmoplegia (complete weakness of all extraocular muscles and so no movements possible).
- Corneal ulceration.
- Papilledema soon develops.
- Finally it may also cause loss of vision.

It is called as **malignant exophthalmos**. (eventhough it is not malignant nor related to any malignancy).

It needs emergency treatment, i.e. large doses of systemic steroids (Prednisolone) are given along with *orbital decompression*, systemic antibiotics, steroid drops, antibiotic drops.

Cardiac Manifestations
- Tachycardia is common. As per **Crile's grading**.

> **Pulse rate**
> Grade I—90—100
> Grade II—100—110
> Grade III—>110.

Sleeping pulse rate is usually checked for three consecutive nights and average is taken as the value.
- Ectopic.
- Pulsus paradoxus.
- Wide pulse pressure.
- Multiple extrasystoles.
- Paroxysmal atrial tachycardia.
- Paroxysmal atrial fibrillation.
- Persistent atrial fibrillation (not responsive to digoxin).

Myopathy
- Weakness of proximal muscles occurs, i.e. the front thigh muscles, or arm muscles.
- Weakness is more when muscle contracts isometrically either while getting down steps, or lifting a filled bucket.
- Often when it is severe it resembles myasthenia gravis. Once hyperthyroidism is controlled recovery occurs.

Pretibial Myxedema
- **Pretibial myxedema** is often a feature of primary thyrotoxicosis.
- Is usually symmetrical, red, shiny, thickened skin, with coarse hair.
- In severe cases skin of whole leg below the knee with foot and ankle is involved.
- It is due to deposition of myxomatous tissues (mucin like deposits) in skin and subcutaneous plane.
- It might or might not regress completely after treatment for toxicity.
- It is associated with exophthalmos with high levels of thyroid stimulating antibodies.

Thyroid Acropachy

Thyroid acropachy is clubbing of fingers and toes in primary thyrotoxicosis.

TOXIC NODULE
- It is a solitary overactive nodule.
- There is an autonomous hypertrophy and hyperplasia of the part of gland where there is a nodule [it is not due to thyroid stimulating antibody (TsAb)].
- Here high levels of circulating thyroid hormones suppress TSH secretion, and so normal thyroid tissue surrounding the nodule is itself suppressed and inactive.

Once patient becomes euthyroid by drugs, surgery (hemithyroidectomy) or radioactive iodine therapy I^{131} in a therapeutic dose of 5 mcurie is given orally.

Because normal gland is inactive, radioactive iodine affects only the autonomous nodule, allowing the normal gland to remain intact,

The man who has no inner life is a slave to his surroundings

	Differentiating points between primary and secondary hyperthyroidism	
	Primary thyrotoxicosis	**Secondary thyrotoxicosis**
1.	Symptoms appear first, then swelling.	Swelling appears first.
2.	Goiter is diffuse, smooth, firm or soft, both lobes are involved.	Swelling is large nodular, obvious.
3.	There is thrill and bruit.	—
4.	Features are much more severe compared to that of secondary toxicosis.	Symptoms appear after long time, which is less severe and slowly progressive compared to primary toxicosis.
5.	Eye signs and exophthalmos are common.	Cardiac features are more common.
6.	As it is an autoimmune disease, there may be hepato-splenomegaly. *Histologically, there is hyperplasia of acini, lined by columnar epithelium, often containing vacuolated colloid.*	Eye signs are not common.

which later gets activated, and functions normally.

Drugs are used initially, only for a temporary period to make the patient euthyroid.

Investigations for Thyrotoxicosis

❖ *Thyroid function tests:*

Type of disease	T4	T3	TSH
Conventional hyper-thyroidism	In-creased	In-creased	Undetect-able
T_3 hyper-thyroidism	→	In-creased	Undetect-able
Subclinical hyper-thyroidism	→	→	Undetect-able

Serum T_3 and T_4 levels are very high. TSH is very low or undetectable. Sometimes, only T_3 level is increased and is called as T_3 *toxicosis*. Here in T_3 toxicosis, *free T_3 estimation is important.*

❖ Radioisotope study by I^{131} (diagnostic dose—5 microcurie is used) shows more up take, i.e. *hot nodules* or hot areas. This is very useful in autonomous solitary toxic nodule.

❖ TRH estimation.

❖ ECG—to look for cardiac involvement and if required opinion from cardiologists is taken and cardiac problems are managed.

❖ Total count and neutrophil count are very essential baseline investigations before starting antithyroid drugs (as it may cause agranulocytosis).

Treatment

1. Antithyroid drugs.
2. Surgery.
3. Radioiodine therapy.

1. ANTITHYROID DRUGS

Indications for antithyroid drugs:

❖ Toxicity in pregnant women—Propylthiouracil is preferred.
❖ Toxicity in children and young adults.
❖ Before subtotal thyroidectomy, to make the patient euthyroid.
❖ After radioactive I^{131} therapy for 6 to 12 weeks (effects of radiotherapy starts only in 6 to 12 weeks).

a. **Carbimazole**
   - Is the commonest drug used.
   - Dose is 5–10 mg, exactly 8th hourly (as $T_{1/2}$ of carbimazole is 8 hours).
   - Usually given for 12–18 months.

*Life is a long lesson in humility—**James M Barrie***

- Peak plasma level should be maintained in optimum concentration to have a proper benefit.
- Often triiodothyronine 20 microgram 4 times daily or thyroxine 0.1 mg daily is given in combination with antithyroid drugs, to prevent iatrogenic thyroid insufficiency or to prevent the increase in size of goiter.
- It acts by blocking thyroid hormone synthesis. Carbimazole also suppresses the autoimmune process in thyroid in Graves' disease.

b. **Methimazole:** Similar like carbimazole. Dose is 5 to 20 mg daily. *Methimazole is long acting and more potent*; given as once a day dose. It is not used in pregnancy.

c. **Propylthiouracil:**
- It acts by blocking thyroid hormone synthesis as well as by blocking peripheral conversion of T_4 to T_3.
- It also decreases the thyroid autoantibody levels.
- It can be given in hyperthyroidism in children and pregnancy.
- Dose is 200 mg 8th hourly.

Antithyroid drugs are continued during and after surgery, for 7–10 days and after radioactive iodine therapy for 6 weeks to 12 weeks.

Studying HLA status and TsAb level can assess response to treatment and possibility of relapse in primary thyrotoxicosis.

Propranolol
- Dose is 40 mg tid.
- It reduces the cardiac problems and also blocks the peripheral conversion of T_4 to T_3, as it is the T_3 which is the principle active agent in periphery.
- Contraindications are bronchial **a**sthma, heart **b**lock, **c**ardiac failure.

Note:
Lugol's iodine (5% iodine + 10% potassium iodide): It decreases the vascularity of the gland and makes it more firmer and easier to handle during surgery. Dose is 10–30 drops/day (minims) for 10 days prior to surgery. Potassium iodide tablets 60 mg tid also can be given instead of Lugol's iodine. But its use at present is disqualified. (One minim = one drop. One mL = 16 drops).

Advantages of antithyroid drugs
- Avoids surgery and its complications.
- Avoids radiotherapy.

Clinical improvement occurs in 2 weeks. Biochemical improvement occurs in 6 weeks.

Disadvantages of antithyroid drugs
- Prolonged course of treatment for 18 months and in spite of this cannot predict the remission or relapse. Relapse rate is 40%.
- Size of swelling may not regress.
- It may lead to *agranulocytosis and thrombocytopenia*, liver damage, hair loss.
- Sore throat is the earliest presentation of agranulocytosis. If it is so, drug has to be stopped; total count has to be done. If it is less, agranulocytosis is confirmed. High doses of injection benzyl penicillin 10–20 lacs, 6th hourly, IV has to be started to prevent infection. If required, blood transfusion has to be done. Patient usually recovers by this. To control toxicity, Tablet Propranolol 40 mg tid has to be started. Rarely they need bone marrow transplantation.

2. **SURGERY**

Indications:
- Failure of drug treatment in primary thyrotoxicosis in young patients.
- Autonomous toxic nodule.
- Nodular toxic goiter.
- When malignancy cannot be ruled out.

Surgery done is *subtotal thyroidectomy*—both lobes with isthmus are removed and a tissue equivalent to pulp of finger is retained in lower pole of the gland on both sides—8 grams.

Life shrinks and expands in proportion to one's courage

Choice of therapies

Condition	Age	Treatment
Diffuse toxic goiter		
a. Small goiter b. Large goiter	Over 45 years Under 45 years	Antithyroid drugs for 18 months. Radioiodine therapy. Surgery (*subtotal thyroidectomy*).
Toxic nodular goiter		Surgery (subtotal thyroidectomy). Initially antithyroid drugs are given to make the patient euthyroid before surgery.
Toxic solitary nodule	Under 45 years Over 45 years	Radioiodine. Surgery (hemithyroidectomy)
Recurrent thyrotoxicosis after surgery	Under 45 years Over 45 years	Antithyroid drugs. Radioiodine therapy.
Failure of antithyroid drugs or radioiodine therapy		Surgery.

In autonomous nodule, *hemithyroidectomy* is done—entire lateral lobe with whole of isthmus is removed.

Advantages:
- Rapid cure and high cure rate.
- Patient should be euthyroid before undergoing surgery (it should be confirmed by repeated estimation of T_3 and T_4 levels).

Disadvantages:
- Recurrent thyrotoxicosis (5%).
- Thyroid insufficiency 20–45%. It is revealed in 6 months to 2 years and confirmed by doing T_3 and T_4 and TSH estimation. Hypothyroidism is better than recurrent thyrotoxicosis. It is treated by tablet L-thyroxine 0.1 mg daily (OD) for life long.
- Complications of thyroid surgery itself.

3. RADIOIODINE THERAPY
Indications:
- Primary thyrotoxicosis after 10 years of age.
- In autonomous toxic nodule.
- In recurrent thyrotoxicosis.
    - Radioiodine destroys the cells and causes the complete ablation of thyroid gland. It is given only after the age of 45 years, as the chances of genetic mutation (damage), leukemia, carcinomas are high in younger individual.
    - Usual dose is 5 to 10 millicurie, or 160 microcurie/g of thyroid.
    - It takes 3 months, to get full response, and so until then, the patient has to take antithyroid drugs. Often additional one or two doses of radioiodine are required to have complete ablation. Eventually they go for hypothyroidism and so require maintenance dose of L-thyroxine 0.1 mg daily.
    - To give therapeutic dose, patient should be admitted and isolated for 7 days (half life) to prevent irradiation. It is given orally soon after getting from the manufacturer without much delay to have optimal efficacy.

Advantages:
- No surgery.
- No prolonged drug therapy.

Disadvantages:
- Availability of facilities.
- Proper follow-up is essential.

Contraindications:
- Pregnancy.
- Breastfeeding.
- Chronic smokers.
- Patients with severe ophthalmopathy.

Love the life you live. Live the life you love—**Bob Marley**

TOXIC THYROID IN PREGNANCY

- *Radioiodine therapy is an absolutely contraindicated* in pregnancy (high-risk to fetus).
- Antithyroid drugs can be administered carefully.
- But, the problem here is that both TSH and antithyroid drugs crosses the placental barrier and baby born may be hypothyroid and goitrous.
- Propylthiouracil is preferred in pregnancy.
- Subtotal thyroidectomy can be done in second trimester.

TOXIC THYROID IN CHILDREN

Radioiodine therapy is *absolutely contraindicated* in children because of high-risk of developing thyroid carcinoma. Recurrence rate is also very high after surgery. So proposed treatment is, initially antithyroid drugs are given until adolescent period and then subtotal thyroidectomy is done.

THYROCARDIAC

- Severe cardiac damage resulting from hyperthyroidism (may be partly or wholly due to same), usually secondary type, requires proper opinion from cardiologists and treatment with Propranolol. Subtotal thyroidectomy is the treatment.
- In a patient **with thyrotoxicosis, with recent onset of proptosis** early thyroidectomy has to be avoided. Because early surgery may precipitate malignant exophthalmos. Here the patient has to be treated initially with antithyroid drugs and if required with steroids, until the proptosis has remained static for six months. Then subtotal thyroidectomy is done.
- Since half life of L-thyroxine is 7 days, Propranolol and antithyroid drugs has to be continued for 7 days after thyroidectomy.

T_3 THYROTOXICOSIS

It should be suspected if the clinical picture is suggestive of toxicosis, but routine tests for thyroid function are within normal range.

RADIOACTIVE IODINE

It is used both as a diagnostic as well as a therapeutic agent.
1. I^{131}—*is used for radioactive iodine therapy.*
2. I^{123}—*is used for diagnostic studies.*
   - For diagnostic purpose I^{123} is given orally on previous day *(Dose—5 microcurie; $T_{1/2}$ (half life) of I^{123} is 13 hours* and so it is suitable for diagnostic purpose).
   - Patient should not take L-thyroxine for 7 days prior to radioisotope study.
   - Thyroid treats this I^{123} similar to inorganic I^{127}. This I^{123} enters the thyroid from the circulation and gets incorporated into T_3, T_4 and later released into circulation as protein bound iodide (PBI). *Normal value of PBI is 8 µg%.*
   - Using *Gieger Muller's gamma ray counter* scanning of thyroid gland is done to visualize gland.
      - *Hot* area suggests more uptake.
      - *Warm* area suggests normal uptake.
      - *Cold* area suggests no uptake.

I^{123} radioisotope can be safely used in children and pregnancy for only diagnostic purpose (5 microcurie) as the dose is low.

Indications for diagnostic radioactive iodine study
• Doubtful toxicity. • Ectopic thyroid. • Autonomous toxic nodule. • After total thyroidectomy, to look for secondaries in follicular carcinoma thyroid. • Retrosternal thyroid.

Radioisotope study is done to see the secondaries by doing whole body scanning (total body scintigraphy). For diagnostic

It takes 26 muscles to smile, and 62 muscles to frown

radioactive study Technetium 99 pertechnetate can also be used but it is not as good as I^{123}.

Therapeutic Uses

- In primary thyrotoxicosis after 10 years.
- In autonomous toxic nodule after 10 years, it is useful as remaining gland still will function adequately after radiotherapy (as during radiotherapy radioisotope will not be taken up by this retained normal gland as it is suppressed in the presence of toxic nodule which will function later adequately).
- In follicular carcinoma of thyroid, after total thyroidectomy, if there are secondaries elsewhere in the body, as in bone or lungs, then radioiodine therapy is given. I^{131} is given as its half life is 8 days. Patient should be isolated for this period. It is given orally in a dose of 5 milli curies (160 microcurie/g of thyroid).

	Half life
I^{123}	— 13 hours.
I^{131}	— 8 hours.
I^{132}	— 2.3 hours.
Tc 99 scan	— 6 hours.

THYROID NEOPLASM

A. **Benign**
   - Follicular adenoma.
   - Hurthle cell adenoma.
   - Colloid adenoma.
   - Papillary adenoma.
B. **Malignant** (Dunhill classification):
   a. ***Differentiated***
      - Papillary carcinoma (60%).
      - Follicular carcinoma (15%).
      - Papillofollicular carcinoma behaves like papillary carcinoma of thyroid.
      - Hurthle cell carcinoma behaves like follicular carcinoma.
   b. ***Undifferentiated***
      Anaplastic carcinoma (13%).

   c. ***Medullary carcinoma*** (6%).
   d. ***Malignant lymphoma*** (4%).
   e. ***Secondaries*** in thyroid (rare).

DIFFERENTIATED THYROID CARCINOMA

- Differentiated thyroid carcinoma (DTC) is a spectrum of disease derived from follicular cells. Both papillary and follicular carcinomas are grouped under this. 90% of thyroid malignancies are differentiated one. Papillary, follicular and Hurthle cell carcinomas are DTCs.
- AGES (Mayo clinic, Hay); AMES (Lahey clinic); MACIS; *Sloan Kettering* scoring— are different scoring systems used for DTCs. Sloan Kettering scoring includes low, intermediate and high-risk groups. First three scoring systems have low and high-risk groups.
- Papillary spreads through nodes; follicular through blood. FCT causes pulsatile vascular secondaries.
- Incidence of thyrotoxicosis in DTCs is 2%.
- Galectin-3, RET/PTC rearrangements, CD44 are the probable tumor markers under evaluation.
- **TNM staging for DTCs (AJCC, 2018) are**: T-Tumor: Tx – Primary cannot be assessed; T0 – No evidence of primary tumor; T1–<2 cm (T1a <1 cm; T1b 1–2 cm); T2–2–4 cm; T3a–>4 cm limited to thyroid; T3b – Gross extrathyroidal extension invading strap muscles only from a tumor of any sized; T4a – Gross extrathyroidal extension invading into subcutaneous tissue, larynx, trachea, esophagus and recurrent laryngeal nerve; T4b – Gross extrathyroidal invasion to prevertebral fascia, carotid encasement or involvement of mediastinal vessels. Suffix 's' is added for solitary nodule; 'm' added to multiple nodules. **N-Regional nodes** (central/lateral neck compartment/ superior mediastinal): Nx – regional nodes cannot be assessed. N0 – no nodes;

Success usually comes to those who are too busy to be looking for it—**Henry David Thoreau**

N0a – One or more cytologically or histologically confirmed benign nodes; N0b – No radiological or clinical evidence of locoregional nodes. N1a – Spread to level VI (pre/paratracheal, prelaryngeal) and level VII (mediastinal) nodes, unilateral or bilateral. N1b – Nodal spread unilateral or bilateral or contralateral lateral lymph nodes of level I, II, III, IV, V or retropharyngeal nodes. Suffix 'san' is sentinel node; 'f' is FnAC or core biopsy.
M - Metastases: cM0 – No distant spread. cM1 – Distant spread present. pM1 – Distant spread microscopically confirmed.
Note: Age is included in staging which is an important factor. Age at diagnosis: <55 years OR >55 years.

- Total/near total thyroidectomy, central compartment dissection ± MRND, suppressive L-thyroxine radioactive iodine therapies are different modalities of treatment.
- They usually carry good prognosis.
- Tall/columnar cell, trabecular, scirrhous, solid types of papillary carcinoma; oxyphilic, insular types of FCT carry poor prognosis (Fig. 18.14).

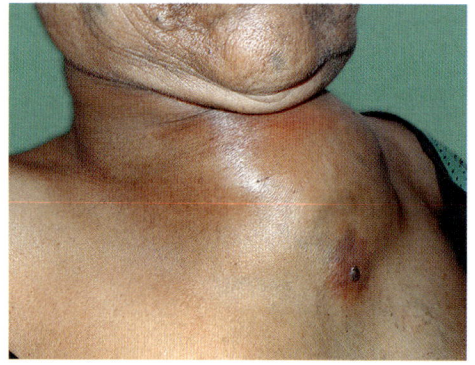

Fig. 18.14: Carcinoma thyroid—advanced stage.

Etiology of Thyroid Malignancy

- Radiation either external or radioiodine can cause papillary carcinoma thyroid. There is increased incidence of thyroid carcinoma among children following exposure to ionizing radiation after the Chernobyl nuclear disaster in Ukraine in 1986. Earlier radiotherapy was the treatment for acne, tonsillar diseases, adenoids, thymus enlargement or hemangiomas which in turn predisposed papillary carcinoma of thyroid.
- Pre-existing multinodular goiter. It turns into follicular carcinoma of thyroid.
- Medullary carcinoma thyroid is often familial.

PAPILLARY CARCINOMA

- It is 60% common.
- Common in females and young age group.
- TSH levels in the blood of these patients are high and so it is called as *hormone dependent tumor*.
- It is a slowly progressive and less aggressive tumor.
- It is commonly multicentric.
- It spreads within the gland through intrathyroidal lymphatics to other lobe, comes out of the capsule and spreads to lymph nodes.
- Usually there is no blood spread.

Types

1. Occult (<1.5 cm).
2. Intrathyroidal.
3. Extrathyroidal.

Gross

It can be soft, firm, hard, cystic. It can be solitary or multinodular. It contains *brownish black fluid*.

Microscopy

It shows cystic spaces, papillary projections with *psammoma* bodies, malignant cells with 'Orphan Annie eye' nuclei (intranuclear cytoplasmic inclusions).

I never see what has been done; I only see what remains to be done—**Buddha**

Clinical Features

- Soft or hard or firm, solid or cystic, solitary or multinodular thyroid swelling.
- Compression features are uncommon in papillary carcinoma thyroid.
- Often discrete lymph nodes in the neck are palpable.

Diagnosis

- Fine needle aspiration cytology.
- Radioisotope scan shows cold nodule.
- TSH level in the blood is higher.

Treatment

- Near total, or total thyroidectomy.
- *Suppressive dose* of L-thyroxine 0.3 mg OD life long.
- *Block dissection (functional block)* is required if lymph nodes are involved.
- *Radioactive iodine therapy* (I^{131}) is indicated if tumor is more than 4 cm; if there is extrathyroid spread or lymph node involvement or multicentric.
- Occasionally if small lymph nodes are present, 'Berry picking' may be done (not accepted now).

Prognosis

Prognosis is good and it is one of the curable malignancies.

AMES scoring
A: Age. Age less than 40 years has got better prognosis.
M: Distant metastasis.
E: Extent of the primary tumor.
S: Size of the tumor. Size less than 4 cm has got better prognosis.
AGES scoring
A: Age less than 4 cm has got better prognosis.
G: Pathologic grade of the tumor.
E: Extent of the primary tumor.
S: Size of the primary tumor. Size less than 4 cm has got better prognosis.

Psammoma bodies are seen in
- Papillary carcinoma thyroid.
- Meningioma.
- Serous cystadenoma of ovary.

Berry's in thyroid
- Berry ligament.
- Berry sign.
- Berry picking.

FOLLICULAR CARCINOMA (FIG. 18.15)

- It is 15% common.
- It is common in females.
- It can occur either de novo or in a pre-existing multinodular goiter.
- It is a more aggressive tumor.
- It spreads mainly through blood into the lung, bones, and liver.
- Bone secondaries are typically vascular, warm, pulsatile, localized, commonly in skull, long bones, ribs (Figs. 18. 16A and B).
- It can also spread to lymph nodes in the neck occasionally.

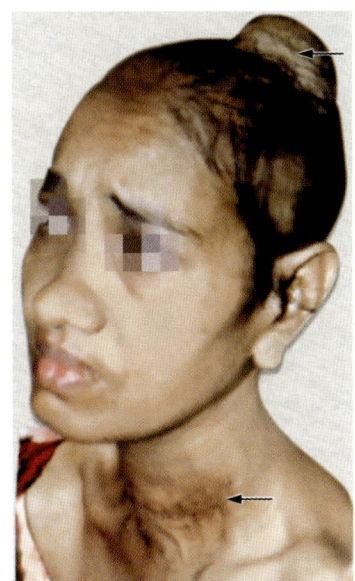

Fig. 18.15: Follicular carcinoma thyroid with skull secondaries.

---

*If you really look closely, most overnight successes took a long time—***Steve Jobs**

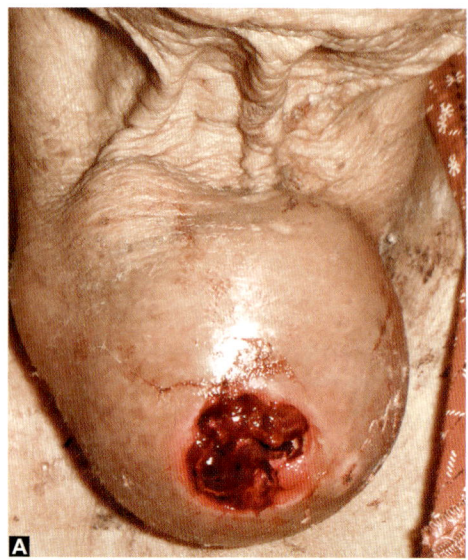

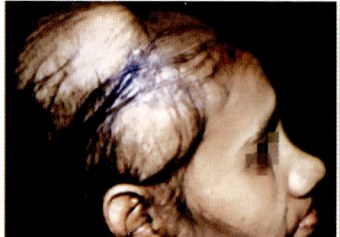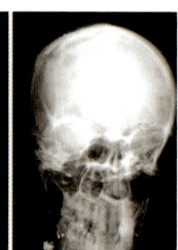

Fig. 18.17: X-ray skull showing secondaries from follicular carcinoma thyroid.

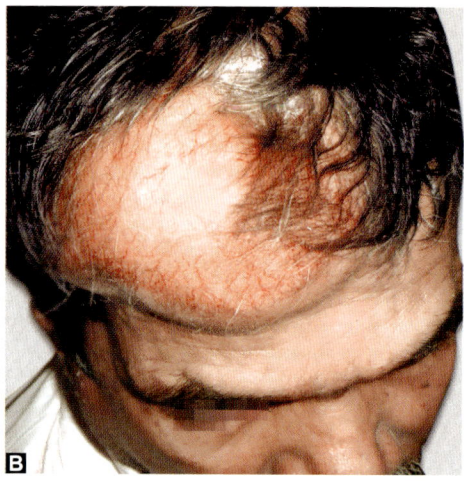

Figs. 18.16A and B: (A) Fungating follicular carcinoma thyroid in a female; (B) Pulsatile vascular skull secondaries from FCT in a male patient.

Clinical Features

- Swelling in the neck, firm or hard and nodular.
- Tracheal compression and stridor.
- Dyspnea, hemoptysis, chest pain when there are lung secondaries.
- Recurrent laryngeal nerve involvement causing hoarseness of voice, +ve 'Berry's sign' signifies advanced malignancy (infiltration into the carotid and so absence of carotid pulsation).
- Pulsatile secondaries in the skull, and long bones (Fig. 18.17).

Investigations

- Most often FNAC is inconclusive, because capsular and angioinvasion which is the main feature in follicular carcinoma cannot be detected by FNAC.
- Frozen section biopsy is very useful.
- Ultrasound abdomen, chest X-ray, X-ray bones are the other investigations required.

Treatment

Total thyroidectomy is done, along with block dissection (MRND) whenever lymph nodes are enlarged.

Maintenance dose of L-thyroxine 0.1 mg OD is given life long.

Follow-up

- It is by radioisotope I^{123} scan done at regular intervals (6 months) to look for secondaries.
- **Thyroglobulin estimation** is a good follow-up method to decide for radioisotope study.

Further Treatment

- If secondaries are detected therapeutic dose Ra I^{131} is given. L-thyroxine has to

The most important thing that you wear is the expression on your face

be stopped 7 days prior to RT, and then required dose of Ra I^{131} is given.
* Secondaries in bone are treated by *external radiotherapy*. Internal fixation should be done whenever there is pathological fracture.

Note:
* **Hurthle cell carcinoma** is a variant of follicular carcinoma of thyroid which contains abundant oxyphill cells. It spreads more commonly to regional lymph nodes than follicular carcinoma of thyroid. It carries *poor* prognosis.
* There is *no role* of chemotherapy for follicular carcinoma thyroid.

ANAPLASTIC CARCINOMA (FIG. 18.18)

* It is a very aggressive tumor of short duration, presents with a swelling in thyroid region which is rapidly progressive causing:
    - Stridor and hoarseness of voice.
    - Dysphagia.
    - Fixity to the skin.
* Swelling is hard, with involvement of isthmus and bilateral lateral lobes.
* FNAC is diagnostic.
* Tracheostomy and isthmectomy has got a role to relieve respiratory obstruction temporarily.
* Treatment is *external radiotherapy*.
* However prognosis is poor.

MEDULLARY CARCINOMA OF THYROID

* It is uncommon (5%) type of thyroid malignancy.
* It is arises from the *parafollicular 'C' cells* which is derived from the ultimobronchial body (Fig. 18.19).
* It contains characteristic *'amyloid stroma'* wherein malignant cells are dispersed.
* In these patients blood levels of *calcitonin* both basal as well as that following calcium or pentagastrin stimulation is high, a very useful tumor marker.
* Tumor also secretes 5-HT (serotonin), prostaglandin and vasoactive intestinal polypeptide (VIP).
* It spreads mainly to lymph nodes.
* It may be associated with MEN II syndrome and pheochromocytoma with hypertension.
* There may be mucosal neuromas in lips, oral cavity.

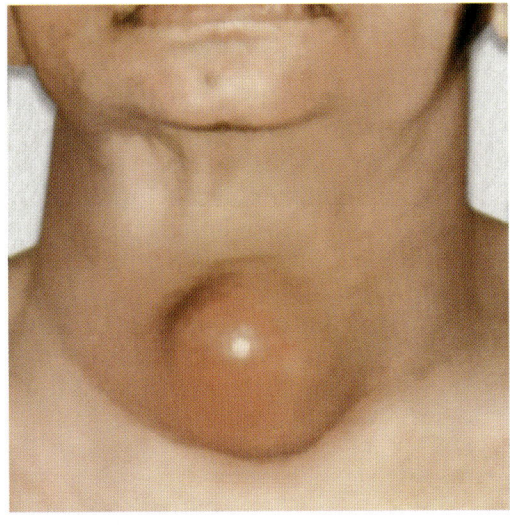

Fig. 18.18: Anaplastic carcinoma of thyroid.

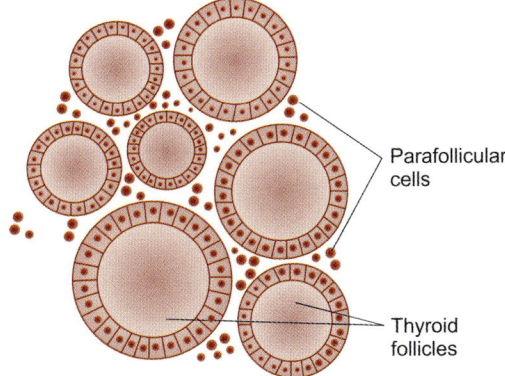

Fig. 18.19: Note the parafollicular cells. Cell of origin of medullary carcinoma thyroid.

*The secret of success is to do the common thing uncommonly well—**John D Rockefeller Jr***

Features

- Thyroid swelling often with enlargement of neck lymph node.
- Diarrhea, flushing.
- Hypertension, pheochromocytomas and mucosal neuromas when associated with MEN II syndrome.
- Sporadic and familial types occur in adulthood whereas conditions associated with MEN syndrome II occur in younger age groups.
- **Types**
  - Sporadic.
  - Medullary carcinoma of thyroid (MCT) with MEN II syndrome.
  - Familial MCT.
- **Investigations**
  - FNAC: It shows amyloid deposition with dispersed malignant cells and 'C' cell hyperplasia.
  - Tumor marker: Calcitonin level will be higher.
  - Ultrasound neck—thyroid region.

Treatment

- *Total thyroidectomy* + central node dissection + maintenance dose of L-thyroxine.
- Neck lymph node block dissection whenever lymph nodes are involved.
- Adriamycin is drug used for chemotherapy.
- No role of suppressive hormone therapy or radioactive iodine therapy.

All family members of the patient should be evaluated for serum calcitonin and if it is high they should undergo prophylactic total thyroidectomy (Can also be assessed by genetic evaluation).

Prognosis

- Sporadic MCT and MCT with MEN II are aggressive.
- Familial MCT not associated with MEN II has got better prognosis.

MALIGNANT LYMPHOMA

- It is non-Hodgking lymphoms (NHL) type. Occurs in a pre-existing Hashimoto's thyroiditis (not proved well).
- FNAC is useful to diagnose the condition.
- Chemotherapy is the main treatment.
- Often total thyroidectomy is done to enhance the results.

HASHIMOTO'S THYROIDITIS

- Also called as diffuse nongoitrous thyroiditis.
- It is an autoimmune thyroiditis, common in women.
- There is hyperplasia initially, then fibrosis, eventually infiltration with plasma cells and lymphocytic cells.

Features

- Painful, diffuse, enlargement of usually both lobes of thyroid which is firm, tender and smooth (occasionally one lobe is involved).
- Initially they present with toxic features but later, they manifest with features of hypothyroidism.
  - Hyperplasia   Hyperthyroid
  -                          Euthyroid
  - Fibrosis   Hypothyroid
- There may be hepatosplenomegaly.
- It is often associated with other autoimmune diseases.
- In 85% cases significant rise in the thyroid antibodies (microsomal, thyroglobulin, or colloid antibodies) is observed.
- It can predispose to *papillary carcinoma* of thyroid.
- Often condition may be associated with or may predispose to *malignant lymphoma* also. It is at present not well-proved.

Investigations

- FNAC, T_3, T_4, TSH. Thyroid antibodies assay.

There are no secrets to success. It is the result of preparation, hard work, and learning from failure—**Colin Powell**

- Usually ESR is very high (over 90 mm/hour).

Treatment

- L-thyroxine therapy.
- Steroid therapy often is helpful.
- If goiter is large and causing discomfort, then subtotal thyroidectomy is done.

DE QUERVAIN'S SUBACUTE GRANULOMATOUS THYROIDITIS

It is due to viral etiology either mumps or coxsackie viruses causing inflammatory response with infiltration of lymphocytes, neutrophils, multinucleated giant cells.

Clinical Features

- Presents with diffuse pain, swelling in thyroid which is tender.
- Commonly seen in females.
- Initially there will be transient hyperthyroidism with high T_3 and T_4 but poor radioiodine uptake.
- It is usually a self-limiting disease.

REIDEL'S THYROIDITIS (0.5% common)

- A very rare benign entity wherein thyroid tissue is replaced by fibrous tissue which interestingly infiltrates the capsule into muscles, paratracheal tissues, carotid sheath.
- It is often associated with retroperitoneal and mediastinal fibrosis ('Woody thyroiditis,' 'Ligneus thyroiditis').

Features

- Hard, fixed, swelling with stridor, often Berry's sign may be positive, i.e. absence of carotid pulsation.
- **Differential diagnosis:** Anaplastic carcinoma of thyroid.

- **Investigations:**
  - T_3, T_4 may be low due to hypothyroidism.
  - Radioisotope scan will not show any uptake.
  - FNAC to rule out carcinoma.
- **Treatment:**
  - Isthmectomy is done to relieve compression on the airway.
  - They require L-thyroxine replacement later, as hypothyroidism is common.

THYROIDECTOMY

Types

1. *Hemithyroidectomy*: Along with removal of one lobe, entire isthmus is removed. It is done in benign diseases of only one lobe.
2. *Subtotal thyroidectomy* commonly done in toxic thyroid either primary or secondary and also often for nontoxic multinodular goiter. Here about 8 grams, or a tissue size of pulp of finger is retained on lower pole, on both sides and rest of the thyroid gland is removed.
3. *Partial thyroidectomy* is removal of the gland in front of trachea after mobilization. It is commonly done in nontoxic multinodular goiter.
4. *Near total thyroidectomy*: Here both lobes except the lower pole which is very close to recurrent laryngeal nerve and parathyroid is removed. It is done in case of papillary carcinoma of thyroid.
5. *Total thyroidectomy*: Entire gland is removed. It is done in case of follicular carcinoma of thyroid, and medullary carcinoma of thyroid.

Procedure

Position:
Under general anesthesia patient is put in supine position with neck extended by placing a sand bag under shoulder—with table tilt of 15° head up to reduce venous congestion.

Love means making the other happy, even from a distance

Incision:
Horizontal crease incision is done, two finger breadth above the sternal notch, from one sternomastoid to the other (Fig. 18.20).

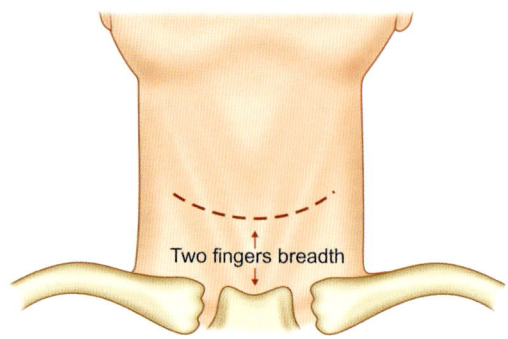

Fig. 18.20: Note the incision for thyroid surgery.

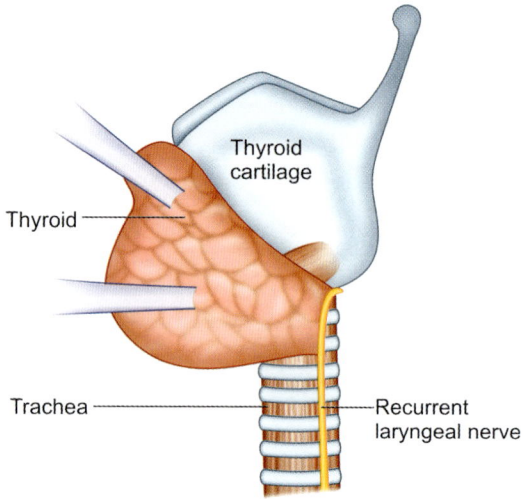

Fig. 18.21: Note the relation of recurrent laryngeal nerve.

Procedure:
Skin and platysma are incised—upper flap raised up to thyroid cartilage, lower flap up to sternoclavicular joint. Deep fascia is opened vertically in the midline. Strap muscles are retracted or cut in between two Kocher's forceps. Pretracheal fascia is opened to mobilize the thyroid. First, short stout middle thyroid vein is ligated, then superior thyroid pedicle is ligated close to the gland so as to avoid injury to external laryngeal nerve. Inferior thyroid artery is ligated away from the gland so as to avoid injury to recurrent laryngeal nerve (Fig. 18.21). Mobilized gland is removed. Bed is sutured with catgut so as to prevent bleeding. Drain is placed. The wound is close in layers (Fig. 18.22).

Thyroid steal:
Patient is taken to operation theater for few days before doing surgery so as to reduce the anxiety of the patient.

Complications of Thyroidectomy

Hemorrhage:
It may be due to slipping of ligatures either superior thyroid artery or other pedicles. It will cause tachycardia, hypotension, breathlessness, and compression over the

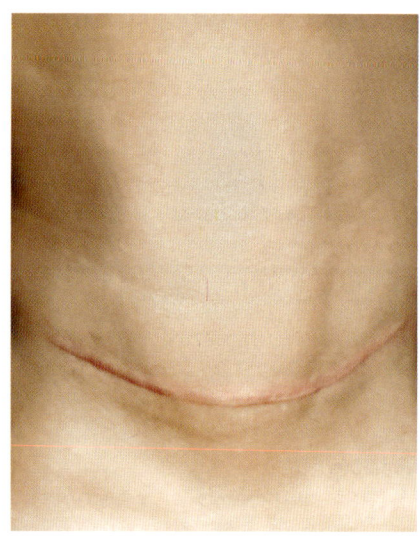

Fig. 18.22: Typical thyroidectomy—postoperative scar.

trachea may cause severe stridor, respiratory obstruction. As a first aid, immediate release of sutures including that of deep fascia has to be done and pressure over the trachea is released. Then patient is shifted to operation theater, and under general anesthesia exploration is done

The only limit to our realization of tomorrow will be our doubts of today—**Franklin D Roosevelt**

and bleeders are ligated. Blood transfusion may be required.

Respiratory obstruction:
It may be due to hematoma (if it is so, the hematoma has to be evacuated), or due to laryngeal edema. For laryngeal edema, *immediate emergency endotracheal intubation* is done along with steroid injections. Often emergency tracheostomy may be required as a life-saving procedure.

Recurrent laryngeal nerve palsy:
It can be transient or permanent. Transient is 3% common. They usually recover in 3 weeks to 3 months. Often they require steroid supplement and speech therapy. Permanent paralysis is rare.

Hypoparathyroidism:
It is rare, 0.5% incidence. Mostly it is temporary due to vascular spasm of parathyroid glands, occurs in 2-5th postoperative day. Present with weakness, +ve Chvostek's sign, carpopedal spasm, convulsions. Serum calcium estimation has to done and then 10 mL of 10% calcium gluconate is given IV eighth hourly, and later supplemented by oral calcium 500 mg 8th hourly. After 3-6 weeks, patient is admitted, drug is stopped and serum calcium level is repeated (Fig. 18.23).

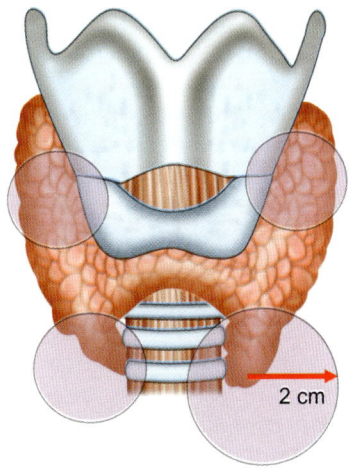

Fig. 18.23: Note the location of parathyroid glands.

Complications of thyroidectomy		
Metabolic	**Nerve injuries**	**Other complications**
Hypoparathyroidism	• External laryngeal nerve injury—pitch of the voice is lost	• Respiratory obstruction
• Temporary hypoparathyroidism	• Recurrent laryngeal nerve injury	• Skin flap necrosis—rare
• Temporary hypocalcemia without hypoparathyroidism (hungry bone syndrome)	**Vascular complications**	• Infection
• Permanent hypoparathyroidism	• Hemorrhage—primary and reactionary	• Discharge and sinus formation
• Spurious hypoparathyroidism (total calcium is less but ionized calcium is normal)	• Hematoma formation	• Wound granuloma
Thyroid crisis	• Compromised tracheoesophageal blood supply	• Keloid formation
Hypothyroidism/thyroid failure/myxedema		
Intraoperative	**Immediate postoperative**	**Late postoperative**
• Hemorrhage	• Hematoma	• Hypothyroidism
• Nerve injuries	• Laryngeal edema	• Recurrent nodule
	• Respiratory obstruction—strider	• Recurrent toxicity
	• Hypoparathyroidism	• Wound infection
	• Recurrent laryngeal nerve injury and its problems	• Granuloma/keloid

We do not remember days, we remember moments

Thyrotoxic crisis (Thyroid storm):
- Occurs in a thyrotoxic patient inadequately prepared for thyroidectomy and rarely a thyrotoxic patient presents in a crisis following an unrelated operation or stress. They present in 12-24 hours with severe dehydration due to circulatory collapse, hypotension, hyperpyrexia, and often cardiac failure.
- Treatment is injection hydrocortisone, oral antithyroid drugs, tepid sponging of whole body, beta blocker injection, oral iodides, large amount of IV fluids for rehydration, digitoxin, cardiac monitor, often ventilator support, and observation. It has got high mortality rate with critical period of 72 hours. Fluid and electrolyte management, cardiac management are important aspects to be monitored and treated.

Injury to external laryngeal nerve:
It causes weakness of cricothyroid muscle leading to alteration in pitch of voice.

Hypothyroidism:
Revealed clinically after 6 months.

Others:
- Wound infection, stitch granuloma formation.
- Keloid formation.

EMIL THEODOR KOCHER

He was the *first surgeon to get Nobel Prize.*
He did extensive work on thyroid surgeries and designed present technique of thyroid surgeries. He was from Switzerland.
He was the founder of:
- Kocher's vein.
- Kocher's forceps (has got tooth in the tip).
- Kocherization (duodenal mobilization).
- Kocher's incision (right subcostal for cholecystectomy).
- Kocher's thyroid incision.
- Kocher's test.
- Kocher's method for reduction of shoulder dislocation.
   He died in 1917.

Note

Other surgeons who got nobel prizes are Alexis Carrell (for his work on vascular anastomosis), Christiaan Barnard (for heart transplantation), Charles Huggins (Urologist, for management of carcinoma prostate).

HYPOTHYROIDISM

Causes

- Agenesis or dysgenesis.
- Enzyme deficiency.
- Iodine deficiency.
- Hashimoto's thyroiditis.
- Antithyroid drugs.
- Radioiodine.
- Drugs: Lithium, amiodarone.
- After thyroidectomy.

Features (Fig. 18.24)

- *General*: Tiredness, weight gain, cold intolerance, goiter, hyperlipidemia.
- *Cardiovascular*: Bradycardia, angina, cardiac failure, pericardial effusion.
- *Hematological*: Anemia.

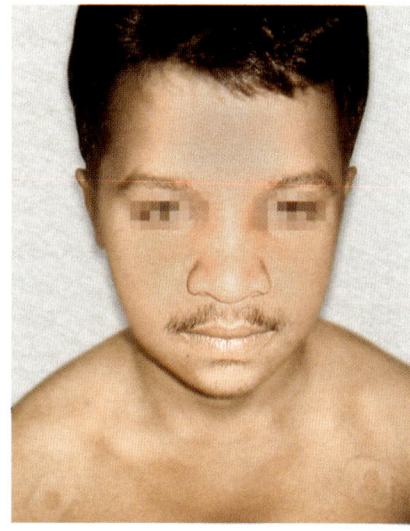

Fig. 18.24: Typical myxedema patient.

Smile, it is the key that fits the lock of everybody's heart—**Anthony J D'Angelo**

- *Dermatological*: Dry skin, vitiligo, alopecia, erythema.
- *Reproductive*: Infertility, menorrhagia, galactorrhea, etc.
- *Gastrointestinal*: Constipation, ileus.
- *Developmental*: Growth and mental retardation, delayed puberty.
- *Other features*: Carpal tunnel syndrome, myalgia, hoarseness, deafness, ataxia, depression, psychosis (myxedema madness).
- **Investigations**
  - T_3, T_4 estimation.
  - TSH level estimation which is higher.

Treatment

- Replacement with L-thyroxine 100 to 150 ug/day.
- In old patients with ischemic heart disease initial therapy is with 25–50 μg/day and then gradually increased up to the required dose.

CRETINISM

- It is fetal/infantile hypothyroidism due to inadequate thyroid hormone production during fetal and neonatal period. It may be due to agenesis, inborn error of thyroid metabolism, dyshormonogenesis or dietary deficiency (endemic).
- Typical hoarse cry, macroglossia, umbilical hernia, thickened skin are the features.
- TSH will be raised; T_3 and T_4 will be low.
- Incidence is 1:4000 live births.
- It is treated with L-thyroxine once a day morning orally.

Narrowing of trachea is seen in:
• Scabbard trachea in long-standing multinodular goiter.
• Retrosternal goiter.
• Carcinoma of thyroid.
• Riedel's thyroiditis.

One joy scatters a hundred grieves

CHAPTER 19

Parathyroid and Adrenal Glands

Chapter Outline

- Anatomy of Parathyroid
- Hyperparathyroidism
- Tetany
- MEN Syndrome (MEA Syndrome)
- Adrenal Glands

ANATOMY OF PARATHYROID

Parathyroids are endocrine glands situated behind the thyroid gland. They are four in number, two on each side (Fig. 19.1).

- Two upper glands are constant in position. Superior is behind recurrent laryngeal nerve. They develop from 4th pharyngeal pouch, hence called as *parathyroid IV*.
- Two lower glands are variable in position. They develop from endoderm of 3rd pharyngeal pouch hence called as *parathyroid III*. It is usually in front of the lower part of recurrent laryngeal nerve.
- Each gland weighs 50 mg. It is brownish (khaki colored) firm gland, which sinks in the fluid unlike fat, which floats. It is usually adjacent to the anastomosis between superior and inferior thyroid arteries posteriorly.
- **Inferior thyroid artery** supplies *both* superior and inferior parathyroid glands. So ligation of this artery prior to branching into parathyroid gland may cause hypoparathyroidism with hypocalcemia.
- Glands (chief cells) secrete parathormone (PTH), which controls the calcium metabolism.

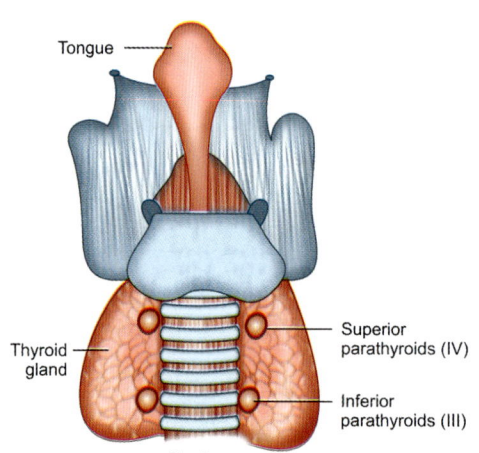

Fig. 19.1: Anatomical location of parathyroids.

Parathyroid hormone
• Increases absorption of the calcium from the gut.
• Mobilizes calcium from the bone.
• Increases the calcium reabsorption from the renal tubules.

Those who can't hear the music think the dancer's mad

> **DiGeorge's syndrome**
> - Absence of parathyroids.
> - Thymic aplasia with immunodeficiency.
> - Cardiac defects.

HYPERPARATHYROIDISM

Types
- Primary
- Secondary
- Tertiary.

Primary is unstimulated inappropriate high PTH secretion due to hyperplasia or adenoma.

Secondary is due to chronic renal failure or due to malabsorption, i.e. due to chronic hypocalcemia.

Tertiary is due to autonomous hyperplasia.

> - Adenoma: 75–90%.
> - Hyperplasia: 20–24%.
> - Carcinoma (rare): 1%.

Carcinoma of parathyroid is one of the most aggressive tumor known, but fortunately rare. May present as a nodule and can have blood born metastasis.

Clinical Features

Clinical vignette of hyperparathyroidism—**"bones, stones, abdominal groans and psychic moans."**
- Hyperparathyroidism is common in middle-aged women.
- Presentation may be *asymptomatic hypercalcemia (commonest—50%)*
- *Nonspecific symptoms and psychiatric symptoms with* behavioral problems (they are most often named as neurotics).
- The bone presents with *osteitis fibrosa cystica* **(von Recklinghausen disease)**, which shows single or multiple cysts or *pseudotumor* in the jaw, skull or middle phalanges.
- The first bony change is seen in lamina dura of tooth.
- In the kidney, there may be bilateral multiple *renal stones (25%) or nephrocalcinosis* (may go for renal failure).
- It may be associated with the *peptic ulcer, pancreatitis, MEN I syndrome*.
- They are more prone for skin necrosis, band keratopathy, pseudogout, myalgia, arthralgia, polyuria, glycosuria, and hypertension.

> **Acute hyperparathyroidism (Crisis)**
>
> It is rare but dangerous presentation (crisis) wherein patient presents with severe, acute abdominal pain, vomiting, dehydration, oliguria and death. Serum calcium is very high.
> **Treatment**
> - Rehydration.
> - Steroids.
> - Clodronate sodium.
> - Drugs to reduce calcium level, i.e. *Mithramycin, Calcitonin, Prednisolone, Biphosphonates*. Biphosphonates like Disodium Pamidronate 60 mg is given slow intravenously as single dose, which prevents mobilization of calcium from the bone and so controls hypercalcemia.
> - Condition has got high mortality rate.

Investigations

> **For confirmation of the hyperparathyroidism**
> - Serum calcium, albumin, phosphorus, PTH, alkaline phosphatase.
> - X-ray skull, jaw, phalanges.
>
> **For localization of the parathyroid glands**
> - US neck, CT neck and mediastinum.
> - Thallium Technetium scan.
> - Thallium 99m labeled Sestamibi scan.
>
> **To look for associated problems**
> - US abdomen.
> - Slit-lamp examination of eye.
> - To find out association of MEN syndrome.

- High serum calcium—>10 mg/100 mL.
- Decreased serum phosphorus.
- Increased urinary calcium—>250 mg/24 hours.

For every minute you are angry you lose sixty seconds of happiness

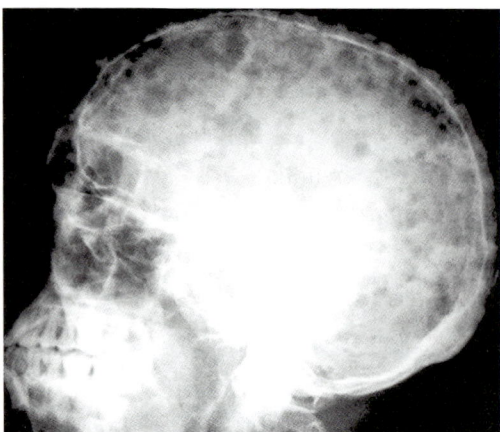

Fig. 19.2: Plain X-ray skull. Note the characteristic salt-pepper appearance of the skull bones.

- Increased serum alkaline phosphatase.
- Increased PTH level in the serum is diagnostic — >0.5 pg/L.
- X-ray skull shows *salt-pepper appearance* (Fig. 19.2).
- X-rays phalanges and jaw are specific.
- Ultrasound abdomen to find out problems in kidney, pancreas.
- Ultrasound neck and CT scan neck and mediastinum.
- Selective venous sampling for PTH is also very useful.
- Thallium–Technetium scan shows *hot spots*, which is diagnostic of parathyroid adenoma.
- *Technetium-99m labeled Sestamibi isotope* scan is better and sensitive (80%) than Thallium-Tc scan. As it is very expensive, it is used in parathyroid re-exploration. It is often combined with single photon emission computerized tomography (SPECT).
- Urinary cAMP level increases in 90% cases.

Note: Serum albumin should also be assessed to get accurate calcium level.

Corrected serum Ca in mmol/L = Measured serum Ca + (40 – Albumin) × 0.02.

Differential diagnosis for hyperparathyroidism

- Secondaries in the bone.
- Multiple myeloma.
- Vitamin D intoxication.
- Sarcoidosis.
- Functioning carcinoma.

Treatment

Surgical:

Indications for parathyroidectomy

- Severe symptoms.
- Young age group.
- Markedly reduced bone density.
- Serum calcium more than 11 mg%.
- Urinary calculi.
- Neuromuscular presentations.
- Urinary calcium more than 400 mg/24 hours.

- Surgical removal of the glands and implantation of fragments of the gland in forearm muscle mass (brachioradialis or sternomastoid) or neck.
- If it is carcinoma, additional hemithyroidectomy with postoperative radiotherapy is required.

Medical:

- Medical treatment of primary hyperparathyroidism is usually ineffective and not popular. However, it is being advocated occasionally as initial therapy and in acute crisis.
- Estrogens, Progestogens, Raloxifene (estrogen receptor modulator), Mithramycin, Calcitonin are the few drugs used. Mithramycin is used once a week but it is hepatotoxic and causes thrombocytopenia.

I have learned silence from the talkative, toleration from the intolerant and kindness from the unkind; yet strange, I am ungrateful to these teachers—**Kalil Gibran**

Surgical aspects in parathyroidectomy

- Single adenoma—excision
- Carcinoma—removal of entire four glands with thyroidectomy.
- Hyperplasia—all four glands are removed with autotransplantation of 1/3rd of one gland over sternomastoid muscle in the neck or over brachioradialis muscle in the forearm.
- Postoperative follow up by doing regular estimations of serum calcium and parathormone.
- Parathyroidectomy is technically difficult. Parathyroid glands are dark-brown in color, which should be confirmed by frozen section biopsy. It should be differentiated from fat and lymph nodes. Fat is yellow in color and floats in water. Lymph node is light brown or pale in color.
- Parathyroid *sinks* in water.

Problems in parathyroidectomy

- Permanent hypoparathyroidism.
- Recurrent hyperparathyroidism-hypercalcemia 12 months after parathyroidectomy.
- Recurrent laryngeal nerve injury.
- Often needs additional thyroidectomy.
- Variations in positions of the gland especially lower, may be in mediastinum.
- Sudden drop in calcium level after surgery due to increased absorption of calcium by bones—*hungry bone syndrome*. There is sudden drop in serum calcium level with features of severe tetany. It should be treated initially by continuous slow intravenous calcium infusion usually for 2–4 days later with oral calcium supplements.

TETANY

It is a condition due to decreased level of calcium in blood causing its effects.

Causes

- After thyroidectomy (it is decreased level of parathormone in the blood causing hypocalcemia). It is usually temporary lasting for 4–6 weeks. It is the commonest cause of hypoparathyroidism. Other causes of hypoparathyroidism are neck dissection, hemochromatosis, Wilson's disease and DiGeorge's syndrome.
- Severe vomiting, hyperventilation associated with respiratory alkalosis.
- Metabolic alkalosis like in pyloric stenosis.
- Rickets, osteomalacia.
- Chronic renal failure.
- Acute pancreatitis.

Decreased PTH causes decrease in calcium level in the blood leading to:

- *Circumoral paresthesia*, paresthesia of neck, fingers and toes.
- Twitching and weakness of tongue muscles, muscles of forearm, hand, foot and digits—*carpopedal spasm.*
- *Chvostek's sign:* Tapping above the angle of the jaw to stimulate branches of facial nerve causes the twitching of the angle of mouth and eyelids.
- Applying the sphygmomanometer to the arm and inflating the pressure more than systolic pressure of the patient for three minutes can demonstrate carpal spasm *(Trousseau's sign).*
- *Stridor* and difficulty in breathing due to paralysis of respiratory muscles.
- Generalized weakness and twitching all over the body in severe cases mimicking *convulsions.*

Management

- Serum calcium estimation is done. It should be less than 7 mg%.
- IV calcium gluconate 10%, 10 mL sixth to eighth hourly is given slowly over 10 minutes.
- Later oral calcium with vitamin D supplementation.
- Follow up at regular intervals by doing serum calcium level.

MEN SYNDROME (MEA SYNDROME)

- Commonly inherited as *autosomal dominant.*
- Cells involved have got common features of *APUD cells (apudomas)* (Amine Precursor Uptake and Decarboxylation).

Everytime something good happens to you, make something good happen to someone else

Types

- **Type I**: Parathyroid hyperplasia or adenomas; pituitary tumor; pancreatic tumor (Endocrine—insulinoma, gastrinoma, glucagonoma, vipoma). It is also called as *Wermer's syndrome*.
- **Type II**: It is also called as *Sipple's disease*:
  - II A includes medullary carcinoma of thyroid + pheochromocytoma + parathyroid hyperplasia (50%).
  - II B includes medullary carcinoma of thyroid + pheochromocytoma + mucosal neuromas in lips and eyelids with bumpy-lumpy lesions, with marfanoid face, megacolon.

ADRENAL GLANDS

SURGICAL ANATOMY OF ADRENAL GLANDS

The adrenal glands are named in relation to the kidneys. The term "adrenal" comes from Latin—*ad* means "near"; and *renes* means - "kidney". Suprarenal is derived from Latin—*supra* means "above" and *renes* means "kidney". Adrenal glands are essential endocrine glands (Figs. 19.3A and B).

Two suprarenal endocrine adrenal glands are located in the retroperitoneum along the upper pole and medial part of the kidneys in front of the crus of diaphragm opposite 12th rib and vertebral end of 11th intercostal space. Each adrenal gland is 5 × 3 × 1 cm in dimensions weighing 5 grams. Adrenal gland is within renal fascia but separated by a fascial septum from kidney. Right gland is *triangular* in shape (top hat); left one is *semilunar* (cocked hat). Gland is yellow or mahogany (reddish-brown) or *golden orange* in color. Right adrenal is relatively higher than left adrenal (right kidney is at lower level than left kidney). Between two adrenal gland structures present are—crura, the aorta and celiac arteries, celiac plexus and inferior vena cava. Kidney may be ectopic or ptotic but adrenal will be in the original position. But fusion of kidney like horse shoe kidney may have fusion of adrenal glands also.

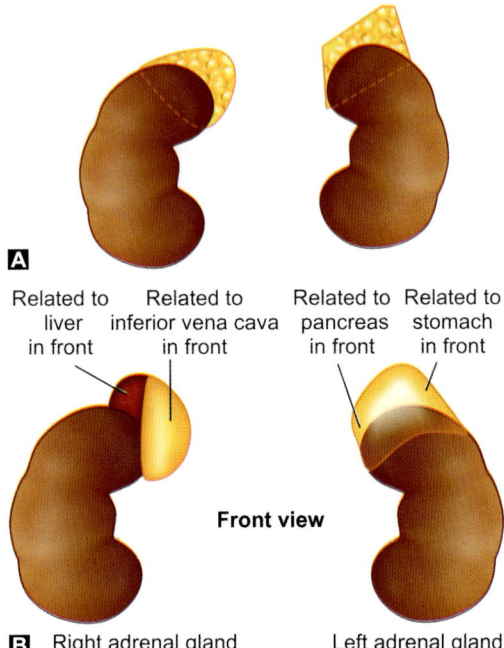

Figs. 19.3A and B: Anatomy of adrenal glands. (A) Adrenal anatomy posterior view; (B) Adrenal anatomy anterior view.

Right Adrenal Gland

It has got a base, an apex, anterior and posterior surfaces, anterior, medial and lateral borders. Anterior surface is related to inferior vena cava (IVC) medially, bare area of the liver laterally and duodenum below. It is devoid of peritoneum. Posterior surface is related to right crus of diaphragm above and right kidney below. Hilum of right adrenal is near upper end. Apex is related to bare area; base is related to upper pole of right kidney. Three arteries supplying the right adrenal gland course behind the IVC. Right adrenal vein arises near upper part of the hilum.

Life itself is the most wonderful fairy tale—**Hans Christian Andersen**

Left Adrenal Gland

It has got narrow upper end and round lower end. Upper end is related to posterior end of spleen; hilum of left adrenal gland is near lower end through which left adrenal vein exits. Anterior surface is related to cardiac end of stomach, splenic artery and pancreas. Gastric related part only is covered with peritoneum/omental bursa. Posterior surface is related to left kidney laterally, left crus of diaphragm medially. Medial convex border is related to left celiac ganglion, left inferior phrenic artery, left gastric artery. Lateral concave border is related to the stomach.

Arterial Supply

Adrenal gland is one of the most vascular organ (gram of tissue) like thyroid (so metastases are common). It is supplied by superior adrenal artery, a branch of inferior phrenic artery; middle adrenal artery, a branch of aorta; and inferior adrenal artery, a branch of renal artery.

Venous Drainage

Venous drainage is not accompanied by adrenal arteries. Adrenal gland is drained by one single vein which begins at the adrenal hilum. *Right adrenal vein* is short (<1 cm) and stout drains from the anteromedial part of the gland from upper part of its hilum into inferior vena cava on its posterolateral aspect directed above downward obliquely. *Left adrenal vein* is long and is directed downward perpendicular to the renal vein and medially to drain into left renal vein after crossing the left renal artery in front. It is on the anterior surface of the gland. Tearing or avulsion of adrenal vein from IVC or left renal vein can occur during dissection causing torrential hemorrhage.

Lymphatics

Adrenal gland is drained into lumbar and lateral aortic nodes. Lymphatic plexus are present under the capsule and in medulla. Subcapsular plexus drains with the arteries; medullary plexus drains with the veins. Right adrenal drains into paraaortic nodes, right renal nodes and nodes at right crus of diaphragm. Left drains into nodes adjacent to left renal artery and para-aortic nodes. Lymph may also drain into the posterior mediastinum through lymphatics along the inferior phrenic artery. Lymphatics from the upper pole of right adrenal gland may communicate with lymphatics of the liver.

Nerve Supply

Adrenal medulla has got myelinated preganglionic sympathetic fibers. Celiac and renal plexus give branches to adrenals.

Structure

Adrenal gland has got outer thick cortex and inner thin medulla. Two are independent in development, structure and function. Cortex has got *outer* zona glomerulosa secreting mineralocorticoids; *middle* zona fasciculata secreting glucocorticoids; *inner* zona reticularis secreting sex hormones. Adrenal medulla contains chromaffin cells in groups, autonomic ganglion cells with capillaries.

Embryology

Adrenal cortex develops from *intermediate mesoderm* of coelomic epithelium; medulla is from *neural crest* cells. Fetal adrenal gland is 20 times larger in relation to body weight than adult adrenal gland. In fetus at 4 months of gestation, adrenal gland is 4 times larger than kidney size of that age. During birth, adrenal gland becomes 1/3rd of the kidney size.

ADRENOCORTICAL TUMORS

Benign Tumors

- They are usually adenomas.
- It may be functioning (secrete hormones) or nonfunctioning.

I am a great believer in luck and I find the harder I work, the more I have of it

- Incidentalomas (3–5%) are tumors (adenomas) which are identified incidentally during US/CT/MRI abdomen done for evaluating the abdomen for some other purpose. Nonfunctioning incidentalomas more than 4 cm; all functioning incidentalomas are operated by adrenalectomy.

Adrenocortical Carcinoma

- It is 1% common; very aggressive tumor.
- It presents with pain, mass abdomen, functioning tumor as Cushing's syndrome.
- CT/MRI is diagnostic. Hormone evaluation is essential to find out functional status of the tumor.
- Secondaries are common in lungs and so CT chest is a must in these patients.
- *Treatment* is—adrenalectomy with adjuvant chemotherapy using Mitotane (Op-DDD) with Cisplatin, Etoposide and Doxorubicin.
- Laparoscopic adrenalectomy is not advised in adrenocortical adenocarcinoma.

CUSHING'S SYNDROME

- It is syndrome complex due to excessive glucocorticoid level in the body.
- It can be excessive intake of steroids or excessive secretion from the adrenal glands.
- It may be due to excess adrenocorticotropic hormone (ACTH) secretion from pituitary by an adenoma or by a functioning tumor from the adrenal gland itself.
- It causes obesity, central redistribution of fat, buffalo hump, proximal muscle wasting, hypertension, diabetes, skin changes.
- 24 hours free cortisol level is raised. CT/MRI may show adrenal tumor.
- *Treatment*: Drugs like Metapyrone, Aminoglutethimide, Mitotane; Adrenalectomy bilateral or unilateral; pituitary ablation.

CONN'S SYNDROME

- It is excessive secretion of the aldosterone due to primary hyperaldosteronism with reduced plasma renin activity.
- It is commonly due to aldosterone secreting adrenocortical adenoma. It can be idiopathic.
- *Features*: Hypertension, hypokalemia, hypernatremia, metabolic alkalosis.
- *Investigations*: Serum potassium, renin, aldosterone estimation; CT abdomen; selective adrenal venous sampling.
- *Treatment*: Adrenalectomy; spironolactone.

NEUROBLASTOMA

- It is *commonest childhood tumor* arising from adrenal medulla.
- It is malignant adrenal medullary tumor, it usually occurs in less than 5 years age.
- It is equal in both sexes.
- Extra-adrenal neuroblastoma also can occur.
- It can be *Pepper* type (right side with liver secondaries); *Hutchinson's* type (left side skull and orbit secondaries).
- It can be *low/intermediate/high* risk group.
- It can be stroma rich or stroma poor tumor histologically (*Shamida*).
- *Features*: Mass in the loin which does not move with respiration, nonmobile, crosses midline, knobby and nodular. Hypertension, fever, diarrhea, sweating, dancing eye syndrome, opsomyoclonus, *Racoon's eye sign*, hypokalemia are other features.
- It should be differentiated from Wilm's tumor (kidney).
- *Investigations*: CT/MRI abdomen; urinary VMA (vanillylmandelic acid) and homovanilic acid (HVA) estimation.
- *Treatment*: Adrenalectomy; chemotherapy using Carboplatin, Doxorubicin, Cyclophosphamide.

Don't be distracted by criticism. Remember—the only taste of success some people get is to take a bite out of you—**ZigZiglar**

PHEOCHROMOCYTOMA

- It is a tumor arising from chromaffin tissue of adrenal medulla commonly and extradrenal gland occasionally (10%, *organ of Zuckerkandl*).
- It secretes catecholamines like noradrenaline and often ACTH, vasoactive intestinal peptide (VIP) and other polypeptide.
- It can be benign or malignant. It can be functioning or nonfunctioning.
- *Features*: Severe headache, palpitation, dyspnea, blurred vision, paroxysmal hypertension; adrenal mass which is nonmobile, does not have intrinsic mobility, blood pressure may fluctuate while palpating. It may cause cardiac arrhythmias or cerebral hemorrhage.
- It may be associated with MEN syndrome II.
- *Investigations*: 24 hour urinary estimation; MRI abdomen, plasma free Metanephrine estimation, metaiodobenzylguanidine (MIBG) scan.
- *Treatment*: Adrenalectomy. Prior to surgery, blood pressure should be controlled *first by α blocking agent* like phenoxybenzamine; then by propranolol. During surgery, sodium nitroprusside is used. Adequate fluid therapy is important. Adrenal vein should be ligated first.

Pheochromocytoma
· 10% malignant.
· 10% extra-adrenal.
· 10% bilateral.
· 10% familial.
· 10% childhood.
· 10% multiple.
· 10% calcified.
· 10% not associated with hypertension.

Life is what happens when you're busy making other plans—***John Lennon***

CHAPTER 20

Salivary Glands

CHAPTER OUTLINE

- Anatomy
- Sialography
- Salivary Calculus
- Sialosis
- Sialectasis
- Sialadenitis
- Parotid Abscess (Acute Suppurative Sialadenitis of Parotid)
- Parotid Fistula
- Sjögren's Syndrome
- Mikulicz Disease
- Salivary Neoplasms
- Management of Malignant Salivary Tumors
- Minor Salivary Gland Tumors
- Parotidectomy
- Frey's Syndrome (Auriculotemporal Syndrome, Gustatory Sweating)

GENERAL CONSIDERATIONS

Salivary glands are parotid, submandibular and sublingual. Parotid is in front of the ear lobule. Submandibular gland is in submandibular triangle opposite the floor of the mouth. Sublingual gland is located on each side in the anterior aspect of the floor of the mouth in relation to mucosa, mylohyoid muscle and body of the mandible. Sublingual gland duct drains into mucosa directly into the submandibular duct. Minor salivary glands are around 450 in number and are distributed in lips, cheek, palate and floor of the mouth.

Ectopic salivary gland is also called as aberrant salivary gland; is juxtaposed gland in relation to submandibular salivary gland. *Stafne bone cyst* (Edward C Stafne, dental surgeon, Mayo clinic) is the commonest one which is juxtaposed submandibular salivary gland which gets invaginated into the mandible bone on its lingual side.

SALIVA

- 1500 mL of saliva is secreted daily which contains lingual lipase from tongue glands and α amylase from salivary glands.
- 20% of saliva is from parotid (serous and watery); 70% from submandibular gland (mucus and viscous); 5% from sublingual (mucous and viscous); 5% from minor salivary glands.
- pH of resting saliva is 7.0; of active saliva is 8.0.
- Saliva contains mucin, glycoprotein, IgA, lysozyme, lactoferrin.

Whoever is happy will make others happy too—Anne Frank

- Saliva facilitates swallowing, speech, keeps mouth moist, clean and rinsed. It is antibacterial, neutralizes gastric acid and serves as solvent for taste buds.

ANATOMY

PAROTID GLAND (PARA—AROUND, OTIS—EAR)

Parts of the Parotid Gland (Figs. 20.1 to 20.4)

- *Superficial part*
  - It lies over the posterior part of the ramus of mandible.
- *Deep part*
  - It lies behind the mandible and medial pterygoid muscle.

  Accessory parotid is prolongation of the gland along the parotid duct.

  Parotid duct (*Stensen's*) is 2–3 mm in diameter, begins behind the angle of the mandible, passes through the buccinator muscle, and opens into the oral mucosa opposite upper second molar tooth.

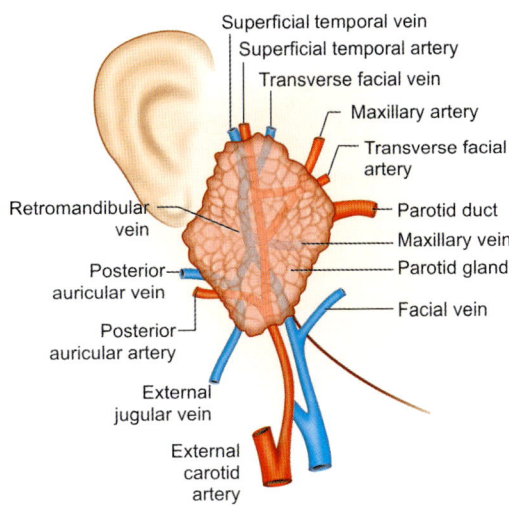

Fig. 20.2: Vascular plane of the parotid.

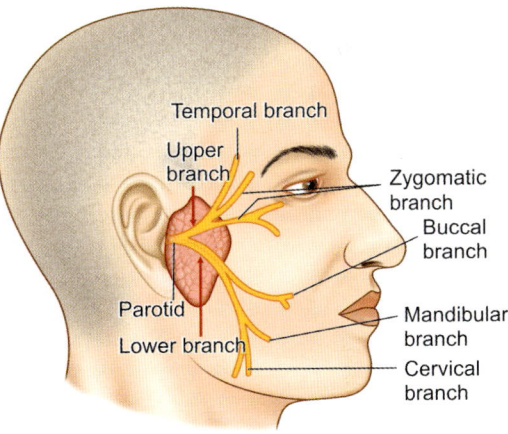

Fig. 20.3: Pes anserinus.

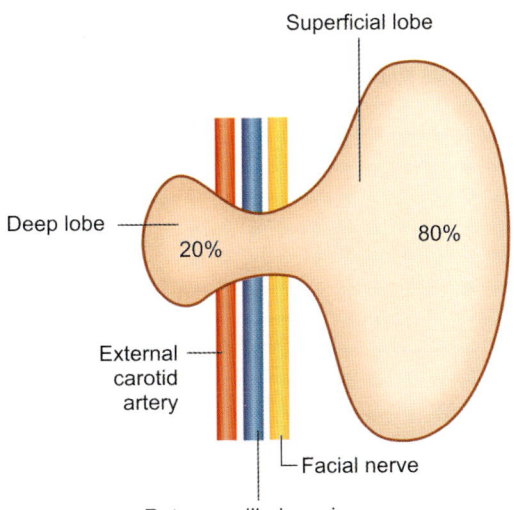

Fig. 20.1: Lobes of the parotid. 80% of the gland is superficial. Note the faciovenous plane of Patey in parotid gland.

FACIAL NERVE

- ***Facial nerve*** emerges from the stylomastoid foramen lying between external auditory meatus and mastoid process.
- It passes around the neck of the condyle of mandible and becomes superficial, later dividing into *temporofacial and cervicofacial branches,* which in turn divides into many branches.
- Some of these may be interconnected *as pes anserinus.*

Kindness is a language which the dumb can speak, the deaf can understand

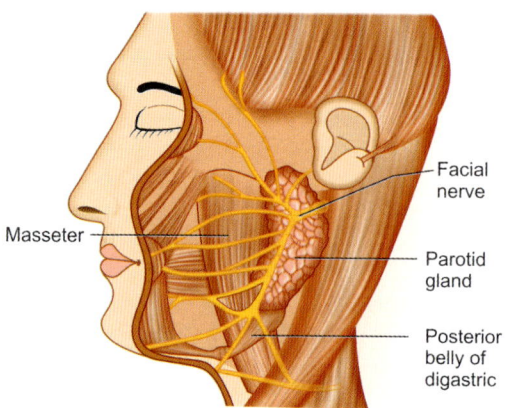

Fig. 20.4: Anatomical relations of the parotid gland.

SUBMANDIBULAR SALIVARY GLAND

Parts (Figs. 20.5 and 20.6)

1. *Superficial part*:
   It lies in submandibular triangle, superficial to mylohyoid and hyoglossus muscles, between the two bellies of digastric muscles.
2. *Deep part*:
   It lies in the floor of the mouth and deep to the mylohyoid.

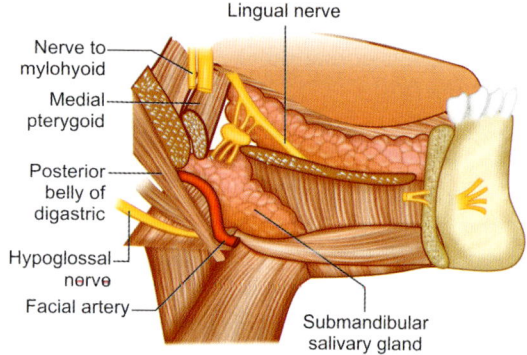

Fig. 20.5: Anatomical relations of the submandibular gland.

- While exiting the skull through stylomastoid foramen (it is accompanied by stylomastoid branch of posterior auricular artery which enters the same foramen), it gives posterior auricular nerve and motor nerves to posterior belly of digastric and stylohyoid. Trunk is initially 1cm from posterior medial surface (*extraglandular*) and *intraglandular* for 1cm before giving divisions.

Branches are:
- *Temporal* (auricularis anterior and superior part of frontalis);
- *Zygomatic* (frontalis and orbicularis oculi);
- *Upper and lower buccal branches* (buccinator, orbicularis oris, lip elevators); mandibular (lower lip muscles);
- *Cervical* (platysma).

FACIOVENOUS PLANE OF PATEY

- This plane contains retromandibular vein and posterior facial vein.
- Facial nerve is superficial to this plane.
- External carotid artery dividing into superficial temporal artery and maxillary artery is deeper to venous plane.

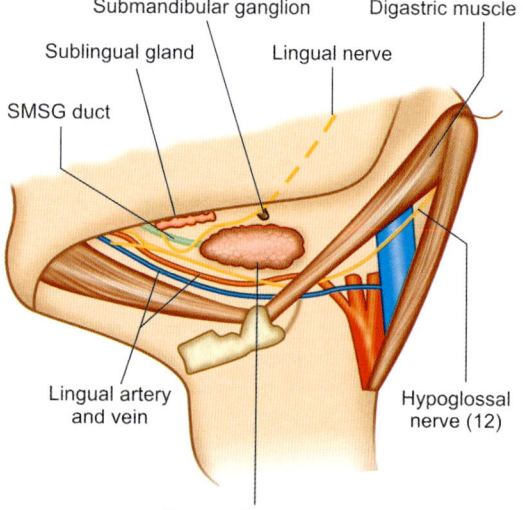

Fig. 20.6: Relations of the submandibular salivary gland (SMSG).

It is during our darkest moments that we must focus to see the light—**Aristotle**

- Submandibular duct (*Wharton's*) (5 cm), comes from the deep part of the gland, enters the floor of the mouth, on a papilla beside the frenum of the tongue.
- Lingual nerve and submandibular ganglion are attached to upper pole of the gland.
- Facial artery emerges from under surface of the stylohyoid muscle, enters the gland from posterior and deep surface reaching its lateral surface crossing the lower border of mandible to enter the face.
- Venous drainage is to anterior facial vein.

SIALOGRAPHY (FIG. 20.7)

Indications
- Salivary fistulas.
- Sialectasis.
- Congenital conditions.
- Extraglandular masses.

Dye used is lipiodol or sodium diatrizoate (hypaque).

24 gauge cannula is passed into either Stensen's duct or Wharton's duct and X-ray is taken after injecting 1 mL of the dye into the duct.

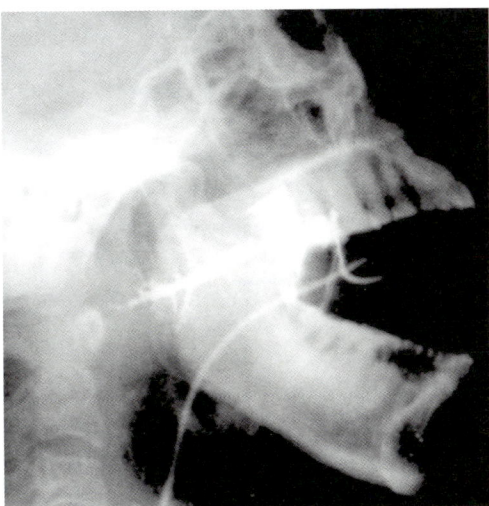

Fig. 20.7: Sialogram X-ray done to visualize the ductal pattern in parotid.

Findings
- Narrowing (stricture).
- Grape-like cluster appearance (sialectasis).
- Dilatations.
- Communications (fistulas).
- Mass lesions.

Sialography should never be performed in acute inflammation. Only 1 mL of dye is injected, if more dye is injected it will cause *extravasation, and chemical sialadenitis.*

SALIVARY CALCULUS

- 80% submandibular.
- 80% radiopaque.
- It is commonly calcium phosphate and calcium carbonate stones.
- Calculi are more common in submandibular gland, because the secretion of the gland is viscous, contains more calcium and also its drainage is nondependent, leading to stasis.
- Secretion from parotid is serous, contains less calcium and so stones are not common.

Presentation

Acute features
- Pain, swelling, tenderness is seen in submandibular region and floor of the mouth.
- Duct is inflamed and swollen.

Features in chronic cases
- Pain is more during mastication due to stimulation.
- Salivary secretion is more during mastication causing increase in gland size.
- Firm, tender swelling is bidigitally palpable.
- When stone is in the duct, it is palpable in the floor of the mouth as a tender swelling with features of inflammation in the duct. Pus exudes through the duct orifice.
- In submandibular salivary gland, the stones are multiple, associated with inflammation of gland *(sialadenitis)* (Fig. 20.8).

Human beings, by changing the inner attitudes of their minds, can change the outer aspects of their lives

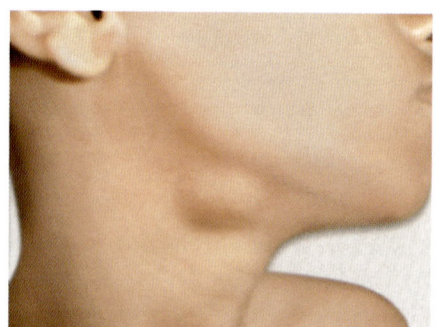

Fig. 20.8: Submandibular sialadenitis in a young boy who required excision of gland.

Differential Diagnosis

- Submandibular lymphadenitis.
- Salivary neoplasm.

Investigations

- Intraoral X-ray (dental occlusion films) to see radiopaque stones (Fig. 20.9).
- FNAC of the gland to rule out other pathology.
- Total count and ESR in acute phase.

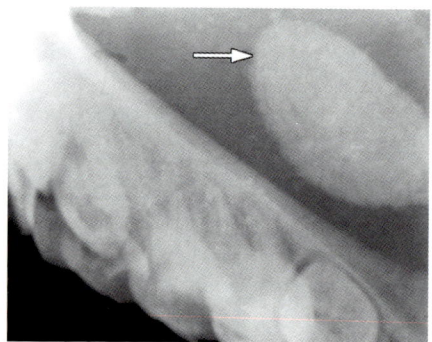

Fig. 20.9: X-ray showing large stone in duct of submandibular salivary gland, which is radiopaque (*Courtesy:* Dr Jagadish, Mangaluru).

Treatment

- *If it is a ductal stone*, removal of the stone is done intraorally, by making an incision on the duct. Incised duct is not sutured as it may result in stricture.
- *If stone is in the gland*, excision of *submandibular* gland is done.

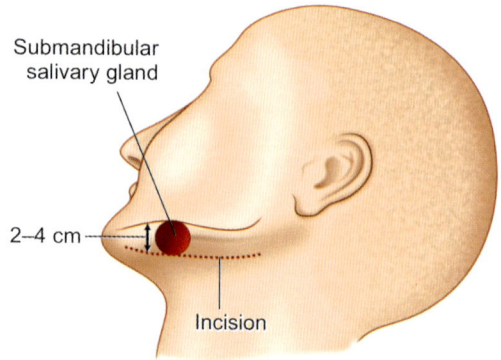

Fig. 20.10: Incision for excision of submandibular salivary gland. It should be 2 cm below the margin of the mandible to avoid injury to marginal mandibular nerve.

Submandibular salivary gland excision
Technique:
Approach is from submandibular region (outside). Skin incision is made in submandibular region, about 5–8 cm length, parallel to and 2–4 cm below the mandible (Fig. 20.10). Incision is deepened through the deep fascia until the gland is visualized without raising the flaps (so as to avoid injury to marginal mandibular nerve, branch of facial nerve). Facial artery is ligated twice. Lingual nerve and hypoglossal nerves are taken care of. Mylohyoid is retracted so as to remove the deep portion of the gland. Drain is placed after removal of the gland.

Complications of surgery
- Hemorrhage.
- Infection.
- Injury to marginal mandibular nerve, lingual nerve, hypoglossal nerve.

Rule of two in submandibular salivary gland
• Two parts divided by mylohyoid muscle.
• Two conditions affect it—tumor and stone.
• Two superficial nerves—cervical and mandibular branch of facial nerves.
• Two deep nerves—lingual and hypoglossal nerves.
• Incision—2 cm below the mandible.
• Ligate facial artery at 2 places.

Life is either a daring adventure or nothing at all—Helen Keller

Salivary calculi	
Submandibular gland	Parotid
80% *common*.	20% incidence (rare).
80% radiopaque.	Radiolucent.
Seen in plain X-ray (intraoral).	Not seen in plain X-ray.
Sialogram is not needed.	Identified by sialogram.

Calculi are common in submandibular salivary gland

- Viscous nature and mucin content.
- Calcium content.
- Nondependent drainage.
- Stasis.

SIALOSIS

- It is enlargement of the salivary gland due to fatty infiltration as a result of various metabolic causes like diabetes, acromegaly, obesity, and liver disease.
- **Clinical features**:
  - Bilateral diffuse enlargement of parotids, which is smooth, firm and nontender.
- **Treatment**:
  - The cause is treated.

SIALECTASIS

- It is an aseptic dilatation of salivary ductules causing grape-like (*cluster-like*) dilatations.
- It is a disease of unknown etiology with destruction of gland parenchyma accompanied by stenosis and cyst formation in the ducts.
- It is common in parotids; often bilateral.
- Presents as a smooth, soft, fluctuant, nontransilluminating swelling, which increases in size during mastication. It is tender initially. It lasts for many days with a long symptom-free period of the disease.
- Sialogram is diagnostic.
- Treatment is conservative (nonsurgical).

SIALADENITIS

- It is inflammation of the salivary gland. It is common in parotid and submandibular salivary glands.
- Viral, allergic, drug-induced are common in parotid. Bacterial is common in submandibular salivary gland. Specific infections like tuberculosis, syphilis, toxoplasmosis, HIV, can occur in both. Irradiation and postoperative dehydration also can cause sialadenitis.
- Sialadenitis can be acute or chronic.
- **Acute** is common in parotid usually due to *mumps* (paramyxovirus) virus infection. Mumps spread by direct/airborne contact/saliva. It causes generalized swelling of both parotids with acute onset of pain swelling which is tender with fever. It is usually seen in children. Fever, myalgia is common. It disappears in 7 days usually. It can cause viral pancreatitis and orchitis especially in adult (after childhood). Usually lifelong immunity is achieved after one infection. Treatment is usually symptomatic.
- *Acute bacterial suppurative sialadenitis* occurs often in parotid due to staphylococcus infection which may cause trismus, respiratory distress or rupture into auditory canal. It needs proper surgical drainage under general anesthesia.
- **Chronic** sialadenitis is common in submandibular salivary gland; usually associated with salivary calculi in the gland or duct which requires either the extraction of the stone from the duct or excision of the submandibular salivary gland under general anesthesia.

PAROTID ABSCESS (ACUTE SUPPURATIVE SIALADENITIS OF PAROTID)

- It is result of an acute bacterial sialadenitis of parotid gland.

Great people talk about ideas; average people talk about things; small people talk about other people

- It is an ascending bacterial parotitis, due to reduced salivary flow and poor oral hygiene.
- Causative organisms are *Staphylococcus aureus, Streptococcus viridans*, and often other gram-negative and anaerobic organisms.

Causes of acute parotitis (Differential diagnosis of suppurative parotitis)

- Viral—mumps.
- Bacterial—*Staphylococcus aureus*.
- Allergic.
- HIV infection.
- Radiotherapy.
- Specific infections like syphilis.

Clinical Features

- Pyrexia, malaise, pain and trismus.
- Red, tender, warm, well-localized, firm swelling is seen in the parotid region.
- Tender lymph nodes are palpable in neck.
- Features of bacteremia are present in severe cases.
- Pus or cloudy turbid saliva may be expressed from the parotid duct opening.

Investigations

- Ultrasound of parotid region.
- Pus collected from duct orifice is sent for culture and sensitivity.
- Needle aspiration from the abscess to confirm the formation of pus.

Note:
Sialogram is contraindicated in acute phase, as it causes retrograde infection leading into bacteremia.

Treatment

- Antibiotics are started depending on culture report.
- When it is severely tender, localized, incision and drainage have to be done under G/A. Skin is incised in front of the tragus vertically (**Blair's incision**) (Fig. 20.11) and then parotid sheath is (pyogenic membrane) opened horizontally. Pus is drained using sinus forceps and sent for culture study. Antibiotics are continued.

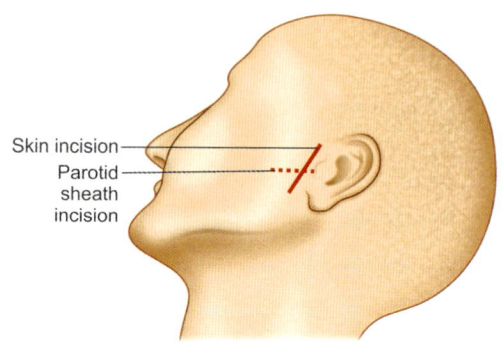

Fig. 20.11: Blair incision used to drain the parotid abscess.

- Adequate hydration, mouthwash with chlorhexidine or potassium permanganate solution and proper oral hygiene are important.

Complications of suppurative parotitis and abscess

- Septicemia.
- Severe trismus.
- Rupture into the external auditory canal.

Note:
In suppurative parotitis, patient may develop severe laryngeal or pharyngeal edema and may require steroids, tracheostomy and critical care.

PAROTID FISTULA

- Parotid fistula may arise from parotid gland or duct or ductules. It may open inside the mouth as internal fistula; or open outside onto the skin as external fistula. Fistula from the duct has profuse discharge. Fistula from the gland often shows only minimal discharge.
- Incidence of salivary fistula is 0.2–3%.

*Never let the fear of striking out keep you from playing the game—**Babe Ruth***

Types

1. *Duct fistula* forms after superficial parotidectomy. It is profuse and often persisting. So duct should be ligated using nonabsorbable suture as far as possible, anteriorly to allow normal saliva drainage from deep lobe. If common duct is ligated deep lobe atrophies without causing any fistula.
2. *Gland fistula* occurs from the raw surface after superficial parotidectomy. It is mild and symptom subsides in a month with anticholinergic drugs. Jacobsen tympanic neurectomy completely stops the secretion from the fistula in this type.

Causes

- After superficial parotidectomy.
- After drainage of parotid abscess, ruptured abscess.
- After biopsy, trauma.
- Recurrence of malignant tumor.

Features

- Discharging fistula in the parotid region of the face, and discharge is more during eating.
- Tenderness and induration; trismus.

Diagnosis

Sialography to find out the origin of the fistula whether from parotid gland or duct or ductules; fistulogram or CT fistulogram; discharge study; MRI.

Treatment

- Anticholinergics—hyoscine bromide (probanthine); radiotherapy is tried.
- Often exploration of fistula is required; repair or reinsertion of the duct into the mucosa is done.
- *Newman Seabrock's operation*—a probe is passed into the parotid duct through the opening in the mouth. Another probe is passed through the fistula. Duct and fistula are dissected over the probe. After removal of the fistula track severed duct ends are identified; and ends are trimmed. Probes are removed. A tantalum wire is passed into the duct across the severed ends and duct is sutured over it using
- 4-0 Vicryl. Tantalum stent is removed after 3 weeks.
- Total conservative parotidectomy is done in failed cases.

SJÖGREN'S SYNDROME

It is an autoimmune disease causing progressive destruction of salivary and lacrimal glands, leading to *keratoconjunctivitis sicca (dry eyes), and xerophthalmia (dry mouth)*.

Types

- Primary.
- Secondary.

Primary Sjögren's Syndrome

- Severe dry mouth.
- Severe dry eyes.
- Widespread dysfunction of exocrine glands.
- Incidence of developing lymphomas is high.
- There is no association of connective tissue disorders.

Secondary Sjögren's Syndrome

- Dry mouth.
- Dry eyes.
- With association of connective tissue disorders like.
  - Primary biliary cirrhosis (near 100%).

If the only tool you have is a hammer than treat everything like a nail

- Systemic lupus erythematosus (30%).
- Rheumatoid arthritis (RA) (15%).

Clinical Features

- It is common in middle-aged females who present with dry eyes, dry mouth, enlarged parotids and enlarged lacrimal glands.
- Often they are tender.
- Super added infection of the mouth, with *Candida albicans* is common.

Investigations

- Autoantibody estimation—rheumatoid factor, antinuclear factor, salivary duct antibody.
- Sialography.
- Estimation of salivary flow.
- Slit-lamp test of eyes.
- Schirmer test—to detect lack of lacrimal secretion.
- Fine needle aspiration cytology (FNAC) of parotids and lacrimal glands.
- ^{99}Technetium pertechnetate scan for gland function.

Treatment is Conservative

- Artificial tears.
- Artificial saliva.
- Frequent drinking of water.
- Treat the cause.

MIKULICZ DISEASE

- It is a clinical variant of Sjögren's syndrome.
- It is an *autoimmune disorder* of salivary and lacrimal glands, resulting in infiltration of the glands with round cells.

Triad

- Symmetrical enlargement of all salivary glands.
- Narrowing of palpebral fissures due to enlargement of the lacrimal glands.
- Parchment like dryness of the mouth.

SALIVARY NEOPLASMS

Etiology

- *Genetic:* Loss of alleles of chromosomes in 12q, 8q, 17q. Eskimos are more prone for salivary neoplasm.
- *Infective:* Mumps, Epstein-Barr virus, chronic sialadenitis may be the cause; but not proved emphatically. Recurrent inflammation can cause duct dysplasia and carcinoma.
- *Radiation:* It is more common in survivors of atomic bomb explosion; mucoepidermoid carcinoma is more in these patients.
- *Smoking:* Adenolymphoma of Warthin's shows 40% risk in smokers.
- *Sex:* Benign tumors and many malignancies are common in females; Warthin's and some malignancies are common in males.
- *Environment and diet:* Arctic eskimos show dietary deficiency of vitamin A and develop salivary tumor. Industrial agents like nickel, cadmium, hair dyes, silica, and preservatives may increase the risk of salivary tumors.

Classification

a. *Epithelial (90%)*
   1. *Adenomas*
      - Pleomorphic adenoma.
      - Monomorphic adenomas.
      - Adenolymphoma *(Warthin's tumor)*.
      - Oxyphil adenomas.
   2. *Carcinomas*
      - Mucoepidermoid carcinoma—commonest malignancy.
      - Acinic cell carcinoma (1%).
      - Adenoid cystic carcinoma—very aggressive (10%).
      - Adenocarcinoma.
      - Squamous cell carcinoma (2%).
      - Carcinoma in ex pleomorphic adenoma.
      - Undifferentiated carcinoma.

*You will face many defeats in life, but never let yourself be defeated—**Maya Angelou***

b. *Nonepithelial*
   - Hemangioma—commonly seen in infants, usually in parotid. Spontaneous regression is common.
   - Lymphangioma.
   - Neurofibromas and neurilemmomas.
c. *Malignant lymphomas*.

Clinical features of parotid tumor
• Raised ear lobule (Figs. 20.12A and B).
• Cannot be moved above the zygomatic bone.
• Deviation of uvula and pharyngeal wall towards midline in case of deep lobe.
• Facial nerve, masseter, skin, lymph node and bone involvement in case of malignancy.

Incidence

- About 75–80% salivary neoplasms are in the parotids (Fig. 20.13) of which 80% are benign.
- 80% of these are pleomorphic adenomas (Figs. 20.14 to 20.15).
- 15% of salivary tumors are in the submandibular salivary gland, of which 60% are benign.

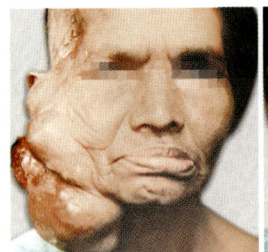
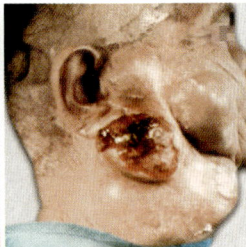

Fig. 20.13: Carcinoma parotid which is fungating.

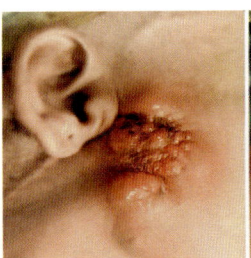
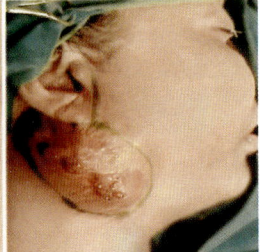

Fig. 20.14: Recurrent carcinoma parotid.

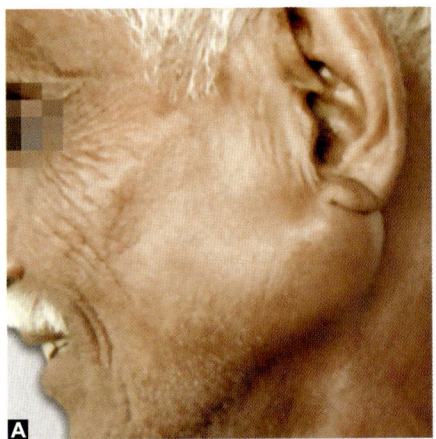
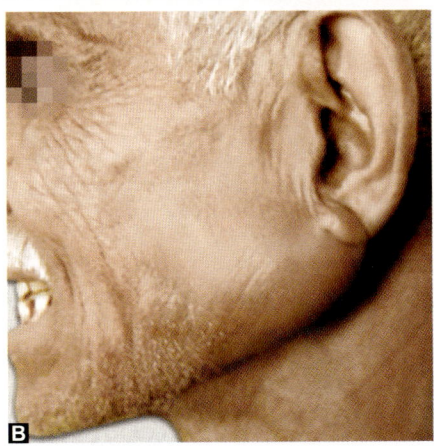

Figs. 20.12A and B: Typical parotid swelling with earlobe raise. Facial nerve should be tested by clenching the teeth.

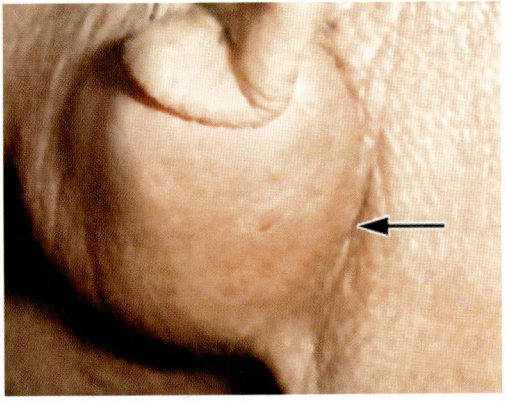

Fig. 20.15: Parotid tumor showing typical raise in earlobe.

*Start each day with a positive thought and a grateful heart—**Roy T Bennett***

- 95% of these are pleomorphic adenomas.
- 10% of salivary neoplasms are in the minor salivary glands—palate, lips, cheeks, and sublingual glands. Of these, only 10% are benign.

PLEOMORPHIC ADENOMAS (FIG. 20.16) (MIXED SALIVARY TUMOR)

- Commonest of the salivary gland tumor. It is 80% common.
- More common in parotids.
- It is mesenchymal, myoepithelial and duct reserve cell origin.

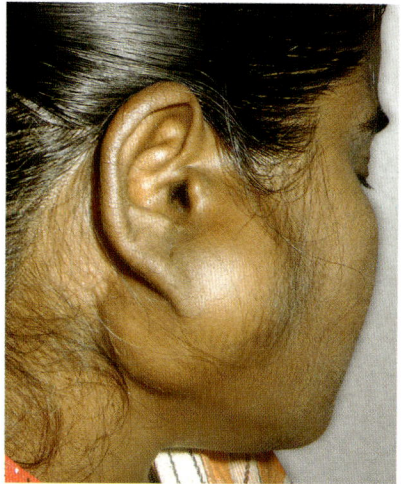

Fig. 20.16: Typical pleomorphic adenoma of the parotid gland.

Grossly
It contains cartilages, cystic spaces, and solid tissues.

Histologically, it shows:
- Epithelial cells.
- Myoepithelial cells.
- Mucoid material with myxomatous changes.
- Cartilages.
- Even though it is capsulated, tumor may come out as *pseudopods* and may extend beyond the main limit of the tumor tissue.

- When disease occurs in parotid, commonly it involves superficial lobe or superficial and deep lobe together.
- But sometimes only deep lobe is involved and then it presents as swelling in the lateral wall of the pharynx, soft palate and posterior pillar of the fauces. There may not be any visible swelling in the preauricular region—*Dumbbell tumor*. This tumor is in relation to styloid process, mandible, stylohyoid, styloglossus, stylopharyngeus muscles.

Clinical Features

- It is in 1:1 male to female ratio. 80% common.
- Occurs in any age group. Usually unilateral.
- Present as a single painless, smooth, firm lobulated, mobile swelling in front of the parotid with *positive curtain sign* (as the deep fascia is attached above to the zygomatic bone, it acts as a curtain, not allowing the parotid swelling to move above that level. Any swelling superficial to the deep fascia will move above the zygomatic bone).
- The ear lobule is lifted.
- When deep lobe is involved, swelling is commonly located in the lateral wall of pharynx, posterior pillar and over the soft palate.
- Facial nerve is not involved.

Long standing pleomorphic adenoma may turn into carcinoma (carcinoma in ex pleomorphic adenoma). Its features are:
- Recent increase in size.
- Pain and nodularity.
- Involvement of skin.
- Involvement of masseter.
- Involvement of facial nerve (Fig. 20.17)—lower facial nerve palsy (difficulty in closing eyelid, difficulty in blowing and clenching teeth).
- Involvement of neck lymph node.

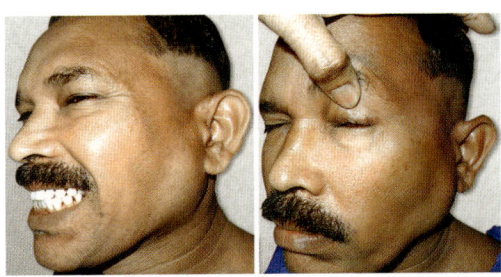

Fig. 20.17: Parotid tumour. Facial nerve should be examined to rule out its involvement.

Pain in salivary tumors

- Benign tumors are usually painless.
- Sudden onset of pain denotes malignant transformation.
- Pain is dull boring at primary site or referred to ear through auriculotemporal nerve.
- Pain is due to:
  - Capsular distension by tumor.
  - Obstruction to free flow of saliva.
  - Nerve infiltration.
  - Inflammation like in Warthin's.
  - Tumor necrosis.

Investigations

- FNAC is very important and diagnostic.
- CT scan to know the status of deep lobe.

Open biopsy is contraindicated in parotid tumors due to

- Seedling and high recurrence chance.
- Chance of injury to facial nerve.
- Chance of parotid fistula formation.

Treatment

- *Surgery*—First line of treatment.
- If only superficial lobe is involved, then *superficial parotidectomy* is done wherein parotid gland superficial to facial nerve is removed.
- If both lobes are involved, then *total conservative parotidectomy* is done by retaining facial nerve.

❖ Enucleation *is avoided*, as the recurrence is high.

Note
- Enucleation is avoided as it causes high recurrence due to extension of *tumor outside as pseudopods* across the capsule.
- Incomplete excision, 10% of tumors which are highly cellular are other causes for recurrence.
- RT is given after surgery even though it is benign.
- Inexplicable metastasis can occur even though it is benign.
- Tumor may implant due to spillage while surgical removal into retained residual parotid (deep lobe in superficial parotidectomy).
- *Recurrence after parotidectomy* in pleomorphic adenoma is 5%. It is due to spillage, improper technique, inadequate margin, retained pseudopods, multicentricity. Recurrent tumor is multinodular without any capsule. Expression of MUC1/DF3 in the tumor is marker to predict recurrence.

ADENOLYMPHOMA (WARTHIN'S TUMOR, PAPILLARY CYSTADENO-LYMPHOMATOSUM) (FIG. 20.18)

❖ It is a benign tumor that occurs only in parotid, usually in the lower pole.
❖ Common in males. It is often bilateral.
❖ It is said to be due to trapping of jugular lymph sacs in parotid during developmental period.

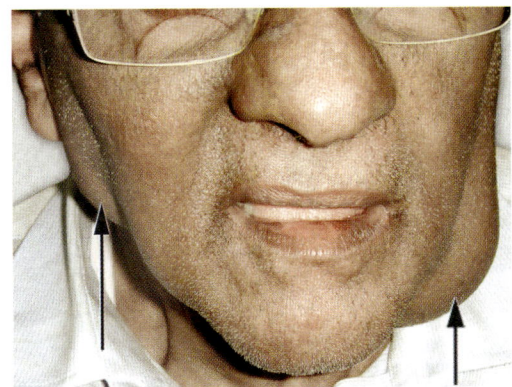

Fig. 20.18: Warthin's tumor of parotids. It is common in males; often bilateral; common in elderly.

Be brave to stand for what you believe in even if you stand alone—**Roy T Bennett**

- It composed of *double layered columnar epithelium*, with papillary projections into cystic spaces with lymphoid tissues in the stroma.

Clinical Features
- It presents as a slow growing, smooth, soft, cystic, fluctuant swelling, in the lower pole, often bilateral, and is nontender.
- It is common in males. It is 10% common.

Investigations
- Adenolymphoma produces *a 'hot spot'* in ^{99}Technetium pertechnetate scan—*it is diagnostic*.
- FNAC.

Note:
Adenolymphoma does not turn malignant.

Treatment
Superficial parotidectomy.

ONCOCYTOMA (OXYPHIL ADENOMA)
- It is <1% of salivary tumors.
- Usually benign, originating from oncocytes (oxyphilic cells).
- Radiation and occupational hazards are the causes.
- Common in parotid; but rarely can occur in submandibular salivary gland.
- Gross—small, *tan colored*, well circumscribed encapsulated solid tumor.
- Microscopy—*large oncocytes* with *swollen granular cytoplasm* due to abundant mitochondria. Tyrosine crystals are present in glandular spaces.
- Predilection for Tc99 with hotspots and FNAC are the investigations.

MUCOEPIDERMOID TUMOR (FIG. 20.19)
- It is the commonest malignant salivary gland tumor (in parotid glands).
- It is slowly progressive, often attains a large size, and spreads to neck lymph nodes.
- It contains malignant epidermoid and mucus secreting cells.

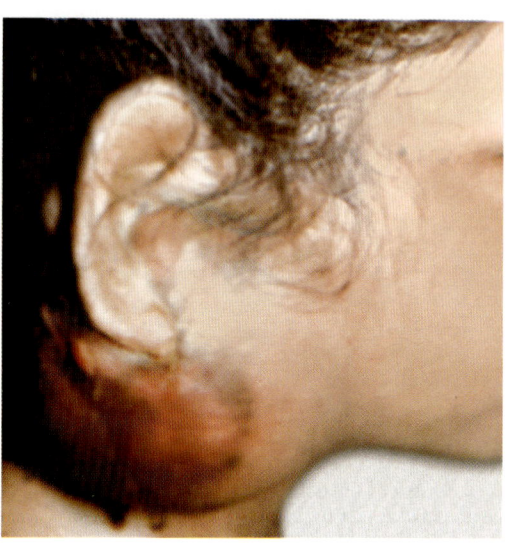

Fig. 20.19: Mucoepidermoid tumor.

Types
- *Low grade.*
- *High grade.*
  Facial nerve involvement is rare or very late in mucoepidermoid carcinoma of parotid.

Clinical Features
- Swelling in the salivary gland (parotid or submandibular) region, slowly increasing in size, eventually attaining a large size, which is hard, nodular, often with involvement of skin and lymph nodes.
- Facial nerve is usually not involved.

ADENOID CYSTIC CARCINOMA
- It is *most common* tumor in submandibular and sublingual salivary glands. 50% of cases occur in minor salivary glands— *palate*.
- It is also called as *cylindromatous* carcinoma.

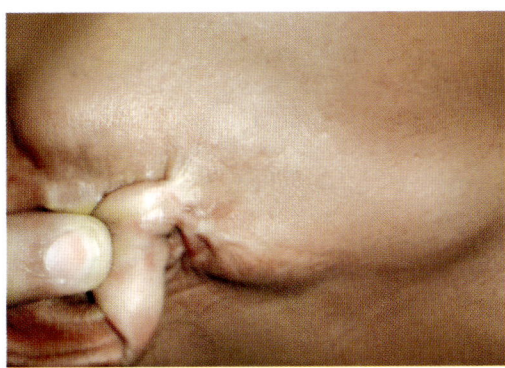

Fig. 20.20: Recurrent parotid tumor right side. Note the scar of previous surgery. It was adenoid cystic carcinoma. Recurrence has occurred after 6 years. Patient underwent radical parotidectomy.

- It is second most common malignant salivary tumor; but it is rare in parotid (2% of parotid tumors, 15% of malignant parotid tumors) (Fig. 20.20).
- It is common in females (3:2). Common in 5th and 6th decades.
- It is *slow growing but highly malignant* with remarkable capacity for recurrence. But it is classified under *low grade* malignancy.
- *Microscopy:* Cribriform, tubular, and solid are three types. *Cribriform* type shows cells in nests separated by round or oval spaces—*'Swiss-cheese'* pattern. Myo and duct epithelial cells with lace-like pattern are also seen. It *invades* periosteum and bone medulla early and spreads extensively.
- It has got high affinity for *perineural spread* (both axially and circumferentially; antegrade and retrograde fashion) along mandibular and maxillary divisions of trigeminal (*common*) nerve and facial nerve. It infiltrates nerve more proximally for long distance. Tumor may reach *Gasserian* trigeminal ganglion, pterygopalatine ganglion and cavernous sinus.
- Blood spread can occur to *lungs*, bones and liver. Lung secondaries may remain *dormant for many years* and so is not a contraindication for surgery of primary tumor. Blood spread can occur decades after removal of primary tumor.
- Radical parotidectomy/wide or radical excision of submandibular and sublingual glands with neck nodal dissection and postoperative RT is the treatment of choice.
- Positive margin, perineural spread, solid type on microscopy carry poor prognosis. Lung metastasis will not affect the prognosis.
- Local recurrence is common. 5 years survival is 70%.
- Regional nodal spread can occur but is rare.

MALIGNANT MIXED TUMOR (MMT)

- It is 10% of salivary malignancy in incidence with epithelial and mesenchymal elements (Fig. 20.21).
- It carries worst prognosis.

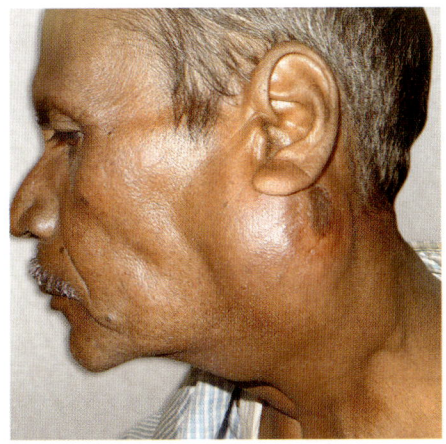

Fig. 20.21: Malignant salivary gland tumor; note the skin changes and ulceration.

Types

- *Carcinoma ex pleomorphic adenoma:* It is the commonest type. Previous long standing parotid swelling shows rapid change, fixity, facial nerve spread, neck nodal involvement

*To belittle, you have to be little—**Kalil Gibran***

are typical. Transformation is 2% in 5 years tumor; 10% in 15 years tumor. It is the most aggressive salivary malignancy. Radical parotidectomy is the treatment.
- *Primary malignant mixed tumor:* It is also called *as carcinosarcoma* which arises as de novo. It shows components of both carcinoma and sarcoma with metastatic potential both through lymph nodes and blood.
- *Metastasizing mixed tumors:* It contains structures typical of benign mixed tumor both at primary and at metastases sites.
- *In situ noninvasive carcinoma* in pleomorphic adenoma: There is no evidence of capsular invasion. Lesion with less than 8 mm invasion in depth shows 100% of 5 years survival; >8 mm invasion carries <50% of 5 years survival.

ADENOCARCINOMA OF SALIVARY GLANDS

- It is 3% of parotid and 10% of submandibular and minor salivary gland tumors.
- It is equal in both sexes.
- It is common in children.
- It can be tubular, papillary and undifferentiated.
- 20% involve facial nerve clinically.
- Undifferentiated type is aggressive.

SQUAMOUS CELL CARCINOMA OF SALIVARY GLANDS

- It is rare in salivary glands.
- In salivary glands, parotid is the common site.
- It is almost never seen in minor salivary glands.
- It is classified as high grade tumor.
- It is common in men (3:1).
- It occurs in 6th or 7th decade. It is aggressive nonencapsulated tumor arising from ductal system.
- It grows rapidly causing pain, facial palsy, skin fixity, ulceration.
- It spreads commonly to neck nodes.
- It carries poor prognosis.
- Radical parotidectomy and RT is the treatment of choice.

ACINIC CELL TUMOR

It is a rare, slow growing tumor that occurs almost always in parotid and is composed of cells alike serous acini. It is more common in women. It occurs in adult and elderly.

General features of malignant salivary tumors
• Fixation.
• Resorption of adjacent bone.
• Pain and anesthesia in the skin and mucosa.
• Muscle paralysis.
• Skin involvement and nodularity.
• Involvement of jaw and masticatory muscle.
• Nerve involvement (facial nerve in parotid or hypoglossal nerve in submandibular salivary gland).

- It can involve facial nerve or neck lymph nodes.
- Clinically, it is of variable consistency with soft and cystic areas.

SUBMANDIBULAR SALIVARY GLAND TUMORS

Benign tumors
- Commonly pleomorphic adenomas, are smooth, firm or hard, bidigitally palpable, without involving adjacent muscles or hypoglossal nerve or mandible bone.
- Diagnosis is by FNAC, orthopantomogram (OPG), and CT scan.
- Excision of both superficial and deep lobes of the gland is done.

Malignant tumors (Fig. 20.22):
- They are hard, nodular, often get fixed to skin, muscles, hypoglossal nerve, and mandible.
- Diagnosis is by FNAC of primary tumor and of lymph nodes when involved, CT scan and OPG.

Never let yesterday use up too much of today

Chapter 20 : Salivary Glands

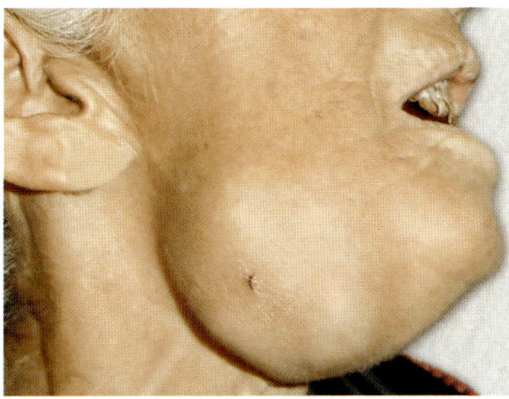

Fig. 20.22: Submandibular salivary gland tumor which is malignant. Patient underwent wide excision.

Treatment

- Wide excision, with removal of adjacent muscle, soft tissues, and mandible (Fig. 20.23).
- If lymph nodes are involved, block dissection of neck (classical neck dissection) is done.

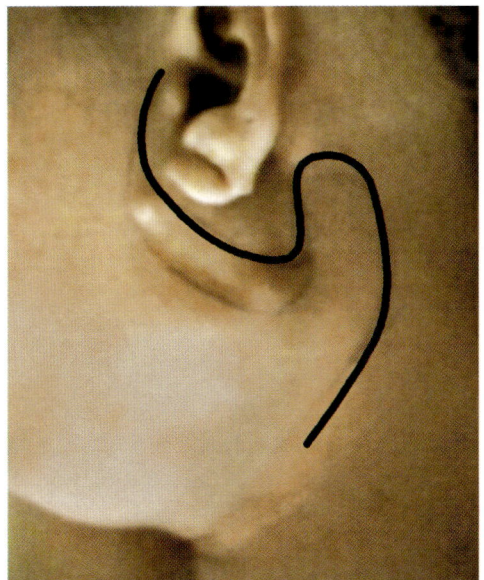

Fig. 20.23: Incision for parotid tumor. Note the lazy S incision involving the skin over the tumor within the incision.

MANAGEMENT OF MALIGNANT SALIVARY TUMORS

Specific investigations
- FNAC.
- CT scan to see the deep lobe of the parotid; to look for the involvement of bone, extension into the base of the skull; relation of tumor to internal carotid artery, styloid process.
- Orthopantomogram (OPG).
- Blood grouping and cross matching; required quantity of blood is kept ready.
- FNAC of lymph node.
- MRI shows better soft tissue definition than CT scan.

Sialogram is not useful in assessment of tumor.

TNM staging of malignant salivary tumors

TNM Staging of Malignant Salivary Tumors (AJCC, 8th Edition, 2018, Clinical Staging)

T—Tumor
Tx —Tumor cannot be assessed.
T0 —No evidence of primary tumor.
Tis - Carcinoma in situ.
T1 —Tumor <2cm without extraparenchymal spread.
T2 —Tumor 2–4 cm without extraparenchymal extension
T3 —Tumor >4 cm or with extraparenchymal spread but no facial nerve spread.
T4—T4a: Spread to facial nerve, skin, mandible, ear canal. T4b: Spread to base of skull, pterygoid plates and encased external carotid artery.
Note: Extraparenchymal extension is clinical or macroscopic evidence of invasion of tissues. Microscopic evidence alone does not constitute extraparenchymal extension.

N—Nodal spread
Nx—Nodes cannot be assessed.
N0—No regional lymph node spread.
N1—Regional single node <3 cm with ENE (-).
N2—N2a: Single ipsilateral node <3 cm with ENE (+); OR single ipsilateral node 3–6 cm with ENE (-).
N2b: Multiple ipsilateral nodes <6 cm in size and ENE (-). N2c: Bilateral or contralateral nodes <6 cm with ENE (-).

Contd...

---

*May you live every day of your life— **Jonathan Swift***

Contd...

N3—N3a: Single ipsilateral node >6 cm with ENE (-).
N3b: Single ipsilateral node >3 cm with ENE (+) OR multiple ipsilateral or contralateral or bilateral any sized nodes with ENE (+) OR single contralateral node of any size with ENE (+).
Note: **ENE** means extra-nodal extension; ENE_{mi} is microscopic metastases <2 mm; ENE_{ma} is macroscopic >2 mm. Suffix – ***sn*** is for SLN biopsy; ***f*** is for FNAC or core biopsy; ***u*** is nodes above lower border of the cricoid; ***l*** is nodes below the lower border of cricoid.

M—Distant metastases
cM0—Distant spread not present.
cM1—Distant metastases present.
pM1—Distant metastases, microscopically confirmed.

Staging
Stage 0—Tis N0 M0
Stage I—T1 N0 M0
Stage II—T2 N0 M0
Stage III—T3 N0 M0; T0,T1,T2,T3 N1 M0
Stage IV—IVA: T4a N0/N1 M0; T0,T1,T2,T3,T4a N2 M0. Stage IVB: Any T N3 M0; T4b Any N M0. Stage IVC: Any T Any N M1.

Treatment

In parotid:

Indications for surgery

- T1, T2, T3 tumors of low grade—total conservative parotidectomy (Fig. 20.24).
- T4 tumors, high grade tumors, SCC—radical parotidectomy.

It includes facial nerve sacrifice, may involve resection of skin, mandibular ramus, masseter muscle, infratemporal fossa dissection, subtotal petrosectomy.
Note: In T1 low grade, superficial parotidectomy is often practiced; but not ideal.

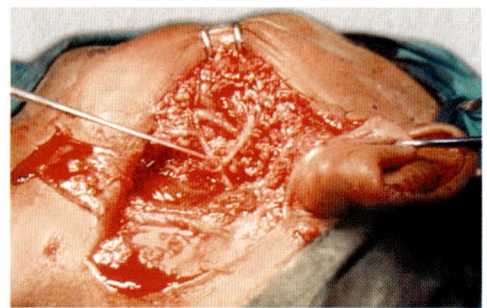

Fig. 20.24: Ontable exposure of facial nerve branches after superficial parotidectomy for a benign tumor.

Indications for facial nerve sacrifice

- Prep-operative weakness/paralysis of nerve.
- Intraoperative evidence of gross invasion even in presence of normal preoperative function.
- Tumors transgressing through facial nerve from superficial to deep lobe.
- Nerve stump is checked by frozen section for negative margins, if positive mastoidectomy and nerve dissection in temporal bone is needed.

Surgery:
- *Radical parotidectomy* is done which includes removal of both lobes of parotid, soft tissues, part of the mandible with facial nerve.
- Facial nerve is reconstructed using greater auricular nerve, or sural nerve.
- Often lateral tarsorrhaphy or temporal sling reconstruction is done.

Complications of surgery

- Hemorrhage.
- Infection.
- Fistula.
- Frey's syndrome.
- Facial nerve palsy.

Postoperative radiotherapy:
It is quiet useful to reduce the chances of relapse. Usually external radiotherapy is given. It is given in all carcinomas, but more useful in adenoid cystic and squamous cell carcinomas.

Chemotherapy:
It is also given. Drugs given here depend on tumor type. Intra-arterial chemotherapy is beneficial.

Preoperative radiotherapy:
It is given in large tumors to reduce the size and make it better operable, i.e. to down stage the disease.

If lymph nodes are involved:
Confirmed by FNAC, radical neck dissection is done.

*Pursue what catches your heart, not what catches your eyes—**Roy T Bennett***

In submandibular salivary gland:
Wide excision is done, with removal of mandible, and soft tissues around. If lymph nodes are involved, then block dissection of the neck is done.

Indications for radiotherapy in malignant salivary gland tumors

- All adenoid cystic and adenocarcinomas.
- T3 and T4 tumors.
- Recurrent tumors.
- Poorly differentiated tumors.
- Tumors with lymph node involvement.
- As preoperative radiotherapy.
- Recurrent benign pleomorphic adenomas.
- Spillage during surgery in case of pleomorphic adenomas.

MINOR SALIVARY GLAND TUMORS

- It is 10% of salivary tumors.
- It is common in:
  - *Palate (40%).* The commonest site (Fig. 20.25).
  - *Lip*
  - *Cheek*
  - *Sublingual glands.*
- 10% are benign—*commonly pleomorphic adenomas.*
- 90% are malignant—*commonly adenoid cystic carcinomas.*
- They present as swelling with ulcer over the summit.

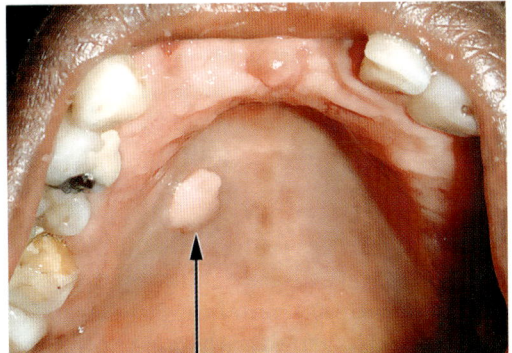

Fig. 20.25: Minor salivary gland tumor of hard palate.

- If it is malignant, then extension into the palate, maxilla, pterygoids can occur often with involvement of lymph node.
- **Differential diagnosis:** Squamous cell carcinoma of oral cavity.

Investigations

- Incision biopsy.
- CT scan.
- X-ray maxilla.
- FNAC of lymph node.

Treatment

- Wide excision often with palatal excision or maxillectomy is done.
- Reconstruction by dental plates, skin grafting, or flaps are done.
- Lymph node block dissection of the neck is done, if involved.

Points to be remembered

- Salivary gland tumors are usually benign in an adult.
- It is rare in children but when it occurs, it is commonly malignant.
- Clinical and FNAC are diagnostic methods.
- *Open biopsy is contraindicated.*
- *Sialogram is not useful in salivary tumors.*
- CT or MRI is often needed.
- Nerve should be preserved in benign lesions.
- Nerve can be sacrificed to achieve clearance in malignancies.

PAROTIDECTOMY

Procedure

Lazy 'S' incision is used; skin flaps are raised up to the anterior margin of the parotid using sharp dissection and bipolar cautery. Facial nerve identification markers are—tip of the tragal cartilage; dissection of the posterior belly of the digastric, sternocleidomastoid muscle, stylomastoid branch of the posterior auricular artery. Nerve travels horizontally

Laughter is the sun that drives away the winter from the human face

from the stylomastoid foramen as a thick whitish structure which later divides into two branches. Parotid is dissected carefully off the nerve using fine hemostat and bipolar cautery. Injuring branches of the facial nerve should be avoided. Deep lobe is removed if needed separately after retracting the exposed facial nerve branches. Wound is closed with a suction drain (Figs. 20.26 and 20.27).

Types

* **Superficial/lateral parotidectomy (Patey):** It is removal of superficial lobe of the parotid in front of the faciovenous plane of Patey.
* **Partial (functional) parotidectomy:** It involves resection of parotid pathology with normal parotid tissue, done in benign pathology and low grade malignancies. Here main facial nerve trunk is identified but there is no need to dissect the branches.
* **Total conservative parotidectomy:** Here both superficial and deep lobes of the parotid are removed preserving the facial nerve. Dissection along the faciovenous plane is carried out to identify the branches of the facial nerve retaining the isthmus/tumor-bearing area. Nerve branches are retracted aside to reach the deep lobe which is removed entirely by dissecting off the branches of facial nerve carefully without injuring them. This is the right technique even though many advocate removing superficial lobe initially then deep lobe separately. Retromandibular vein is ligated here.
* **Radical parotidectomy:** Involves removal of both lobes of parotid with facial nerve, fat, fascia, masseter, pterygoid, buccinator along with neck lymph node dissection. Facial nerve is sacrificed. Its branches whenever possible can be saved as additional advantage of survival not thereby removing uninvolved branches. On table frozen section biopsy of cut ends of nerve are needed. Ends of the cut nerve branches are tagged by fine sutures for eventual nerve grafting using great auricular nerve or sural nerve. Often radical parotidectomy is combined with removal of temporomandibular joint, mastoid process and external auditory meatus with less additional benefit. Mastoidectomy is done to visualize the clear proximal part of the facial nerve. Reconstruction

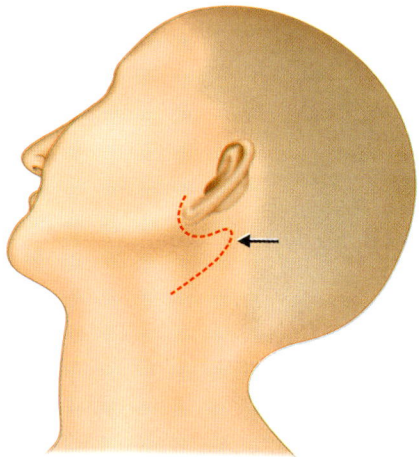

Fig. 20.26: 'S' (Lazy S) shaped incision for parotidectomy.

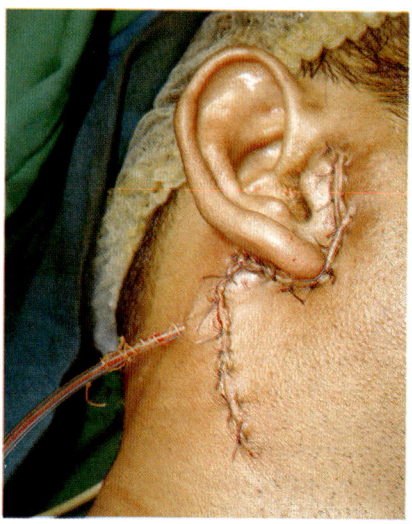

Fig. 20.27: Postoperative sutured wound with suction drain.

*Make improvements, not excuses. Seek respect, not attention—**Roy T Bennett***

of the main trunk, marginal mandibular, temporal and buccal branches are done to maintain eye closure and good oral competence.
- **Extended total parotidectomy:** Removal of the superficial and deep parotid gland also may be extended to involve adjacent structures.
- **Suprafacial extracapsular parotidectomy:** It is done for benign tumor (pleomorphic adenoma) at lower pole wherein all branches of facial nerve need not be dissected. Under general anesthesia, with preauricular incision *superficial muscular aponeurotic system layer (SMAS) is a fibrous network that invests the facial muscles, and connects them with the dermis; platysma inferiorly; zygomatic arch superiorly; facial nerve courses deep to the SMAS and the platysma*) is exposed with subplatysmal plane. Flap is raised 1 cm beyond the tumor area. Tumor circumference is marked and cruciate incision is placed over the fascia; incision is deepened to raise four flaps. Blunt and careful sharp dissection is done away from the tumor capsule with a margin of 3 mm; normal parotid is retracted all around and dissection is carried out. Facial nerve branches whenever visible carefully dissected off the field without injuring it. Tumor capsule should not be ruptured to avoid spillage. Entire tumor is removed with 2–3 mm margin. Fascia is sutured back; suction drain is placed; wound is closed in layers. This technique reduces the chances of facial nerve injury and Frey's syndrome.

Complications of Parotidectomy

- Facial nerve injury.
- Hemorrhage.
- Salivary fistulas.
- Infection.
- Frey's syndrome.
- Flap necrosis is common.
- Sialocele and numbness over the face and ear.

Conservative surgeries are becoming popular for malignancy but they are not universally accepted.

FREY'S SYNDROME (AURICULOTEMPORAL SYNDROME, GUSTATORY SWEATING)

- It occurs in 10% of cases.
- It is due to injury to the auriculotemporal nerve, wherein postganglionic parasympathetic fibers from the otic ganglion become united to sympathetic nerves from the superior cervical ganglion *(Pseudosynapsis)*.

Causes

- Surgeries or accidental injuries to the parotid.
- Surgeries or accidental injuries to temporomandibular joint.
- Rarely birth trauma.

Clinical Features

- Flushing, sweating, pain and hyperesthesia in the skin over the face innervated by the auriculotemporal nerve, whenever salivation is stimulated (i.e. during mastication).
- Involved skin is painted with iodine and dried. Dry starch applied over this area will become blue due to more sweat in the area in Frey's syndrome—**starch iodine test.**
- Condition causes real inconvenience to the patient.

Treatment

- Initially conservative and reassurance. Most of the time they recover.
- Occasionally they require surgical division of the tympanic branch of the

Nothing great was ever achieved without enthusiasm

glossopharyngeal nerve below the round window of middle ear (i.e. intratympanic parasympathetic neurectomy).

Treatment of Frey's syndrome

- Reassurance.
- Jacobsen neurectomy (tympanic).
- Injection of botulinum toxin to the affected skin.
- Antiperspirants like aluminum chloride.
- Syndrome can be prevented ontable by placing muscle (sternomastoid) or fascial (temporalis) flaps or artificial membranes over parotid bed.

FACIAL NERVE PALSY

- Facial nerve palsy after parotidectomy is lower facial nerve palsy.
- Features are inability to close eyelid, exposure keratitis, difficulty in clinching teeth and blowing air, masseter weakness and drooping of the angle of the mouth.
- Often it could be due to neuropraxia due to handling of the nerve during surgical technique. In such occasion, steroids will be beneficial.
- Classic nerve injury if identified, nerve repair is done immediately. Nerve can be reconstructed using nerve grafts from sural nerve, great auricular nerve.
- Nerve cross suturing is done often by suturing hypoglossal/spinal accessory/ phrenic nerves to distal branches of the facial nerve.

In late cases, either static or dynamic procedures are done.

Surgeries for facial nerve palsy

Static
- Suspension surgeries of lip, cheek and angle of mouth using temporal fascia, palmaris longus or synthetic materials.
- Correction of medial canthus to reduce epiphora.
- Lateral tarsorrhaphy to treat exposure keratitis.
- Upper lid weights.

Dynamic
- Muscle transfer—temporal to masseter with nerve and vessel.
- Free muscle graft.
- Cross facial nerve transplant using sural nerve from normal facial to paralyzed facial nerve.
- Nerve grafts.
- Neurovascular gracilis muscle graft using microscope.

You talk when you cease to be at peace with your thoughts—**Kalil Gibran**

CHAPTER 21

Oral Cavity

Chapter Outline

- Retromolar Trigone
- Ranula
- Sublingual Dermoids
- Cancrum Oris (Noma)
- Leukoplakia
- Erythroplakia
- Oral Submucosal Fibrosis
- Premalignant Conditions of the Oral Cavity
- Oral and Upper Aerodigestive Cancers
- Carcinoma Cheek (Buccal Mucosa)
- Neoplasm of Lip
- Carcinoma of Lip
- Tongue
- Carcinoma Tongue
- Nasopharyngeal Carcinoma
- Maxillary Tumors
- Carcinoma Hard Palate

SURGICAL ANATOMY

Lips

Lips are two fleshy folds lined by skin outside and mucous membrane inside. Upper lip is bounded by nose and nasolabial groove. Lower lip is bounded by cheek and labiomental groove. Orbicularis oris forms the muscular bulk of the lip which encircles the lip and is supplied by facial nerve. *Frenulum* in the midline joins the upper and lower lips to the gums. *Vermilion border* is red border of the lip where skin part merges gradually into the mucous membrane part. It contains wet line inside and a dry line outside. Small rounded nodule at the center of the lowest part of the upper lip is called as tubercle. A depression running from tubercle to nostrils is called as *philtrum*. The corners where upper and lower lips meet at right and left angles are called as *commissures* of lip. 5 mm elevation of mucous membrane posterior to commissure is called as *commissural papule*. Upper lip drains into upper deep cervical nodes. Center of lower lip drains into *submental nodes* then to upper deep cervical nodes. Lateral part of lower lip drains into submandibular lymph nodes then *to middle cervical nodes*. Lymph from angles of mouth drains into both nodes of upper and lower lips. Lips are red or reddish brown in young. It is often brownish in smokers.

Cheek

It is large fleshy flap one on each side covering the vestibule. It contains skin, superficial fascia with facial muscles, parotid duct, mucus glands, buccinator with buccopharyngeal fascia, submucosa and mucous membrane. Buccal pad of fat lies on the buccinator partly deep and partly in front of masseter.

Money is a good servant, but a dangerous master

RETROMOLAR TRIGONE

- *Retromolar trigone* is oral mucosal part of the anterior surface of the ascending ramus of the mandible; it is a triangular area bounded by temporal crest on the medial side, anterior border of ramus on the lateral side and base posterior to the socket for the third molar. Lateral boundary of retromolar triangle in its upper 1/3rd provides attachment to superficial fibers of temporalis muscle. The medial boundary of the triangle in its upper 2/3rd provides attachment to deeper fibers of temporalis muscle. The medial border near its lower end was crossed by lingual nerve and in its middle was crossed by buccal nerve and artery. Deep to the medial border, medial pterygoid muscle was seen. Along anterior border of medial and anteromedial to the triangle, pterygomandibular raphe gives attachment to buccinator anteriorly and superior constrictor muscle posteriorly.
- **Base is inferior behind the lower 3rd molar and apex is superior at the tuberosity of the maxilla**.
- Mucosa is densely adherent to muscle/tendons and bone underneath. Medially mucosa blends with anterior tonsillar pillar; laterally with buccal mucosa.
- Retromandibular fossa and retromandibular foramen is related to the trigone. It is also called as *coffin corner/sump area*.
- *Malignancy here denotes advance nature*. It can spread medially and behind towards pharynx; laterally towards temporal fossa; high chances of perineural invasion and spread; bone involvement is common; extension above to skull based is possible.

Gingivae or Gums

They are mucous membrane covering the alveolar process of the jaws. It is pink in color in healthy person. It is spotted with brown melanin pigment in dark skin people and people from Mediterranean region. It is pigmented in smokers, pan chewers. Gingival margin is occlusal border at which gingiva meets teeth. *Free gingiva* is gingival part encircling the tooth forming a gingival sulcus. *Attached gingiva* is mucosa which is firmly bound to the underlying bone. *Alveolar mucosa* is movable vascular mucosa and less attached to bone. Lips should be everted properly to inspect the gums. Proper light is needed. Gums recede as age advances.

Tongue

Tongue is a muscular, glandular and vascular flat organ. Anterior 2/3rd is termed as body; posterior 1/3rd is base/root. Superior surface *is dorsum of the tongue*. It is an essential organ of taste. Tongue is important in speech, mastication and swallowing. *Filiform papillae* are located in anterior 2/3rd of the dorsum of tongue and are numerous, fine, hair-like. *Fungiform papillae* are mushroom-shaped, deep red, larger, sparsely located near the tip of the tongue. Large, red, leaf-like *foliate papillae* are located in posterior third of tongue on lateral aspect which contains taste buds. *Circumvallate papillae* are 8–12 in number, mushroom-shaped, arranged in large-V shaped, row near posterior third of the dorsum tongue and contains plenty of taste buds. Small circular opening just posterior to this V row in the midline is called as *foramen cecum* which is the remnant of thyroglossal duct. Shallow groove just behind the circumvallate papilla on either sides of the foramen cecum is called as *terminal sulcus*. Numerous mucin glands and lymph follicles in the posterior third of the dorsum of tongue are called as lingual tonsils. *Posterior third of the tongue is difficult to inspect*; it needs head light, and spatula. It is better felt than seen. *Ventral surface* is smooth, has a median fold, *frenulum linguae* and deep lingual veins on either side. *Lingual frenulum* is attached about 10–15 mm below the mandibular central incisor tooth. *In tongue*

In three words I can sum up everything I've learned about life: it goes on—**Robert Frost**

tie, it is only 3-4 mm below the central incisor. It is congenital short frenulum; which is better seen when tip of the tongue is rolled upward.

Floor of the mouth: It is U-shaped area bounded by lower gum and oral tongue. It ends posteriorly at the insertion of anterior tonsillar pillar into the tongue. Sublingual papilla is present on each side of the frenulum; on summit of which is the opening of the duct (Wharton's) of submandibular salivary gland. Laterally and behind this papilla, sublingual fold is present which overlies the sublingual gland. Genioglossus and geniohyoid muscles are deeper to it. On either side, mylohyoid muscles form the muscular part of the floor of the mouth. It arises from mylohyoid ridge of the mandible extending up to the 3rd molar tooth. Submandibular salivary gland rests on the external surface of mylohyoid muscle; only small deeper part extends into the internal surface. Submandibular salivary duct runs about 5 cm between sublingual gland and genioglossus to end in papilla. Lingual and hypoglossal nerves are closely related to gland and duct. Alveolingual sulcus is valley shaped space between tongue and mandibular alveolar bone. Tip of the tongue should be kept upward to touch the palate to inspect the floor of the mouth.

Palate

Roof of the mouth is formed by hard palate and soft palate.

Hard palate is firm anterior part of the roof of the mouth ending opposite 3rd molars, anterior to fovea palatine. *Soft palate* is mobile posterior part of the roof of the mouth. Junction between hard and soft palate is called as *vibrating line*. Small rounded elevation of tissue in the midline behind the central incisors is called as *nasopalatine papilla* which lies over incisive foramen through which nasopalatine nerve traverses to supply anterior hard palate. Slightly elevated central line is called as palatine raphe. Here mucosa is firmly adherent to underneath periosteum without any fat and so it is harder area of hard palate. Sides of hard palate contain fat and minor salivary glands (there are around 350 minor salivary glands in posterior hard palate). Series of elevations in hard palate are called as *palatine rugae,* useful for food positioning and aiding tongue to produce specific sounds. Hard palate is partition between nasal and oral cavity. Anterior 2/3rd is formed by palatine process of maxillae; posterior 1/3rd is by horizontal plates of palatine bones. Anterolateral margins continue with alveolar arches and gums. Posterior margin attaches to soft palate.

Soft palate is more red than hard palate due to its vascularity. There is no bone in soft palate behind vibrating line. Soft palate vibrates or moves. It is mobile muscular fold. It has got anterior and posterior surfaces, superior and inferior margins. Uvula is small fleshy part projecting from center of the posterior margin of the soft palate. Pair of pits on either side of the center of the soft palate just behind the vibrating line is called as *fovea palatini* to which palatine mucous glands open. Side of the uvula has got anterior and posterior folds. Anterior palatoglossal arch contains palatoglossus muscle ends as anterior pillar of fauces (in front of tonsils). Posterior palatophayngeal arch contains palatopharyngeus muscle ends as posterior pillar of fauces (behind tonsils). Soft palate contains mucous glands and taste buds. Soft palate contains following muscles—tensor veli palati; levator veli palati; musculus uvulae; palatoglossus; palatopharyngeus. All muscles except tensor palati are supplied through pharyngeal plexus through cranial part of accessory nerve; tensor palati is supplied by the mandibular nerve. General sensory nerves are derived from middle and posterior palatine nerves which are branches of maxillary nerve and from glossopharyngeal nerve. Gustatory

The way to get started is to quit talking and begin doing—**Walt Disney**

special sensations are carried through lesser palatine nerve → greater petrosal nerve → geniculate ganglion of facial nerve → nucleus of solitary tract. Secretomotor fibers are derived from superior salivatory nucleus through greater palatine nerve and lesser palatine nerves. Paralysis of the soft palate (vagus nerve lesions) causes nasal regurgitation of liquids, nasal twang in voice, flattening of palatal arch.

RANULA

(*Rana = Frog*, **ranula looks like belly of frog, hence the name**).

Ranula is an *extravasation cyst arising from sublingual gland.* Only occasionally it arises from the submandibular salivary gland.

Features (Fig. 21.1)

- *It presents as*—bluish, smooth, well localized, nontender, soft, fluctuant, brilliantly transilluminant swelling in the lateral aspect of the floor of the mouth adjacent to ventral surface of the tongue.

- It often extends into the submandibular region through the deeper part of the posterior margin of mylohyoid muscle and is called as *plunging ranula. Plunging ranula* is *cross-fluctuant* across mylohyoid muscle. Swelling will be seen and felt both in the floor of the mouth in oral cavity and in the submandibular region of neck. If one side (floor of the mouth) of the swelling is pressed, elevation/raise will be felt in the fingers placed on the other side (neck). It is *bidigitally* palpable.
- Ranula has a delicate fibrous capsule and is lined by a layer of macrophages. It contains clear fluid.

Clinical features of ranula
• Bluish swelling in the floor of the mouth.
• Laterally placed, nontender.
• Fluctuant and cross fluctuant.
• Brilliantly transilluminant.

Differential Diagnosis

- Lymph cyst.
- Sublingual dermoid.

Treatment

- Initially *marsupialization* can be done and later when the wall of the ranula gets thickened, it is excised.
- If ranula is small, it can be excised directly.
- Sublingual salivary gland excision may be needed often. It is done under general anesthesia through intraoral approach. One should avoid injuring lingual nerve and submandibular salivary gland duct. Only when there is a need to excise submandibular salivary gland approach through neck is used.

Note:
Marsupial means pouch where baby is kept, carried and sucked on the mother's belly in kangaroo.

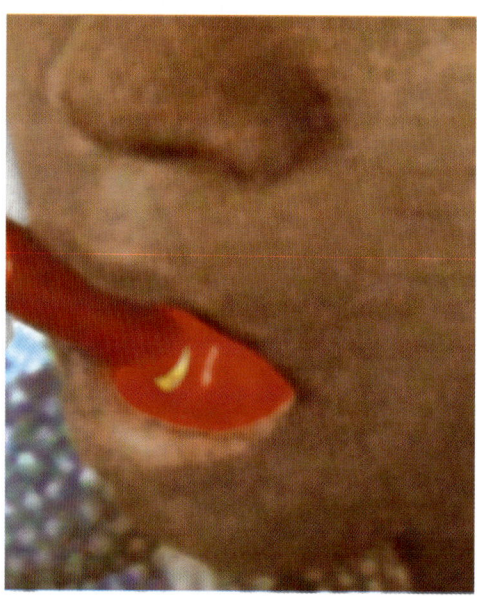

Fig. 21.1: Ranula—it is brilliantly transilluminant.

Wisdom in the man, patience in the wife, brings peace to the house and a happy life

SUBLINGUAL DERMOIDS

They are *sequestration dermoids* lined by squamous epithelium containing keratin.

Types

1. ***Median sublingual dermoid***:
   - It is derived from epithelial cell rests at the level of fusion of *two mandibular arches*.
   - It is located between two genial muscles, above the level of mylohyoid muscle.
   - It is a midline swelling which is smooth, soft, cystic, nontender, nontransilluminant.
   - **Treatment** is excision through per oral approach.
   - Complication is abscess formation.
2. ***Lateral sublingual dermoid***:
   - It develops in relation to submandibular duct, lingual nerve and stylohyoid ligament.
   - It is derived from *first branchial arch*.
   - It forms a swelling in the lateral aspect of the floor of the mouth.
   - **Treatment:** Small dermoids are removed per orally; larger one, through submandibular incision.

STOMATITIS

It is inflammation of oral mucosa by trauma, radiotherapy, chemicals, nutritional deficiency or infection.

- *Traumatic stomatitis* may be due to dentures, teeth bite, and brushing of teeth harshly which presents as painful thin covering of furr with increased salivation. Proper mouthwash will cure the condition.
- *Aphthous stomatitis* is seen in malnutrition, debility, steroid usage. Presentation is as multiple hyperemic painful vesicles later forming deep round painful ulcers. It is treated with mouthwash and if needed by antibiotics. Recurrent aphthous stomatitis with ulcers is often familial, more common in women, common in lip, cheek, tongue which are very painful with more salivation. It heals spontaneously. But during active period, it interferes with speech, swallowing distressfully. It is treated by many drugs like Levamisole, antibiotics, vitamin B and C, local applications of anesthetics (Xylocaine)/choline salicylate/ benzalkonium chloride.
- *Candida stomatitis* (Monilia thrush) is due to fungal infection, *Candida albicans* which is seen in diabetics, individuals on steroid therapy, long-term antibiotics, patients who are bedridden, on prolonged ICU care, in infants, debility. Initially appears as multiple red spots in the tongue and buccal area which are painful, which later turn into curdy white patches. Often it extends into pharynx and esophagus causing dysphagia. It is treated with antifungal drugs like Clotrimazole or Fluconazole. *Rhagades* occur at corners of mouth in congenital syphilis leaving radiating scar and furrow.
- *Vincent's ulcerative st*omatitis (*Vincent's angina/trench mouth) is* due to infection by Gram –ve anaerobic *Borrelia vincentii and Fusiformis fusiformis*. It is common in adolescents and young adults below the age of 35 years. Presents with fever, excessive salivation, red swollen gums with painful ulcers covered with yellow slough (*pseudomembrane*) which can be removed like *membrane—ulcerative gingivitis*. From the gums it spreads to cheek, palate, and pharynx. Tongue involvement is uncommon. Tender neck lymph nodes are palpable. *Musty foetor oris* is typical. Edentulous patients will not develop this infection. Infection in tonsillar crypts is called as *Vincent's angina*. It is confirmed by swab culture. It is treated by antibiotics (penicillin group); peeling of membrane, mouthwash, supportive measures, vitamin B and C.
- *Nutritional stomatitis* is due to—(1) vitamin B deficiency like nicotinic acid (pellagra), riboflavin deficiency. It is common in

*We are all like the bright moon, we still have our darker side—**Kalil Gibran***

tongue presenting as red area with atrophy of papillae. (2) Vitamin C deficiency is commonly seen as bleeding gums and loosening of teeth. (3) Iron deficiency anemia causes superficial glossitis, mainly in females.

* *Angular stomatitis* is superficial lengthy red brown fissures/ulcers in and around the angle of the mouth with cracks. Candida and streptococcal infections are common. It is often called as *cheilosis/perleche*. It is treated with vitamin B, C, iron and protein supplements with adequate oral hygiene. Perleche is seen in children who suck their finger.

CANCRUM ORIS (NOMA)

* It is an infective gangrene, a severe form of Vincent's acute ulcerative gingivitis and stomatitis.
* Seen in poorly nourished, ill child due to *Borrelia vincentii* and *Fusiformis bacteriae*.
* It starts in gums, spreads into cheek, bone, soft tissues and skin causing extensive tissue loss with severe toxemia.
* There will be other secondary infection also.

Treatment

* Systemic antibiotics, high dose Penicillins, Metronidazole.
* High protein and vitamin rich diet, through nasogastric tube.
* Wound irrigation and liberal removal of the dead tissue.
* Blood transfusion, total parenteral nutrition (TPN).
* Later patient requires flaps to cover the defect.

It has got high mortality.

LEUKOPLAKIA

It is a white patch in the mucosa of the oral cavity that cannot be characterized clinically or pathologically to any other disease. It is a premalignant condition.

Types

1. *Homogenous*.
2. *Nodular*—more potentially malignant.
3. *Speckled*—more potentially malignant.

Clinically the lesion appears as white or grayish colored, well-localized patch in the cheek, tongue, palate or other areas of the oral cavity (Fig. 21.2).

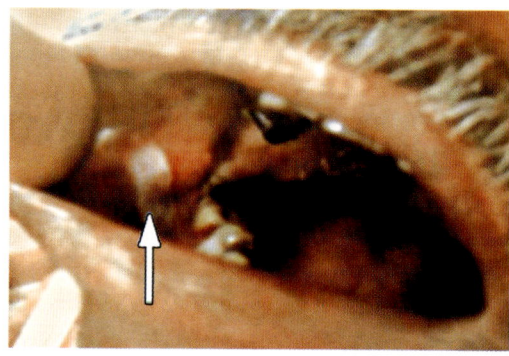

Fig. 21.2: Leukoplakia cheek. Note the typical white patch. It is a premalignant condition.

Common causes
• Smoking.
• Spirit.
• Sepsis.
• Superficial glossitis.
• Syphilis.
• Spices.
• Sharp tooth.
• Susceptibility.
• *Pan* chewing using areca, tobacco, slaked lime.
• Chronic hypertrophic candidiasis (long standing candidial infection).

Incidence

* *Incidence of* leukoplakia in those who smoke or chew pan is 20%, whereas incidence in non-smokers is 1%.
* *Incidence of* leukoplakia turning into malignancy is 2–4%. It increases with age, duration of the pan chewing, smoking.

Every man is the master of his own fortune

Histology

Parakeratosis with widening of rete pegs.

Histological staging
• Acanthosis.
• Parakeratosis.
• Widening of retepegs.
• Dyskeratosis.
• Dysplasia.
• Carcinoma in situ.

Biopsy confirms the diagnosis as well as rules out the carcinoma.

Treatment

- Pan chewing and smoking has to be stopped.
- Excision, if required skin grafting has to be done.
- Regular follow up is necessary.

ERYTHROPLAKIA (FIG. 21.3)

- It is *red velvety* appearance of the mucosa, which cannot characterize any recognized condition.
- It is 17–20 times more potentially malignant than leukoplakia.
- Histologically *parakeratosis with severe epithelial dysplasia* is the typical feature.
- Diagnosis is by biopsy.

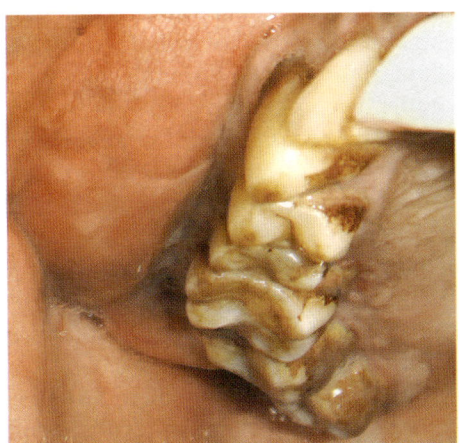

Fig. 21.3: Erythroplakia of cheek.

Treatment

Biopsy and surgical excision.

ORAL SUBMUCOSAL FIBROSIS

- It is a progressive fibrosis deep to the mucosa of the oral cavity, which causes *trismus and ankyloglossia.*
- The mucosa of cheek, gingivae, palate and tongue shows a *mottled/marbled pallor* (Fig. 21.4).
- It is common in Asians and Indians.

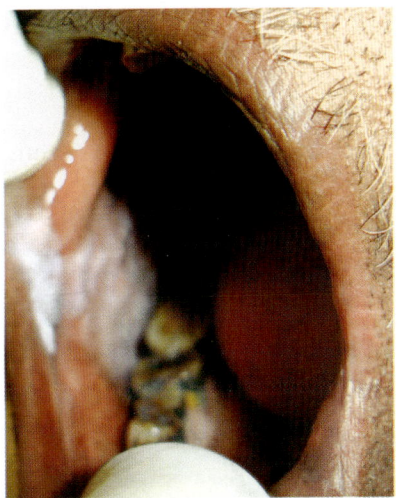

Fig. 21.4: Submucosal fibrosis of right cheek. Note the stiff fibrotic bands and scarring.

Etiology

- Hypersensitivity to chilli, betelnut, tobacco and vitamin deficiencies probably alter the collagen metabolism leading to juxtaepithelial fibrosis, epithelial atrophy and dysplasia.
- **4.5–7.6%** of oral submucosal fibrosis can turn into *malignancy.*

Treatment

- Precipitating factors have to be avoided.
- Surgical excision when required, followed by skin grafting has to be done.

*We choose our joys and sorrows long before we experience them—**Kalil Gibran***

PREMALIGNANT CONDITIONS OF THE ORAL CAVITY

High risks: These are lesions with definite risk of malignant change.
- Leukoplakia.
- Erythroplakia.
- Chronic hyperplastic candidiasis is due to *Candida albicans* infection.

Medium risks: Premalignant but not associated with higher incidence of carcinoma.
- Oral submucosal fibrosis.
- Syphilitic glossitis.
- Sideropenic dysphagia.

Equivocal risk lesions
- Oral lichen planus.
- Dyskeratosis congenita.
- Discoid lupus erythematosus.

Premalignant conditions of oral cavity
- Leukoplakia.
- Erythroplakia.
- Chronic hyperplastic candidiasis.
- Oral submucosal fibrosis.
- Syphilitic glossitis.
- Sideropenic dysphagia.
- Oral lichen planus.
- Discoid lupus erythematosus.
- Dyskeratosis congenita.

ORAL AND UPPER AERODIGESTIVE CANCERS

- It is one of the commonest cancers in Asian countries and India (40%).
- All 'S' mentioned probably are the causative agents. Smoking, quid of chewing pan are important causes. Tobacco, betel nut, alcohol, *human papilloma virus* (*present in 80% of oral cancers*; present in 40% normal individual), Epstein-Barr virus, vitamin A deficiency, Plummer Vinson syndrome, bad dental hygiene, denture irritation are etiologies. Risk is 8 times in tobacco users; 10 times with quid users; 30 times with night quid users.
- Alcohol increases the solubility of carcinogen and suppresses the DNA repair.
- Incidence of oral cancer in India is 28 per 1,00,000 population. Commonest oral cancer in India is of buccal mucosa (more than 70%).
- In West, in oral cavity—it is common in tongue (50%), buccal mucosa (25%), floor (15%), gums and others (10%).
- Leukoplakia (*commonest*), erythroplakia, chronic hyperplastic candidiasis are *precancerous lesions*; submucosal fibrosis, syphilitic glossitis, sideropenic dysphagia are *precancerous conditions*. Oral lichen planus, discoid lupus, dyskeratosis congenita are doubtful associated lesions. *Precancerous lesion* is one where cancer is more likely to occur; *precancerous condition* is one where there is increased risk of cancer.
- Upper aerodigestive cancers include that of oral cavity, larynx, and pharynx. Depending on anatomical location, they present with different features other than common features—trismus, ear pain, hoarseness of voice, dysphagia, ankyloglossia.
- Usually they are locoregional disease with high affinity to involve regional lymph nodes. Distant spread is *rare except* in nasopharyngeal carcinoma. Tongue has *highest* incidence of nodal spread, then floor of the mouth, lower alveolus, cheek, upper alveolus and palate.
- Multiple *synchronous* (at same time, 10%) de novo sites and or *metachronous* (at different periods, 15%) multiple sites may be seen.
- Cancers in posterior third of tongue and floor of the mouth are often missed on clinical examination—*coffin corner or sump area*.
- Primary may be very small to be detected clinically in places like fossa of Rosenmuller, pyriform fossa, nasopharynx, posterior

A man who does nothing never has time to do anything

third tongue but present clinically as hard lymph node secondaries in neck called as *secondaries with unknown primary*. Hard secondaries in neck confirmed by fine needle aspiration cytology (FNAC) but all investigations including blind biopsies, CT head and neck region and endoscopies could not identify the primary lesion creates a situation called as secondaries in neck nodes with an *occult primary (30%)*.

- *Trismus* (pterygoid muscle involvement), *ear pain* due to auriculotemporal nerve involvement, *eye pain* in nasopharyngeal carcinoma, *dysphagia* due to tongue involvement mainly the posterior third, *hearing loss* due to spread to Eustachian tube can occur.
- Bronchopneumonia, aspiration are common problems.
- Biopsy, endoscopy, CT neck, magnetic resonance imaging (MRI), chest X-ray are different investigations needed, depending on anatomical location of lesion.
- Staging will help to plan the treatment and predict prognosis.
- Surgical wide excision and radiotherapy are main modalities of treatment. Chemotherapy is used as an adjuvant. Curative treatment in early growth aims at preservation of functions like swallowing, speech, cosmesis; but with adequate oncological clearance is the principle of surgical approach. Radiotherapy is also used as curative therapy.
- Palliative chemotherapy, radiotherapy and surgery can be done depending on location of the lesion.
- Involvement of mandible, neck nodes—number, size, and fixity alters the prognosis and treatment schedule.
- Outcome also depends on the anatomical location of the malignancy. Lip carries better prognosis; tongue has poor prognosis.
- General principles used in approaching oral cancers are as follows (however, it depends on grading and staging of the tumor):

  - If only primary is present which is mucosal with size less than 2 cm without nodal spread, then wide local excision with supraomohyoid block dissection of same side is done (N0); primary also may be treated with curative brachytherapy or external beam teletherapy. If nodes are histologically positive then radical neck dissection is done.
  - Larger mucosal primary with similar features are also treated similarly; but postoperative radiotherapy or/and chemotherapy is added depending on grading of the tumor.
  - In all these types of lesions, if there are positive mobile neck nodes which are confirmed by FNAC, then radical neck dissection should be done.
  - If primary lesion extends into adjacent soft tissue with mandibular involvement then mandibular resection (marginal mandibular/segmental/partial/hemimandibulectomy) is needed. Part is reconstructed using plates or bone graft taken from iliac crest or opposite 11th rib. 2.4 mm reconstruction plate with pectoralis major myocutaneous flap (PMMF) or nonvascularized bone graft (iliac crest cancellous chips) or vascularized bone graft from fibula/iliac crest/scapula are the present recommendations. Skin covering is done by split skin graft inside to mucosa or by appropriate flaps depending on the need and feasibility of the donor area (PMMF/DP flap/forehead flap). Neck is addressed similarly. Postoperative external beam radiotherapy (EBRT) and chemotherapy is needed either concurrent or sequential.
  - If primary is advanced then chemotherapy with EBRT is used. If lesion reduces in size and becomes operable it is then operated accordingly.
  - In fixed primary or secondary, RT with chemotherapy is used; palliation to relieve pain, fungation, sepsis.

*The smallest act of kindness is worth more than the greatest intention—**Kalil Gibran***

- In advanced stage, terminal events may be severe malnutrition, bleeding, sepsis, and bronchopneumonia.
- Posterior lesions have got poor prognosis than anterior lesions. Lip carries best. Prognosis depends on anatomical location, grading, lymph node status, soft tissue involvement and response of therapy.

Carcinoma of Gingivobuccal Complex

- It is cancer squamous cell carcinoma (SCC) involving *buccal mucosa and gingiva* etiology of which is keeping tobacco quid in gingivobuccal sulcus.
- It is often called as *Indian oral cancer* as it is most commonly seen in India.
- Buccal mucosa extends from upper to lower alveolus; from commissure in front to retromolar region behind.
- Features and management are same. Marginal mandibulectomy/segmental resection is commonly needed.
- Adjuvant RT and chemotherapy is useful.

CARCINOMA CHEEK (BUCCAL MUCOSA)

- *Squamous cell carcinoma is the most common type of carcinoma of the cheek* (Fig. 21.5).
- Occasionally it can be adenocarcinoma arising from the minor salivary glands or mucous glands. Rarely it can also be melanoma.

Sites of carcinoma in oral cavity in order	
In India (Fig. 21.6)	In Western countries
• Cheek—*commonest*	• Tongue
• Floor of the mouth	• Floor of the mouth
• Palate	• Lip
• Lips	• Cheek

Malignancies of the oral cavity
• *Squamous cell carcinoma—commonest.*
• Minor salivary gland tumors.
• Melanomas.
• Adenocarcinomas—rare.
• Sarcomas—rare.

Precipitating factors:
All *'S'*—*Smoking, Spirit, Syphilis, Sharp tooth, Sepsis, Spices.*

Premalignant conditions	
• Leukoplakia.	• Submucosal fibrosis.
• Erythroplakia.	• Hyperplastic candidiasis.

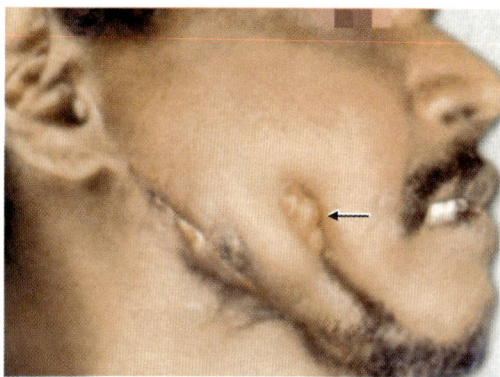

Fig. 21.5: Recurrent carcinoma cheek (postsurgical).

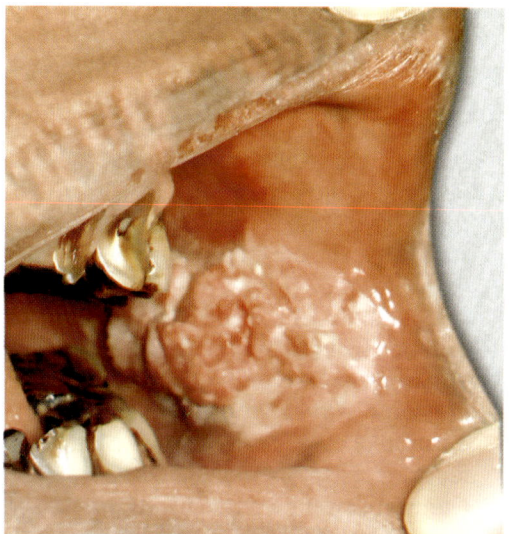

Fig. 21.6: Carcinoma buccal mucosa. It is commonest oral cancer in India.

To read without reflecting is like eating without digesting

Betel nut chewing (pan, with pan quid kept in cheek pouch for a long time) is an important causative factor of carcinoma cheek.

Types
Ulcerative; Proliferative (exophytic); Verrucous.

Verrucous carcinoma (Fig. 21.7):
- It occurs as a superficial proliferative exophytic lesion with minimal deep invasion.
- Lesion has got white, dry, velvety or warty, keratinized surface.
- It is of low grade, very well-differentiated squamous cell carcinoma, which is locally malignant without any lymphatic spread.
- It is a curable malignancy.
- After biopsy, treatment is *wide excision*. *Radiotherapy is not given* as it may lead to anaplastic transformation.

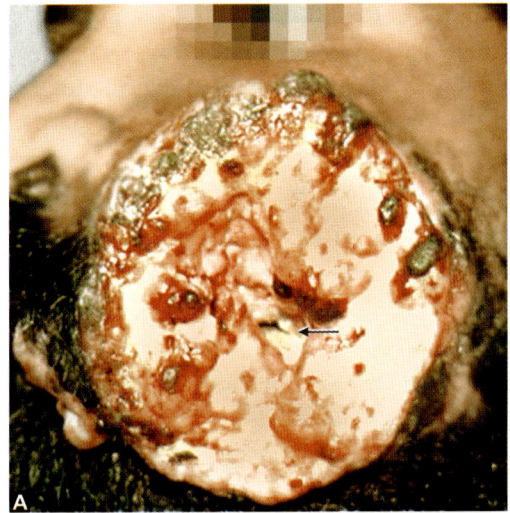

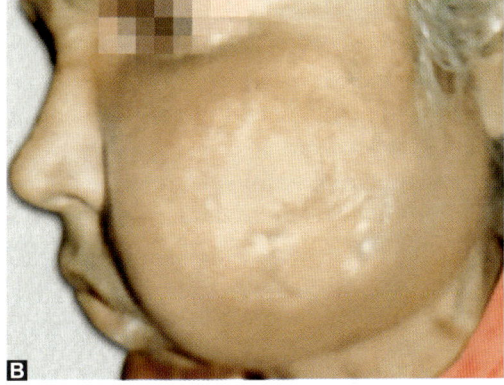

Figs. 21.8A and B: Advanced carcinoma cheek in two different patients. In first male patient there is fungation with orocutaneous fistula.

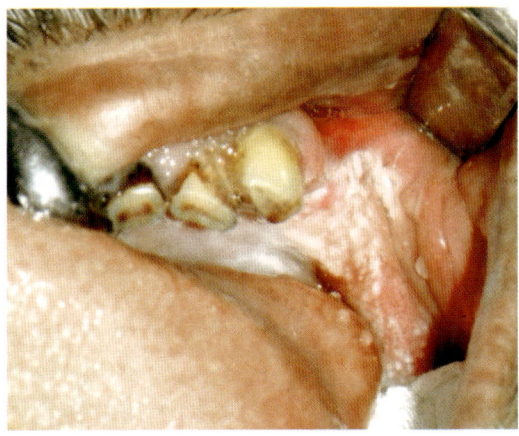

Fig. 21.7: Verrucous carcinoma of oral cavity at gingiobuccal sulcus with leukoplakia.

Biological Behavior of Carcinoma Cheek (Figs. 21.8A and B)
- Carcinoma cheek is more common in posterior half of cheek than anterior.
- It spreads into the deeper plane to involve buccinator, pterygoids; into the retromolar trigone, base of the skull, pharynx.
- It spreads outward to involve the skin causing fungation, ulceration, orocutaneous fistula formation.
- Mandible is commonly involved either by direct extension or through subperiosteal lymphatic plexus, which communicates freely with oral lymphatics.
- Lymph nodes commonly involved are submental, submandibular, and deep cervical and often lateral pharyngeal groups.
- Infection of the tumor area and soft tissues around is common; causing fever, foul smelling ulcer, and halitosis.

*Make improvements, not excuses. Seek respect, not attention—**Roy T Bennett***

- Respiratory infection is common in these patients.
- Dysphagia occurs when tumor extends into the retromolar region, soft palate, pharynx.

Clinical Features

- *Ulcer* in the cheek which gradually increases in size in a patient with history of chewing pan or smoking.
- *Pain* occurs when it involves the skin, bone or if secondarily infected. Referred pain into the ear signifies involvement of lingual nerve.
- *Involvement of retromolar trigone* indicates that it is an advanced disease, as the lymphatics here communicate freely with the pharyngeal lymphatics.
- *Everted edge, induration* are the typical features of the ulcer. Induration occurs in the edge and base.
- Bidigital examination of mandible is done to look for thickening, tenderness, and sites of fracture.
- *Trismus and dysphagia* signify involvement of pterygoids, or posterior extension.
- Occasionally, it may extend into the *upper alveolus and to the maxilla* causing swelling, pain and tenderness.
- Submandibular lymph nodes and upper deep cervical lymph nodes are involved which are hard, nodular, initially mobile but later get fixed to each other and then to deeper structure.
    - Once lymph nodes get fixed, it may infiltrate into hypoglossal nerve (tongue deviates toward the same side), spinal accessory nerve (defective shrugging of shoulder) and cervical sympathetic chain (*Horner's syndrome*).
    - Compression over external carotid artery causes absence of superficial temporal artery pulsation.
    - Eventually it causes fungation and bleeding from major vessels—***carotid blowout***.

TNM staging for oral cavity cancers (AJCC 2018 edition)

T – Primary tumor
Tx – Primary tumor cannot be assessed.
Tis – Carcinoma in situ.
T1 – Tumor ≤2 cm with DOI (depth of invasion) ≤5 mm.
T2 – Tumor <2 cm with DOI >5 mm OR tumor 2–4 cm in size with DOI ≤10 mm.
T3 – Tumor 2–4 cm with SOI >10 mm OT tumor >4 cm with DOI ≤10 mm.
T4a – Moderately advanced local disease: Tumor >4 cm with DOI >10 mm OT tumor invading adjacent structures only like cortical bone of mandible or maxilla or involves the maxillary sinus or skin of the face. Note: Superficial erosion of bone/tooth socket by a gingival primary is not sufficient to classify as T4.
T4b – Very advanced local disease: Tumor invades masticator space, pterygoid plates or skull base and/or encasing the internal carotid artery.
Note: DOI is Depth Of Invasion NOT tumor thickness.
N – Nodal spread
Nx – Nodes cannot be assessed.
N0 – No regional lymph node spread.
N1 – Regional single node <3 cm with ENE (–).
N2 – N2a: Single ipsilateral node <3 cm with ENE (+); OR single ipsilateral node 3–6 cm with ENE (–). N2b: Multiple ipsilateral nodes <6 cm in size and ENE (–). N2c: Bilateral or contralateral nodes <6 cm with ENE (–).
N3 – N3a: Single ipsilateral node >6 cm with ENE (-). N3b: single ipsilateral node >3 cm with ENE (+) OR multiple ipsilateral or contralateral or bilateral any sized nodes with ENE (+) OR single contralateral node of any size with ENE (+).
Note: ENE means extra nodal extension; ENE_{mi} is microscopic metastases <2 mm; ENE_{ma} is macroscopic >2 mm. Suffix – *sn* is for SLN biopsy; *f* is for FNAC or core biopsy; *u* is nodes above lower border of the cricoid; *l* is nodes below the lower border of cricoid.
M – Distant metastases
cM0 – Distant spread not present.
cM1 – Distant metastases present.
pM1 – Distant metastases, microscopically confirmed.

Diseases of the soul are more dangerous than those of the body

Staging groups

Stage 0 – Tis N0 M0
Stage I – T1 N0 M0
Stage II – T2 N0 M0
Stage III – T3 N0 M0; T1,T2,T3 N1 M0
Stage IV – **IVA:** T4a N0/N1 M0; T1,T2,T3,T4a N2 M0.
IVB: Any T N3 M0; T4b any N M0. **IVC:** Any T Any N M1.

Features of advanced carcinoma cheek (Fig. 21.9)

- Involvement of retromolar trigone.
- Extension into the base of skull and pharynx.
- Fixed neck lymph nodes.
- Extension to the opposite side.

- FNAC from lymph nodes (no biopsy from lymph nodes).
- CT scans—to assess the extension of tumor and its secondaries.
- Orthopantamogram to look for the involvement of mandible—destruction and fracture sites (Fig. 21.10).

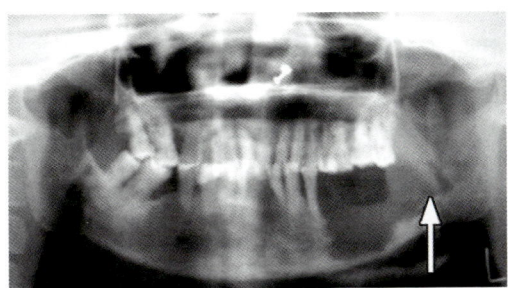

Fig. 21.10: Orthopantomogram showing secondaries in mandible.

Treatment

Treatment may *be curative or palliative.*

Treatment strategy

- **Surgery** (Fig. 21.11): Wide excision, hemimandibulectomy, neck lymph nodes block dissection.
- **Radiotherapy**: Curative or palliative; external or brachytherapy.
- **Chemotherapy**: Intra-arterial, IV or orally.

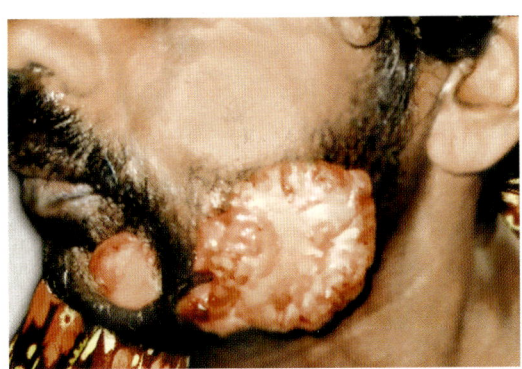

Fig. 21.9: Advanced stage 4 carcinoma cheek.

Investigations

- *Wedge biopsy* usually taken from two sites. Biopsy has to be taken from the edge as it contains active cells; not from the center as it is the area of necrosis.
  Malignant *squamous cells with epithelial pearls (Keratin pearls)* are the histological features.

Broder's histological grading

1. Well-differentiated — >75% epithelial pearls.
2. Moderately differentiated — 50–75% epithelial pearls.
3. Poorly differentiated — 25–50% epithelial pearls.
4. De-differentiated — <25% epithelial pearls.

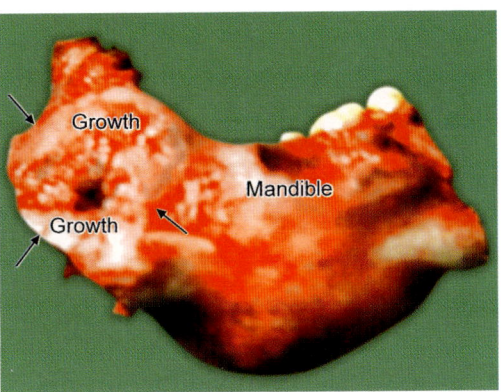

Fig. 21.11: Resected specimen after hemimandibulectomy.
(*Courtesy:* Dr Jagadishchandra, MDS)

Never lose hope. Storms make people stronger and never last forever—**Roy T Bennett**

- **Early growth without bone involvement**:
    - *Curative radiotherapy* using Cesium¹³⁷ needles or Iridium¹⁹² wires, i.e. brachytherapy.
      Advantages are that:
        - Surgery is avoided.
        - No surgical mutilation and parts are retained.
        - As it is a squamous cell carcinoma, primary is radiosensitive.
    - Other option is *wide excision with 1–2 cm clearance*. Often, the approach to the tumor is by raising the cheek flap (outside). After the wide excision, the flap is placed back (**Patterson operation**).
    - Presently advanced technology in radiotherapy, facilitates the use of external radiotherapy also. The incidence of dreaded complication like *osteoradionecrosis of mandible* has reduced due to better RT methods.
- **Growth with mandible involvement (Figs. 21.12 to 21.14)**: Here along with wide excision of the primary tumor, hemimandibulectomy or segmental resection of the mandible or marginal mandibulectomy (using rotary electric saw) is done.
- **Operable growth with mandible involvement and mobile lymph nodes on same side** (confirmed by FNAC): Along with wide excision of the primary, hemimandibulectomy and radical neck lymph node dissection is done (*Commando-like operation*) (Fig. 21.15).
- **Operable growth with mandible involvement; mobile lymph nodes on same side and opposite side**: Along with wide excision of the tumor, hemimandibulectomy, radical neck lymph node dissection on same side and functional block dissection on opposite side are done, retaining the internal jugular vein, sternomastoid, spinal accessory nerve.
- **Operable primary tumor with mobile lymph nodes on same side but without mandibular involvement**: Wide excision

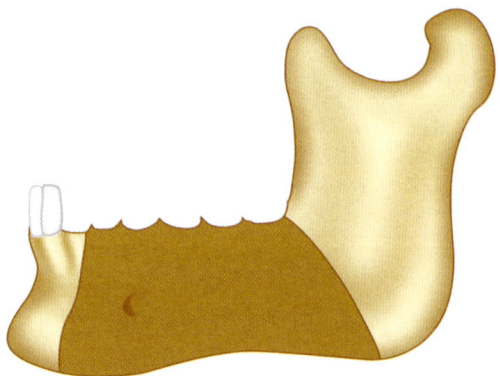

Fig. 21.13: Segmental resection of the mandible.

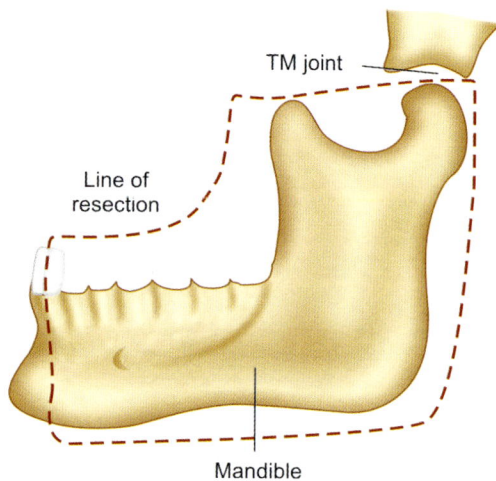

Fig. 21.14: Hemimandibulectomy.

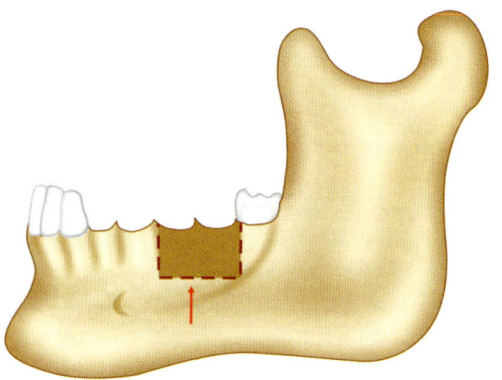

Fig. 21.12: Marginal mandibulectomy.

*Maturity is when you stop complaining and making excuses, and start making changes—**Roy T Bennett***

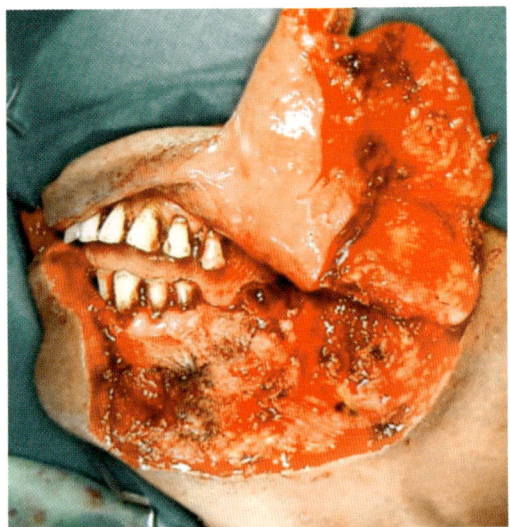

Fig. 21.15: Carcinoma cheek, ontable wide excision. It requires pectoralis major myocutaneous flap for reconstruction.

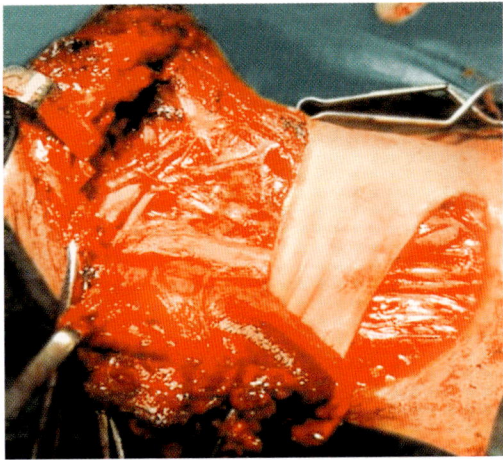

Fig. 21.16: Radical neck dissection for secondaries in neck through McFee incision.

of primary tumor and radical neck lymph node dissection on same side are done. Mandible is not removed (Fig. 21.16).
- **Fixed primary tumor or advanced neck lymph node secondaries**: Only palliative *external radiotherapy* is given to palliate pain, fungation and to prevent anticipated torrential hemorrhage.

- ❖ **Preoperative radiotherapy is often used in fixed lymph nodes to downstage** the disease so as to make it operable.
- ❖ **Postoperative radiotherapy is given in T_3 and T_4 tumors**; N_2 and N_3 nodal status to reduce the recurrence and to improve the prognosis.
- ❖ **Prophylactic block dissection has become popular**.
  Reasons are—even though clinically, lymph nodes are negative there may be microscopic involvement of lymph nodes (25–65%). Clinically detectable disease in lymph nodes of the patient signifies extracapsular spread, which has got poor prognosis. Recurrence rate is less after prophylactic block compared to block dissection with clinically positive nodes because there is no extracapsular spread in the former even if there is microscopic spread of tumor in many cases. Block dissection is an acceptable surgery as there is negligible mortality and less morbidity.
- ❖ **If growth is extending to upper alveolus**: Partial maxillectomy or total maxillectomy may be required.
- ❖ **Role of chemotherapy**: Drugs used are Methotrexate, Vincristine, Bleomycin, Adriamycin.
  Often it is given intra-arterially through external carotid artery using *arterial pump* or by increasing the height of the drip more than 13 feet so as to attain a pressure more than systolic pressure. Chemotherapy can also be given IV or orally.

Reconstruction after surgery (Figs. 21.17 to 21.20)

- Split skin graft.
- Deltopectoral cutaneous flap-based on 2nd perforator of internal mammary artery.
- Forehead flap-based on anterior branch of superficial temporal artery.
- Pectoralis major myocutaneous flap-based on thoracoacromial artery.
- Mandible reconstruction by cortical bone graft or rib, fibula or synthetic material.
- Free flaps (microvascular).

The mill gains by going, not by standing still

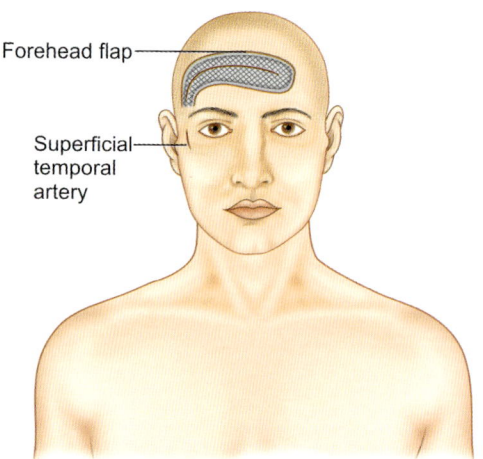

Fig. 21.17: Forehead flap is used after wide excision of carcinoma cheek. It is based on anterior branch of superficial temporal artery.

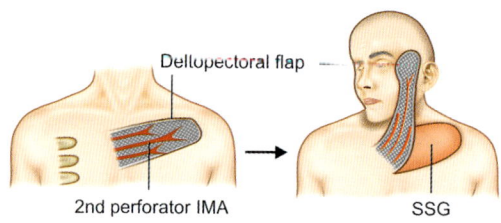

Fig. 21.18: Deltopectoral flap used to cover defect after surgical clearance in carcinoma cheek. It is based on 2nd perforator, a branch of internal mammary artery (IMA). (SSG: split-skin graft)

Problems with surgery
- (Surgical) mutilation.
- Anesthesia complications.
- Requirement for reconstruction.
- Mortality.
- Morbidity.

Problems with radiotherapy
- When mandible is irradiated, chances of the dreaded problem, osteoradionecrosis are high which requires the removal of mandible.
- Loss of taste and dryness.
- Infection.
- Skin excoriation.
- Trismus may get aggravated.
- Can itself cause dysphagia, laryngeal edema.

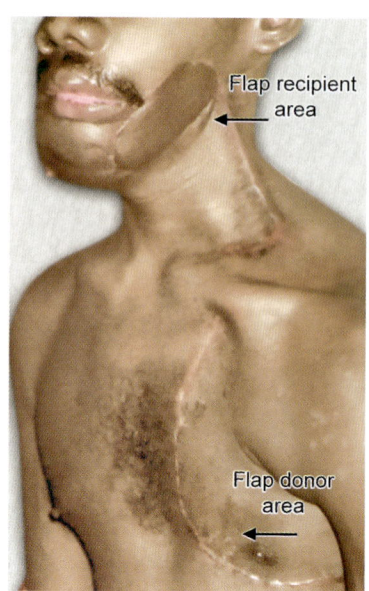

Fig. 21.19: Carcinoma cheek operated with radical neck dissection of same side lymph nodes. Reconstruction done using pectoralis major myocutaneous flap.

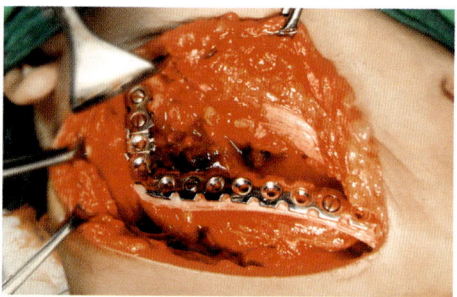

Fig. 21.20: Reconstruction of the mandible after hemimandibulectomy using plate and opposite rib fixation (*Courtesy:* Dr Jagadishchandra, MDS).

Problems with chemotherapy
- Bone marrow suppression.
- Megaloblastic anemia.
- GIT symptoms.
- Hepatotoxicity and renal toxicity.
- Alopecia.

LIP

❖ Lip begins at vermilion border. It has got upper lip, lower lip and oral commissure.

Fire proves gold, adversity proves men

Squamous cell carcinoma (SCC) is the commonest lip cancer (90%). SCC is common in lower lip; basal cell carcinoma (BCC) is common in upper lip. Other cancers in lip are spindle cell carcinoma, adenoid squamous carcinoma, malignant melanoma, minor salivary gland tumor.

- *Mucus cyst* of lip is a common condition. It can occur in upper or lower lip. It is a retention cyst derived from mucus glands of the lip. It presents as bluish, soft, fluctuant often transilluminating well-localized swelling. It may resolve on its own. If it does not, it should be excised under local anesthesia. Absorbable suture is used to appose the wound starting from vermilion margin. Usually vertical elliptical incision is used to excise. Sutured wound heals rapidly with very limited scar.
- *Macrocheilia* is enlargement of lip mass in other than neoplastic conditions. Lymphangioma is the commonest cause. Hemangioma, inflammatory conditions also can cause macrocheilia.
- Papilloma, lipoma, pyogenic granuloma, keratoacanthoma, minor salivary tumors are other swellings which can occur in lip.
- *Cheilitis* often associated with stomatitis is common in vitamin deficiency, malnutrition, sepsis, drug induced, RT induced presents as redness, pain, diffuse swelling. In chronic cases, there will be linear ulcers especially at commissure. *Actinic cheilitis* is a premalignant lesion. Cause is treated (Fig. 21.21).
- *Pigmentation* of lip occurs in Peutz Jegher's syndrome (brown), Addison's disease (black).
- *Herpes labialis* is formation ulcers in lip due to herpes simplex virus. Repeated multiple ulcers develop in lip. It is contagious by kissing. So kissing should be avoided including in children. Touching repeatedly can transfer the virus to eye causing herpes keratitis.
- Cleft lip is a common congenital condition.

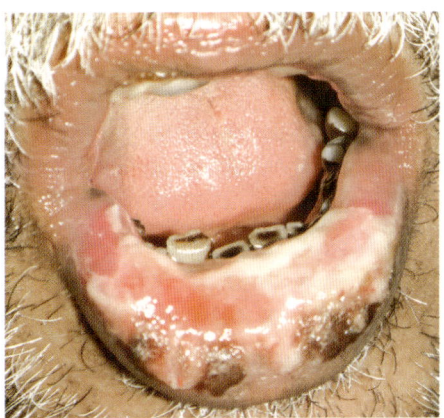

Fig. 21.21: Lip infection—cheilitis.

NEOPLASM OF LIP

- *Minor salivary gland tumors* are common in *upper lip*. They are usually *pleomorphic adenomas*.
- In lower lip, squamous cell carcinoma is common.

Note:
Lip is the commonest site of oral cancer.

CARCINOMA OF LIP

- Incidence is 10% (Figs. 21.22 and 21.23).
- It is more common in men (90%). Common in *lower lip (90%)*.

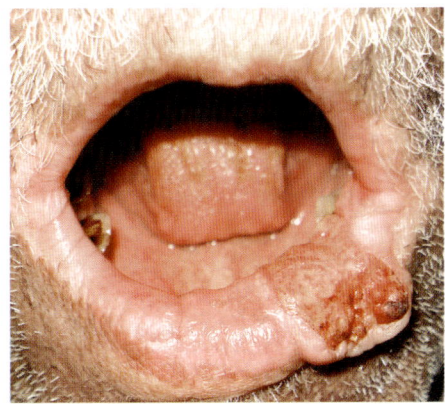

Fig. 21.22: Carcinoma lower lip (SCC is the commonest in lower lip).

Success isn't always about greatness; it's about consistency; Consistent hard work leads to success; Greatness will come— **Dwayne Johnson**

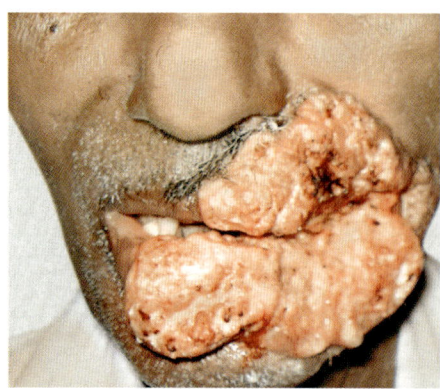

Fig. 21.23: Carcinoma lip. Note the proliferative lesion. Lower lip is commonly involved by squamous cell carcinoma.

- Commonly due to exposure to sunlight (ultraviolet rays).
- Initially starts as a red, granular dry lesion, which eventually gets ulcerated and forms an ulceroproliferative lesion. Occasionally it occurs at the angle of mouth. Verrucous carcinoma also can occur in lip.
- It spreads to submental nodes and later to other neck nodes on both sides.
- Usually it is a *well-differentiated squamous cell carcinoma*.

Causes

- Ultraviolet rays, smoking.
- Leukoplakia.
- *Agriculturists who are commonly exposed to sunlight get carcinoma lip more often and so it is called as countryman's lip.*
- **Khaini chewers** (tobacco + lime).

Clinical features of carcinoma lip

- Nonhealing progressive ulcer, painless to begin with.
- Everted edge with indurations.
- Growth moves with the lip.
- Submental, submandibular and upper deep neck nodes may get enlarged.
- In half of the cases, lymph nodes are enlarged due to infection or as reactive.
- Fungation, bleeding.

Differential Diagnosis

- Keratoacanthoma.
- Basal cell carcinoma, melanoma.
- Minor salivary gland tumors.
  Often carcinoma of lip is an extension from carcinoma of cheek.

Diagnosis

Wedge biopsy, FNAC of lymph nodes.

Treatment

- If lesion is less than 2 cm, then curative *radiotherapy is given*, either brachytherapy or external beam radiotherapy. It gives a good cure. Dose: 6000 cGy units.
- If tumor is more than 2 cms, *wide excision* is done. Excision up to one-third of lower lip can be sutured primarily in layers keeping vermillion border in proper apposition without causing any microstomia. Excision of more than one-third of the lip requires reconstruction using different flaps (Fig. 21.24).

Methods

- *Abbe-Estlander's rotation flap* is used for either upper or lower lip lesions of less than ½ of lip located at the angle based on labial artery (Figs. 21.25 and 21.26). Here base may or may not be divided at a later stage, even though it may cause some microstomia.
- *Fries' modified Bernard facial flap:* It is reconstruction using lateral facial flaps. It is used when defect is more than ½ of lip and midline.
- *Nasolabial flap* is used when defect is more than ½ of lip laterally or defect is in the floor of the mouth.
- *Abbe switch flap* is used for upper or lower lip lesions at the midline or at the site other than angle based on labial artery. Here base of the flap should be released at a later stage, once flap is taken over (Fig. 21.27).

*Knowing yourself is the beginning of all wisdom—**Aristotle***

Chapter 21 : Oral Cavity

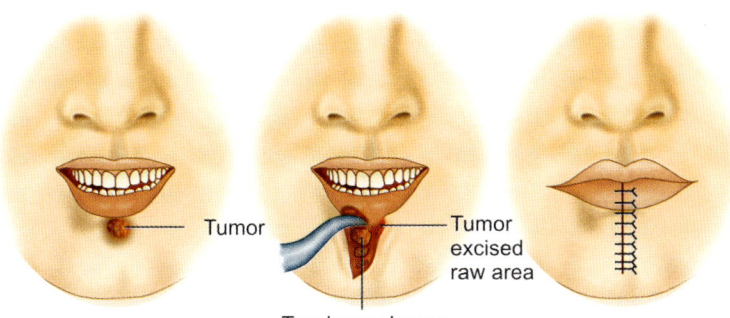

Fig. 21.24: Primary repair of lip after wide excision of small tumor. One-third of the lip can be sacrificed. Lip is sutured in layers. First layer with absorbable sutures for mucomuscular layer. Second layer is skin with non-absorbable monofilament sutures like polypropylene.

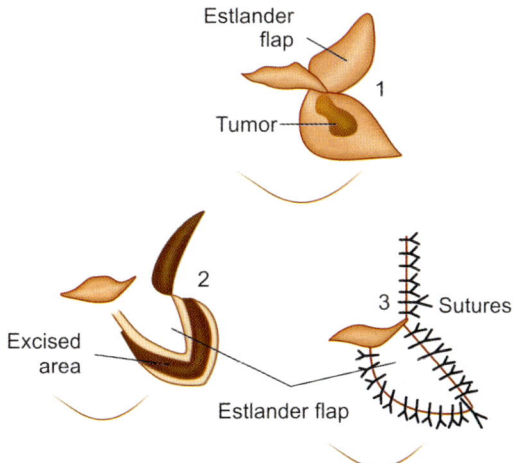

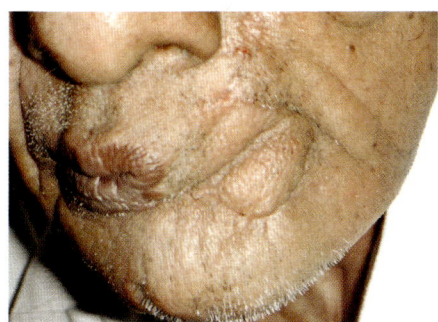

Fig. 21.26: Abbe Estlander flap.

Prognosis

Good. 5-years survival is 70%.

Fig. 21.25: The upper lip flap based on upper labial artery can be used in lower lip tumor after excision when primary suturing is not possible.

- Other methods:
  - Microvascular flaps.
  - Cheek flap; free radial artery flap.
  - W flap; Gillies fan flap.
  - Karapandzic flap; Johansen stepladder procedure.
  - Forehead/deltopectoral flaps.
- Lymph nodes are dealt by radical neck dissection on one side and functional block or suprahyoid block dissection on other side.
- Postoperative radiotherapy is given if tumor is large or if lymph nodes are involved.

TONGUE

LYMPHATIC DRAINAGE OF THE TONGUE

- Tip drains into submental lymph nodes.
- Lateral margin drains to submandibular lymph nodes and then into upper deep cervical lymph nodes. Many lymphatic vessels pass as subperiosteal lymphatics of mandible. So carcinoma can involve the bone through this route.
- Lymphatics in the midline of tongue freely cross communicate with each other and so, spread of malignancy can occur to bilateral neck lymph nodes.

An error gracefully acknowledged is a victory

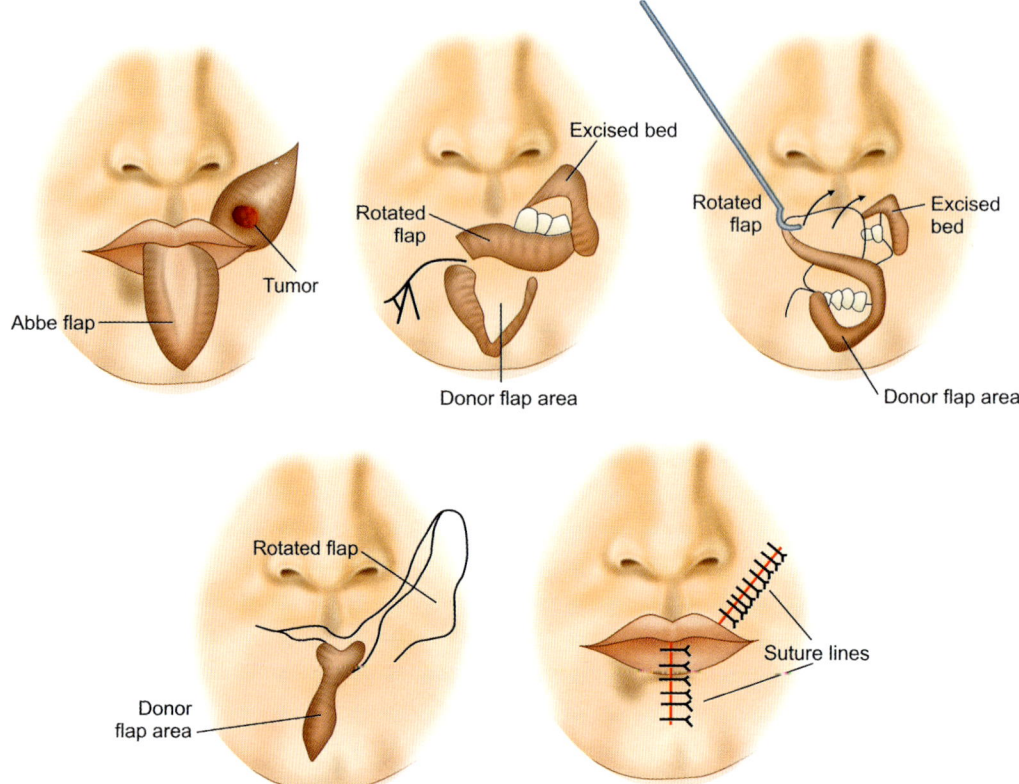

Fig. 21.27: For upper lip tumor when primary repair is not possible, then lower lip flap based on inferior labial artery can be rotated to upper lip.

- Lymphatics from posterior third of tongue drain into pharyngeal group of lymph nodes, as well as to the upper deep cervical lymph nodes. Early spread to the pharyngeal lymph nodes from carcinoma of posterior third of tongue has a poor prognosis (Figs. 21.28A and B).
  Lymphatic vessels are named as:
  - Apical vessels.
  - Central vessels.
  - Marginal vessels.
  - Basal vessels.

DEVELOPMENT AND NERVE SUPPLY OF THE TONGUE

- *Anterior two-third* develops from first branchial arch through two lingual swellings and one tuberculum impar. It is supplied by lingual nerve for general sensation and by chorda tympani for taste sensation.
- *Posterior one-third* develops from third arch from cranial half of hypobranchial eminence. It is supplied by glossopharyngeal nerve for both general and taste sensations.
- *Posterior most part* develops from the fourth arch. It is supplied by vagus nerve (internal laryngeal nerve).
- *Muscles of the tongue* are derived from occipital myotomes and are supplied by hypoglossal nerve except palatoglossus, which is supplied by cranial part of accessory nerve.

*Do what is right, not what is easy nor what is popular—***Roy T Bennett**

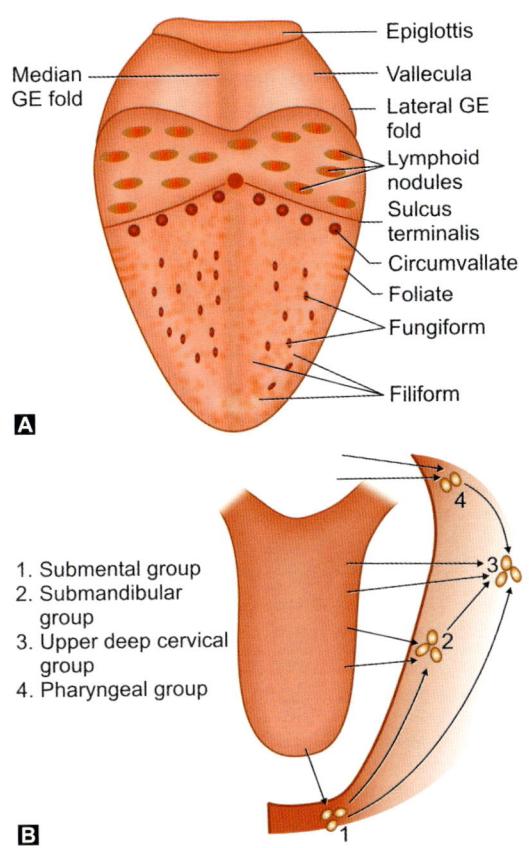

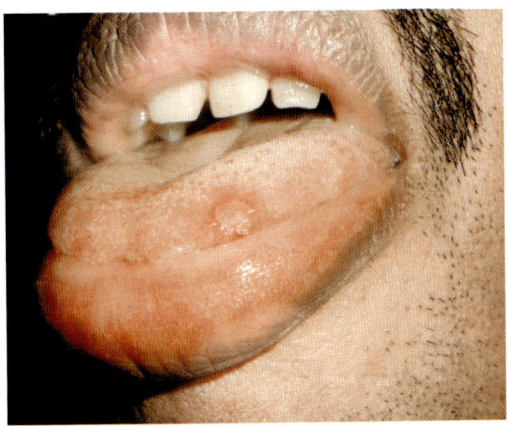

Fig. 21.29: Aphthous ulcer tongue.

Figs. 21.28A and B: Anatomy and lymphatic drainage of tongue. (GE: glossoepiglottic)

DIFFERENTIAL DIAGNOSIS OF TONGUE ULCERS

Dental Ulcer

It is common in sides of tongue due to sharp tooth, denture, and broken tooth. Usually it is acute in onset painful, self limiting ulcer. Occasionally repeated trauma forms an indolent chronic ulcer which mimics carcinoma; it should be excised to rule out carcinoma and to cure the ulcer.

Aphthous Ulcer (Fig. 21.29)

It can be:
1. *Minor* aphthous ulcers come in crops, common in menstruating women as a crop with painful, round, yellow base and, red margin. It regresses spontaneously in 2 weeks.
2. *Major* aphthous ulcers, large and deep which often becomes chronic and takes more time to subside with a scar. Chlorhexidine gluconate, local application of triamcinolone acetate, choline salicylate gel are different local applicants used to promote healing.
3. *Behcet's syndrome* is genital ulcer, conjunctival ulcer and multiple oral ulcers. *Reiter's syndrome* is urethritis, arthritis, periarteritis nodosa, conjunctivitis, and oral ulcers.
4. *Herpetiform aphthous ulcer* is not due to herpes simplex. They are small, 1–2 mm diameter ulcers occur in crops which heal by usual drugs mentioned above.

Syphilitic Ulcer

Extragenital chancre often occurs in tongue in *primary syphilis* which is painless with shotty, submental and submandibular lymph nodes. *In secondary syphilis*, multiple shallow snail track ulcers in the margins and undersurface; mucous patches on the tongue and fauces; Hutchnson's condyloma wart in midline of tongue can occur. *In tertiary syphilis*, gumma-

A fault once denied is twice committed

tous ulcer occurs in anterior 2/3rd of tongue as a deep punched out painless ulcer as gumma with wash leather slough. Endarteritis is the cause for punched out look. *Interstitial glossitis* with loss of papillae causing longitudinally fissured bald lobulated tongue in tertiary syphilis. In carcinoma arising from syphilitic ulcer, RT is *questionable* as blood supply is precarious due to endarteritis; RT further compromises it leading to tongue necrosis.

Tuberculous Ulcer

It is undermined shallow often multiple painful ulcer. Ulcer can occur in margins, tip or anterior 2/3rd of tongue. Neck nodes may be involved. Larynx and lung tuberculosis may be present.

Herpetic Lingual Ulcer

It is involvement of lingual nerve presenting as acute neuralgia with vesicles which form multiple superficial painful ulcers.

Other Ulcers

Multiple ulcers in smokers due to glossitis (*smoker's ulcer*), ulcers due to vasculitis, eosinophilic granuloma. Post-pertussis ulcer in whooping cough occurs on upper part of frenum linguae and under the tip of tongue.

Differential diagnosis for tongue ulcers	
• Dental ulcers.	• Syphilitic ulcers.
• Aphthous ulcers.	• Tuberculous ulcers.
• Ulcers in lichen planus.	• Malignant ulcers.

BENIGN TUMORS OF THE TONGUE

Fibroepithelial Polyp

It is due to repeated trauma at one place may be due to teeth (incisor) forming a thickened submucous scar which gets pulled out like a stalked polyp due to sucking and swallowing mechanism. It commonly enters the gap between the lower incisor teeth.

Granular Cell Myoblastoma

It is a benign noncapsulated firm mobile mass in the tongue showing pseudoepithelial hyperplasia of mucosa of tongue with eosinophilic granular cells in deeper plane. It is often mistakenly diagnosed as carcinoma of tongue. It is treated by excision.

Benign tumors of the tongue
• Papilloma.
• Fibroepithelial polyp.
• Hemangioma and lymphangioma.
• Neurofibroma.
• Lipoma.
• Granular cell myoblastoma.

TONGUE FISSURE

❖ Congenital fissures are transverse which run laterally from midline with normal papillae in between. Candida infection can occur on this (Fig. 21.30).

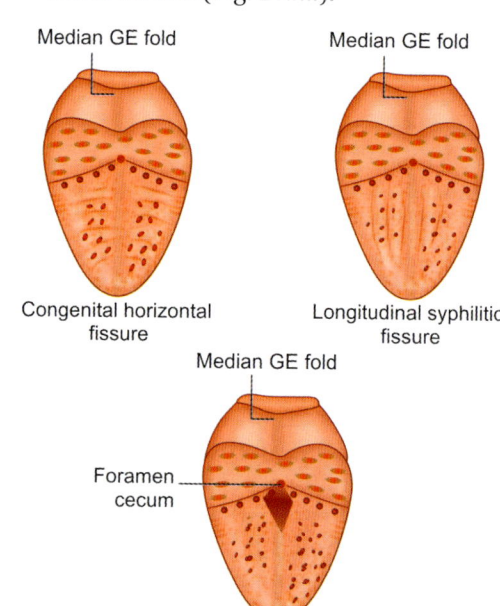

Fig. 21.30: Congenital fissures of tongue are transverse; syphilitic fissures are longitudinal. Median rhomboid glossitis is persistent tuberculum impar. (GE: glossoepiglottic)

Through hard work, perseverance and a faith in God, you can live your dreams—Ben Carson

❖ Syphilitic fissures are deep bald and longitudinal.

GLOSSITIS

Median Rhomboid Glossitis

❖ It is smooth, lobulated, triangular firm patch anterior to foramen cecum of tongue in midline with deeper color.
❖ Candida infection can occur in it.
❖ It mimics carcinoma. Biopsy rules out malignancy. Carcinoma is uncommon in midline.

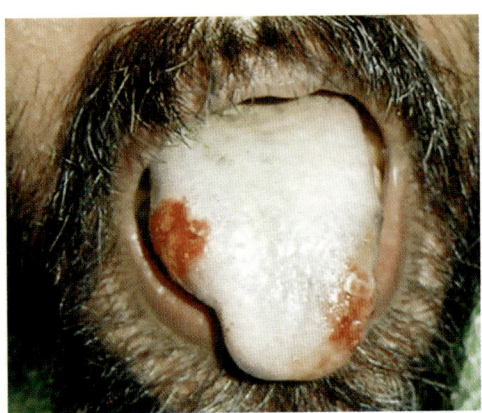

Fig. 21.31: Severe superficial glossitis.

Glossitis Migrans (Geographic Tongue)

❖ It begins as benign small red patches with white furred margin which spread and recede in an irregular way to appear as fresh patches.
❖ White margin contains keratinized epithelium and inflammatory cells over filiform papillae.
❖ It is often seen in patients with congenital heart diseases and acute gastrointestinal diseases. Etiology is unknown.

Other Glossitis

❖ *Hunter's glossitis* is seen in pernicious anemia.
❖ *Hairy tongue* is overgrowth of filiform papillae with black/brown stain on it due to bacteria, fungi, tobacco or drugs. It is a misnomer. There are no hair. Cessation of causative agent, mechanical scraping, cleaning are the treatment methods.
❖ Agranulocytosis glossitis.
❖ Nonspecific glossitis.
❖ *Pellagra glossitis,* due to deficiency of nicotinamide (B_3).
❖ Chronic superficial glossitis in malnutrition, iron and vitamin B deficiencies (Fig. 21.31).

TONGUE TIE (FIGS. 21.32A AND B)

❖ It is short, thick, fibrous frenum linguae.
❖ During protrusion, lateral margin and tip of the tongue is everted with dorsal mid part heaping.
❖ It causes speech defect, difficulty in cleaning the inner part of lower teeth.
❖ It is treated surgically under local anesthesia (or general in child). Tongue lifted upward with a stay suture at the tip; fibrous frenum is divided using fine scissor; linear wound is closed longitudinally using fine catgut from the tip of the tongue toward the margin of the floor of the mouth.

Macroglossia (Fig. 21.33)

It is painless diffuse enlargement of tongue

Causes
1. *Lymphangioma*—soft, painless enlarged tongue with ulcers.
2. *Hemangioma*—soft, fluctuant, compressible, bleeding, red/blue lesion.
    i. Both are treated by sclerotherapy (ethonalamine oleate)/partial excision.
    ii. Angiogram/MR angiogram must be done in hemangioma.
    iii. Ligation of lingual artery/ECA on both sides may be needed in large lesions.
3. *Neurofibroma*—partial excision is done.
4. *Tongue muscular hypertrophy*—partial excision is done.

Condition your mind and remain cool under all conditions

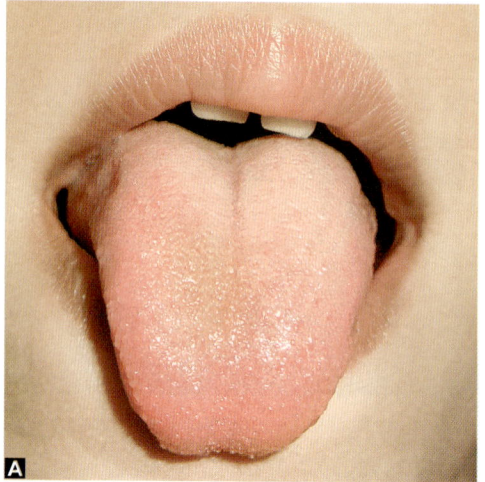
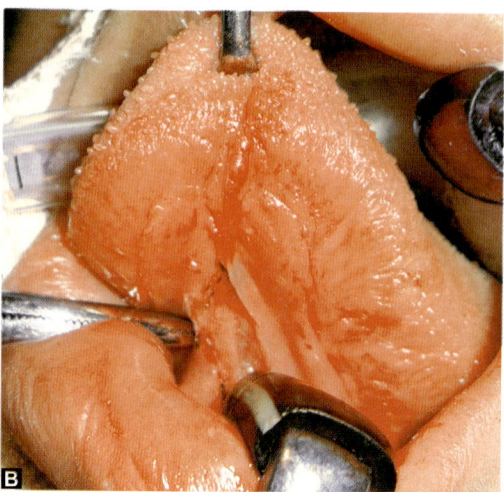

Figs. 21.32A and B: Tongue tie on-table photograph.

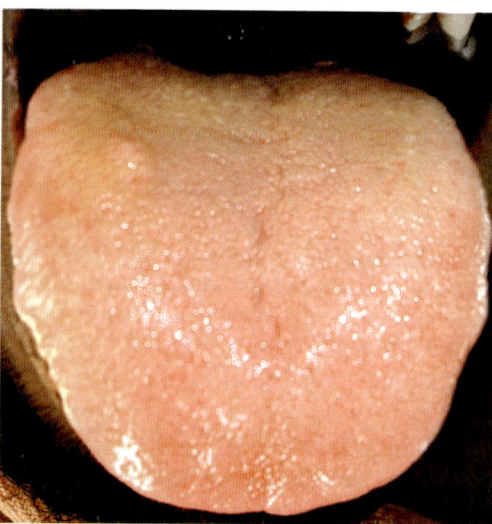

Fig. 21.33: Macroglossia.

CARCINOMA TONGUE

Incidence is equal in both sexes. Presently, its incidence is increasing in females due to increase in number of female smokers.

Etiology

- Leukoplakia.
- Erythroplakia.
- All S's.
- Premalignant conditions mentioned earlier.

Types (Figs. 21.34A and B)

Gross:
- Papillary.
- Ulcerative or ulceroproliferative.
- Fissure with induration (Fig. 21.35).
- Lobulated, indurated mass.

Histologically:
- Squamous cell carcinoma—commonest.
- Adenocarcinoma may be from minor salivary glands or mucous glands.
- Melanomas.

Sites:
- Lateral margin—commonest—47-50%.
- Posterior third—20%.
- Dorsum—6.5%.
- Ventral surface—9%.

Clinical Features

- *Painless ulcer*/lesion in the tongue which later may become painful. Eventual pain will be present due to infection/ulceration or due to involvement of lingual nerve

If life were predictable it would cease to be life, and be without flavor—Eleanor Roosevelt

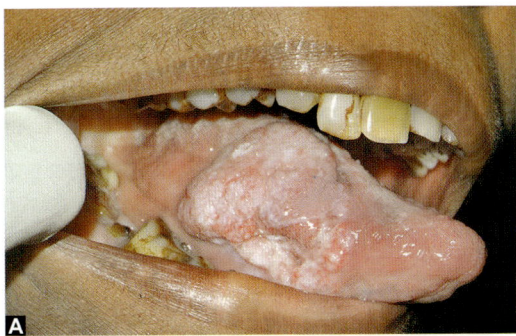

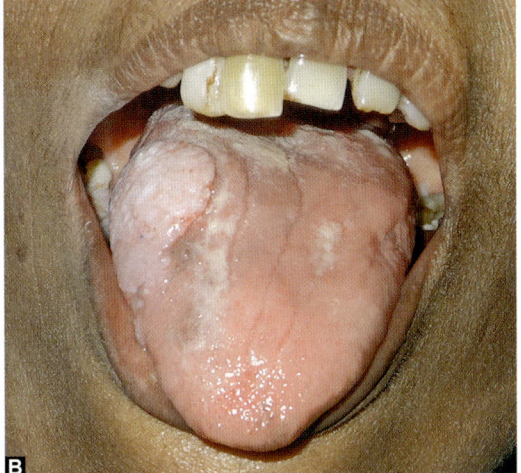

Figs. 21.34A and B: Carcinoma tongue. Commonest site is lateral margin.

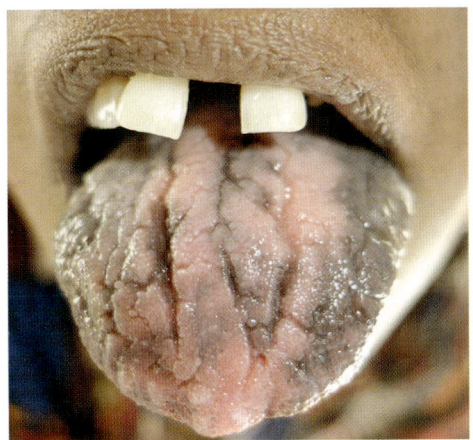

Fig. 21.35: Fissure in the anterior aspect of the tongue midline. It is a premalignant condition or it itself can be malignant.

(causes radiation pain to ear through auriculotemporal nerve). Pain on swallowing often occurs in case of carcinoma of posterior third of the tongue.
- Excessive salivation.
- *Dysphagia* either due to fixed tongue or due to the involvement of genioglossus or growth in the posterior third of the tongue.
- *Visible ulcer* in anterior two-thirds of tongue. Growth or ulcer in posterior third, is usually not visible. Ulcer with *everted edge, indurated base* and *induration* extends *much beyond* the visible margin. Often ulcer or indurated area may cross the midline.
- *Ankyloglossia*.
- Inability to articulate.
- *Foetor* (Halitosis). Due to infection and necrosis in the oral cavity.
- *Change in voice*: Occurs in posterior third tumors. Tumor in posterior third area is more aggressive.
- Palpable *lymph nodes* in the neck which are hard, nodular and may get fixed in advanced stages.
- Features of bronchopneumonia.

Spread of Carcinoma Tongue (Fig. 21.36)

Local spread:
In case of growth in anterior two-thirds of tongue, the spread occurs to genioglossus muscle, floor of the mouth, opposite side and mandible. In case of growth in posterior third of tongue, it spreads locally to tonsil, lateral side of pharynx, soft palate, epiglottis, larynx and cervical spine.

Lymphatic spread:
From tip of tongue, it spreads to submental nodes. From lateral margin, it spreads to submandibular lymph nodes and later to deep cervical lymph nodes. Lymphatics in the tongue are freely communicating, and so involvement of bilateral neck lymph nodes is common. From posterior third, it spreads to

Success means growth and growth means change

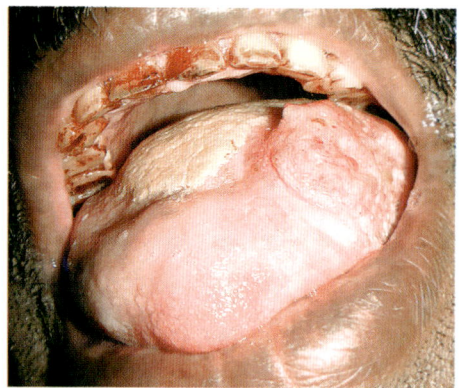

Fig. 21.36: Carcinoma tongue with leukoplakia.

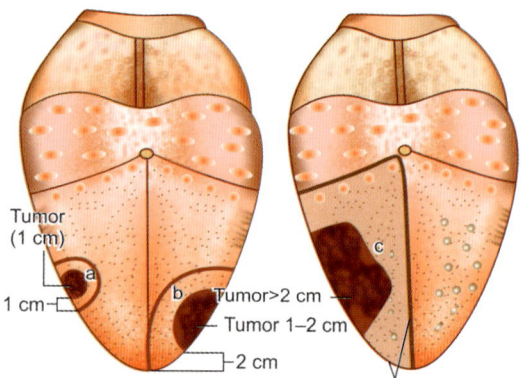

Fig. 21.37: (a) Wide excision is done in small lateral margin tumor of 1 cm size with 1 cm clearance; (b) Tumor between 1 and 2 cm size is treated by partial glossectomy with 2 cm clearance; (c) Tumor larger than 2 cm requires hemiglossectomy.

pharyngeal nodes and upper deep cervical lymph nodes.

Investigations

- Edge biopsy: Biopsy from posterior third growth should be done under general anesthesia.
- FNAC of lymph nodes.
- Indirect and direct laryngoscopy to see posterior third growth.
- CT scan to see the extension of posterior third growth or to see the status of advanced secondaries.
- Chest X-ray to see bronchopneumonia.

Treatment

Surgery, Radiotherapy, Chemotherapy.

Surgery:
- Tumor which is less than 1 cm size is treated with *wide excision* with 1 cm margin of clearance; tumor of 1–2 cm in size is treated by wide with 2 cm clearance of margin as *partial glossectomy*; tumor which is more than 2 cm is treated with *hemiglossectomy* (Fig. 21.37).
- Larger primary tumor can be given preoperative radiotherapy, and then later hemiglossectomy is done.
- Same side palpable, mobile lymph nodes are removed by *radical neck block dissection*.
- *Bilateral mobile lymph nodes* are dealt with *one side radical block and other side functional block dissection with essentially retaining internal jugular vein* (on opposite side) to maintain the cerebral venous blood flow. Other option is same side radical neck dissection and suprahyoid block dissection can be done on opposite side.
- *Wide excision is done when* growth is in the tip.
- Posterior third growth can be approached by lip split and mandible resection, so as to have *total glossectomy*.
- When mandible is involved *hemimandibulectomy* is done.
- The procedure that involves wide excision or hemiglossectomy, hemimandibulectomy and radical neck dissection together is called as *Commando operation*.
- Reconstruction of tongue and other area after surgery:
  - By deltopectoral flap, forehead flap, pectoralis major muscle flap, skin grafting.

Always remember that you are absolutely unique. Just like everyone else—Margaret Mead

- Prophylactic block dissection is becoming popular at present.

Postoperative management:
- Control of infection.
- Edema.
- Regular mouthwash.
- Maintaining the airway.
- Prevention of aspiration.

Radiotherapy:
- In small primary tumor—curative radiotherapy (brachytherapy using cesium or iridium needles).
- Large primary tumor—initial radiotherapy is given to reduce the tumor size so that the later resection will be better.
- Advanced primary as well as secondaries in the neck can be controlled by palliative external radiotherapy.
- Postoperative radiotherapy is given in large tumors to reduce the chances of relapse.
- In case of growths in the posterior third of tongue, radiotherapy is of curative as well as palliative mode.

Complications of radiotherapy
• Loss of sensation like taste.
• Trismus and ankyloglossia.
• Infection.
• Pharyngeal and laryngeal edema.
• Dermatitis and skin infection.

Chemotherapy:
Given in postoperative period and also for palliation.
- **Price-Hill regimen** is commonly used. Drugs are Methotrexate, Vincristine, Adriamycin, Bleomycin and Mercaptopurine.
- It is given either intraarterially, as regional chemotherapy through external carotid artery using arterial pump or through IV. It can also be given orally.
- For melanoma, Melphalan and Dacarbazine (DTIC) are used.

Complications of chemotherapy:
- Megaloblastic anemia.
- Bone marrow suppression.
- Alopecia.
- Sepsis.

Terminal events
• Inhalational bronchopneumonia.
• Hemorrhage from erosion of lingual artery. In posterior third of the tongue, erosion into internal carotid artery can occur.
• Cancer cachexia.
• Asphyxia due to pressure on air passages or due to edema glottis.

Prognosis

5-year survival for females is 50%, for males is 25%.

Nodal prognostic factors
• Positive histology in node reduces the survival.
• Level III and IV have poor prognosis.
• Bilateral/contralateral nodes carry poor prognosis.
• Extracapsular spread/size >3 cm carry poor survival.
• >3 in number of nodes involved is poor sign.

Prognostic Factors

- Size of the tumor—>4 cm carries poor prognosis.
- Site of tumor (posterior third has got poor prognosis).
- Tumor crossing the midline has poor prognosis.
- Lymph nodes status.
- Differentiation.
- Bone involvement.

CARCINOMA OF POSTERIOR ONE-THIRD/BASE OF THE TONGUE

- Lesion may remain asymptomatic for long-time.
- Clinically may be missed easily.

Turn your stumbling blocks into stepping stones

- Earlier symptoms are features mimicking sore-throat and throat discomfort.
- Dysphagia and change in voice (hot potato voice) occurs later.
- Referred pain in the ear, bleeding from mouth, visible mass in posterior third of tongue are late local features.
- Induration on palpation in posterior third is diagnostic of the carcinoma.
- As posterior third tongue has got abundant lymphatics which cross-communicate on either side, lymph node spread is common (70%). Bilateral nodal spread is common. Massive nodal involvement and involvement of jugulodigastric node are also common.
- Infiltration into the tongue muscles like genioglossus, epiglottis, pre-epiglottic space, tonsillar pillars and hypopharynx are common.
- Carcinoma posterior third of the tongue is commonly poorly differentiated and so carries poor prognosis.
- Blood spread can occur into bones, liver and lungs in posterior third cancers.
- *Palpation under anesthesia* will give better idea about the tumor, its spread and also allows the biopsy.
- CT scan is always needed to plan the staging and therapy.
- T_1, T_2, N_0 and N_1 diseases are treated by surgical wide excision often total glossectomy using midline mandibulotomy incision (mandible split) with neck dissection on both sides (MRND one side). Postsurgery radiotherapy is needed, if it is a poorly differentiated type or nodal status is more than N_1.
- Advanced lesions need palliative radiotherapy or chemotherapy.
- T_4 lesions are often treated by total glossectomy with laryngectomy and neck dissection but overall outcome is not good.
- In many centers, primary curative radiotherapy is used.
- Lymphoepithelioma and transitional cell carcinoma can occur in posterior third tongue (rarely).

Carcinoma floor of the mouth:
- It is usually aggressive tumor.
- It is rare in India.
- It is 2nd common site of oral carcinoma (SCC) in western countries.
- It invades hyoglossus, mylohyoid, genioglossus and anterior mandible early.
- Bilateral neck nodes are commonly involved.
- Rim resection of mandible with wide excision of tumor with muscles and soft tissues and bilateral neck dissection is necessary.
- Often visor anterior approach with anterior mandible resection followed by proper reconstruction with bone graft and plates is needed.
- Postoperative radiotherapy and later chemotherapy is used to prevent recurrence.
- Prognosis is poor and also has poor cosmetic results.

Carcinoma alveolus:
- It is squamous cell carcinoma arising from gums.
- It is common in males.
- It is common in India.
- It is commonly due to tobacco/pan chewing.
- Features and precipitating factors are similar to other oral carcinomas.
- There will be invariable bone involvement by direct extension.
- Nodal spread is also common.
- Wide excision with mandibulectomy and block dissection of neck is the treatment.

NASOPHARYNGEAL CARCINOMA

- Nasopharynx lies above the level of the soft palate which divides it from oropharynx below.
- It is also called as postnasal space or epipharynx. Eustachian tube opens on its anterolateral wall. Fossa of Rosenmüller is located above and behind the opening of the Eustachian tube as a small depression.
- It is common in China but rare in India.
- Squamous cell carcinoma is commonest type (85%). Lymphoma, lymphoepithe-

*Keep smiling, because life is a beautiful thing and there's so much to smile about—**Marilyn Monroe***

lioma, melanoma, rhabdomyosarcoma can occur rarely.
- Grossly it can be proliferative, ulcerative or infiltrative type.

Features

- Epistaxis, nasal speech, postnasal discharge and nasal obstruction.
- Pain in the ear, with unilateral deafness due to compression of Eustachian tube along with fluid collection in the middle ear.
- Elevation and immobility of soft palate on the same side.
- Pain in the area of distribution of trigeminal nerve due to direct infiltration of the nerve at foramen lacerum.
- Palpable secondaries in upper deep cervical lymph nodes (70%)—most common presentation.
- It is most common in China and Taiwan.
- Its incidence in China is 18–25%. In India, it is only 0.5%. Male to female ratio is 3:1.
- Vitamin C deficiencies, burning of wood, salted fish use and *Epstein-Barr virus* are the common etiological factors.
- VI cranial nerve palsy is most common palsy in nasopharyngeal carcinoma.

Trotter's triad

- Unilateral deafness (conductive deafness).
- Immobile elevated soft palate.
- Pain in the distribution of trigeminal nerve.

Differential Diagnosis

- Lymphoma.
- Lymphoepithelioma.
- Minor salivary gland tumor.

Investigations

- Biopsy from the primary site.
- FNAC from the neck lymph nodes.
- X-ray of the skull to visualize erosions.
- CT scan skull.
- MRI to confirm intracranial extension.

Histological type: Squamous cell carcinoma.

Treatment

- External irradiation for primary.
- Radical block dissection of cervical lymph nodes.
- Systemic chemotherapy using Methotrexate, Vincristine or Adriamycin or Bleomycin.

MAXILLARY TUMORS

- *Maxillary sinus is the commonest site for malignancy of paranasal sinuses.* Ethmoids, frontal and sphenoids are next in order.
- It is common in people working in furniture industries, mustard gas industries, and leather industries. It is common in Bantus in South Africa where snuff with nickel and chromium is commonly used (Fig. 21.38).

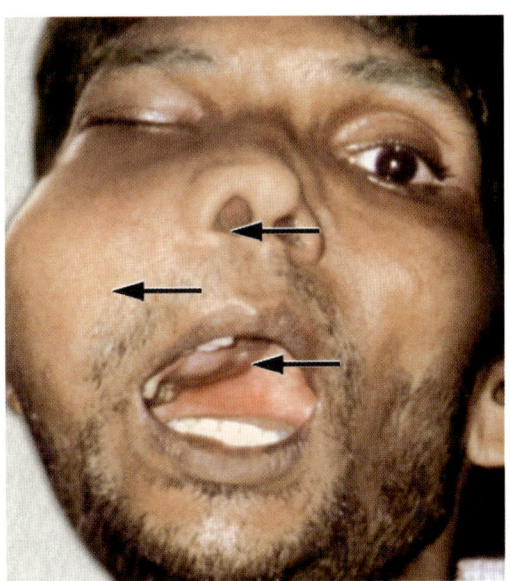

Fig. 21.38: Carcinoma maxillary antrum. Note the involvement of nostril, palate and skin over the maxilla.

In between goals is a thing called life, which has to be lived and enjoyed

Types

1. Squamous cell carcinoma (80%).
2. Adenocarcinoma.
3. Transitional cell carcinoma.
4. Salivary gland tumors.
5. Sarcomas and melanoma.
6. Burkitt's lymphoma.

Behavior and Presentation

* Initially may be asymptomatic, or may present with *epistaxis or features of chronic sinusitis*.
* When it spreads to the floor, loosening of the teeth, necrosis, antro-oral fistula can occur.
* Extension medially causes nasal block, fungation, bloody nasal discharge, blockage of nasolacrimal duct *(epiphora)*.
* Extension anteriorly causes pain, anesthesia and swelling in the cheek, ulceration and fungation in the skin of cheek.
* Spread above into the orbit causes ocular pain, epiphora, diplopia, proptosis.
* *Posterior spread is most dangerous* as it is not revealed easily. It causes postnasal discharge, pain, trismus, limitation of movement of temporomandibular joint. Extension into the base of skull can occur.
* Involvement of upper deep cervical lymph nodes in later stage is common.

Classification

1. **Ohngren's classification (Fig. 21.39)**
An imaginary plane is drawn extending between medial canthus of eye and the angle of mandible. Growth situated above this plane is called as *suprastructural* which has got poor prognosis. Growth below this plane is called as *infrastructural*. It has got better prognosis.

2. **Lederman's classification (Fig. 21.40)**
Two horizontal lines are used, one passes through the floor of the orbit, another passes through the floor of the antra. These lines are called as *line of Sebileau*.
   i. *Suprastructure type*: In this type, olfactory area of nose, ethmoidal, sphenoid, and frontal sinuses are involved.
   ii. *Mesostructural type*: This involves maxillary sinus and nasal respiratory part are involved.
   iii. *Infrastructural type*: This type involves alveolar process.

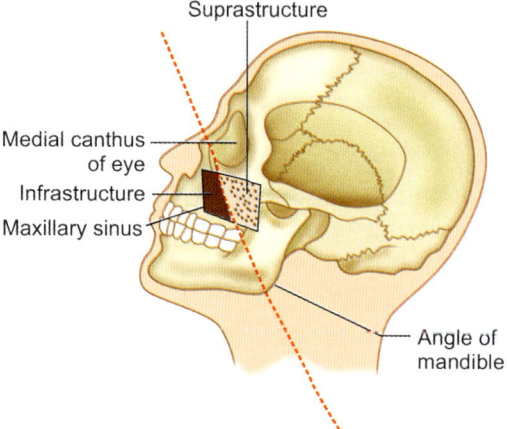

Fig. 21.39: An imaginary plane is drawn extending between medial canthus of eye and the angle of mandible and line in this plane is called as *Ohngren's line*.

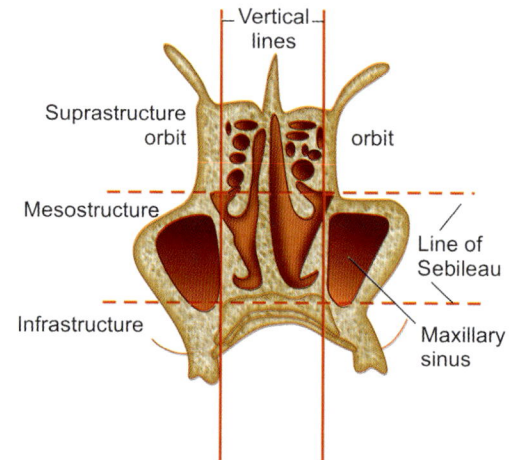

Fig. 21.40: Diagrammatic representation of Lederman's classification.

*You have brains in your head. You have feet in your shoes. You can steer yourself any direction you choose—***Dr Seuss**

Lederman's classification is further divided by two vertical lines over medial walls of the orbit to separate ethmoid sinuses and nasal fossa from maxillary sinuses.

TNM staging of maxillary tumors

T – Primary tumor
Tx – Primary tumor cannot be assessed.
Tis – Carcinoma in situ.
T1 – tumor limited to maxillary sinus mucosa with no erosion or destruction of bone.
T2 – Tumor causing bone erosion or destruction including extension into the hard palate and or middle nasal meatus except extension to posterior wall of the maxillary sinus and pterygoid plates.
T3 – Tumor invades either the bone posterior wall of the maxillary sinus, subcutaneous tissue, floor or medial wall of the orbit, pterygoid and ethmoid sinuses.
T4 – T4a: Moderately advanced local disease – Tumor invading anterior orbital contents, skin of cheek, pterygoid plates, infratemporal fossa, cribriform plate, sphenoid and frontal sinuses. T4b: Very advanced local disease – Tumor invading orbital apex, dura, brain, middle cranial fossa, cranial nerves other than maxillary division of trigeminal nerve, nasopharynx or clivus.
N – Nodes: Same as oral cavity.
Staging
Stage 0: Tis N0 M0.
Stage I: T1 N0 M0.
Stage II: T2 N0 M0.
Stage III: T3 N0 M0; T1, T2, T3 N1 M0.
Stage IV: ***IVA***: T4a N0/N1 M0; T1, T2, T3, T4a N2 M0.
Stage IVB: Any T N3 M0; T4b Any N M0. ***Stage IVC***: Any T Any N M1.

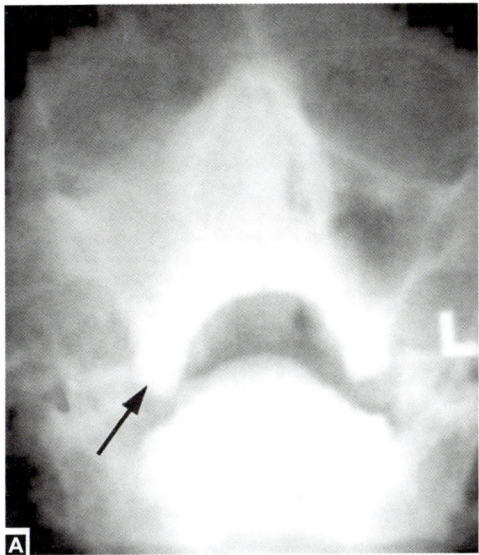
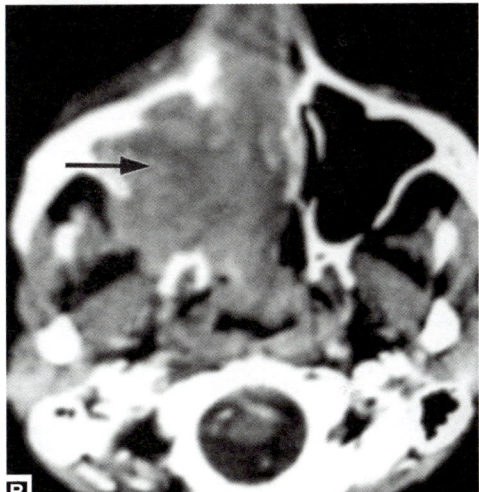

Figs. 21.41A and B: X-ray picture showing haziness and irregularity in the maxillary sinus suggestive of carcinoma. CT picture shows extensive involvement of the maxilla.

Differential Diagnosis

Chronic sinusitis.

Diagnosis

- X-ray of the part—opacity of the involved sinus with destruction of bony walls is seen (Fig. 21.41A).
- CT scan (Fig. 21.41B).
- Biopsy is done through nasal/oral or on early stage through Caldwell-Luc operation (Fig. 21.42).
- Sinus endoscopy for detailed examination of sinus and for biopsy.

Treatment

- *Preoperative megavoltage radiotherapy* is given. After six weeks, *total maxillectomy*

You can become strongest in your weakest place

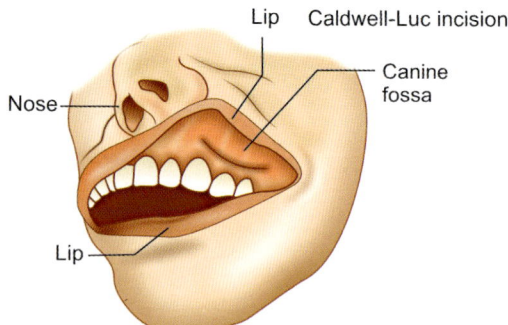

Fig. 21.42: Incision for Caldwell-Luc operation which is used for taking biopsy from maxillary tumor. Incision is not used for definitive therapy for carcinoma maxilla. Incision is also used in benign conditions to approach maxillary sinus. Gingivobuccal mucosa is incised and mucoperiosteum is raised. Bone of canine fossa is cut to reach the maxillary antrum.

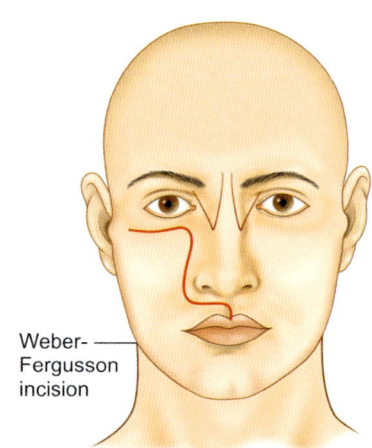

Fig. 21.43: Weber-Fergusson incision used for total maxillectomy.

is done. Reconstruction of maxilla along with dental reconstruction is required (Fig. 21.43).
- When lymph nodes are involved radical neck lymph nodes dissection is done.
- Postoperative radiotherapy and chemotherapy is given as an adjuvant therapy.
- Overall prognosis is 30–40%.

CARCINOMA HARD PALATE

- Minor salivary gland tumors are more common in palate (Fig. 21.44).
- In males *in reverse smokers,* squamous cell carcinoma is seen in palate due to repeated thermal injury.
- Malignant tumors may spread to periosteum, bone, maxilla, sinus, or nose.
- Salivary gland tumors are commonly malignant and are of adenoid cystic type. Other types also can occur. It presents as a single solid, smooth, swelling with ulcer over the summit.
- Squamous cell carcinoma is ulcerative with raised and everted edge (Fig. 21.45).
- Upper deep cervical lymph nodes are involved in 25% of patients.
- Investigations are edge biopsy, FNAC lymph node and CT scan to see extensions.
- *Treatment* is wide excision with removal of the underlying palatal bone. Often partial or total maxillectomy (*Weber-Fergusson incision*) may be required. Myocutaneous flap with dental prosthesis is essential to reconstruct after surgery. Postoperative radiotherapy and neck block dissection are often required.

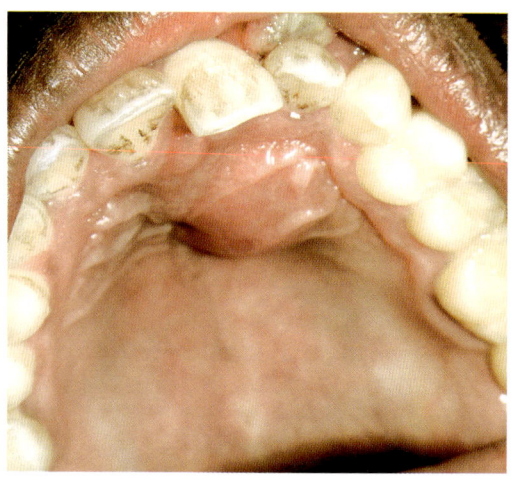

Fig. 21.44: Palatal tumor.

The days that make us happy make us wise

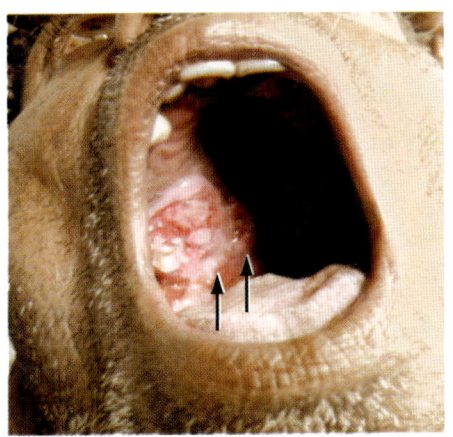

Fig. 21.45: Carcinoma hard palate extending laterally.

Treatment strategy for oral malignancies

- Wide excision with adequate clearance.
- Hemimandibulectomy when bone is involved.
- Proper reconstruction after surgery.
- Maintenance of functions like swallowing, speech.
- Neck nodal dissection radical/modified radical.
- Adjuvant therapy—chemotherapy/radiotherapy.
- Curative radiotherapy for early cases, palliation in late cases, and in postsurgery cases.
- Regular follow up with clinical methods along with investigations.

Prognostic factors in oral carcinomas

- Stage of the disease—stage I and II has got 80% 5-years survival.
- Stage III and IV has got less than 20% 5-years survival rate.
- T_3 and T_4 lesions has got poor survival rate.
- Carcinoma lip has got best prognosis.
- Carcinoma posterior 1/3rd tongue have got worst prognosis.
- Cheek, floor of the mouth and palate has got intermediate prognosis.
- Histologically positive nodes decrease the survival rate by 50%.
- Level III and IV, node >3 cm, bilateral nodes extracapsular nodal spread are poor prognostic factors.
- Grading (differentiation) of the tumor.
- Tumor thickness >6 mm has got poor prognosis.
- Exophytic tumor is better than infiltrating type.

Problems with oral carcinomas

- Upper airway obstruction and bronchopneumonia.
- Feeding difficulties and severe malnutrition.
- Immunosuppression.
- Secondary sepsis, uncontrollable bleeding.
- Fixity of secondaries, fungation and disability.
- Psychological trauma.

TRISMUS

- It is inability to open the mouth adequately.
- Causes are—submucosal fibrosis, carcinoma buccal and gingivobuccal complex, post-radiotherapy sequelae, infection like tetanus, parotitis, dental or peritonsillar abscess.
- In carcinoma, tumor invasion of pterygoids, buccinator, masseter, temporalis causes trismus.
- *Grading of trismus*: Inter incisor distance more than 3.5 cm is—normal; Grade I is between 3.0–3.5 cm; Grade II is between 2.0–3 cm; Grade III is less than 2 cm.
- It is often clinically assessed by placing fingers perpendicularly between two jaws at incisor level. More than 3 fingerbreadth is considered as normal.
- *Problems with trismus* are—inability to put fingers or spoon into mouth; difficulty in cleaning the mouth; infection; difficulty in assessing the tumor/pathology clinically. During surgery, intubation is difficult and so tracheostomy may be needed in these patients.
- *Management* is by treating the cause; release of soft tissue in case of fibrosis; draining the abscess and antibiotics for infection.

When love and skill work together, expect a masterpiece

CHAPTER 22

Laryngeal Tumors

CHAPTER OUTLINE

- Surgical Anatomy of Larynx
- Benign Lesions of Larynx
- Malignant Tumors
- Care after Total Laryngectomy
- Total Laryngectomy

SURGICAL ANATOMY OF LARYNX

Larynx lies in the anterior midline of neck extending from trachea to the root of tongue; in front of the 3rd to 6th cervical vertebrae; but in females and children it will be higher than males. Larynx is 3.5 to 4.5 cm in size.

Larynx is made up of cartilages, joints, muscles and membranes; lined by mucous membrane (anterior surface and upper part of posterior surface of epiglottis, upper part of aryepiglottic folds and vocal folds are lined by stratified squamous epithelium; remaining lower part is by ciliated columnar epithelium).

Laryngeal Cartilages (Figs. 22.1 and 22.2)

They are 9 in number; 3 paired; 3 unpaired.

Unpaired	Paired
• Thyroid—1	• Arytenoids—2
• Cricoid—1	• Corniculates—2
• Epiglottic—1	• Cuneiforms—2

Thyroid cartilage is **V**-shaped with right and left quadrilateral laminae. Laminae are situated obliquely which meets in front with 90°

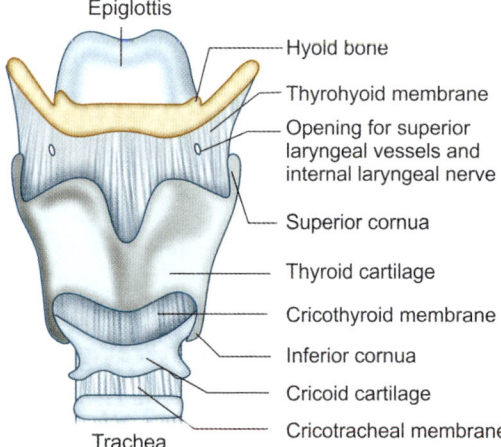

Fig. 22.1: Laryngeal cartilages and related membranes.

in males and 120° in females. Lower anterior fused part forms laryngeal prominence; upper part shows thyroid notch. Free posterior margin extends above on each side as superior cornu which is attached to greater cornu of hyoid bone through lateral thyrohyoid ligament; its lower extension is inferior cornu, one on each side, articulates with cricoid cartilage through

The eyes sees only what the mind is prepared to comprehend

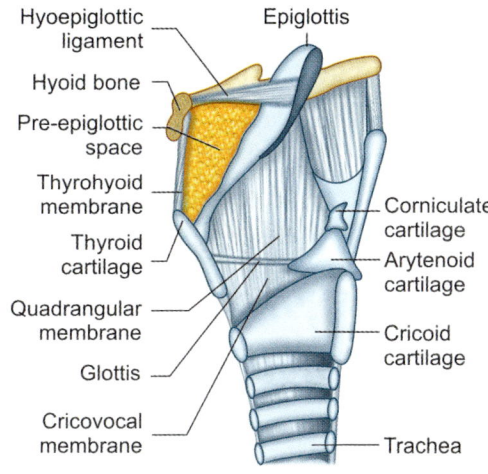

Fig. 22.2: Sagittal cut section of larynx.

cricothyroid joint. An oblique line is present on the outer surface of the thyroid cartilage extends from superior thyroid tubercle near root of the superior cornu to inferior thyroid tubercle near middle of lower border which gives attachment to thyrohyoid and inferior constrictor muscle of pharynx.

Cricoid cartilage is thicker, stronger **ring**-shaped, located below the thyroid cartilage which is having narrow anterior arch with broad posterior lamina. Projected upward part of the lamina articulates superiorly with arytenoid cartilage. Cartilage also connects to thyroid cartilage at inferior cornu through cricothyroid joint.

Epiglottic cartilage is **leaf**-shaped cartilage located in the anterior wall of the upper part of the larynx. Its free broad upper end projects upwards behind hyoid bone and tongue. Lower stalk end is attached to upper end of angle between two laminae of the thyroid cartilage. It is attached to tongue through median glossoepiglottic fold and hyoepiglottic ligament.

Arytenoids cartilages are 2 in number. It is pyramidal in shape lies in the upper border of the cricoid cartilage below and corniculate cartilage above. Concave base articulates with cricoid lamina. It has got anterior vocal process and lateral muscular process.

Corniculate (Santorini) and cuneiform (Wrisberg) cartilages are situated ventral to arytenoids situated in aryepiglottic fold.

Laryngeal Intrinsic Muscles

Cricothyroid is the only muscle which lies outer part of the larynx. It arises from lower lateral part of cricoid running above and behind to insert into lower border and inferior cornu of thyroid cartilage. It has got vertical and oblique fibers. It is supplied by external laryngeal nerve. It is tensor of vocal cord.

Posterior cricoarytenoid is a triangular muscle originates from posterior part of lamina of cricoid to insert above and laterally into the muscular process of the arytenoids. It is the only abductor of vocal cord.

Lateral cricoarytenoid originates from lateral part of upper part of arch of cricoid running upwards and backwards to insert into the muscular process of the arytenoids. It is adductor of vocal cord along with transverse and oblique arytenoids.

Transverse arytenoid is the only unpaired muscle of larynx runs horizontally from posterior surface of one arytenoid to other. It is adductor of vocal cord.

Oblique arytenoids are two strip muscles which arise from muscular process of one arytenoid running obliquely to insert into the apex of the opposite arytenoid. It is adductor of vocal cord. *Aryepiglotticus* is part of it runs along the aryepiglottic fold towards epiglottis. Aryepiglotticus closes the inlet of larynx.

Thyroarytenoid originates from posterior part of the angle of the thyroid cartilage and adjacent cricothyroid ligament running upwards and backwards to insert into anterolateral surface of arytenoid cartilage. It is relaxor of vocal cord. Its upper fibers run as *thyroepiglotticus* along aryepiglottic fold to reach epiglottis. Some of its fibers form *vocalis* muscle by attaching into vocal ligament.

Count your age by friends, not years. Count your life by smiles, not tears—John Lennon

Nerve Supply

Motor:
- Cricothyroid—external laryngeal nerve.
- All other muscles—recurrent laryngeal nerve.

Sensory:
- Above the vocal fold—internal laryngeal nerve.
- Below the vocal fold—recurrent laryngeal nerve.

Lymphatic Drainage of Larynx

- *Above the vocal cords*, lymphatics travel through thyrohyoid membrane to upper deep cervical lymph nodes.
- *Below the vocal cords*, it drains into prelaryngeal, pretracheal, lower deep cervical and mediastinal lymph nodes.

Laryngeal joints
- Cricothyroid (synovial)
- Cricoarytenoid (synovial)—it causes *normal laryngeal crepitus* by its gliding and rotatory movements.

Laryngeal ligaments
Extrinsic
- Thyrohyoid membrane is between hyoid and thyroid cartilage. It has got median and lateral thyrohyoid ligaments. It is pierced by internal laryngeal nerves and superior laryngeal vessels.
- Hyoepiglottic ligament.
- Cricotracheal ligament.

Intrinsic
Fibroelastic membrane with *quadrate membrane* above and *conus elasticus* below. **Quadrate membrane** extends from arytenoid cartilage to epiglottis with its lower free border becoming vestibular fold (*false vocal cord*) and upper border forms aryepiglottic fold. **Conus elasticus** is also called as cricovocal membrane extends from arch of cricoid cartilage upwards and medially forming thick anterior cricothyroid ligament and upper free border as vocal fold (*true vocal cord*).

Actions of larynx
- *Abduction* of vocal cord—*only posterior cricoarytenoid*
- *Adduction* of vocal cord—lateral cricoarytenoid, transverse and oblique arytenoids

Contd...

Contd...

- *Tensor* of vocal cord—cricothyroid—maintains pitch of voice
- *Relaxor* of vocal cord—thyroarytenoid
- *Closing* of laryngeal inlet—aryepiglotticus
- *Opening* of the laryngeal inlet—thyroepiglotticus
- *Elevation* of larynx—thyrohyoid, mylohyoid
- *Depression* of larynx—sternothyroid, sternohyoid

Spaces of larynx
- Pre-epiglottic space of Boyer
- Paraglottic space
- Reinke's space behind the vocal process of the arytenoid and in front of anterior commissure. Edema here causes fusiform Reinke's edema with swelling.

Cavity of Larynx

- Laryngeal cavity extends from inlet of larynx to cricoid cartilage.
- Inlet of larynx is bounded by epiglottis in front, interarytenoid fold behind, aryepiglottic fold on each side. Between upper vestibular folds of mucous membrane space rima vestibule and lower vocal folds rima glottidis are present. Anterior 3/4th of rima glottidis is intermembranous and posterior 1/4th is intercartilaginous.
- Part above the vestibular fold is vestibule of larynx—*supraglottis/supraglottic*.
- Part between vestibular and vocal folds is ventricle of larynx.
- Space between vocal cords in front and vocal process and base of arytenoids behind is called as *glottis/glottic*.
- Part below the vocal folds is *infraglottic-subglottic* (Fig. 22.3).

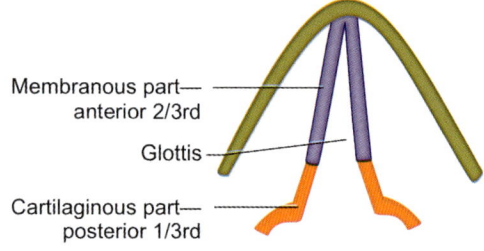

Fig. 22.3: Parts of vocal cord.

---

*The secret of life, though, is to fall seven times and to get up eight times—**Paulo Coelho***

Functions of the Larynx

1. Respiration
2. Phonation
3. Lower airway protection

BENIGN LESIONS OF LARYNX

Non-neoplastic

It is due to infection/trauma/degeneration. They are more common than true benign neoplasms.

1. **Vocal (singer's/screamer's) nodule**
   - It is vocal trauma nodule due to unnatural prolonged low tone speak or high intensity speech.
   - Site is at the junction of anterior 1/3rd and posterior 2/3rd of the vocal cord as it is the point of maximum vibration during speech.
   - It is usually of pinhead sized; common in singers, teachers, actors and more talkative people.
   - It is bilateral.
   - *Laryngoscopy* is diagnostic.
   - Nodule is initially reddish, edematous and soft but later forms white in color. Hyperplasia with inflammatory edema is obvious.
   - *Presentation* is—pain while talking, hoarseness, voice fatigue.
   - *Treatment*—voice rest, excision using operating microscope or laser.
2. **Vocal polyp**
   - It is soft, smooth, often pedunculated unilateral polyp that occurs due to sudden shout which leads to localized hemorrhage and edema formation.
   - Smoking, allergy, vocal abuse—are other factors.
   - It causes hoarseness of voice, diplophonia, dyspnea and stridor.
   - It is treated by excision using operating microscope.
3. **Reinke's edema**
   - It is fluid collection in Reinke's subepithelial space due to smoking and abuse.
   - It is bilateral and looks like diffuse polyposis.
   - *Treatment*—is vocal cord stripping. One side is operated first. Re-epithelialization of mucosa occurs later. Smoking should be stopped.
4. **Other conditions**
   - *Contact ulcer:* It occurs in vocal processes due to hammering of arytenoids with each other.
   - *Intubation granuloma:* It occurs after undergoing general anesthesia. It is treated by endoscopic excision.
   - *Keratosis/leukoplakia:* It is white/warty plaque on the upper surface of one or other or both vocal cords due to epithelial hyperplasia. It is due to chronic irritation of vocal cords. It is considered as 'precancerous' condition. It is treated by vocal cord stripping. Specimen should be sent for histology.
   - *Amyloid tumor* of the larynx.
   - *Cystic lesions of the larynx:* Retention ductal cysts occurs in mucosa of valleculae, aryepiglottic fold, false vocal cords and pyriform fossa. *Saccular cyst* occurs due to blockage of the orifice of saccule causing retention cyst. It may be anterior or lateral. *Laryngocele* is air filled sac with dilatation of the saccule which can be external or internal.

Neoplastic (Benign Neoplasms)

1. **Papilloma**
   - Laryngeal papilloma is the commonest type (80%).
   - It is usually *squamous* papilloma.
   Types
   A. Juvenile/childhood papilloma
      - They are *multiple*; and of *viral* origin.
      - They are seen in epiglottis, true and false vocal cords; but can occur anywhere.
      - They are friable, sessile or pedunculated, irregular glistening white lesions.

Art is long, life short, judgement difficult, opportunity transient

- They may disappear spontaneously.
- Present as hoarseness of voice, cough, dyspnea and stridor.
- *Treatment*: Endoscopic excision; cryosurgery; laser (CO_2); microelectrocautery; podophyllin application. Laser is better.
- They are known to recur; so multiple laryngoscopies are needed. Interferon therapy is used to prevent recurrence.

B. Adult papilloma
- It is usually, *single*; common in males.
- It occurs in anterior commissure of vocal cord.
- It may be premalignant.
- *Treatment*—endoscopic excision; CO_2 laser; cryosurgery.

2. **Others**
- Chondromas.
- Hemangiomas.
- Granular cell tumor arising from Schwann cells and is submucosal.
- Glandular tumor like pleomorphic adenoma, oncocytoma.
- Rhabdomyoma, neurofibroma, neurilemmoma, lipoma, fibroma.

Childhood papilloma	Adult papilloma
Multiple of viral origin (Papova).	Single of neoplastic origin.
Can occur in glottic, supra- and infraglottic region.	Glottic only.
Not premalignant.	Premalignant.
Recurrence common. Excision is difficult.	Not common after complete excision.
Causes more dyspnea, *stridor*, cough. May require tracheostomy.	Easier removal. Hoarseness only.

Note: Stridor can be inspiratory, expiratory or biphasic.

Types
Ulcerative; proliferative.

Anatomical Types (Fig. 22.4)

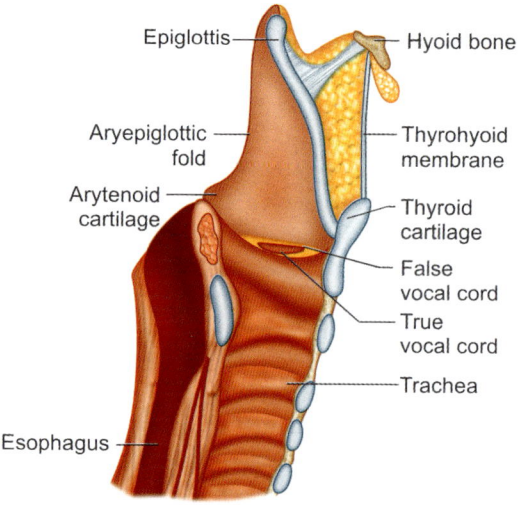

Fig. 22.4: Anatomy of larynx showing supraglottic, glottic, subglottic regions.

MALIGNANT TUMORS

Etiology

- Smoking, tobacco.
- Alcohol intake.
- Occupational/industrial exposure to chemicals like mustard gas, asbestos, benzopyrones, petroleum products.
- Previous radiation.
- Genetic—Russians develop familial laryngeal cancers.
- Papilloma, virus, keratosis, malnutrition.
  - Squamous cell carcinoma is commonest (95%).
  - Common in males (10:1).
  - Common in 5th/6th decade.
  - Common in India.

* **Supraglottic (25%):**
  - It arises from infrahyoid part of epiglottis, ventricles, and arytenoids.
  - It spreads to neck lymph nodes early (40%) due to rich lymphatics in this area.
  - Throat pain, dysphagia, palpable neck nodes and referred pain are common features.
  - Hoarseness of voice, loss of weight, respiratory obstruction, halitosis are late features.

*In the end, it's not the years in your life that count. It's the life in your years—**Abraham Lincoln***

- Carcinoma in epiglottis causes bilateral nodal spread.
- Local spread occurs to vallecula, base of tongue and pyriform fossa.

❖ **Glottic (65%) (Fig. 22.5):**
- It is the commonest type.
- It begins from upper part or free edge of vocal cords (mid or anterior) often extending 10 mm below.
- Lymphatic spread is slow (only 4%) as this area has got least lymphatics.
- Opposite vocal cord can involve as *kiss cancer*.
- Vocal cord mobility is unaffected in early cases. Vocal cord fixation signifies thyroarytenoid spread which is a poor prognostic sign.
- It presents very early due to early hoarseness of voice. Eventual cord fixation causes stridor.
- Locally it spreads anteriorly to anterior commissure, posteriorly to vocal process and arytenoids, above to ventricle and false vocal cords, below to subglottis.

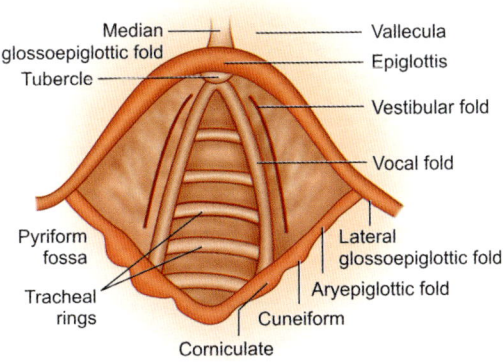

Fig. 22.5: View of larynx as seen through a laryngoscope.

❖ **Subglottic (2%):**
- It is less common involving undersurface of true vocal cords and subglottic space.
- It spreads to deep cervical and paratracheal nodes (20%).
- Upward spread is rather late and so hoarseness is not an early symptom in this type.

- It can spread through cricothyroid membrane or thyroid gland.

Note (Fig. 22.6)
❖ In Indian subcontinent supraglottic tumors are more common than glottic. Glottic type is common in Western countries.
❖ Fixation of cords is due to involvement of thyroarytenoid muscle or cricoarytenoid joint.
❖ **Laryngoscopy is important** (indirect and direct)—to identify the type, extent, appearance of lesion; to check vocal cord mobility. Vocal cord fixation suggests infiltration into the thyroarytenoid muscle or cricoarytenoid joint.

Clinical features	*Investigations*
• Hoarseness of voice.	• Indirect laryngoscopy (ILS) (Fig. 22.7).
• Pain and discomfort.	• Direct laryngoscopy and biopsy.
• Cough, dyspnea, stridor, dysphagia in late cases.	• CT neck-*very useful investigation.*
• Bloody sputum.	• Chest X-ray.
• Palpable neck nodes, which eventually get fixed.	• FNAC of lymph node.
	• Microlaryngoscopy in small lesions to identify and to have proper biopsy.
• Absence of laryngeal crepitus.	• Toluidine blue staining to stain early superficial cancers which facilitate the accurate biopsy.
• Common in males—10:1.	• Hopkin's endoscopy.
	• Flexible, fiberoptic laryngoscopy.

STAGING

Tumor
T1—Tumor confined to one anatomical site in larynx with normal cord mobility.
T2—Tumor confined to one anatomical region within larynx.
T3—Tumor spreads beyond one anatomical region within larynx with cord fixation.
T4—Tumor spreads beyond larynx—thyroid cartilage/neck soft tissues/pharynx/esophagus.

It is what a man thinks of himself that really determines his fate

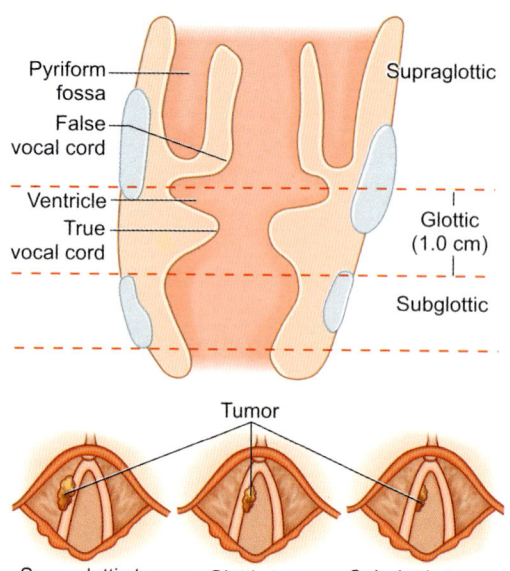

Fig. 22.6: Types of laryngeal carcinoma. Note the typical sites. Glottic is the commonest site. Next is supraglottic. Subglottic is rare.

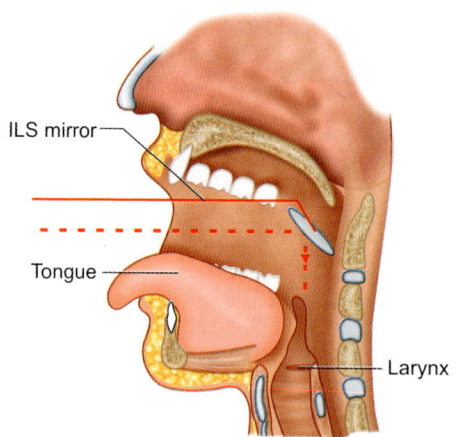

Fig. 22.7: Indirect laryngoscopy (ILS) to visualize larynx and its parts.

Nodal staging is similar to any other oral carcinomas.

TREATMENT

- *Supraglottic:*
  - Stage I—curative radiotherapy is the choice.
  - In stage II and III total laryngectomy and block dissection of neck nodes.

Conservative laryngeal surgery	
Indications • Early growth without fixation especially glottic type. **Types** • Cordectomy through laryngofissure—excision of vocal cord after splitting of larynx. • Partial frontolateral laryngectomy—excision of vocal cord and anterior commissure. • Partial horizontal laryngectomy—excision of supraglottis (epiglottis, aryepiglottic folds, false vocal cords and ventricle).	**Advantages** • Permanent tracheostomy is avoided. • Voice is retained. **Disadvantages** • Inadequate clearance. • Recurrence of the disease.

- *Glottic:*
  - Radiotherapy is the choice as nodes are commonly not involved.
  - Endoscopic laser surgery or open partial laryngectomy can be done.
- *Subglottic:*
  - Total laryngectomy is the treatment of choice with nodal block dissection when needed.
- *In advanced stage IV carcinomas:*
  - Surgery and radiotherapy both are not possible.
  - Here chemotherapy is given using Cyclophosphamide, Cisplatin and Methotrexate.
- *In advanced resectable tumors:*
  - Induction chemotherapy for 3 cycles with Methotrexate and Cisplatin 100 m/sq meter BSA (at 0, 22, 43 days) and total laryngectomy is under trial.
  - Concurrent chemotherapy and radiotherapy are also under trial in these cases.

Role of Radiotherapy in Laryngeal Cancer

- In early growth with no impairment in motility, curative RT is very useful with 90% cure rate with preservation of voice.

*It is better to be hated for what you are than to be loved for what you are not—**Andre Gide***

- It is commonly used in superficial exophytic lesions, growth in tip of epiglottis and aryepiglottic folds.
- In subglottic extension, fixed growths, nodal spread stage, radiotherapy is less effective.

CARE AFTER TOTAL LARYNGECTOMY

- **Speech therapy** by creation of pseudoglottis, aphonic lip speech, battery operated artificial larynx (electro-larynx), transoral pneumatic device, esophageal speech prosthesis. Tracheoesophageal speech prosthesis (TOSP) is ideal (Singer-Blom prosthesis, Panje prosthesis).
- Social and job rehabilitation.
- Care of permanent tracheostomy by avoiding immersion in the water, care during bath and shower use and swimming. Shower covers are available for this purpose.
- Often along with total laryngectomy, total thyroidectomy and removal of parathyroid glands are required. Patient then needs supplementation with thyroxine and calcium for lifetime.

TOTAL LARYNGECTOMY (FIGS. 22.8A TO C)

Indications
- T3 lesions with cord fixation.
- All T4 lesions.
- Bilateral arytenoid spread.
- Thyroid/cricoid spread.
- Transglottic cancers involving ventricle with fixation of the cord.
- Posterior commissure disease.
- Failure of conservative surgery or RT.

Problems
- Mortality of surgery.
- No speech.
- Having permanent tracheostomy and its problems.

Technique (Fig. 22.8A)
- Entire larynx with hyoid bone, pre-epiglottic space, strap muscles, one or more rings of trachea are removed.
- Pharyngeal wall is repaired.
- Lower tracheal stump is sutured to the skin as permanent tracheostomy.
- Often laryngoesophagectomy is done when pharyngeal spread is present. Gastric pull-up is done to maintain GI continuity.
- Technique may be combined with neck nodal dissection both sides.

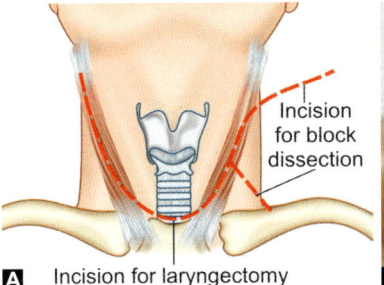
A Incision for laryngectomy

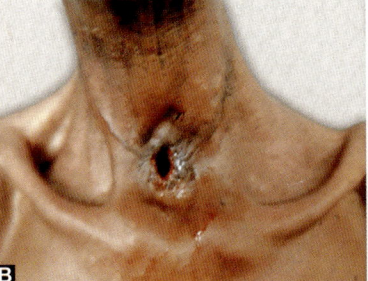
B

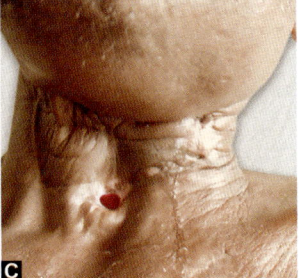
C

Figs. 22.8A to C: (A) Gluck—Sorenson's laryngectomy incision. Extension lines sideward can be used for adding radical neck dissection; (B) and (C) Carcinoma larynx, patient underwent total laryngectomy with permanent tracheostomy.

Happiness lies in the joy of achievement and the thrill of creative effort

CHAPTER 23

Tonsils

Chapter Outline

- Anatomy of the Tonsils
- Acute Tonsillitis
- Chronic Tonsillitis
- Peritonsillar Abscess (Quinsy)
- Tonsillectomy
- Acute Pharyngitis

ANATOMY OF THE TONSILS

- It is a mass of lymphoid tissue, situated on either side of oropharynx. The medial surface exposed to the pharynx is pitted by crypts. It forms a part of Waldeyer's ring. It is located between anterior and posterior pillars. Laterally it is covered by a well-defined capsule which is on the tonsillar bed (Fig. 23.1).
- *Tonsillar bed* is formed by (from medial to lateral) pharyngobasilar fascia, superior constrictor muscle and styloglossus, buccopharyngeal fascia, glossopharyngeal nerve and stylohyoid ligament, paratonsillar vein and tonsillar artery. Paratonsillar vein drains into common facial vein and pharyngeal plexus.
- Upper pole extends into soft palate with supratonsillar fossa in between.
- Lower pole extends as anterior tonsillar space which is separated from tongue.
- It is supplied by tonsillar branch of facial artery. Ascending pharyngeal, ascending palatine and descending palatine arteries also supply the tonsil.
- Tonsil drains into upper deep cervical nodes—jugulodigastric lymph nodes.

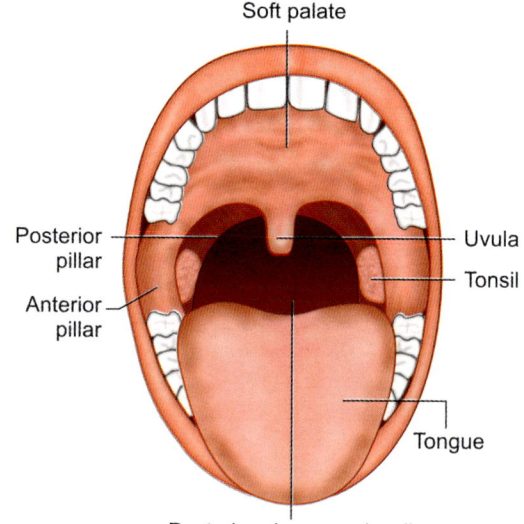

Fig. 23.1: Anatomy of oropharynx.

Once you learn to quit, it becomes a habit

ACUTE TONSILLITIS

It is generalized inflammation of the tonsils, accompanied by inflammation of fauces and pharynx.

Causative Agents

- Viral (Rhino, adeno).
- Bacterial (streptococcus hemolytics, staphylococcus, pneumococcus, *H. influenzae*).

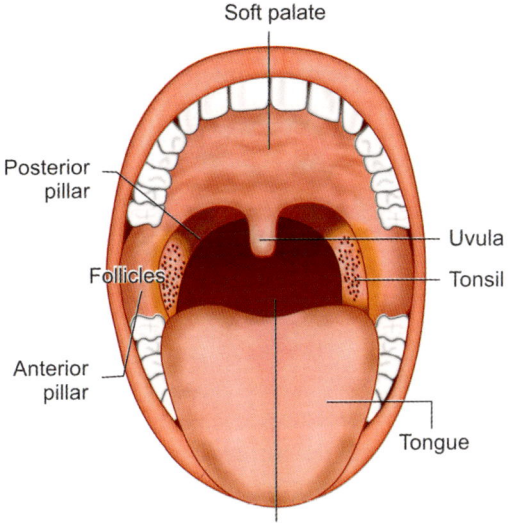

Fig. 23.2: Acute follicular tonsillitis.

Types

Acute catarrhal tonsillitis is seen along with generalized pharyngitis due to viral infection.
Acute follicular tonsillitis (Fig. 23.2) is of bacterial origin with pus filled crypts.
Acute parenchymatous tonsillitis involves tonsil parenchyma which is red and inflamed.
Acute membranous tonsillitis is formation of membrane due to exudates from crypts.

Precipitating Factors

- Malnutrition.
- Exposure to cold.
- Pollution.
- Immunodeficiency status.

Clinical Features

- Sore throat.
- Pyrexia, headache, malaise.
- Difficulty/painful swallowing.
- Earache.
- Tonsils are enlarged, congested, become studded with yellow spots over the crypts, which coalesce to form a patch on the tonsil.
- Tongue is coated and with foul breath.
- Cervical lymph nodes (jugulodigastric) are enlarged.

Complications

- Chronic tonsillitis.
- Peritonsillar abscess.
- Parapharyngeal/retropharyngeal abscess.
- Laryngeal edema.
- Acute otitis media.
- Septicemia, subacute bacterial endocarditis.
- Rheumatic fever, acute glomerulonephritis.

Treatment

- Patient is confined to bed.
- Analgesics nonsteroidal anti-inflammatory drugs (NSAIDs) for pain.
- Antipyretics.
- Antibiotics—Penicillin is the drug of choice. Alternatively Amoxycillin/Ampicillin/Erythromycin can be given.
- Fluids and soft diet are advised.
- Warm antiseptic gargle for smoothening can be given.

CHRONIC TONSILLITIS

It occurs as a complication of acute tonsillitis with microabscesses walled off by fibrous tissue seen in tonsillar lymphoid follicles. It also can occur in chronic sinusitis/caries teeth/recurrent sub-clinical tonsillitis (Fig. 23.3).

Don't be pushed around by the fears in your mind. Be led by the dreams in your heart—**Roy T Bennett**

Clinical Features

- Recurrent sore throat, chronic cough, throat irritation.
- Halitosis, change in voice, dysphagia.
- Difficulty in breathing at night.
- Yellowish beaded pus with cheesy material and congestion over the surface.
- Palpable jugulodigastric lymph nodes in the neck.

Types

- *Chronic follicular tonsillitis* is chronic inflammation wherein yellowish, cheesy materials are present in the crypts.
- *Chronic parenchymatous tonsillitis* is chronic infection of tonsils with enormously enlarged tonsils which interfere with speech, swallowing and breathing. It causes sleep apnea also.
- *Chronic fibroid tonsillitis* is chronic fibrotic inflammation of the gland which is small, firm and fibrotic.

Complications

- Peritonsillar/intratonsillar abscess.
- Tonsillolith—stone in tonsil usually due to chronic infection. It causes foreign body sensation and gritty feeling is typical on palpation. Tonsillectomy is needed.
- Focus of infections like rheumatic fever, glomerulonephritis.

PERITONSILLAR ABSCESS (QUINSY)

- Recurrent attacks of tonsillitis causes obliteration of the clefts resulting in infection spreading towards the peritonsillar space leading to abscess formation. It may be sequelae of acute tonsillitis or de novo to begin.
- *Streptococcus pyogenes, Staphylococcus aureus* and anaerobics are the causative organisms.
- Usually unilateral.

Clinical Features

- Common in adults.
- Severe pain the throat.
- High temperature.
- Dysphagia and otalgia on the same side.
- Dribbling of saliva, voice change (hot potato voice).
- Trismus, torticollis.
- There is marked edema, bulging of the tonsillar, peritonsillar and palatal region on the affected side, with the uvula being pushed to the opposite side.
- Cervical lymph nodes are enlarged and tender.

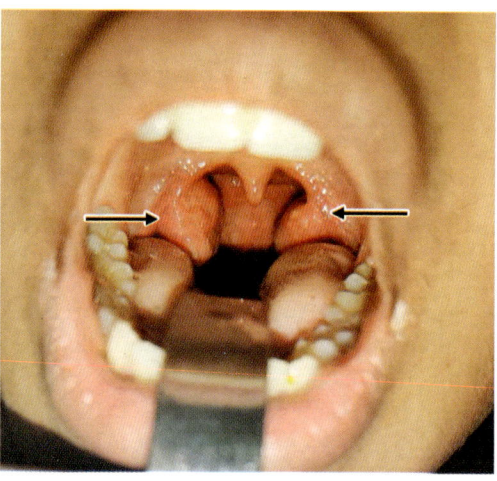

Fig. 23.3: Enlarged tonsils in tonsillitis.

Treatment of chronic tonsillitis

- Conservative treatment using antibiotics, mouthwash, oral hygiene, diet, therapy for causes like sinusitis.
- Tonsillectomy.

Investigations and Treatment (Fig. 23.4)

- Total count (raised); erythrocyte sedimentation rate (ESR); blood culture if needed. When septicemia is present relevant investigations like platelet count, serum creatinine, liver function tests, etc.

Children, like animals use all their senses to discover the world

- Antibiotics—Injection Penicillin 5L 8th hourly IV/Injection Amoxicillin or higher antibiotics are started.
- Analgesics, antipyretics, IV fluids, warm saline gargling of the mouth.
- *Incision and drainage:*
  - Incision is made on the most fluctuant bulged out area on the palate (just above the upper pole of tonsil).
  - It should be done under general anesthesia as aspiration or bleeding may occur.
  - Pus is drained and sent for culture and sensitivity. Antiseptic mouthwash is given.
- In severe cases occasionally temporary tracheostomy may be a need as a life saving procedure (due to severe respiratory distress).
- Tonsillectomy is advised after 4–6 weeks once the acute phase subsides—*interval tonsillectomy.*

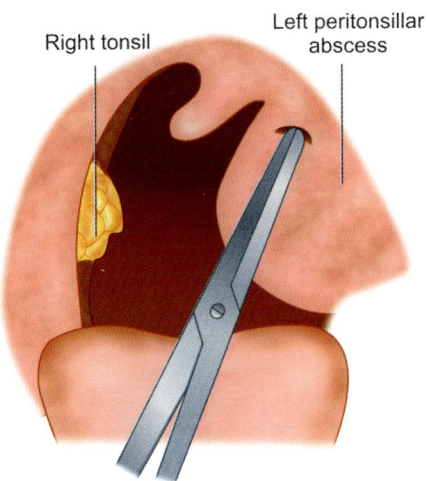

Fig. 23.4: Peritonsillar abscess drainage.

TONSILLECTOMY

Indications
- Recurrent attacks of tonsillitis.
- Following an attack of peritonsillitis.
- Chronic tonsillitis, with recurrent exacerbation.
- Enlarged tonsil causing mechanical obstruction.
- Enlarged tonsil suspicious of malignancy.
- Persistent carrier of streptococcus hemolyticus.

Procedure (Fig. 23.5)

- *Tonsillectomy* is now done by *dissection method* under general anesthesia.
- The patient is laid in supine position with head extended; sand bag being placed under the shoulder.
- A Boyle-Davis mouth gag is used to open and fix the jaw including the tongue.
- A pack is placed in the larynx to prevent aspiration.
- The tonsil are grasped with tonsil holding forceps and stretched medially.
- The mucosa is incised over the upper pole, anterior pillar and part of posterior pillar.
- Using blunt dissection the tonsil is separated from its bed.
- Finally the lower pole of the tonsil is separated with a snare. The bleeding vessel is ligated or cauterized.

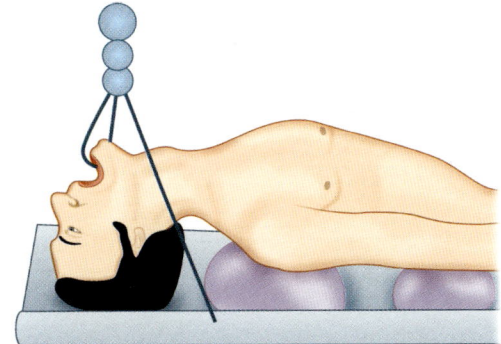

Fig. 23.5: Operative position for tonsillectomy [Guillotine method of tonsillectomy is now obsolete (not used)].

Nursing Care

- Postoperatively the patient is placed in '*tonsillar position*', i.e. made to lie on one side with knee and hips flexed. A pillow

Tell me and I forget. Teach me and I remember. Involve me and I learn—**Benjamin Franklin**

is placed behind him to prevent rolling on the back. Monitoring of BP, PR, RR is done. Any excessive swallowing, especially in children are noted, as it indicates a possibility of postoperative bleeding from the tonsillar bed.
- After 4-5 hours the patient is encouraged to take fluids. So earlier the patient uses the muscles of pharynx, easier it becomes and more rapid is the recovery.
- Analgesics and sedatives.
- Normal diet can be advised from the day 2. Patient is asked to do antiseptic gargle after any food intake.
- Antibiotics are given to prevent any infection.
- Patient should be ambulant from the 2nd day.
- There may be earache in the postoperative period due to referred otalgia. A white slough may be seen over the tonsillar bed due to the healing process. The patient should be reassured regarding these aspects.

Complications

1. **Reactionary hemorrhage:**
 - Commonly seen in the first 5-6 hours of postoperative period. It occurs mainly due to failure to ligate all bleeding points or slipping of ligatures. It is more dangerous in children as it goes unnoticed until hematemesis sets in. The child looks pale with tachycardia and features of shock.

 Management
 - The airway is cleared and the tonsillar fossa is inspected.
 - The clots are removed and a swab is held firmly against the fossa for few minutes, which usually controls the bleeding. If bleeding continues the bleeding points are ligated under anesthesia.
 - Blood transfusion may be necessary.

2. **Secondary hemorrhage:**
 - Occurs after 24 hours of postoperative period, usually between 5th-10th day; in the form of mild bleeding to frank ooze. It mainly occurs due to secondary infection. Slough or infected clot may be seen in the tonsillar fossa.

 Management
 - Patient is asked to have H_2O_2 gargle, which removes the clots/slough and bleeding usually stops.
 - Systemic antibiotics are started.
 - If bleeding persists, then the tonsillar pillars are sutured over a gauze as it is very difficult to ligate the bleeding points due to edema.

3. **Others:**
 - Aspiration pneumonia.
 - Lung collapse.
 - Acute otitis media
 - Palatal injury.
 - Sepsis.

ACUTE PHARYNGITIS

It is acute inflammation of the pharynx commonly associated with common cold, viral infections (measles, influenza).

Clinical Features

- Sore throat, fever, headache.
- Cough and odynophagia.
- Pharyngeal mucosa, tonsils, palate are congested, uvula is edematous.

Investigations

Throat swab for culture and sensitivity.

Treatment

- Bedrest.
- Analgesics.
- Antibiotics—Benzathine penicillin 24L. IM or Erythromycin/Cephalosporin.
- Warm saline gargle.
- Antiseptic lozenges for soothening.

Liberty means responsibility; that is why most men dread it

CHAPTER 24

Cleft Lip, Cleft Palate and Jaw Tumors

Chapter Outline

- Cleft Lip and Cleft Palate
- Diseases of the Palate
- Orthopantomogram
- Preauricular Sinus
- Jaw Tumors
- Epulis
- Ameloblastoma
- Dentigerous Cyst (Follicular Odontome)
- Dental Cyst (Radicular Cyst, Periapical Cyst)
- Osteomyelitis of Jaw
- Alveolar Abscess (Dental Abscess)
- Cherubism
- Fibrous Dysplasia of Bone/Jaw

CLEFT LIP AND CLEFT PALATE

Development of Face

Face is developed from median nasal process, lateral nasal process, maxillary process, mandibular arch, globular arch, olfactory pit and eye. Any changes in the development or fusion of these arches leads to formation of different types of cleft lip or cleft palate.

Etiology

- Familial.
- Protein and vitamin deficiency.
- Rubella infection.
- Radiation.
- Chromosomal abnormalities.

Classification

I. *Cleft lip* alone: Unilateral.
   Bilateral.
   Median.

II. *Cleft of primary palate only*:
   a. Complete—means absence of premaxilla.
   b. Incomplete—means rudimentary premaxilla.
      i. Unilateral.
      ii. Bilateral.
      iii. Median.

III. *Cleft of secondary palate only*:
   a. Complete.
   b. Incomplete.
   c. Submucous.
   It can be:
   – Cleft with soft palate involvement.
   – Cleft without soft palate involvement.

IV. *Cleft of both primary and secondary palates.*

V. *Cleft lip and cleft palate together.*

Defect is often associated with other congenital anomalies of cardiac, gastrointestinal, neurological system, Pierre-Robin syndrome, Klippel-Feil syndrome, trisomy.

The fool doth think he is wise, but the wise man knows himself to be a fool—**William Shakespeare**

Cleft lip

- *Central*—rare in upper lip. Between two median nasal processes (*Hare lip*) (Fig. 24.1).
- *Lateral*—between maxillary and median nasal process. *Commonest*. Can be unilateral or bilateral (Fig. 24.2).
- *Incomplete* cleft lip does not extend into nose.
- *Complete* cleft lip extends into nasal floor.
- *Simple* cleft lip is only cleft in the lip.
- *Compound* cleft lip is cleft lip with cleft of alveolus.

LAHS classification of cleft disorders

- 'L' for lip, 'A' for alveolus, 'H' for hard palate, 'S' for soft palate.
- *Capital* 'LAHS' for 'complete' type
- *Small letters* 'lahs' for ' incomplete types'.
- *Asterisks* 'lahs' for microclefts.
- 'LAHSHAL' for bilateral clefts.

Incidence

- Common in Caucasians.
- In 75% of cases it is unilateral. Commonly occurs on the left side.
- In 50% of cases it is combined cleft lip and palate.
- In 25% of cases it is cleft lip alone.
- In 25% of cases it is cleft palate alone.

Problems in Cleft Disorders (Figs. 24.3 to 24.6)

- Difficulty in sucking and swallowing. This is commonly observed in cleft palate than in cleft lip.
- Speech is defective especially in cleft palate mainly to phonate B, D, K, P, T and G.
- Altered dentition or supernumerary teeth.
- Recurrent upper respiratory tract infection.
- Chronic otitis media, middle ear problems.
- Cosmetic problems.
- Hypoplasia of the maxilla.
- Problems due to other associated disorders.

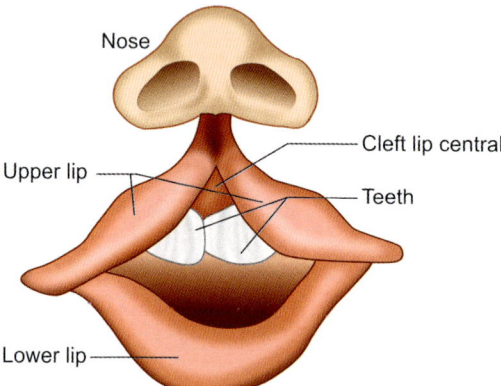

Fig. 24.1: Central cleft lip (Hare lip, Type I cleft lip—it is rare).

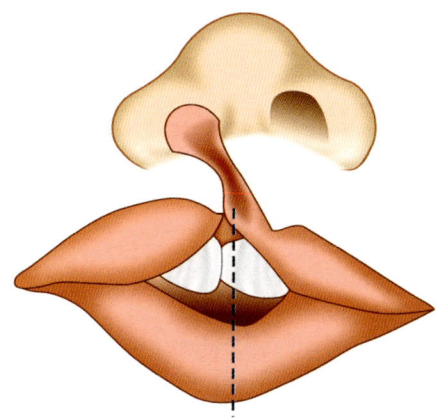

Fig. 24.2: Lateral type of cleft lip (Type II variety—it is commonest). It is due to imperfect fusion of maxillary process and median nasal process. It can be unilateral or bilateral.

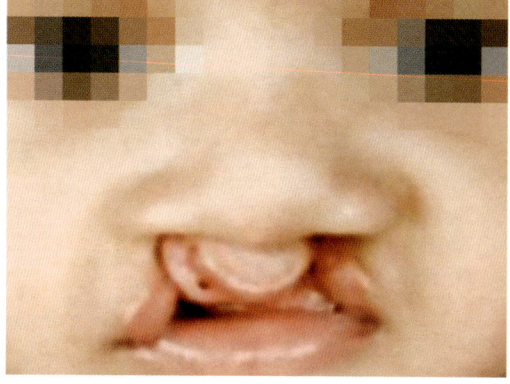

Fig. 24.3: Bilateral cleft lip.

A clear conscience can bear any trouble

Treatment for Cleft Lip (Fig. 24.7)

Millard criteria is used to undertake surgery for cleft lip.

Millard criteria (Rule of 10)
• 10 pound in weight.
• 10 weeks old.
• 10 g Hb%.

a. *Millard cleft lip repair* by rotating the local nasolabial flaps.
b. Management of associated primary or secondary cleft palate deformity.
c. Proper postoperative management like control of infection, training for sucking, swallowing and speech.
d. Tenninson's 'Z' plasty (Tenninson-Randall triangular flap).

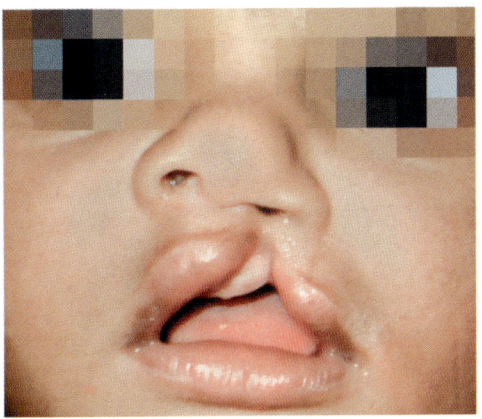

Fig. 24.4: Unilateral cleft lip, lateral type which is the commonest type.

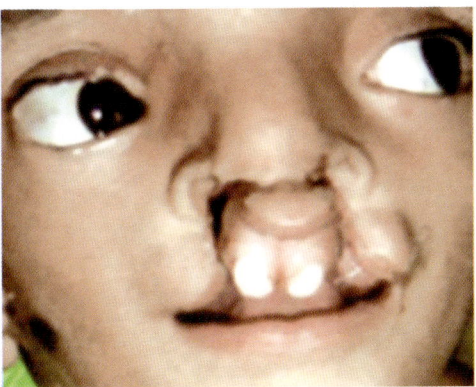

Fig. 24.5: Bilateral cleft lip with involved palate.

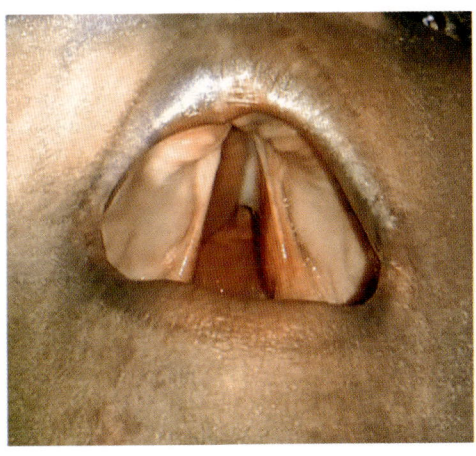

Fig. 24.6: Cleft palate only. Lip is normal.

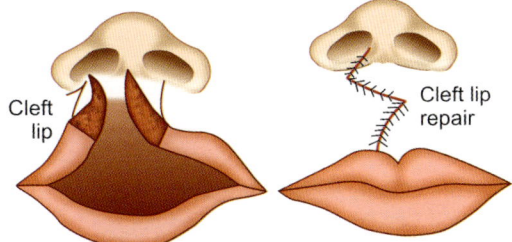

Fig. 24.7: Steps of cleft lip repair.

Principles of cleft lip repair
• "Rule of 10' should be fulfilled.
• Infection should not be there.
• Millard advancement flap is commonly used for unilateral cleft lip repair.
• Bilateral cleft lip repair can be done either as single or two staged (with 6 months gap in each stage) procedure.
• One stage bilateral cleft lip repair is done using Veau III method/Millar's single stage/Black method.
• Proper markings are made prior to surgery and incision should be over full thickness lip.
• Often 1:2,00,000 adrenaline injection is used to achieve hemostasis.
• Three layer lip repair should be done (mucosa, muscle and skin).
• Cupid's bow should be horizontal.
• Continuity of white line should be repaired.
• Vermilion notching should not be there.

*Be the reason someone smiles. Be the reason someone feels loved and believes in the goodness in people—***Roy T Bennett**

Cleft palate

- It is due to failure of fusion of the two palatine processes.
- Defect in fusion of lines between premaxilla (developed from median nasal process) and palatine processes of maxilla one on each side.
- When premaxilla and both palatine processes do not fuse, it leads into complete cleft palate (Type I cleft palate) (Fig. 24.8).
- Incomplete fusion of these three components can cause incomplete cleft palate beginning from uvula towards posteriorly to various lengths. So it could be Type II a—bifid uvula (Fig. 24.9), Type II b—bifid soft palate (entire length) (Fig. 24.10) or Type II c—bifid soft palate and posterior part of hard palate (but anterior part of hard palate is normal) (Fig. 24.11).
- Small maxilla with crowded teeth, absent/poorly developed upper lateral incisors.
- Bacterial contamination of upper respiratory tract with recurrent infection is common.
- Chronic otitis media with deafness may occur.
- Swallowing difficulties to certain extent and speech problems can occur.
- Cosmetic problems can occur (Figs. 24.12A and B show cleft lip and palate in an adult).

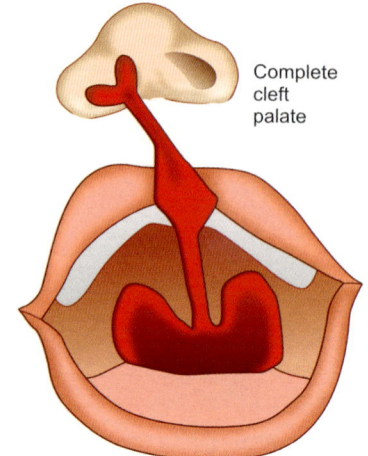

Fig. 24.8: Complete cleft palate type I.

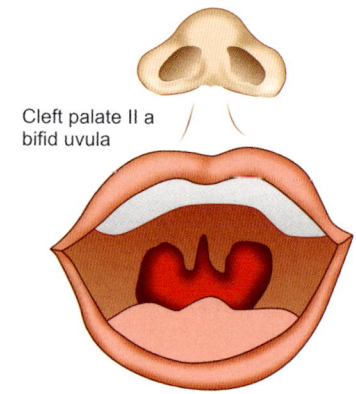

Fig. 24.9: Cleft palate type II a—bifid uvula.

Treatment for Cleft Palate

Criteria for surgery

- 10 kg weight.
- 10 months of age (10–18 months).
- 10 g Hb%.

❖ Cleft palate is usually repaired when baby is 12–18 months. Early repair causes retarded maxillary growth (probably due to trauma to growth center and periosteum of the maxilla during surgery if done early). Late repair causes speech defect.
❖ Both soft and hard palates are repaired.
❖ Abnormal insertion of tensor palati is released. *Mucoperiosteal flaps* are raised in the palate which is sewed together.

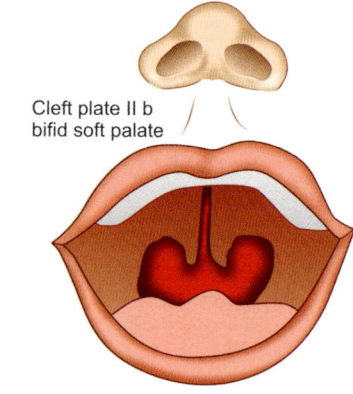

Fig. 24.10: Cleft palate type II b—bifid soft palate (entire soft palate), cleft palate II c—bifid soft palate and cleft posterior hard palate.

The important thing in life is to have a great aim, and the determination to attain it

Chapter 24 : Cleft Lip, Cleft Palate and Jaw Tumors   411

Cleft palate II c—bifid soft palate and cleft posterior hard palate

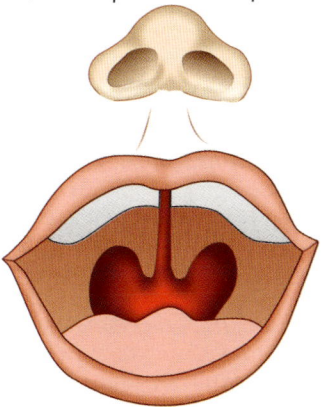

Fig. 24.11: Cleft palate type II c—bifid soft palate entire length with cleft of posterior hard palate (anterior palate is normal).

Principles of palatoplasty (Fig. 24.13)
• Timing is between 10–18 months. • Mucoperiosteum flap is raised. • Palatal defect is closed using 3 layers—nasal, muscle and oral layers. • Hook of pterygoid hamulus is fractured to relax tensor palate muscle to relieve tension on suture line.

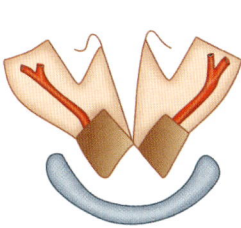 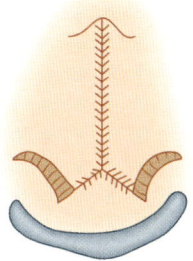

Cleft palate with palatine artery   Cleft palate repair V-Y palatoplasty

Fig. 24.13: V-Y palatoplasty.

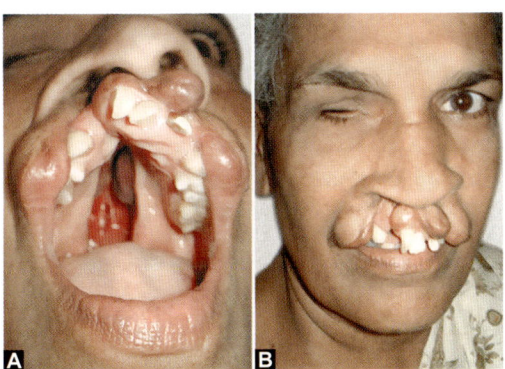

Figs. 24.12A and B: Cleft lip and cleft palate in an adult.

If maxillary hypoplasia is present then *osteotomy of the maxilla* is done. With *orthodontic help teeth extraction and alignment* of dentition is done.
- Regular examination of ear, nose and throat during follow-up period.
- Postoperative speech therapy.
- Often staged surgical procedure is done, whenever complicated problems are present.
- *Wardill-Kilner push back operation*—by raising mucoperiosteum flaps based on greater palatine vessels.

DISEASES OF THE PALATE

- Cleft palate.
- Torus palatinus—*a bony hard swelling in the center of the hard palate.*
- Nasopalatine cysts.
- Epstein's pearls *at the junction of soft and hard palates in the midline in infants due to retained developmental cell rests.*
- Apical cyst or abscess.
- Minor salivary gland tumor—commonest site is palate.
- Maxillary tumor extending into the palate.
- Squamous cell carcinoma of the palate.
- Gummatous perforation in the middle of the palate seen in congenital syphilis.
- Perforation of the palate anywhere in carcinoma palate.

ORTHOPANTOMOGRAM

It is a plain X-ray of the mandible which shows the entire of mandible in a single plane. It is

*It's only after you've stepped outside your comfort zone that you begin to change, grow, and transform—**Roy T Bennett***

better than X-ray mandible lateral view as it highlights proper dentition, inner and outer plates of mandible and joints.

Indications

- Jaw tumors—adamantinoma, dental cyst, dentigerous cyst, osteoclastoma.
- Osteomyelitis of the mandible.
- Fracture mandible.

PREAURICULAR SINUS

- It is due to failure of fusion of anterior tubercles of the auricle creating a sinus.
- Often sinus opening gets sealed forming a preauricular cyst which gets infected forming an abscess.
- Sinus can get infected repeatedly discharging pus through its opening.
- It is often multiple.
- **Investigations:** Sinusogram; discharge study.
- **Differential diagnosis:** Cold abscess; sebaceous cyst.
- **Treatment:** Excision of the sinus with complete track.

Treacher-Collins syndrome

- Mandibulofacial dystosis.
- Hypoplasia of the zygomatic bone and mandible.
- Antimongoloid slant to the palpebral fissure.
- Coloboma of lower eyelid.
- Low ear lobule with deficient middle ears.
- Familial—3rd arch syndrome (mandibulofacial dystosis).

JAW TUMORS

The term '*Jaw tumors*' is a gross terminology which denotes any tumor which arises from jaw either benign or malignant; from upper or lower jaw; from any tissues (layers) of the jaw from mucosa to soft tissues (Figs. 24.14 and 24.15).

Jaw tumors – Classification I

Swelling arising from the gums (Epulis): Congenital epulis, fibrous epulis, pregnancy epulis, giant cell epulis, myelomatous epulis, sarcomatous epulis, carcinomatous epulis.

Swelling arising from the dental epithelium and ectomesenchyme (Odontomes): Ameloblastoma, compound odontome, enameloma, cementoma, dentinoma, odontogenic fibroma and myxoma, radicular odontome, composite odontome. Cysts arising in relation to dental epithelium: Dental cyst, dentigerous cyst.

Swelling arising from the mandible or maxilla: Osteoma and osteoblastoma, torus palatinus and mandibularis, fibrous dysplasia, osteoclastoma (common in mandible), osteosarcoma; secondaries; giant cell reparative granuloma.

Surface tumors: Tumors from the surface which extend into the jaw—ossifying fibroma, osteofibrosis of maxilla, Ivory osteoma of jaw, leontiasis ossea (diffuse osteitis), carcinoma extending into the jaw.

Jaw tumors – Classification II

It can be **odontogenic or non-odontogenic**.

Odontogenic tumors

Odontogenic tumor can arise from: (A) Odontogenic epithelium like—(1) Ameloblastoma; (2) Pindborg's tumor; (3) Clear cell; (4) Squamous cell type. (B) From odontogenic epithelium and ectomesenchyme like—(1) Ameloblastic fibroma; (2) Adematoid odontogenic tumour; (3) Compound odontome; (4) Complex odontome. (C) From odontogenic ectomesenchyme like—(1) Odontogenic fibroma; (2) Myxoma; (3) Benign cementoblastoma.

1. **Epithelial tumors**
   - Ameloblastoma
   - Calcifying odontogenic tumor
   - Odontogenic adenomatoid tumor
   - Composite odontoma, which may be either complex or compound. It is odontogenic hamartoma contains all 4 layers, dentin, enamel, cementum and pulp
2. **Mesodermal tumors:** Odontogenic fibroma, myxoma; cementoma, dentinoma
3. **Malignant odontogenic tumors:** Malignant ameloblastoma; fibrosarcoma

Contd...

The past is a place of reference, not a place of residence; the past is a place of learning, not a place of living—**Roy T Bennett**

Contd...

> **Non-odontogenic tumors**
> 1. Ossifying neoplasm like cemento-ossifying fibroma
> 2. Non-neoplastic bone lesions like fibrous dysplasia, cemento-ossifying dysplasia.
> 3. Cemento-osseous dysplasias like cherubism, central giant cell granuloma.
> 4. Osteoma, osteoblastoma, osteoclastoma, osteosarcoma.
>
> **Other lesions** like hemangioma, neurofibroma also can occur in jaw.

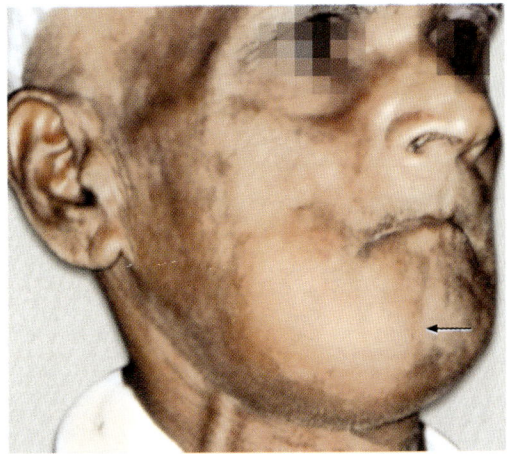

Investigations: Open incision biopsy is preferred. CT of the part; MRI to evaluate soft tissues. CT chest and abdomen are done in malignant cases to assess metastases.

Treatment: Wide excision with part of the bone with 2 cm clearance. Reconstruction is needed with bone graft and reconstruction prosthesis and flaps. Maxillectomy, mandibulectomy are often needed depending on location, size and extent.

Fig. 24.14: Jaw tumor arising from mandible. It could be adamantinoma/osteoclastoma/dentigerous cyst.

* Treatment is wide excision; shows 15% recurrence.

EPULIS (Greek—means upon gum)

Swelling arising from the mucoperiosteum of gums (gingiva). It is gross terminology but still term is used in many conditions (Figs. 24.16A and B).

PINDBORG'S TUMOR

* It is *calcifying epithelial odontogenic tumor (CEOT)*. It arises from epithelial remnant of enamel; it is common in mandibular molar. 50% or more arises from unerupted tooth.
* It presents as painless slow growing jaw tumor. It can be unilocular or multilocular lesion.
* Image shows scattered flaks of calcification with driven snow appearance.

Types

* *Congenital epulis:* It is a benign condition seen in a newborn arising from gum pads (*Neumann's tumor*). It is a variant of granular cell myoblastoma originating from gums. It is more common in girls. It is more common in upper jaw, common in canine or premolar

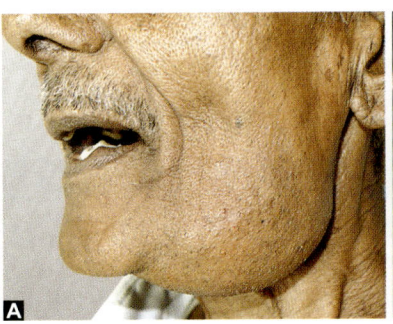
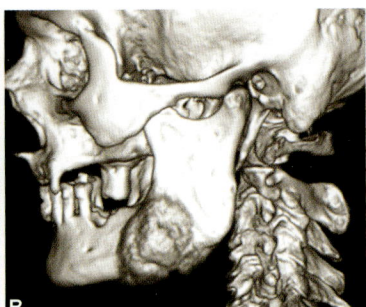
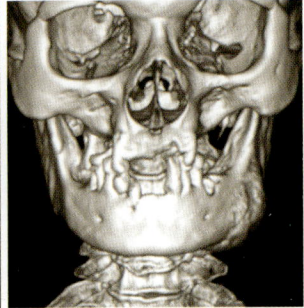

Fig. 24.15A and B: Lower jaw tumor. Reconstructed CT image of the same patient.

Happiness sneaks through the door you didn't know you left open

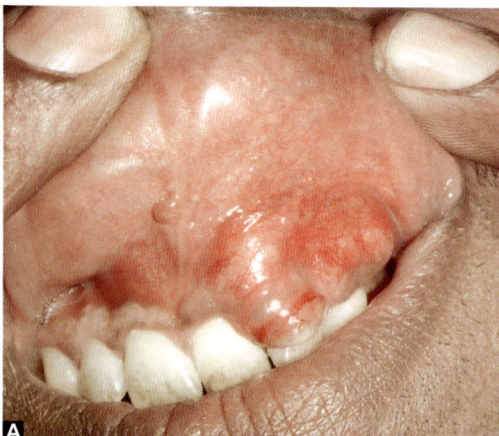 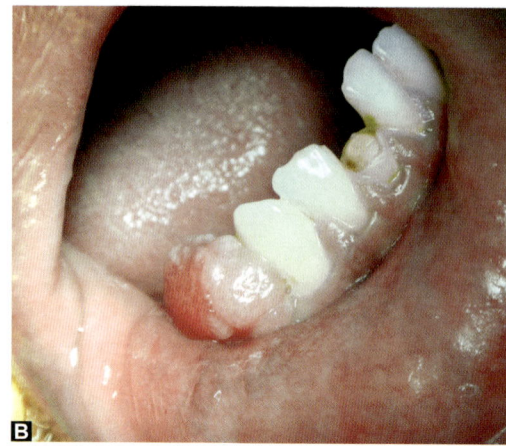

Figs. 24.16A and B: Epulis.

area. It is not a malignant condition. Clinical features are—well localized swelling from the gum which is firm and bleeds on touch. Treatment: Excision.

- **Fibrous epulis:** It is a benign condition, can occur in any individual. It is red, firm/hard, sessile/pedunculated. It is the commonest type. It is fibroma arising from periodontal membrane. Clinical features are—painless, well localized, hard, non-tender, gray pink swelling in the gum which bleeds on touch. Differential diagnosis: Squamous cell carcinoma from the gum. Investigations: X-ray jaw, orthopantomogram (OPG), biopsy from the lesion. Treatment: Excision with extraction of the adjacent tooth. Recurrence can occur if root is not removed properly.
- **Pregnancy epulis:** It occurs in pregnant women due to inflammatory gingivitis. Usually, it occurs during 3rd month of pregnancy. Clinically, it resembles fibrous epulis or pyogenic granuloma. It usually resolves after delivery. Otherwise it should be excised.
- **Epulis fissuratum:** It is a benign hyperplasia of fibrous tissue developing as a reactive lesion to chronic irritation to ill fitting dentures.
- **Myelomatous epulis:** It is seen in leukemic patients. It is investigated for leukemia by peripheral smear, bone marrow biopsy. Treatment is for leukemia.
- **Granulomatous epulis:** It is a mass of granulation tissue in the gum around a caries tooth. It forms a localized soft/firm/fleshy mass in the gum which bleeds on touch.
- **Giant cell epulis:** Osteoclastoma causing ulceration and hemorrhage of gum.
- **Carcinomatous epulis:** Squamous cell carcinoma of the alveolus and gum presenting as localized, hard, indurated swelling with ulceration.
- **Fibrosarcomatous epulis:** Fibrosarcoma arising from fibrous tissue of the gum.

Epulis	
• Congenital.	• Carcinomatous.
• Fibrous—commonest.	• Myelomatous.
• Granulomatous.	• Fibrosarcomatous.
• Pregnancy.	

AMELOBLASTOMA

(Adamantinoma, Eve's disease, Multilocular cystic disease of the jaw).
- It arises from the dental epithelium probably *from the enamel.*

The universe is not hostile, not yet is it friendly. It is simply indifferent.

- It occurs commonly in *mandible* or maxilla.
- Occasionally it is seen in the base of the skull in relation to Rathke's pouch or in tibia.
- Histologically it is a variant of *basal cell carcinoma*.
- It is a *locally malignant tumor*.
- It neither spreads through lymph node nor through blood. Hence it is *curable*.
- It is usually unilateral.
- It can occur in a pre-existing dentigerous cyst.

Features

- Swelling in the jaw usually in the mandible near the angle which attains a large size extending into vertical ramus—*Eggshell crackling*.
- It is gradually progressive, painless, smooth and hard with intact inner table (enlarges externally with *outer table expansion*).
- Lymph nodes are not enlarged.

Differential Diagnosis

- Osteoclastoma of the mandible: Here inner table is not intact.
- Dentigerous cyst.
- Dental abscess.
- *Giant cell reparative granuloma (Jaffe's tumor):* It is a swelling which occurs due to hemorrhage within the bone marrow. It contains vascular stroma, collagen and connective tissue cells. It is common in women. It causes painless enlargement of jaw. It can be treated by calcitonin (100 units/0.5 mg subcutaneously daily for 12 months) or surgical curettage.

Investigations

- Orthopantomogram (OPG) shows multi-loculated lesion—*Honeycomb appearance* (Figs. 24.17A and B).
- Biopsy from the swelling.
- CT scan face and jaw.

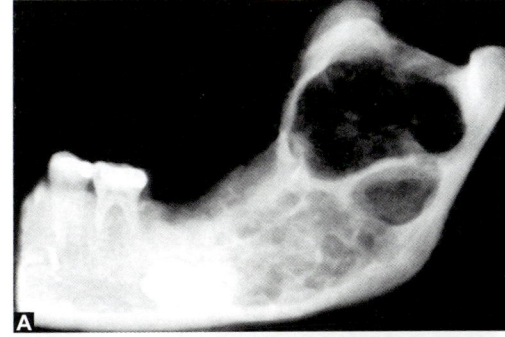
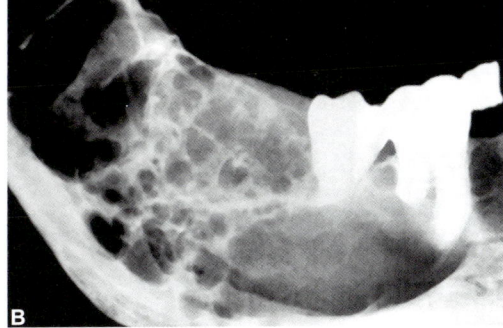

Figs. 24.17A and B: X-ray (two different X-rays) showing typical honeycomb/multiloculated features of adamantinoma (*Courtesy:* Dr Veena Jagadish, MDS).

Treatment

- Segmental resection of the mandible. OR
- Hemimandibulectomy with reconstruction of the mandible.

  Note:
  - Curettage and bone grafting should not be done.
  - It is a curable condition.
  - Recurrent adamantinoma can spread through blood (to lungs).

DENTIGEROUS CYST (FIG. 24.18) (FOLLICULAR ODONTOME)

- It is a unilocular cystic swelling arising in relation to the dental epithelium from an unerupted tooth.

*It is better to remain silent at the risk of being thought a fool, than to talk and remove all doubt of it—**Maurice Switzer***

- Common in lower jaw, but can also occur in upper jaw.
- It occurs over the crown of unerupted tooth. Commonly seen in relation to premolars or molars.
- It causes expansion of outer table of the mandible.

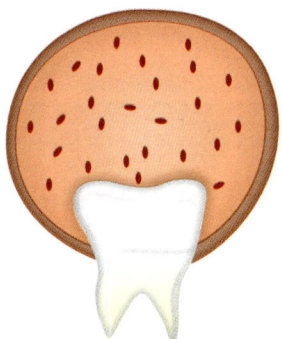

Fig. 24.18: Dentigerous cyst

Features

- Painless swelling in the jaw which is smooth and hard.
- **Differential diagnosis:** Adamantinoma; dental cyst; osteoclastoma.
- **Complication:** It can turn into adamantinoma.
- **Investigations:** Orthopentomogram shows tooth within the cyst, which is well-defined (Fig. 24.19).

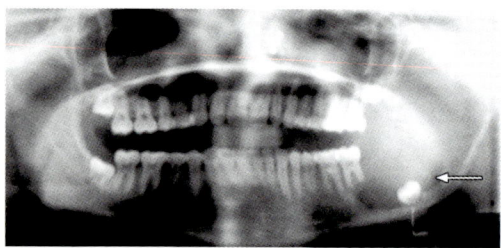

Fig. 24.19: Orthopantomogram showing dentigerous cyst.

Treatment

- If it is small, excision of the cyst is done.
- If it is large, initial marsupialization and later excision is done.
- Unerupted tooth should be extracted.

DENTAL CYST (FIG. 24.20) (RADICULAR CYST, PERIAPICAL CYST)

- It occurs under the root of the chronically infected dead erupted tooth.
- It is lined by squamous epithelium derived by *epithelial debris* of *Malassez*.

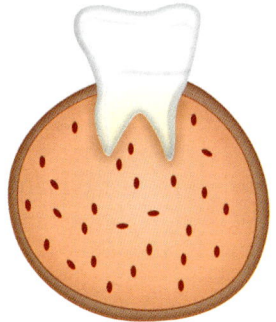

Fig. 24.20: Dental cyst.

Features

- As a smooth, tender swelling in the jaw in relation to caries tooth which causes expansion of the jaw bone.
- **Complication:** It can cause osteomyelitis of the jaw.
- **Differential diagnosis:** Dentigerous cyst.
- **Investigation:** Orthopantomogram.
- **Treatment:** Antibiotics; drainage or excision of the cyst with extraction of the infected tooth is done.

Differences between dental cyst and dentigerous cyst		
	Dental cyst	Dentigerous cyst
Site of occurrence	Erupted tooth under the root	Over the crown of an unerupted tooth
Infection	Common	Not common
Complication	Osteomyelitis	Adamantinoma
Treatment	Excision and extraction of tooth	Marsupialization, excision and then extraction of tooth

No amount of regretting can change the past, and no amount of worrying can change the future—**Roy T Bennett**

Curable malignancies	
• Adamantinoma.	• Papillary carcinoma thyroid.
• Basal cell carcinoma.	• Marjolin's ulcer.
• Verrucous carcinoma.	• Carcinoma colon.

OSTEOMYELITIS OF JAW

It is an inflammatory process in jaw; acute or chronic. It can be in the maxilla or mandible.

Causes

- Alveolar abscess later leading into osteomyelitis.
- Recurrent dental infection; after tooth extraction.
- Trauma; dental/jaw surgeries, after dental extraction.
- Postradiotherapy osteomyelitis (osteoradionecrosis).

Types

Acute

- It is common in children; maxilla or mandible may get involved.
- Swelling, redness, fullness are the features; pus may trickle through nostril if it is in maxilla.

Subacute

- It is the commonest type; common in adult.
- Apical sepsis, endarteritis, bone necrosis is the pathology.
- Common in mandible; rare in maxilla due to existing network vasculature which prevents endarteritis.
- Compression over inferior dental nerve causes numbness in chin in the area of distribution of mental nerve.
- Pain, swelling, tenderness, irregularity, bone thickening are typical.

Chronic

- It is also common in mandible.
- Apical abscess, alveolar abscess, trauma, radiation, chemicals like phosphorus, tuberculosis, syphilis, actinomycosis are the causes.
- Pain, bone thickening, irregularity, discharging sinus, sequestrum in the discharge, discomfort are the features.
- Infection from lower incisor causes median mental sinus.
- X-ray shows features of osteomyelitis with new bone formation and sequestrum.

Management

- X-ray jaw; CT scan of jaw; discharge study; ESR are essential investigations.
- Biopsy from the sinus is needed often.
- It is often difficult to treat. In acute phase, antibiotic coverage, treatment of cause is done. In chronic type, sequestrectomy, mandibulectomy is needed.

ALVEOLAR ABSCESS (DENTAL ABSCESS)

It is due to spread of infection from root of the tooth into the periapical tissue. Initially it forms periapical abscess which later spreads through the cortical part of the bone into the soft tissues around forming an alveolar abscess.

Bacteria: Staphylococci, streptococci, anaerobic bacteria and Gram-negative organisms.

Features

- Deep, throbbing pain in the jaw and adjacent oral cavity with diffuse swelling over the cheek.
- Tender soft tissue swelling in the jaw which eventually bursts spontaneously leading to sinus formation.
- Edema, pain and tenderness in the floor of the mouth

To every disadvantage, there is a corresponding advantage

- Trismus and dysphagia.
- Fever and features of toxemia.
- Tender palpable lymph nodes in the neck.

Investigations

- X-ray of the mandible or maxilla.
- Discharging pus for culture study.

Complications

- Septicemia.
- Spread of infection into other spaces like parapharyngeal spaces.
- Chronic osteomyelitis of the jaw with discharging sinuses.

Treatment

- Antibiotics.
- Drainage of the abscess under general anesthesia.
- Extraction of the tooth at a later period.
- Excision of the sinus whenever required.

CHERUBISM

It is an autosomal dominant condition occurs in first year of life.

Pathology

- Giant cell granuloma with fibrous tissues in the jaw.
- *It is commonly* bilateral.
- *Commonly seen in* angles of the mandible *and also in maxilla.*

Features

- Diffuse enlargement of maxilla and both sides of the mandible.
- Bulging of the cheek causes pull of the lower eyelid. Hence child appears like, as if looking upwards.
- Interference with the development and eruption of the teeth.

Treatment

It is a self-limiting disease. Often requires dental care and treatment for proper dentition.

Pierre-Robin syndrome

- Congenital condition.
- Cleft palate.
- Mandibular hypoplasia.
- Cyanotic episodes.
- Deficiency in transforming growth factor.
- Defective sucking and tongue falling backwards in infants.
- Cryptorchidism.

FIBROUS DYSPLASIA OF BONE/JAW (FIGS. 24.21A AND B)

It is benign self-limiting noncapsulated lesion of bone wherein normal bony architecture is replaced by collagen, fibroblasts, osteoid and calcified tissue. It is often classified as benign tumor with localized developmental arrest, with bone being not differentiated into a mature bone tissue.

It is seen in childhood and adolescents.

Types

It may be polyostotic or monostotic. Condition can occur in long bones, ribs and jaw bones, either mandible or maxilla. Disease is either metaphyseal or in the shaft, never in epiphysis.

1. **Monostotic (70%)**
   - It is equal in both sexes. It occurs in children and adolescents; stops once growth plate is closed.
   - Femur is the commonest bone involved; tibia, ribs, jaw bones, skull and humerus can get involved.
   - It can present as asymptomatic diffuse hard bony swelling or can be painful due to fracture. Discrepancies of the part with asymmetry are common.
   - Monostotic will not turn into polyostotic type.
   - Monostotic will not turn into sarcoma.

Discovery consists of seeing what everybody has seen and thinking what nobody has thought

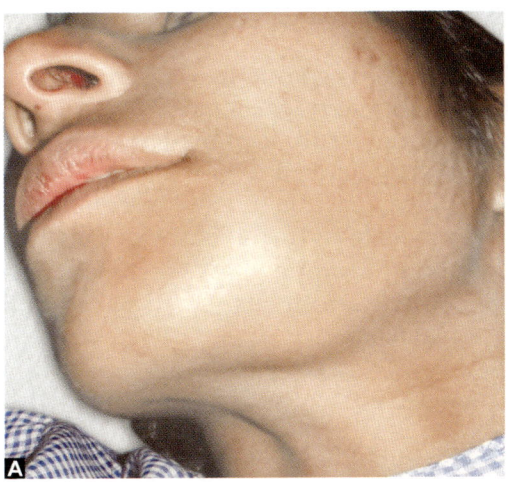 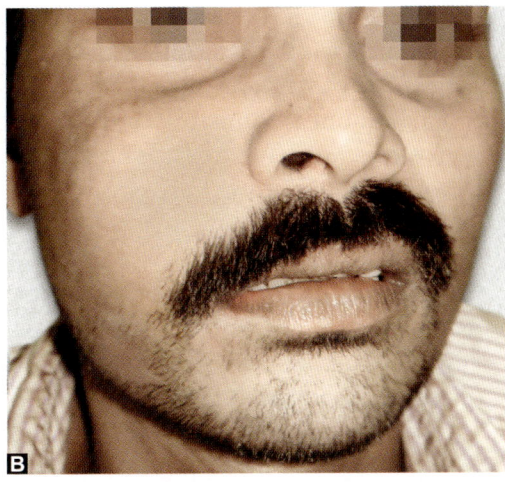

Figs. 24.21A and B: Fibrous dysplasia of mandible and maxilla in two different patients. Mandible is common site in jaw. Overall femur is the commonest site.

2. **Polyostotic fibrous dysplasia (27%) without endocrine dysfunction**
   - It begins in earlier age group than monostotic.
   - It is common in femur, skull, tibia, humerus, ribs, fibula, radius, ulna, mandible and vertebrae. Craniofacial bones are involved in more than 50% of patients.
   - It may continue to grow in adulthood (progressive).
   - There is no evidence of hyperparathyroidism. It should be differentiated from primary hyperparathyroidism of bone.
   - Involvement of shoulder and pelvis causes severe deformity.
   - Severe femur involvement causes 'shepherd crook' deformity.
   - Recurrent spontaneous fractures are common.
   - Polyostotic occasionally turns into sarcoma.

3. **Polyostotic fibrous dysplasia with endocrinopathies (3%)**
   - *Polyostotic fibrous dysplasia with skin pigmentation (Café au lait, on same side of the disease in neck, chest, back, shoulder, pelvis, larger) with sexual precocity in females (McCune Albright's syndrome);* often with hyperthyroidism, growth hormone secreting pituitary adenoma and primary adrenal hyperplasia is 3% common.
   - It is due to mutation of guanyl nucleotide binding protein gene (GNAS gene).

   - Fibrous dysplasia is most common in *femur—shepherd crook deformity;* metaphyseal.
   - In the jaw, mandible is the common site, vertical ramus, outer table expansion.
   - Monostotic is more common.
   - Polyostotic is more problematic—discrepancies, pathological fracture, sarcoma changes.
   - Monostotic ceases with cessation of growth.
   - Surgery should never be done during growing period.

Fibrous Dysplasia of Jaw

- In the jaw, it can occur in maxilla or mandible; but mandible is more common site.
- It presents with diffuse swelling of vertical ramus of the mandible or maxilla. Gritty white, hard cartilages with cysts are the pathology.

*Take responsibility of your own happiness; never put it in other people's hands—**Roy T Bennett***

- Diffuse hard, painless swelling which causes asymmetry is the usual presentation. It progresses with the growth of the bone.
- It is commonly monostotic but can be polyostotic. Monostotic ceases once bone develops completely. Polyostotic may continue to grow.
- Teeth are normal.
- Expansion is towards outer cortex of the mandible.
- Polyostotic occasionally turns into sarcoma (but not monostotic).

Complications of Fibrous Dysplasia

- Deformity and cosmetic problems.
- Pathological fractures.
- Sarcomatous transformation in polyostotic type only.

Differential Diagnosis

- Osteoclastoma, adamantinoma.
- Osteitis fibrosa cystica of primary hyperparathyroidism.

Investigations

- X-ray is diagnostic showing *ground glass/smoke screen* appearance.
- Serum alkaline phosphatase may be slightly elevated.
- Biopsy may be needed to confirm the condition and to rule out other conditions.
- Parathormone assay, serum calcium estimation in suspected parathyroid pathology.

Treatment

- It should not be operated during growing period as if intervened there may be chances that it may turn into osteosarcoma.
- As it is a self-limiting disease it can be left alone once the growth stops or can be corrected by restorative excision to maintain facial contour.
- Thorough curettage with cancellous bone grafting may be done.
- Bisphophonates are often used to relieve pain.

Anything the mind of man can conceive and believe, it can achieve

CHAPTER 25

Maxillofacial Injuries

Chapter Outline

- Primary Care (Early Care) in Maxillofacial Injuries
- Fracture Middle Third Area
- Fracture Mandible
- Complications of Maxillofacial Injuries

Maxillofacial region is a complex bony structure made up of many bones. Often injury involves not just one bone but multiple bones in the complex. Structure is related to the complex and complicated functions of the face, mastication, breathing, and speech and swallowing. So any injury in this region will alter these functions in one way or other (Fig. 25.1).

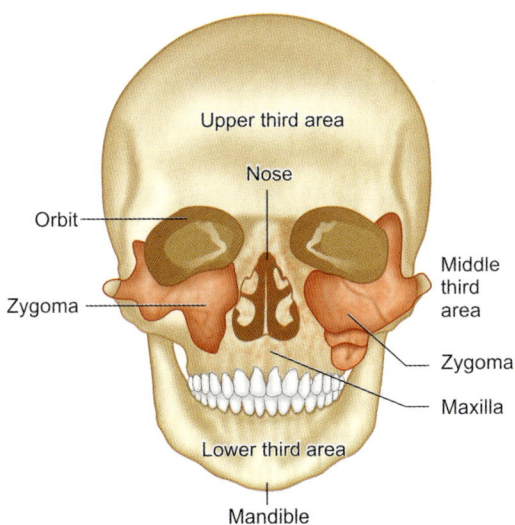

Fig. 25.1: Maxillofacial injuries regions.

Fracture in maxillofacial region can be grouped as:
- Fracture lower third that comprises mandible.
- Fracture middle third that comprises maxilla, zygoma and nose.
- Fracture upper third of the face involving part of the orbit, frontal bones.

Maxillofacial fracture also can be grouped as:
- Fracture of the face, which do not involve the dental occlusion—fractures of zygoma and nose.
- Fracture which involves the dental occlusion-fracture mandible and maxilla.
  Treatment of these fractures always involves restoration and maintenance of correct dental occlusion otherwise it leads into permanent irreversible deformity.

PRIMARY CARE (EARLY CARE) IN MAXILLOFACIAL INJURIES

Injury can be isolated single bone fracture or multiple bone fractures. Any real primary care is usually not required except when there is mechanical respiratory block causing airway obstruction.

Reading make a full man, conference a ready man, and writing an exact man

Respiratory Obstruction

Causes

- Oronasal airway block can occur by blood, clot, vomitus, foreign body, dentures, teeth, saliva, bone pieces, etc.
- Backwards falling of tongue can cause obstruction of the nasopharynx and oropharynx. It is common in bilateral mandibular fracture.
- Occlusion of the nasopharynx and oropharynx can occur in fracture maxilla with posterior and inferior displacement.
- Hematoma in floor of the mouth or posterior oral cavity can cause airway block.
- Laryngeal/pharyngeal edema.
- Surgical emphysema.

Treatment

- Cleaning of the oral and nasal cavities to remove obstructing agents like clot, dentures, teeth or bone. Gauze swabbing and suction.
- Fallen tongue should be placed forward using finger and often temporary alignment of the occlusion may be needed.
- Maxillary disimpaction is done when needed in fracture maxilla.
- Positioning of the patient is important. Prone position with head towards one side is the safest position. If this is not possible then patient may be placed in sitting position, which also improves the breathing. Placing the patient on his back supine position flat should be avoided as much as possible.
- Tracheostomy should be done when needed without delay as it will be life-saving by facilitating the easy airway and breathing.

Control of Pain

Analgesics like nonsteroidal anti-inflammatory drugs (NSAIDs) are used to control pain. Morphine and analogs are not used as they may suppress the respiration. They may mask the pain of alarming severe injury in chest, abdomen or other areas, or they may interfere with pupillary reaction and neurological signs in the presence of intracranial injuries.

Control of Infection

Antibiotics are needed. Tetanus toxoid and often antitetanus globulin (ATG 3000 units IM) are required.

Hemorrhage in Maxillofacial Injuries

Hemorrhage in maxillofacial injuries is usually not life-threatening. But it should be identified and controlled properly. In association with other internal injury, such hemorrhage may be important to cause the circulatory failure.

Hemorrhage may be due to:
- Soft tissue bleeding.
- Bleeding from inferior alveolar artery, palatine vessels.
- Nasal bleeding.

Control of bleeding:
- Blood transfusion, IV fluids, resuscitation.
- Nasal packs.
- Fracture correction.
- Ligation of the bleeder.
- Cauterization.
- Packing the area.
- Under running the bleeding field.
- Embolization.
- External carotid artery ligation above the level of the origin of the superior thyroid artery.

Associated Injuries

All associated injuries should be assessed properly and individually. On priority basis it should be treated.
- Soft tissue injuries.
- Cranial injuries.

*There is a great difference between worry and concern. A worried person sees a problem, and a concerned person solves a problem—**Harold Stephens***

- Orbital injuries.
- Intra-abdominal/thoracic/pelvic injuries.

FRACTURE MIDDLE THIRD AREA

Surgical Anatomy of Middle Third Area

It includes:
- Maxillae, zygomatic bones, palatine bones, nasal bones, lacrimal bones, inferior conchae (one on each side).
- The vomer, ethmoid and its attached conchae, pterygoid plates of sphenoid.

Features

- Middle third articulates with frontal bone and body of the sphenoid at an angle of 45°. It forms an inclined plane inferiorly and posteriorly. It is displaced along the inclined plane in middle third fracture. It can also force mandible downwards producing posterior gagging of the teeth and an anterior open bite (Figs. 25.2 and 25.3).
- In nasoethmoid fracture or LeFort II or III fractures, communition fractures of ethmoid occurs which in turn break the region of cribriform plate of ethmoid leading into CSF rhinorrhea.
- Infraorbital nerve injury can occur in fracture of zygomatic bone leading into anesthesia in the area supplied by the nerve.
- Fracture of orbital floor results in herniation of the orbital contents into the

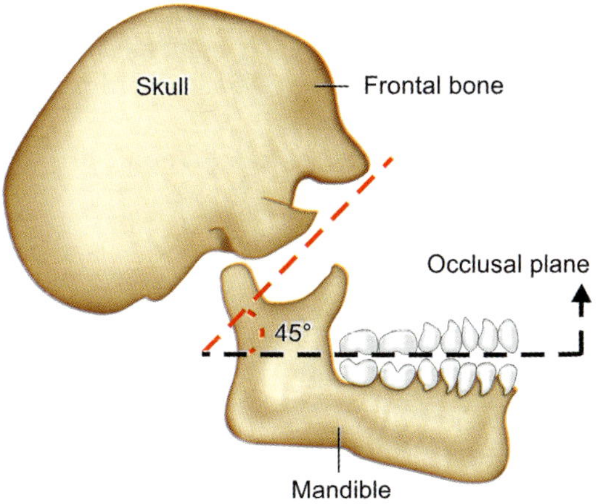

Fig. 25.2: Relation between middle third and cranium in 45° plane.

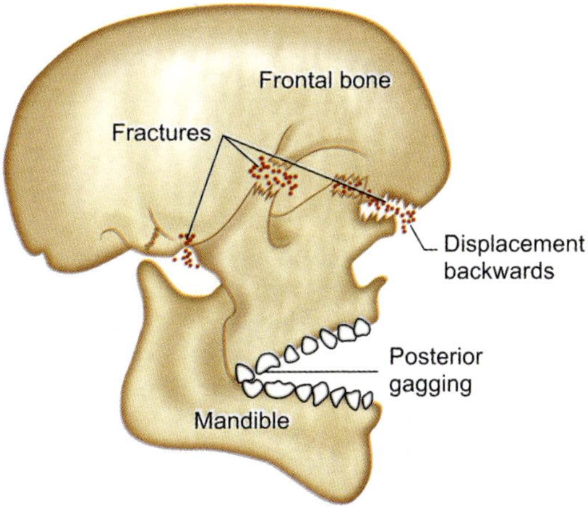

Fig. 25.3: Posterior gagging of occlusion due to displacement backwards of fracture segment in middle third fracture.

Fractures not involving occlusion
Central
- Fracture nasal bones and/or nasal septum.
- Fracture of frontal process of maxilla.
- Fractures of above two extending into ethmoid-nasoethmoid.
- Fractures above three which extends into frontal bone—fronto-orbito-nasal dislocation.

Lateral
- Fractures involving zygomatic bone, arch and maxilla excluding the dentoalveolar component.

Fractures involving occlusion
Dentoalveolar.
Subzygomatic.
- Le Fort I—low level either unilateral or bilateral.
- Le Fort II—pyramidal either unilateral or bilateral.

Suprazygomatic Le Fort III—high level
- Craniofacial disjunction—unilateral or bilateral.

Better alone than in bad company

maxillary sinus which causes diplopia due to restriction of the movements of the inferior rectus and inferior oblique.
* Change in the position of the eye globe/injury to eye globe/optic nerve tear can occur in injury of zygomatic prominence. Fracture middle third includes fracture maxilla, zygoma and nasal bones.

Classification of Fracture Middle Third Area

* Nasoethmoid complex fracture.
* Zygomatic complex fracture.
* Maxillary fracture.

LE FORT CLASSIFICATION (FIGS. 25.4A TO D)

(*Rene Le Fort*—French surgeon classified these fractures by dropping rocks on the face of the cadavers and later dissecting the area for study and research and published paper in 1911).

NASOETHMOID COMPLEX FRACTURE

Classification

* Isolated nasoethmoidal and frontal bone fracture/injury without other facial bone injuries, which can be unilateral or bilateral.
* Combined nasoethmoidal and frontal bone injury with fracture of other bones in middle third face, which can be unilateral or bilateral.

Mode of Injury in Nasal Bone Fracture

* *Lateral violence* on the nose causing nasal bone fracture with deviation, displacement and fracture nasal septum.
* *Head-on-violence* causing backward displacement and splaying of nasal bones creating collapse of nasal bridge and saddle deformity.

Types (Figs. 25.4A to D)	Features
Le Fort I (Guerin's fracture-low level) (floating fracture, horizontal fracture of maxilla) It runs horizontally above the floor of the nasal cavity involving lower third septum, palate, alveolar process of maxilla and lower third of pterygoid plates of maxilla.	• Bleeding from nose. • Posterior gagging of occlusion. • Upper lip swelling. • Palatal ecchymosis. • Occlusion derangement. • Floating maxilla.
Le Fort II (pyramidal fracture) From the nasal bones at topmost, fracture runs laterally towards lacrimal bones, medial wall of orbit, infraorbital margin, through or medial to infraorbital foramen and backwards below the zygomaticomaxillary area through lateral wall of maxillary sinus and pterygoid plates. Zygoma is intact with skull base.	• Edema of middle third face. • Both sides circumorbital and subconjunctival ecchymoses. • Nasal bleeding/obstruction/deformity. • Deformity of face (dish face), diplopia. • Retroposition of maxilla with posterior gagging. • Limitation of ocular movements, CSF rhinorrhea. • Tenderness and separation of infraorbital margin.`
Le Fort III (craniofacial disjunction, high level) Here fracture runs parallel to skull base. It passes through the nasal bone, lacrimal bone, ethmoid bone, optic foramen, inferior orbital fissure, pterygomaxillary fissure and lateral orbital wall with frontozygomatic suture with zygomatic arch.	• Lengthening of face. • Enophthalmos, ocular level depression. • Hooding of eyes, occlusal plane tilting. • Entire facial skeleton moves as a single block. • Tenderness and separation of suture line. • Diplopia. • Trismus, teeth malalignment. *Guerin sign*: Hematoma at greater palatine foramen.

The ultimate measure of a man is not where he stands in moments of comfort and convenience butwhere he stands in times of challenge and controversy—**Albert Einstein**

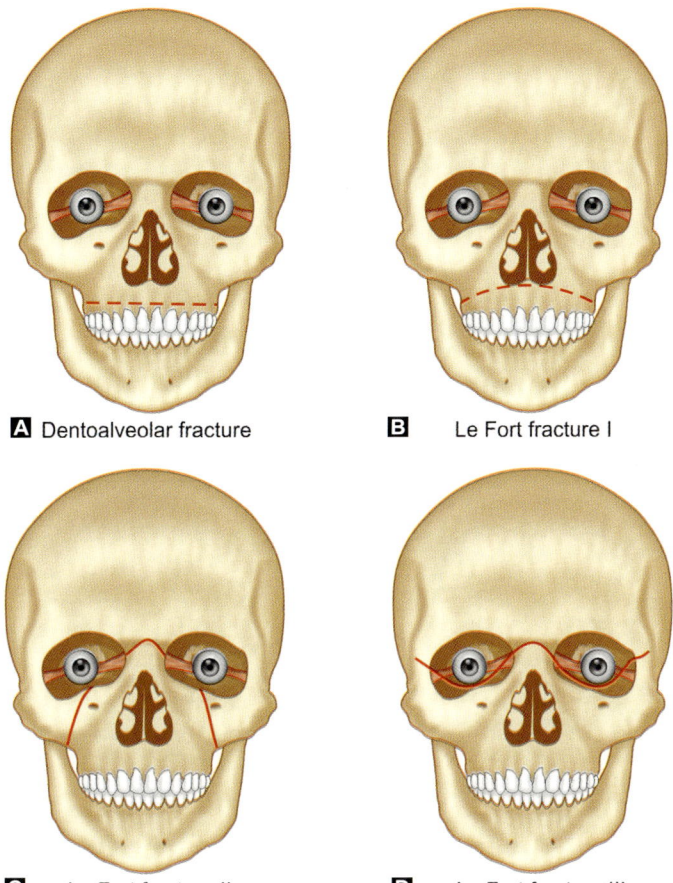

Figs. 25.4A to D: Le Fort classification—different types and also dentoalveolar fracture (For details refer table on previous page).

Features

- Pain, tenderness in nasal and frontal region.
- Swelling in the region with deviation and displacement.
- Bleeding from the nose.
- Subconjuctival hemorrhage.
- Crepitus over nasal bridge.
- CSF rhinorrhea.
- X-ray nasal bone shows fracture.
- CT is done to see other injuries.

Treatment

Fracture is treated on the basis of the clinical examination.

Walsham's forceps is used to reduce the fractured nasal bone. Asch's forceps is used to reduce the nasal septum. Procedure is done under general anesthesia. Alignment is maintained by nasal packs from inside and nasal plaster from outside.

ZYGOMATIC COMPLEX FRACTURE

Classification (Figs. 25.5A to G)

- *Simple fracture which is stable and undisplaced*—here fracture line passes across the infraorbital foramen downwards over anterior wall of the antrum.

Arrogance is the obstruction of wisdom

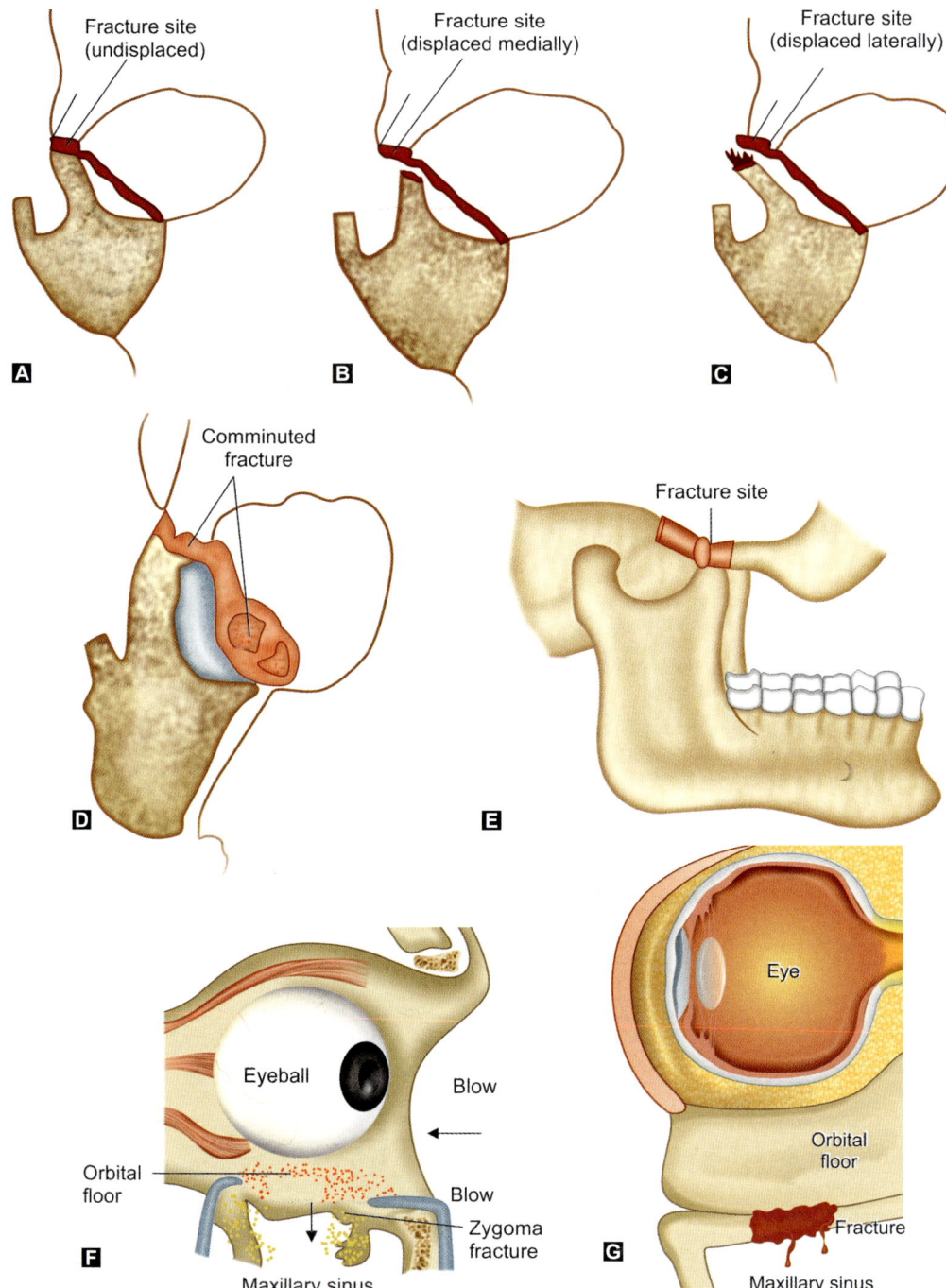

Figs. 25.5A to G: Diagrams showing different types of zygomatic fractures: (A) Undisplaced fracture zygoma; (B) Medially displaced fracture zygoma; (C) Laterally displaced fracture zygoma; (D) Comminuted zygoma fracture; (E) Arch fracture zygoma; (F) Blowout fracture orbit; (G) Orbital floor fracture.

*Be yourself; everyone else is taken—***Oscar Wilde**

- *Simple fracture which is displaced medially.* It may be associated with rotation/tilt in vertical axis, either medial tilt or lateral tilt. Infraorbital nerve may get compressed or branches of superior dental nerve may get torn.
- *Unstable fracture with rotation around horizontal axis* with medial tilt or lateral tilt.
- *Comminuted fracture* extending into the floor of the orbit.
- *Fracture of the zygomatic arch* causes a localized depression of the arch which displaces medially and tends to impinge on the coronoid process of the mandible.
- *'Blowout' fracture* of the orbit is due to direct blunt trauma on the eyeball causing depressed comminuted fracture of the orbital floor with herniation of the orbital fat into the antrum.
- *En bloc dislocation of zygomatic bone* medially/inferiorly/posterolaterally.

Features

- Swelling and bruising in the cheek with subconjunctival hemorrhage.
- Flattening of the cheek prominence.
- Step in the margin of the bony orbit at the infraorbital foramen.
- Sensory loss over the supply of the branches of the superior orbital nerve—teeth on the affected area is anesthetic on percussion.
- Sensory loss over the supply of the infraorbital nerve usually over infraorbital region, upper lip and alar region of the nose.
- Enophthalmos is due to herniation of the orbital fat across the fracture floor of the orbit into the antrum.
- Diplopia is due to entrapment of the inferior rectus muscle preventing upward rotation of the eyeball while looking up.
- Trismus with marked restriction of the lateral movements.
- Epistaxis, lowering of pupil level.
- Infraorbital ecchymosis of the orbit is called as *Panda sign*.

Investigations

- A 30° occipitomental X-ray is used commonly but often obliquity of X-ray may be increased to 60°. In X-ray, findings observed are:
  - Fracture line near infraorbital foramen, zygomatic arch and lateral wall of the antrum.
  - Orbital floor line for fracture.
  - Opacity in the antrum due to blood.
- CT scan is done to see orbital depression and herniation of orbital fat.

Treatment

- *Every patient with zygoma fracture need not require surgical correction.*
- Need for surgery is decided based on clinical features.

Indications for surgery
• Infraorbital anesthesia, trismus.
• Diplopia, enophthalmos.
• Flattening of the cheek.
• Undisplaced fracture with infraorbital anesthesia.

Surgical Approaches

1. Closed reduction of the zygomatic arch through Gillies temporal approach (Fig. 25.6): An oblique skin incision of 2 cm length at temporal region is made between the two branches of the superficial temporal artery. Care is taken to avoid injury to artery. Whitish glistening temporal fascia is identified and incised. Zygoma elevator is introduced beneath the zygoma and fracture fragments are manipulated and elevated into proper position. An audible snap is heard when fracture gets reduced into position. Reduced, disimpacted fracture is always stable. Additional corrections in other parts can be done by different leverage

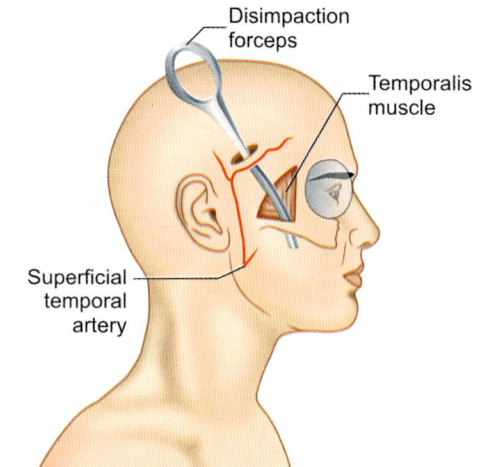

Fig. 25.6: Technique showing method of temporal reduction using disimpaction forceps.

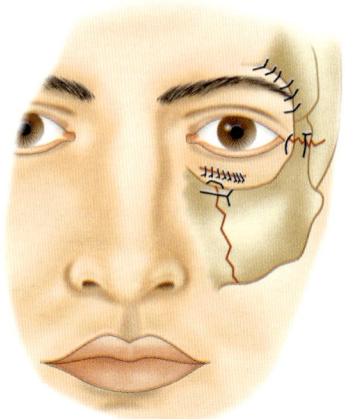

Fig. 25.8: Fracture zygoma showing open reduction and fixation using wires directly. Two types of incisions are shown depending on the site of the fracture.

actions of the elevator. Orbital rim, zygomatic arch are palpated for completion of correction. Skin wound is closed with sutures.

Elevators used are:
- Bristow's periosteal elevator.
- Rowe's zygomatic elevator (Figs. 25.7A and B).

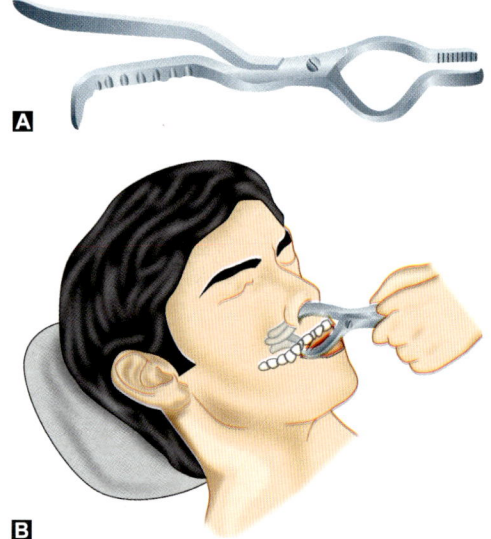

Figs. 25.7A and B: Disimpaction of maxilla using Rowe's disimpaction forceps by downward leverage action.

2. Internal fixation by open reduction and fixation is needed (Fig. 25.8):
- When fracture is unstable or
- Comminuted or
- Zygoma fracture with middle third fractures.

By proper incisions infraorbital and zygomaticofrontal fracture sites are exposed and after open reduction they are fixed using wires/plates and screws.

3. Exploration of the orbital floor is necessary whenever there is:
- Comminuted fracture in orbital floor.
- Orbital fat herniation.
- Diplopia with entrapment of the inferior rectus muscle.

MANAGEMENT OF FRACTURES IN MIDDLE THIRD AREA

Investigations and proper evaluation of the patient by X-ray, CT scan is essential. Approaches and timing of the surgery is decided. Often it requires two or more staged procedures, which should be informed to the patient clearly.

*What lies behind us and what lies ahead of us are tiny matters compared to what lies within us—**Martin Luther King***

Treatment of Middle Third Fracture

Fracture is reduced by manipulation of the fragments into correct dental occlusion to their counterpart on the opposite alveolus. It is maintained in that position until fracture becomes stable. If dental occlusion is correct it is presumed that fracture has been reduced accurately. Stabilization of the fractured bone to unfractured bone is called as *intermaxillary fixation*. Indirect methods are effective in less severe injuries but are inadequate in injuries of circumorbital elements, upper maxilla, glabellar bone and medial orbital wall. Open craniofacial technique like open surgical manipulation and fixation using wires/screws and plates are more ideal and standard way of approach.

'Eyelet' wires and 'arch bars' are used when the teeth are used to fix the fracture segment in reduced position. Gunning splintage is used in old edentulous patients.

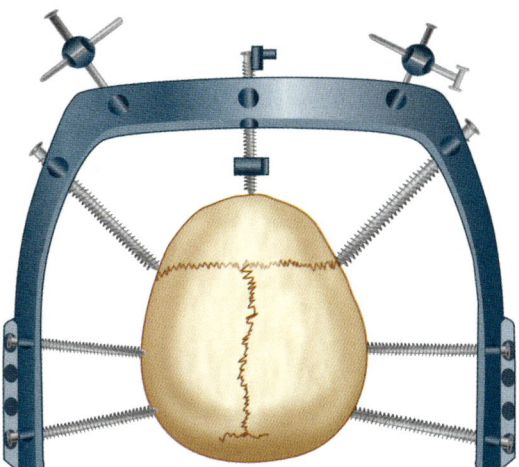

Fig. 25.9: Craniomandibular external fixation of maxilla using halo frame.

Surgical methods are:
- Direct internal fixation
    - Transosseous wiring at fracture site.
    - Stainless plates (steel/titanium).
    - Dynamic/eccentric compression plates.
    - Microplating.
    - Polyglycolic resorbable plates.
    - Transfixation with Kischner wire/Steinman pin.
- *Suppression wires* to mandible—frontal/circumzygomatic/zygomatic/intraorbital.
- *Antral pack/antral balloon* support.
- *Craniomandibular external fixation* of maxilla using box frame/halo frame (Fig. 25.9).
- *Craniomaxillary external fixation of maxilla* using halo frame/supraorbital pins/zygomatic pins.
- *Internal suspension for stabilization* of middle third fractures by circumzygomatic suspension/zygomatic suspension/infraorbital suspension/pyriform aperture suspension/frontal suspension (central or lateral) (Fig. 25.10A).
    - *Circumzygomatic suspension* is used in subzygomatic fractures with intact zygoma and wire is passed around zygomatic arch.
    - *In zygomatic suspension* through buccal sulcus approach, inferior ridge of the zygoma is used for suspension, using wires (Fig. 25.10B).
    - *In infraorbital suspension* a drill hole in the lower border of the orbit is made to pass a wire which is used for suspension. Area is approached through an outer infraorbital, lower orbital margin skin incision or from intraorally through buccal sulcus above the canine fossa. Eyeball should be protected (Fig. 25.10C).
    - *In pyriform aperture suspension*, pyriform bony aperture is approached through a buccal mucosal incision above lateral incisor; drill hole is made to pass suspension wire (Fig. 25.10D).
    - *Frontal suspension* could be lateral or central. *In lateral type* (Fig. 25.10E),

*Something I find profoundly humbling is to note that human genius is limited while human stupidity is not—**Alexandre Dumas***

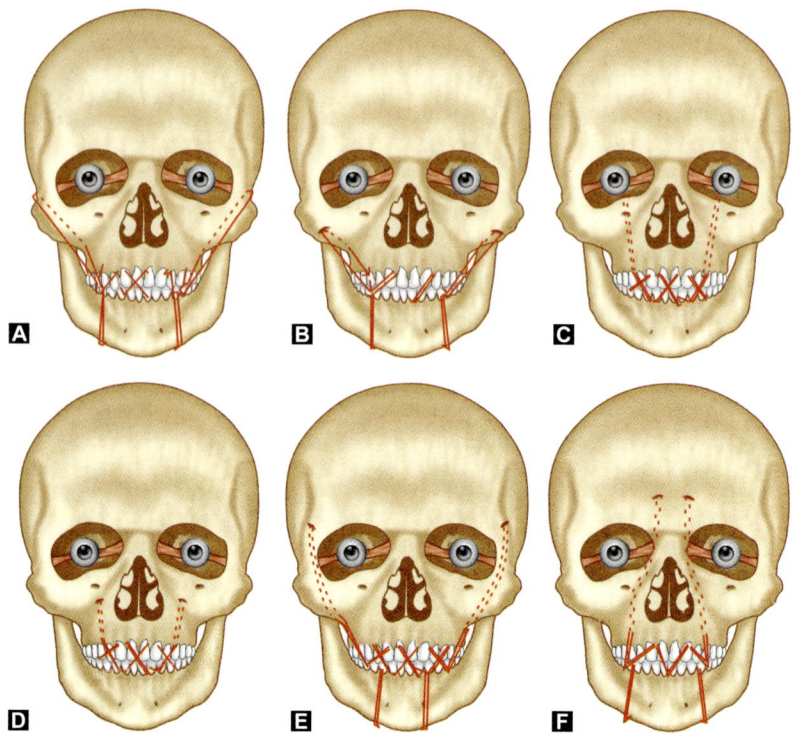

Figs. 25.10A to F: Different types of suspensions for middle third fracture internal fixation: (A) Circumzygotic suspension; (B) Zygomatic suspension; (C) Infraorbital suspension; (D) Pyriform aperture suspension; (E) Frontal lateral suspension; (F) Frontal central suspension.

zygomatic process of the frontal bone just above the frontozygomatic suture line is approached through a lateral eyebrow skin incision and drill holes one on each side are made to pass wires. Each wire on each side is directed towards the buccal sulcus near the 1st molar tooth and wires are used for suspension. *In central type* (Fig. 25.10F), wire is passed through a pin placed on the inner table of frontal bone in the forehead through an incision in the skin above the frontal sinus and is passed across upper canine region, lateral to pyriform margin of nose and lacrimal gland. Procedure is repeated on the other side. After reduction of the fracture segments these wires are fixed to maxillary/mandibular splints.

FRACTURE MANDIBLE

Surgical Anatomy of the Mandible

- Mandible is prominent, mobile horse-shoe shaped bone in the facial skeleton, which is the largest and strongest bone of the face. It has got U-shaped body and two rami one on each side projecting upwards (Figs. 25.11A and B).
- Body of the mandible has got outer surface with symphysis menti, mental protuberance, mental tubercles and mental foramen. External oblique line gives attachment to depressor muscles, buccinator and platysma. Inner surface of the body of mandible has got mylohyoid line for attachment of mylohyoid muscle and superior constrictor muscle of the

*Wisdom ceases to be wisdom when it becomes too proud to weep, too grave to laugh and too selfish to seek other than itself—**Kalil Gibran***

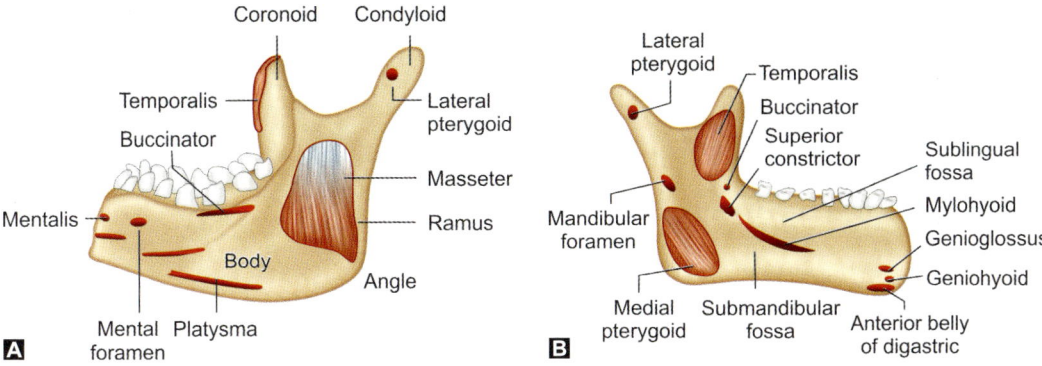

Figs. 25.11A and B: Anatomy of the mandible showing features of external and internal surfaces.

Classification of the fracture mandible (Fig. 25.12)

Depends on the type	Depends on the anatomical site
• Simple. • Compound. • Comminuted. • Pathological. • Greenstick fracture in children.	• Dentoalveolar fracture. • Condylar fracture. • Coronoid fracture. • Fracture ramus of the mandible. • Fracture angle of the mandible. • Fracture in the body of the mandible. • Symphyseal region fracture.

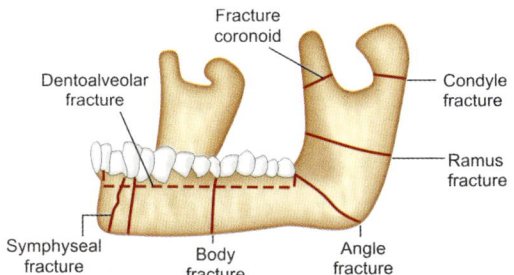

Fig. 25.12: Different sites of fracture mandible.

pharynx. Inner surface has got groove for lingual nerve, submandibular fossa, sublingual fossa, genial tubercles for genioglossus and geniohyoid muscles and mylohyoid groove with mylohyoid vessels and nerve.
❖ Outer surface of the ramus of the mandible gets insertion of the masseter muscle and is related to parotid salivary gland.

❖ Inner surface of the ramus of the mandible has got mandibular foramen which transmits inferior dental/alveolar vessels and nerve. Medial pterygoid muscle is attached to inner surface of the ramus of the mandible.
❖ Coronoid process is flat triangular part with pointed apex which curves and continuous as condyloid process with mandibular notch in between. Temporalis muscle is inserted to this coronoid process.
❖ Condyloid process has got head which forms temporomandibular joint with articulation with temporal bone. Lateral pterygoid muscle is inserted to pterygoid fovea in front of the neck of the coronoid process.
❖ Mandibular notch transmits masseter vessels and nerves.
❖ It is thickest in the body in the region of the mental prominence and third molar region.
❖ Ramus of the mandible has got central core of cancellous bone with two thin layers of cortical bone. Junction between body and vertical ramus is weak structurally.
❖ Neck of the condyle of the mandible is also weaker area.
❖ Teeth in the bone reduce the strength of the mandible and also a constant source of infection.
❖ Medial pterygoid, masseter and temporalis muscles influence the displacements in fracture angle of the mandible.

Our senses don't deceive us; our judgement does

- Mandible is supplied by inferior dental artery centrally and periosteal vessels peripherally. In old people inferior dental arterial supply is poor and blood supply mainly depends on periosteal vessels, which often decides the healing of fracture and also results of open reduction.

(a) Dentoalveolar Fracture

Features

- Horizontal fracture below the alveolar margin.
- Dentoalveolar segment will be freely mobile.
- Tooth may get split vertically/horizontally.
- Derangement in occlusion and alignment.
- Gingival laceration.
- Bleeding.
- Infection and late osteomyelitis of mandible.

Management

- Look for other injuries in face.
- X-ray face to see injuries.
- Dentoalveolar segment reduction and placing jaws in central occlusion position.
- Stabilization using interdental wires or arch bars.
- Liquid diet for 3–4 weeks.

(b) Condylar Fracture (35%) (Figs. 25.13A and B)

In condylar fracture condylar head is pulled forward by the lateral pterygoid muscle. When both condyles are fractured the displacements of both heads causes the patient to gag on his molars producing an open bite. *It is the commonest type of mandibular fracture.*

Classification

- Fracture without displacement.
- Fracture with displacement with anterior overlap/with posterior overlap.
- Fracture with dislocation.

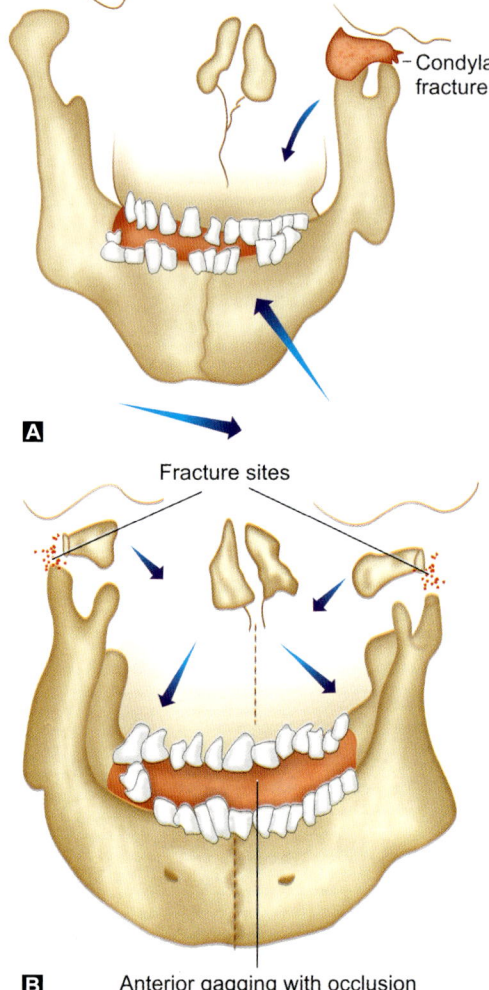

Figs. 25.13A and B: Mandible gets shifted to same side (in figure left side) in unilateral condylar fracture. In bilateral condylar fracture anterior gagging with occlusion occurs.

- Fracture with deviation.
- Extracapsular fracture condyle.
- Intracapsular fracture condyle (Figs. 25.14A and B).

Features

Unilateral (Fig. 25.15)
- Condylar tenderness of the side.
- Decreased condylar movement on the side.

A little may save a deal of friction

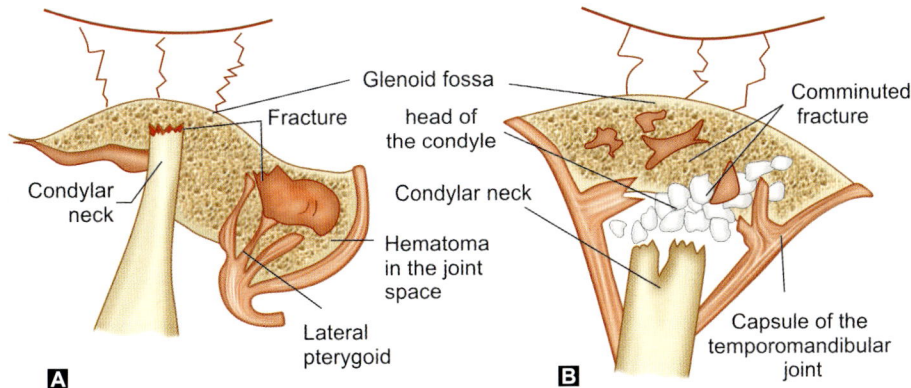

Figs. 25.14A and B: Intracapsular fracture mandible. (A) Shows fracture condyle with hematoma whereas (B) shows comminuted fracture of the condyle.

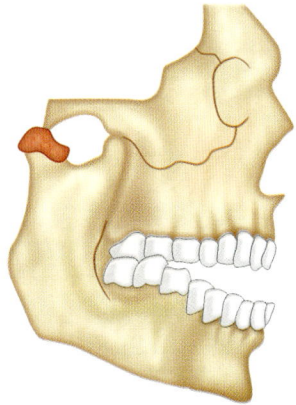

Fig. 25.15: Bilateral condylar fractures can cause an '**open bite**'.

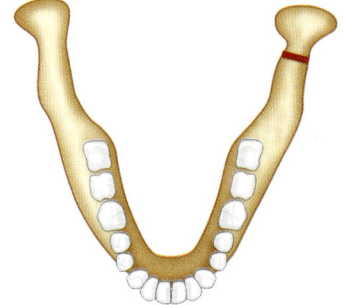

Fig. 25.16: Unilateral condylar fracture.

- Jaw deviation towards fracture site.
- Tear in external meatus and bleeding from ear of the side.
- Preauricular swelling of the side.

Bilateral (Fig. 25.16)
- Condylar tenderness on both sides.
- Absence of condylar movement.
- Bleeding from both ears.
- Preauricular swelling on both sides.
- Anterior open bite.

Management

- *In children* if it is intracapsular fracture, active movements without immobilization is the only treatment. If it is extracapsular, intermaxillary fixation for 10 days, later active movements is needed.
- *In adult* if it is unilateral intracapsular and painful, immobilization is advised for 2 weeks and later active movements are encouraged. If it is bilateral intracapsular condylar fracture intermaxillary fixation for 2 weeks and later fixation with night elastics for another 4 weeks is done. In extracapsular unilateral condylar fracture intermaxillary fixation for 4 weeks is the choice. Bilateral extracapsular fracture condyles are most problematic. It needs intermaxillary fixation for 6 weeks until occlusion is stable. Often it needs proper open reduction.

*I prefer to be a dreamer among the humblest, with visions to be realized, than lord among those without dreams and desires—**Kalil Gibran***

(c) Fracture of the Ramus or Angle of the Mandible

- If fracture is upwards and inwards, it is impacted and undisplaced. It is *favorable fracture* (Fig. 25.17).
- If fracture is downwards and outwards, it gets displaced and it is *unfavorable fracture* (Fig. 25.18).

Clinical Features

- Pain and tenderness in the lower jaw with bruising over the surface.
- Hematoma in the floor of the mouth is called as **Coleman's sign**.
- Difficulty in opening the mouth, speech and swallowing.
- Anesthesia of the lower lip due to compression of inferior dental nerve.
- Deranged dental occlusion (Fig. 25.19).
- Step deformity.

Management

- X-ray of the mandible reveals the fracture site.
- Antibiotics to prevent formation of osteomyelitis of the mandible.
- Open reduction of the fracture and fixation of the fracture segments using titanium/stainless steel plates or wires for 4–6 weeks.

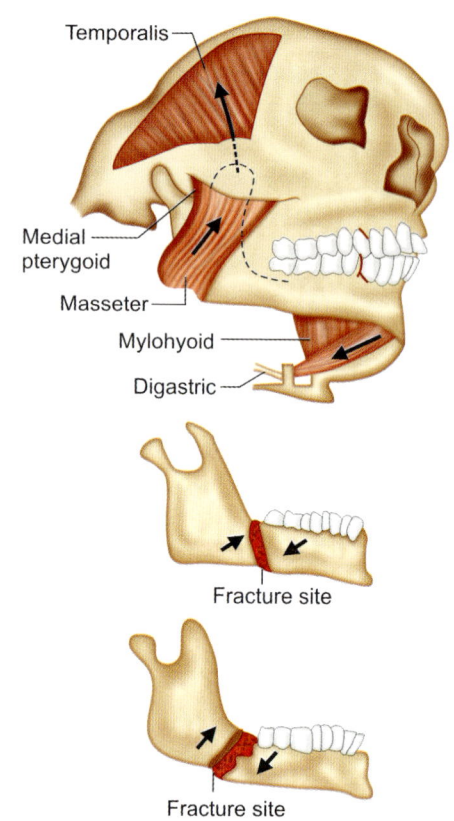

Fig. 25.18: Muscle actions in mandible fracture causing different displacements.

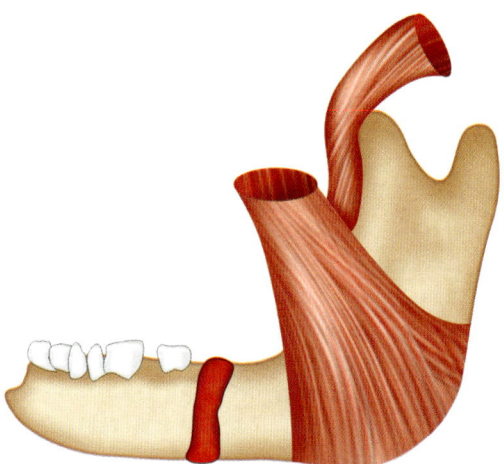

Fig. 25.17: Undisplaced fracture mandible.

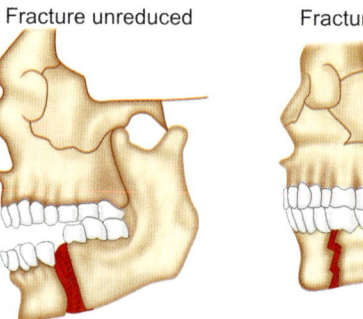

Fig. 25.19: Unreduced and reduced fracture mandible.

Either intraoral buccal sulcus approach or extraoral approach is used.
- Closed reduction of the fracture segments and fixation by:
  - Interdental wiring (Fig. 25.20).

You may be disappointed if you fail, but you are doomed if you don't try

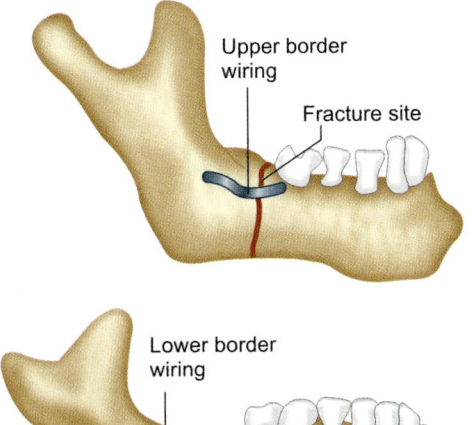

Fig. 25.20: Upper and lower border wiring. It is used to fix the mandibular fractures and is often done together with other fracture fixations in the face.

- Using arch bars.
- Silver alloy or plastic caps.
* Only fluid diet for 6 weeks.
* Irrigation washes to the oral cavity to maintain the hygiene.

(d) Fracture of Symphysis of the Mandible (Figs. 25.21A to C)

It causes:
* Sublingual ecchymosis.
* Step deformity of lower margin of the mandible.
* Difficulty in closing the mouth.
* Occlusion discrepancy.
* Mobile mandible with drooling of saliva.

Types

* Symphysis fracture, central without displacement.
* Symphysis fracture, oblique with displacement.
* Bilateral symphysis fracture.

Treatment

* Closed reduction with intermaxillary fixation for 4 weeks.
* Open reduction and fixation using plates or wires.

Complications of fracture mandible
- Obstruction of the airway.
- Osteomyelitis of the mandible.
- Trismus.
- Speech disturbances.

Management of the Mandibular Fracture

Closed reduction and indirect skeletal fixation using:

Dental Wiring

* Direct interdental wiring (Fig. 25.22).
* Clove hitch wiring.
* Interdental eyelet wiring (Fig. 25.23) is commonly used method for intermaxillary

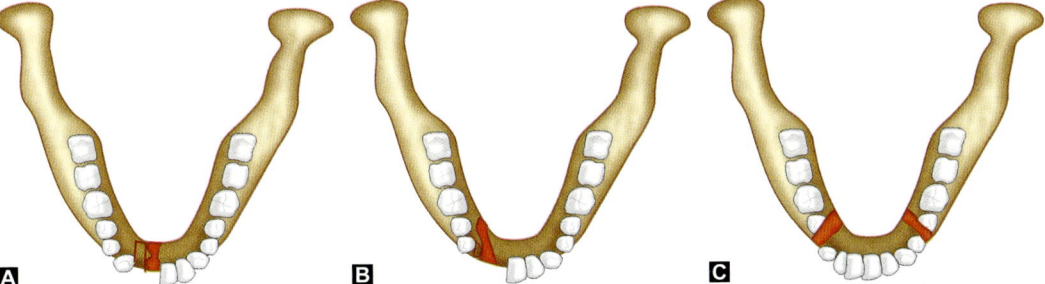

Figs. 25.21A to C: Different types of symphyseal fracture—(A) midline, (B) oblique and (C) bilateral.

A virtuous woman is a splendid prize; a bad...the greatest curse beneath the skies

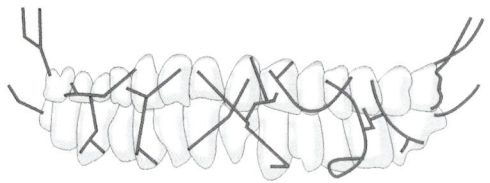

Fig. 25.22: Interdental direct wiring. It is commonly used and accepted method of wiring.

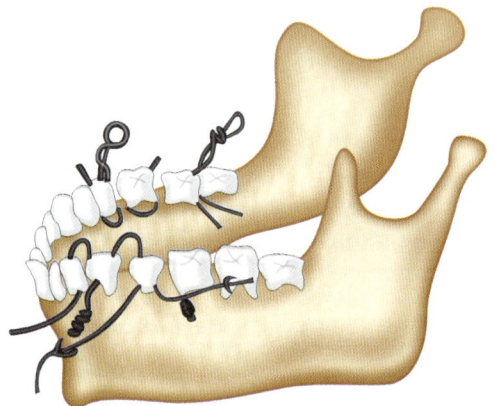

Fig. 25.23: Diagram showing steps in eyelet wiring.

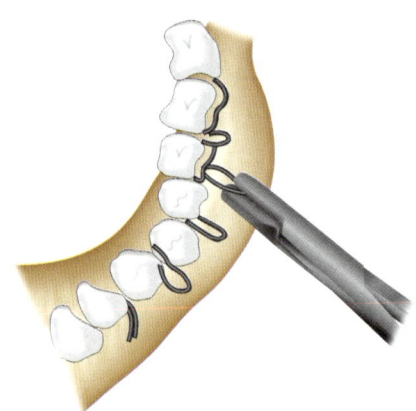

Fig. 25.24: Multiple loop wiring used in mandibular fracture.

fixation. Five eyelets are used in upper and lower jaw.
* Multiple loop wiring (Fig. 25.24).
* Continuous wiring.
* Risdon wiring is used instead of arch bars in midline/paramedian fractures wherein two wires are tied on the posterior teeth.

Arch bars are used in:
* When there are inadequate teeth for wiring
* Dentoalveolar fractures.
* When there is associated middle third area fractures.
* Combination of body and condylar fracture.

Arch bar is done using a malleable metal bar made of flattened soft German silver wire (Fig. 25.25). It is moulded around the alveolar arch on its outer aspect at the level of the necks of teeth to which it is then wired. *Erich arch bar* is modified simple arch bar with cleats along its length. Bar is wired to alveolus and using cleats it is wired to the bar attached to the opposite alveolus.

Gunning splints are used in edentulous patients. Dental impressions are taken and dentures without teeth called as 'gunning splints' are made. They are wired circumferentially to upper and lower jaws and to each other to produce needed fixation (Fig. 25.26). It cannot be used in severe fractured unfavorable fractures.

Cap splints are done when only few teeth are present. It is very lengthy procedure and difficult. Cast silver cap splints or acrylic cap splints are used.

Open Reduction and Direct Skeletal Fixation

* *Transosseous wiring*/osteosynthesis along lower border or upper border.
* *Plating* across fracture segments using either noncompression plates or compression plates (dynamic/eccentric) (Figs. 25.27 and 25.28).
* *Fixation using screw (Fig. 25.29).*
* *Titanium or stainless steel mesh fixation.*

(e) Dislocation of the Mandible

* It occurs at *temporomandibular joint*.
* Unilateral dislocation after trauma is common.
* Bilateral dislocation occurs during yawning and it is recurrent.

Knowledge of self is the mother of all knowledge—**Kalil Gibran**

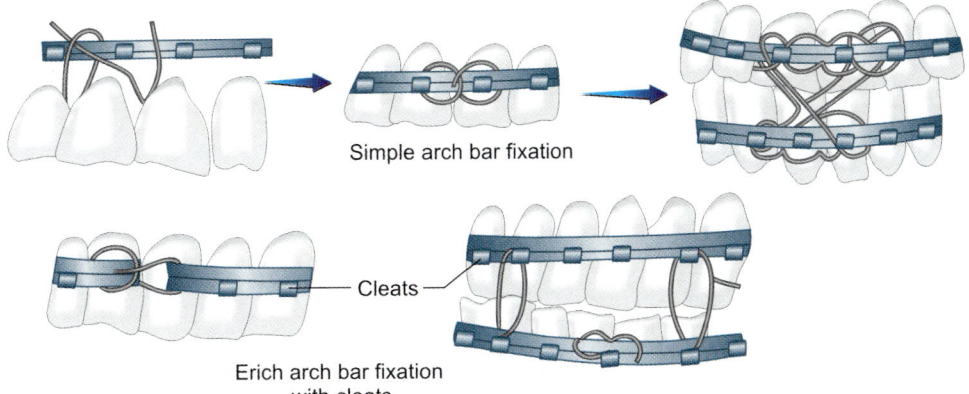

Fig. 25.25: Arch bar wiring. Figure shows both simple and Erich arch bar wiring with cleats to pass wire.

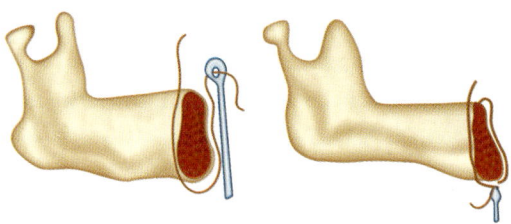

Fig. 25.26: Circum mandibular wiring used in gunning splints.

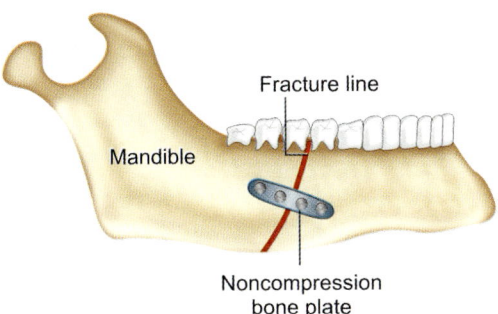

Fig. 25.27: Noncompression bone plating used in mandibular fracture.

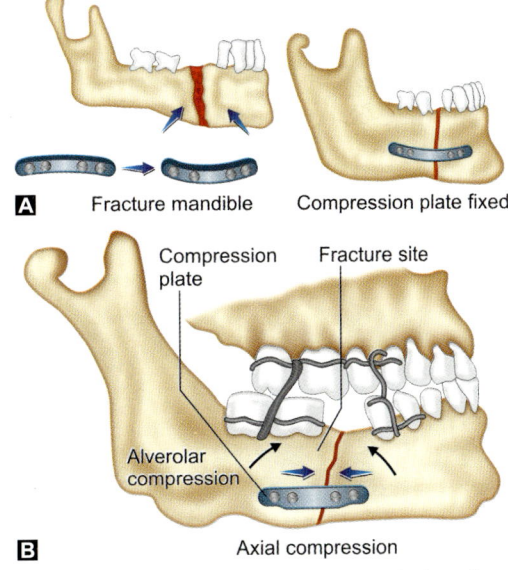

Figs. 25.28A and B: Compression plating of a mandibular fracture. Note the different methods.

Clinical features are difficulty in opening the mouth with pain and tenderness over the joint.

Treatment

- Reduction of dislocation under general anesthesia.
- If there is associated fracture mandible it should be dealt accordingly.

COMPLICATIONS OF MAXILLOFACIAL INJURIES

- Infraorbital nerve anesthesia due to compression/injury of infraorbital nerve in zygoma or middle third area fractures.
- Lower lip anesthesia in fracture mandible due to injury of mandibular nerve.
- Malunion and deformities of face.
- Infection and osteomyelitis.

Don't sit back and take what comes; go after what you want

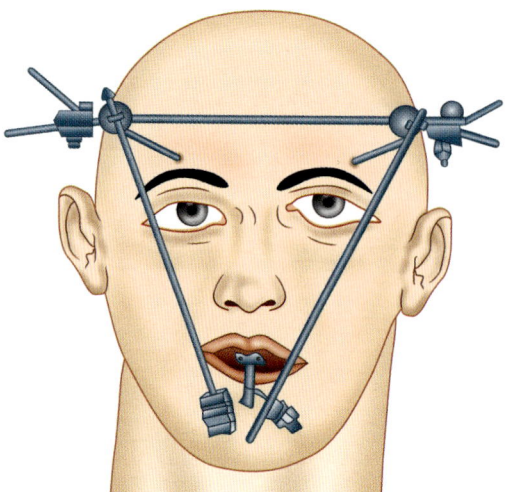

Fig. 25.29: Fixation of the splint to skull. It is often used with gunning splints to fix it to skull.

- Airway block due to posterior pharyngeal edema/backward fall of tongue in mandibular fracture.
- Superior orbital fissure syndrome is seen in zygomatic complex injury due to hematoma in the fissure causing compression of 3rd, 4th and 6th cranial nerves in the fissure. It causes ophthalmoplegia, ptosis, proptosis and dilated pupil.
- Deranged occlusion.
- Nonunion is not as common as malunion. It is due to infection, improper immobilization, systemic diseases and deficiencies, Ankylosis of the temporomandibular joint is common in children, in intracapsular fracture of the condyle and in prolonged immobilization.
- Diplopia/enophthalmos/orbital complications/strabismus.
- Nasal deformity.
- Epiphora due to damage of nasolacrimal duct.
- In comminuted fracture of nasoethmoid complex, cribriform plate is injured causing injury to olfactory nerve leading into loss of smell.
- Alteration in speech is usually temporary.
- Cosmetic disability.

No one has yet realized the wealth of sympathy, the kindness, and generosity hidden in the soul of a child. The effort of every true education should be to unlock that treasure—**Emma Goldman**

CHAPTER 26

Tracheostomy

CHAPTER OUTLINE

- Tracheostomy
- Tracheostomy Tubes

TRACHEOSTOMY

Tracheostomy is making an opening in the anterior wall of trachea and converting it into a stoma on the skin surface.

TYPES

- Emergency tracheostomy.
- Elective tracheostomy.
- Permanent tracheostomy.

High tracheostomy—above the level of isthmus. It can cause tracheal stenosis. It is above 2nd ring.

Midtracheostomy—ideal and commonly used. It through 2nd and 3rd rings behind isthmus. It is approached by dividing thyroid isthmus.

Low tracheostomy—below the isthmus level. It is deep and impinges the suprasternal notch. It can cause torrential bleed which is difficult to control.

TRACHEOSTOMY TUBES (FIG. 26.1)

- ***Fuller's bivalved tracheostomy tube (Fig. 26.2):*** It has got a outer tube and a

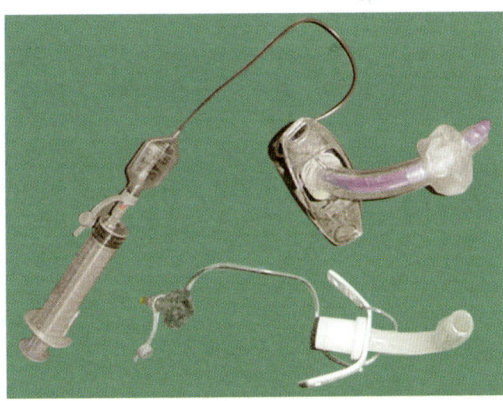

Fig. 26.1: Tracheostomy tube with inflation part and syringe (inflated with air).

inner tube. Outer tube is biflanged and so insertion is easier. Inner tube is longer with an opening on its posterior aspect. Inner tube can be removed and re-inserted easily whenever required.
- ***Jackson's tracheostomy tube (Fig. 26.3):*** It has got outer tube, inner tube and an obturator.
- **Red-rubber tracheostomy tube.**
- **PVC tracheostomy tube.**
- ***Shiley's fenestrated tracheostomy tube:*** It has got outer and inner tube; outer tube has

The greatest glory in living lies in never falling, but in rising every time we fall—**Nelson Mandela**

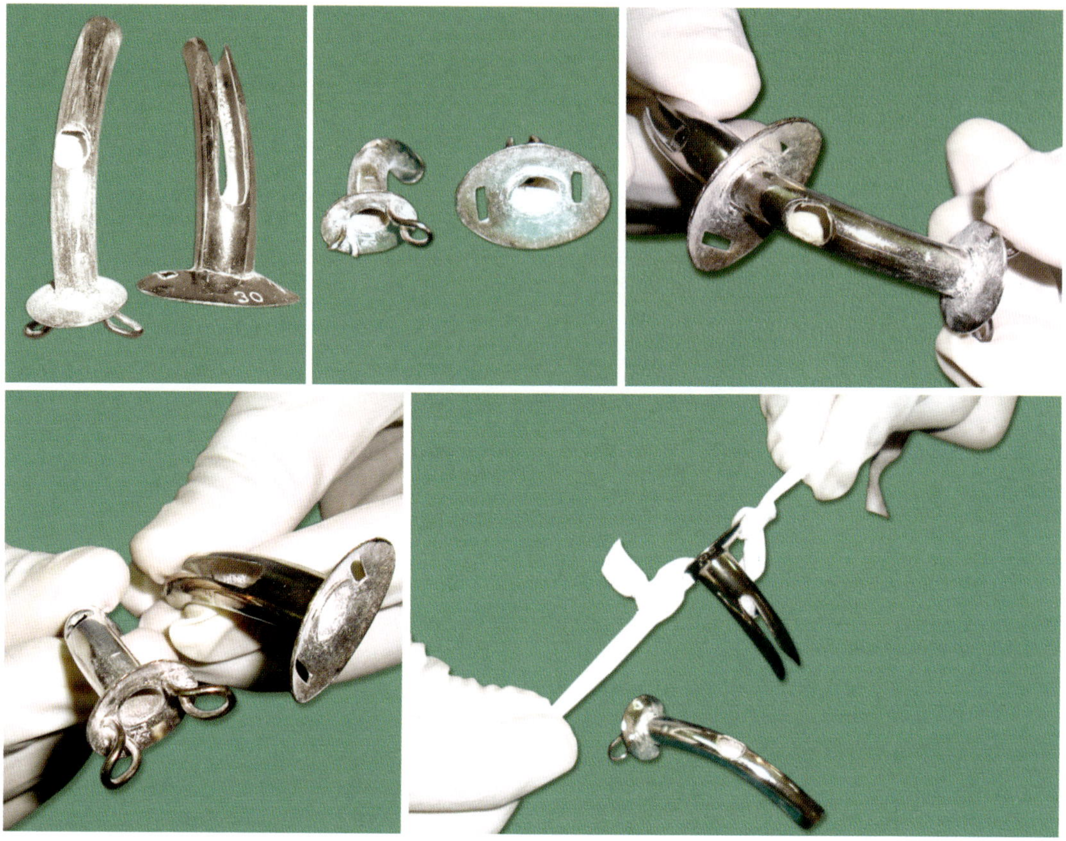

Fig. 26.2: Fuller's biflanged tracheostomy tube.

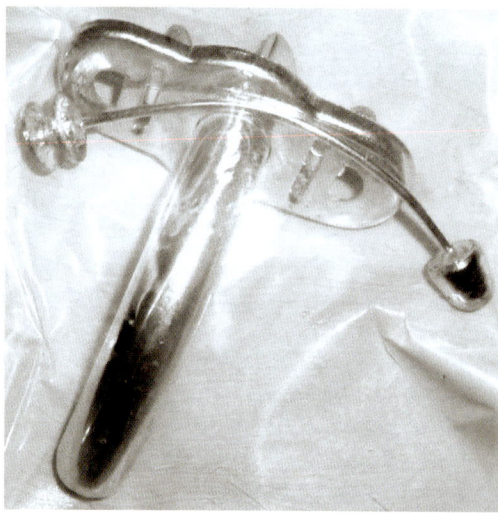

Fig. 26.3: Chevalier Jackson's tracheostomy tube.

got inflatable cuff (when needed); inner tube is changeable and may be fenestrated (for speaking) or nonfenestrated (for mechanical ventilation) (Fig. 26.4).

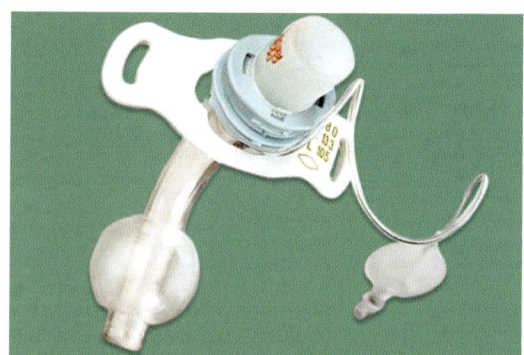

Fig. 26.4: Shiley's tracheostomy tube.

Conduct has the loudest tongue

Modern tracheostomy tubes are made of plastic. They are soft, least irritant and disposable. They have inflatable cuff which makes it easier to give assisted ventilation. Cuff should be deflated at regular intervals to prevent tracheal pressure necrosis (for assisted ventilation, endotracheal tube can be kept for 7 days. Beyond that period patient needs tracheostomy for further ventilation) (Figs. 26.5 and 26.6).

Indications for Tracheostomy

- In head, neck and facial injuries.
- Tetanus.

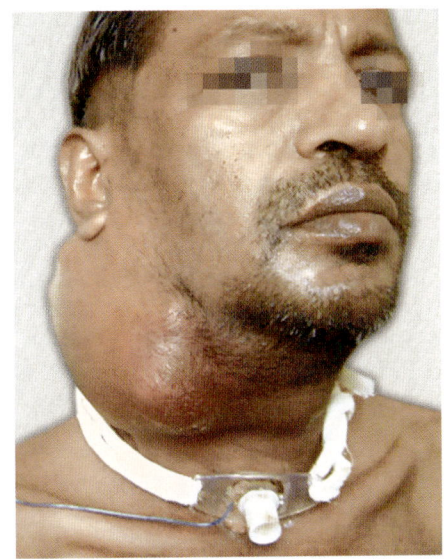

Fig. 26.7: Advanced secondaries in neck with tracheostomy tube to control respiratory stridor.

- Tracheomalacia after thyroidectomy or bilateral recurrent laryngeal nerve palsy.
- Laryngeal edema/spasm.
- Major head and neck surgeries like Commando's operation, block dissection.
- Acute laryngitis as in diphtheria.
- Carcinoma larynx (Fig. 26.7), foreign body larynx, burns mouth, pharynx, larynx.
- Respiratory paralysis like bulbar palsy.
- Respiratory failure due to asthma, acute respiratory distress syndrome (ARDS).

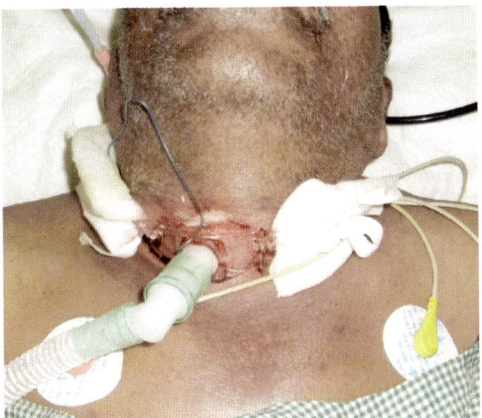

Fig. 26.5: Tracheostomy in position connecting to ventilator.

Technique of Tracheostomy (Fig. 26.8)

Neck of the patient is hyperextended by placing sand bags under the shoulder. Vertical (midline) or horizontal incision is made. Deep fascia is opened. Strap muscles are retracted laterally. Isthmus is divided or retracted upwards. A few drops of lignocaine are instilled into the trachea to suppress the cough reflex. Trachea is fixed with tracheal hook. 2nd and 3rd or 3rd and 4th tracheal rings are opened and circular opening is made. Tracheostomy tube is placed. It is tied around the neck (Fig. 26.9).

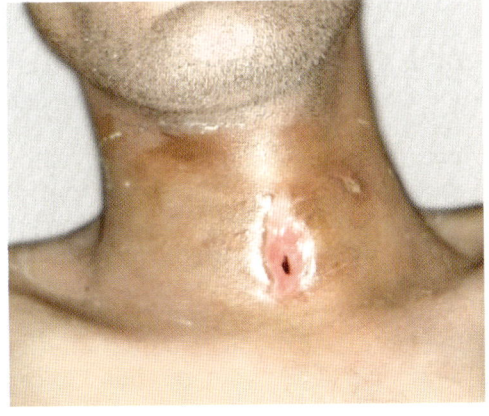

Fig. 26.6: Tracheostomy track without tube in situ.

*Great things happen to those who don't stop believing, trying, learning, and being grateful—**Roy T Bennett***

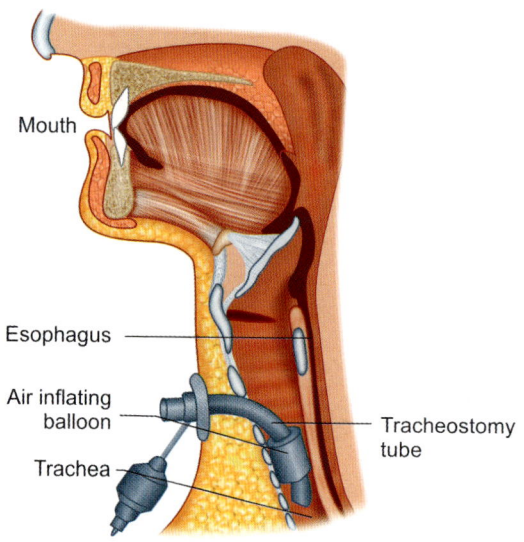

Fig. 26.8: Position of tracheostomy.

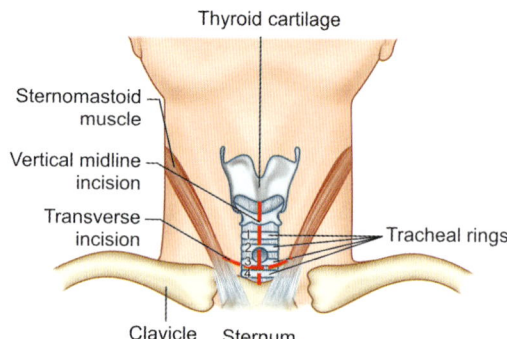

Fig. 26.9: Vertical midline or transverse incisions are used for tracheostomy. **Vertical midline** incision extends from cricoid cartilage to sternal notch. It is used in emergency and often elective tracheostomy. It gives rapid access with less dissection but leads into poor scar. **Transverse incision** can be used in elective tracheostomy. It is placed two finger breadths above the sternal notch with a length of about 5 cm transversely. It gives a better cosmetic scar.

Note:
- First tracheal ring should never be used to do tracheostomy as perichondritis of cricoid cartilage with stenosis can occur.
- Skin should not be sutured or loosely sutured to prevent development of subcutaneous emphysema.
- Cautery should be used during tracheostomy as much as possible to prevent oozing/bleeding from places like muscles, tracheal cut edge. Often torrential hemorrhage known to occur which may need a re-exploration to control bleeding.
- B'Jork flap at the inferior end of the tracheal opening can be done which is sutured to the inferior skin margin.
- Percutaneous approach is done using a needle, cannula, guidewire, and serial plastic dilators then tracheostomy tube is inserted. It is done instead of open method as percutaneous one. One should able to extend the neck of the patient adequately and distant between suprasternal notch to cricoid cartilage should be at least 1 cm. Percutaneous tracheostomy should not be done children younger than 12 years, obese individual and with coagulopathies. Different methods and approaches are used (Figs. 26.10A to D).

Indications for tracheostomy

Respiratory obstruction due to:
- Acute infections causing edema laryx.
- Trauma.
- Neoplasms—benign/malignant.
- Foreign body.
- Bilateral abductor palsy.
- Congenital causes.

Respiratory secretions due to:
- Inability to cough—tetanus, head injury, neurological causes, strychnine poison.
- Painful cough in chest injuries, pneumonia
- Aspiration of secretions.

Respiratory insufficiency due to chronic lung diseases like emphysema, chronic bronchitis, bronchiectasis.

Approaches for tracheostomy

- Vertical.
- Horizontal.
- Percutaneous.

Types

- Temporary.
- Permanent.

Opening can be:
- Circular opening in the trachea.
- B'Jork flap based at lower end of opening.

Charm strikes the sight, but merit wins the soul

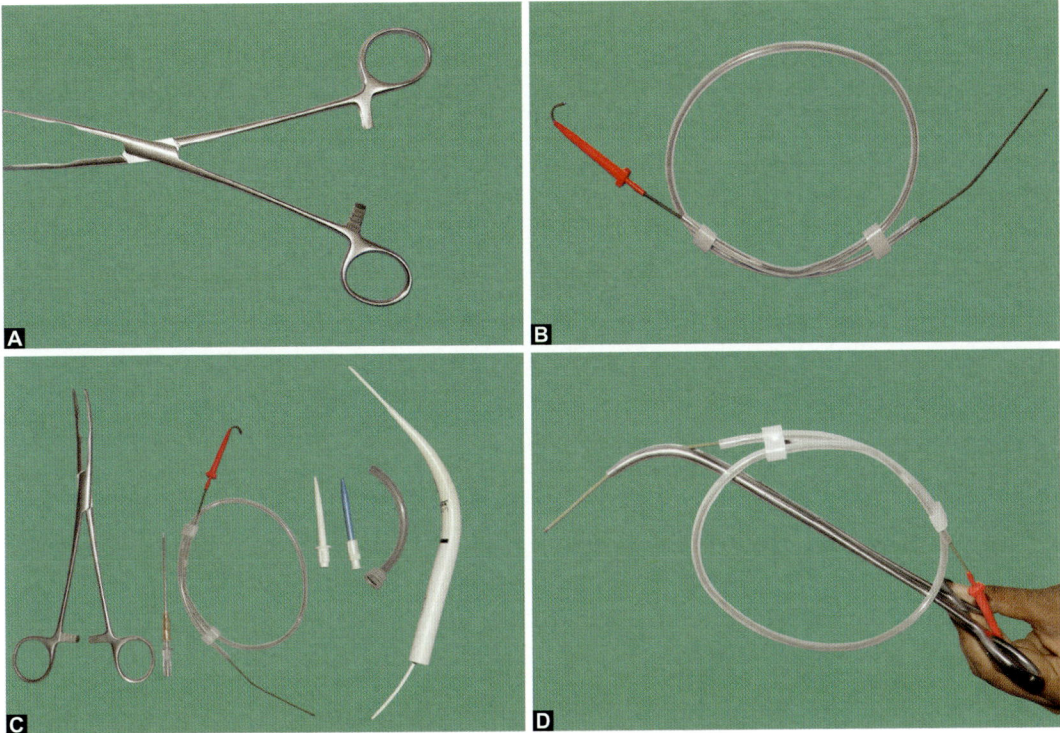

Figs. 26.10A to D: Percutaneous tracheostomy set.

Tracheostomy Care

- Regular suctioning of the tube.
- Cleaning of tracheostomy tube.
- Humidification of the inspired air using normal saline/Ringer lactate/acetylcysteine, (mucolytic agent) to liquefy secretions or crusts so as to prevent blockage.
- Constant observation of the patient for block, bleeding.
- Periodic deflation of the cuff of the tube for short period to prevent pressure necrosis of tracheal mucosa.
- Prevention of infection.
- Decannulation of tracheostomy should be done with care especially in children as sudden respiratory distress can occur and in such occasion emergency reinsertion of the tube should be done.
- Flexible bronchoscopy may be needed to clear the lower airway through the tracheostomy tube.

Functions of the tracheostomy

- Alternate pathway for respiration bypassing the upper airway.
- It decreases the dead space by 50% and reduces the resistance to airflow so as to improve the ventilation.
- It prevents aspiration in bulbar palsy, coma, hemorrhage from larynx/pharynx.
- In injuries of head, chest, abdomen, in respiratory paralysis lower airway is kept clean and patent by doing suction of the secretions through the tracheostomy tube.
- Tracheostomy is better and ideal for intermittent positive pressure ventilation (IPPR).
- To give general anesthesia when endotracheal intubation is not possible.

Complications of Tracheostomy

- Bleeding.
- Aspiration, sudden apnea.

*The future belongs to those who believe in the beauty of their dreams—**Eleanor Roosevelt***

- Pneumothorax.
- Surgical emphysema in the neck.
- Mediastinal emphysema.
- Injury to adjacent structures like esophagus, recurrent laryngeal nerve, thyroid gland.
- Tracheal stenosis.
- Laryngeal stenosis due to perichondritis of cricoid cartilage.
- Tracheitis/tracheobronchitis.
- Displacement/blockage of the tube or erosion of the tube into major vessels.
- Tracheoesophageal, tracheoarterial fistula.

Nursing care

- Consent should be taken.
- Materials like tracheostomy tubes (8.5 size), sterile gown, drapes, gloves, cap, mask, tracheostomy sterile set, gauze, local anesthetic agent, suction apparatus and tubes, connecting tubes to ventilator, sterile syringes should be kept ready.
- During procedure the patient is monitored for vital signs.
- Proper nursing care of the tracheostomy tube is done like, humidifying, cleaning, suction, care of the wound, checking of cuff pressure.
- Tracheal dilator and additional tracheostomy tube should be kept ready at bedside in case of blockage of existing tube/balloon not getting inflated to replace with a new one.
- Absolute asepsis like scrubbing hands, using sterile equipment are essential.
- Sterile suction tubes should be used.
- Care of inner tube is essential in case of metal tracheostomy tube.
- Regular dressing of the wound is needed. Antibiotics are required to prevent pulmonary sepsis.

Treat everyone with politeness and kindness, not because they are nice, but because you are—**Roy T Bennett**

CHAPTER 27

Basic Orthopedics

CHAPTER OUTLINE

- Anatomy of the Bone
- Fracture
- Plaster of Paris
- Arthrodesis
- Arthroplasty
- Osteotomy
- Infections of the Bone
- Paget's Disease of Bone
- Rickets
- Bone Disease of Hyperparathyroidism
- Osteoporosis
- Scurvy
- Osteogenesis Imperfecta
- Achondroplasia
- Tendinitis
- Diaphyseal Achalasia (Multiple Exostoses)
- Enchondromatosis (Ollier's Disease)
- Arthritis
- Rheumatoid Arthritis
- Osteoarthrosis
- Ankylosing Spondylitis
- Kyphosis
- Scoliosis
- Spondylolisthesis
- Intervertebral Disc Prolapse
- Bone Tumors

ANATOMY OF THE BONE

Human skeleton has got 206 bones. It may be long, short, flat, irregular, pneumatic (maxilla, ethmoid, mastoid), sesamoid bones.

Bone can be—***compact lamellar*** bone which is hard and has got bone marrow. It can be ***spongy cancellous bone*** like ends of long bones and flat bones. It can be ***membranous bone*** or ***cartilaginous bone (Fig. 27.1)***.

CARTILAGE

It is hard connective tissue which contains chondrocytes and matrix.

Types

It may be:
a. ***Hyaline*** (articular cartilage, costal, nose, larynx except epiglottis, cuneiform, corniculate, trachea, bronchi. It is avascular and insensitive.

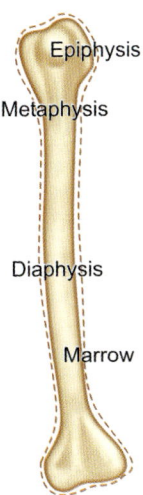

Fig. 27.1: Anatomy of bone showing epiphysis, metaphysis, diaphysis.

Any idiot can face a crisis it's the day to day living that wears you out

b. **White** (intervertebral disk, semilunar, cartilages, symphysis pubis, acetabular and glenoidal labrum). It is vascular but insensitive.
c. **Elastic cartilage** (ear, Eustachian tubes, external auditory meatus, epiglottis, corniculate, cuneiform cartilages). It is avascular and insensitive.

Microscopically bone contains *Haversian canal*, lacunae, lamellae, canaliculi, osteoblasts, osteocytes, osteoclasts.

Bone is covered by thick two layered structure called as *periosteum*. It protects the bone, gives nutrition, allows bone formation by osteogenic activity, and provides attachments to muscles, tendons, ligaments. It is very sensitive due to plenty of nerve networks.

Bone has got three parts—**epiphysis, metaphysis, diaphysis**. Bone gets its blood supply from nutrient artery, metaphyseal vessels, epiphyseal and periosteal vessels.

The process of bone formation which is gradual is called as *ossification*. It may be formed directly from mesenchymal rudiment and is called as **membranous ossification**. Or it may be formed after formation of cartilage from the mesenchymal rudiment and is called as **cartilaginous ossification**.

Primary and secondary *ossification centers* develop during bone formation.

FRACTURE

'**Fracture**' is defined as *break in the continuity of the bone—partial or complete*.

Causes of Fracture

* *Trauma:*
  The commonest cause.
* *Pathological:*
  It is due to underlying pathology like malignancy, secondaries in bone, osteoporosis, osteomyelitis, multiple myeloma, hyperparathyroidism, rickets.
* *Stress fracture:*
  It is due to repeated minor trauma leading to repetitive stress to the bone causing fracture. It is common in second metatarsal of foot, occurs due to repeated marching and stamping. It is also called as *'march fracture'*. It is treated by rest, immobilization with plaster slab of the foot.

Types of Fracture

* *Greenstick fracture:*
  It is seen in children wherein bone breaks incompletely and partially keeping cortex intact. It is treated by rest, immobilization.
* *Closed fracture and simple fracture (Fig. 27.2A)*—wherein fracture does not communicate outside.
* *Open fracture (Fig. 27.2B)*—wherein fracture communicates outside to skin through soft tissues exposing the bone, and allowing infection to get in. It is also called as 'compound fracture'.
* *Transverse fracture (Fig. 27.3A).*
* *Oblique fracture.*

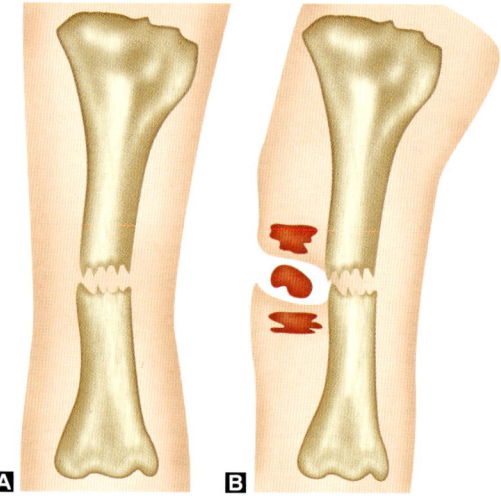

Figs. 27.2A and B: (A) Simple fracture; (B) Open fracture communicating externally.

Do not go where the path may lead, go instead where there is no path and leave a trail—**Ralph Waldo Emerson**

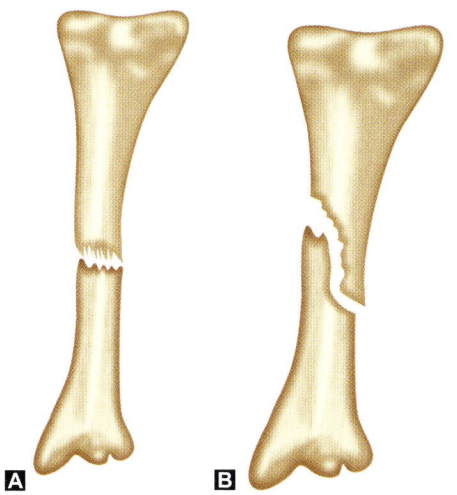

Figs. 27.3A and B: (A) Transverse fracture; (B) Spiral fracture.

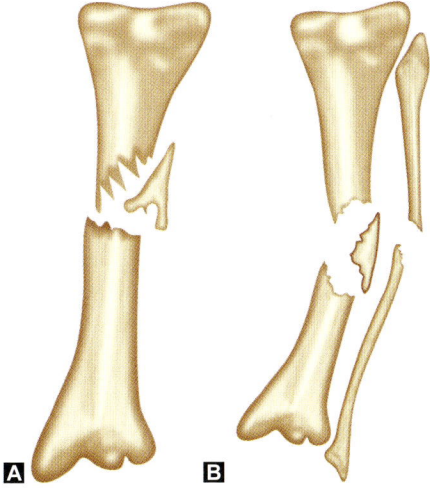

Figs. 27.4A and B: Comminuted fracture.

- Spiral fracture (Fig. 27.3B)
- Comminuted fracture: *Here bone is broken into more than two fragments (Figs. 27.4A and B).*
- *Stellate fracture* begins at one point and radiates towards periphery as a star. It is common in patella and skull.
- *Avulsion fracture* occurs due to powerful contraction of muscle.
- Impacted fracture.

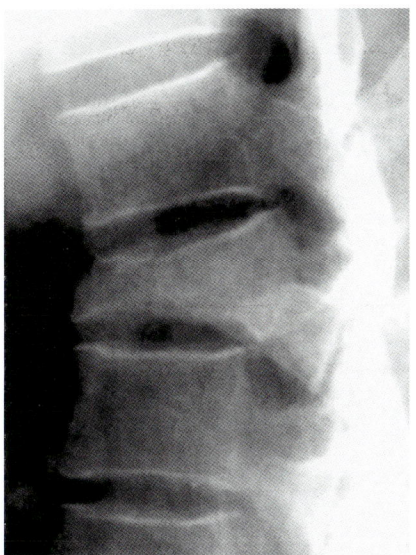

Fig. 27.5: X-ray showing compression fracture spine with wedging of the vertebra.

- *Depressed fracture* is common in skull.
- *Complicated fracture* is a fracture associated with injuries to vessels, nerves, joints.
- Compression fracture (Fig. 27.5).

Mechanism of injury in fracture
· Direct violence. · Indirect violence. · Torsion forces.

Clinical features of fracture
· Pain. · Deformity. · Swelling. · Local bony tenderness. · Shortening of the limb. · Abnormal mobility; crepitus. · Loss of function. · In fractures of femur, tibia there will be features of shock. · Features of associated injuries.

Stages of healing of fracture (Fig. 27.6)
· Stage of hematoma formation. · Stage of granulation tissue formation. · Stage of fibrocartilaginous callus. · Stage of callus formation. · Remodeling phase.

I never see what has been done; I only see what remains to be done—Buddha

Factors affecting fracture healing
• Improper immobilization. • Infection; interposition of soft tissues. • Inadequate blood supply; old age; anemia. • Deficiencies of vitamin C, proteins. • Diabetes, HIV, steroid therapy.

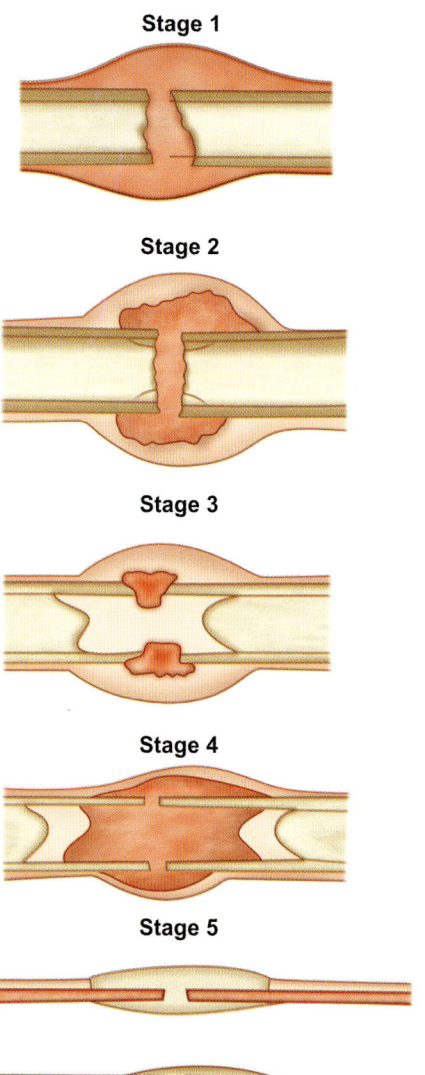

Fig. 27.6: Stages of healing of bone after injury.

Complications of Fracture

Immediate:
- Shock.
- Injury to other structures.
- Compartment syndrome.

Delayed:
- **Fat embolism:** Due to fracture microscopic fat globules from the bone marrow enters the circulation and reaches the lung, brain and skin causing respiratory distress, drowsiness and petechial hemorrhage. Often it is life-threatening.
- Infection.
- Delayed nerve injury.
- Volkmann's contracture.
- 'Myositis ossificans', is common in elbow causing stiffness due to hematoma formation—organization—calcification in front of the elbow joint.
- Disability.

Late:
- Malunion—common in Cole's fracture.
- Nonunion.
- Osteomyelitis of the bone.
- Stiffness and contracture.
- Osteoarthritis of the joint.

Principles of Management of Fracture

- Immediate splinting and first aid.
- Safe transport.
- Assessment of shock, associated injuries, vessel and nerve involvement, type of fracture.
- Resuscitation with blood transfusion, antibiotics, IV fluids, analgesics, splinting, wound debridement.
- X-ray of the part to see fractures. Often MRI is required in spine, hip injuries.
- Proper documentation and case sheet maintenance.
- Reduction of fracture either by closed or by open method (Figs. 27.7A to D).

Idleness rusts the mind

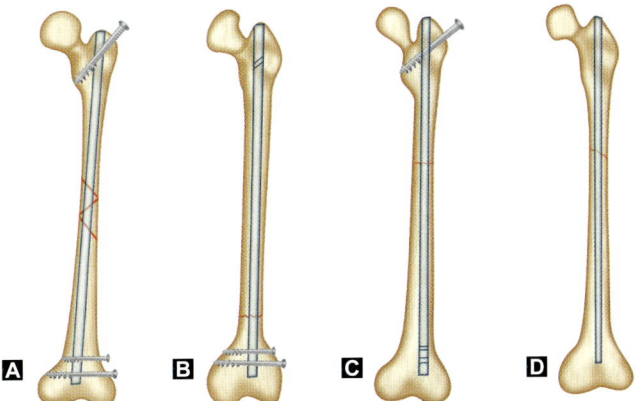

Figs. 27.7A to D: Different methods of interlocking used in fracture shaft of femur: (A) Both ends lock; (B) Distal lock; (C) Proximal lock; (D) Conventional.

- Immobilization.
- Physiotherapy.
- Rehabilitation.
- **Check X-ray** to confirm the proper union of fracture segments.

Principles
• Reduction.   • Rest until recovery.
• Restoration of function.

Reduction:
It means restoration of anatomical alignment. It is done under general anesthesia with muscle relaxation. Simple fractures can be reduced by closed method. Compound fracture requires open surgical method of reduction.

Immobilization:
Once reduced, it should be maintained by proper immobilization using plaster cast. Upper limb fracture unites in 8 weeks. Lower limb fracture unites in 12 weeks. Fracture union is diagnosed by check X-ray.

United fracture site is stiff due to immobilization. Stiffness should be corrected by proper *physiotherapy and rehabilitation.*

Open Reduction by Surgical Method

Indications:
- Compound fracture.
- Distracted fracture.
- Fracture within the joint like fracture neck of femur.
- Fracture near a joint.
- Multiple fractures.
- Pathological fracture.
- Fracture with vascular compression.

Methods of open reduction:
- Screws, screws and plates, wires, intramedullary nails (Figs. 27.8 to 27.10).
- Beware of infection of bone in open reduction.

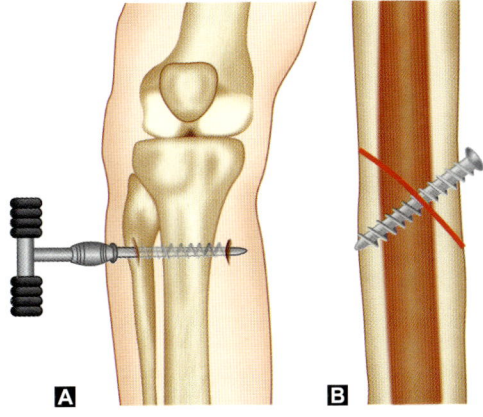

Figs. 27.8A and B: (A) Method of nailing a bone (tibia upper end); (B) Oblique screw placed to an oblique fracture.

Have a strong mind and a soft heart—Anthony J D'Angelo

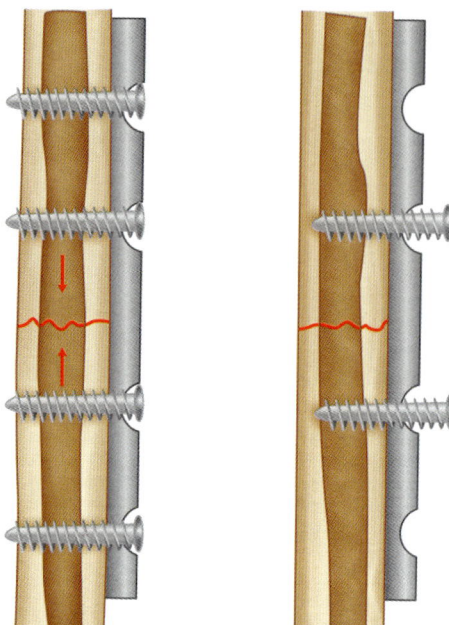

Fig. 27.9: Diagram showing method of compression plate and nail.

PLASTER OF PARIS

Plaster of Paris (POP) is made up of *hemihydrated calcium sulfate*. When water is added, solid hydrated calcium sulfate forms due to exothermic reaction. POP powder can be impregnated with roller bandage. Usually 12–16 layers are required. Now readymade POP bandages and slabs are available. It is dipped in water until air bubbling stops, and then extra water is squeezed gently. POP is thus ready for use as decided. Over that, roller bandage is placed and moulded as required before it sets and solidifies (Fig. 27.11).

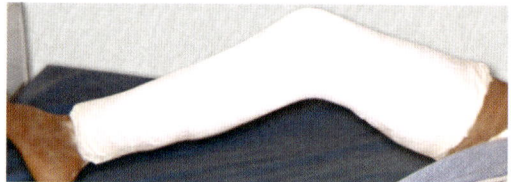

Fig. 27.11: Plaster of Paris cast placed to leg with knee flexion.

Precautions

- After applying the patient is observed for any severe *pain and tenderness, numbness, pallor, duskiness, edema* distally. It signifies that POP is compressing the vessel and requires immediate removal and application of a new POP.
- POP is maintained until fracture unites. If external wound has to be inspected small window cut in the POP over wound area is made to visualize the wound.

Nursing Care

- Nurse should observe the limb for edema, skin color, pulse.
- Weight for the skin traction should be noted.
- Care of bedsore in bedridden patients is important.
- Proper exercise to non-injured limb is essential to prevent stiffness in it.

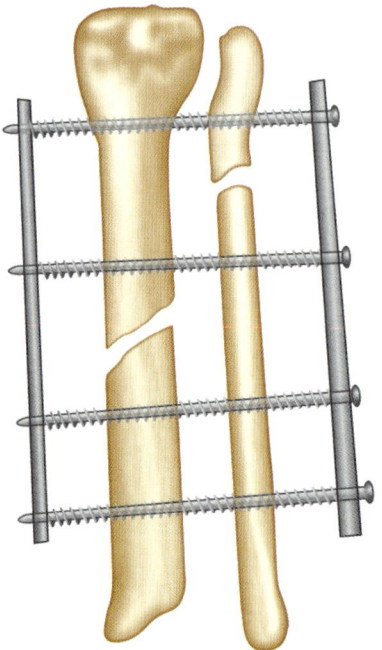

Fig. 27.10: Diagram showing external fixation in fracture tibia and fibula.

You cannot build character and courage by taking away a man's initiative and independence

- Sponge bath, hygiene, nutrition of the patient should be taken care of.
- Soakage and soiling of the dressing or POP should be noted.
- Arranging for dressing as required is essential.
- Care of POP.
- Care of splints. Splints may press certain points in the body and can cause ulceration.
- Both limbs should be positioned properly before placing the skeletal traction.
- Groin rings and pressure points should be taken care of in skeletal traction.
- Care of arthroplasty patient.

ARTHRODESIS

- It is a method used to relieve pain and to achieve stable mechanical system (Fig. 27.12).
- But it permanently restricts the mobility.
- Joint surfaces are excised and raw bony ends are fused together to eliminate the existing joint.
- It is useful in chronic disabled joints like osteoarthrosis, rheumatoid arthritis and other degenerative diseases.

- It is commonly used in spine, toes, hip, and knee joints.
- Patient may not be able to squat and sit on the floor.
- Technique may be intra-articular or extra-articular fixation.

ARTHROPLASTY

It is repair of bone so as to achieve mobile, functioning, painless joint.

Types

a. **Excision arthroplasty (Fig. 27.13):**
   - Both surfaces of the joint are excised and gap is allowed to develop fibrous tissue. It is commonly used in hip, metatarsophalangeal joint.
   - Joint becomes freely mobile and painless. But joint becomes unstable with shortening.
   - Hip—Girdlestone's excision arthroplasty.
   - Great toe—Keller's operation.

b. **Hemiarthroplasty:**
   Here one of the articular surfaces is excised and replaced with prosthesis. Other normal articular surface is left behind. It

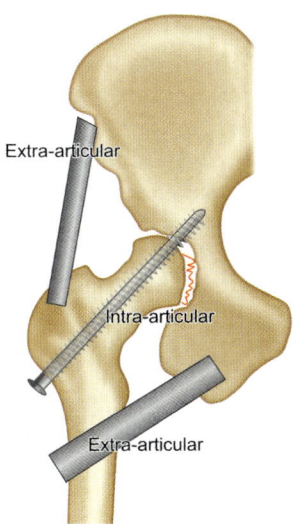

Fig. 27.12: *Types of arthrodesis—extra-articular, intra-articular.*

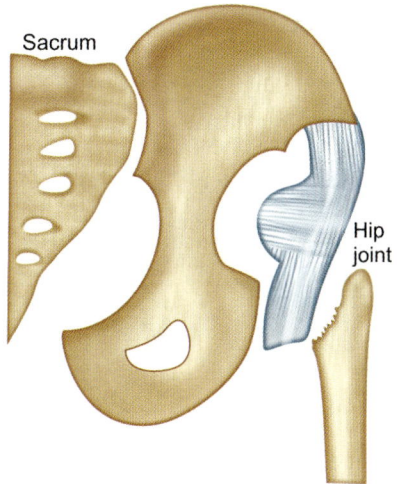

Fig. 27.13: Girdlestone excision arthroplasty.

*Change your thoughts and you change your world—***Norman Vincent Peale**

is commonly done in hip joint wherein femoral head is removed and prosthesis is placed (Fig. 27.14).

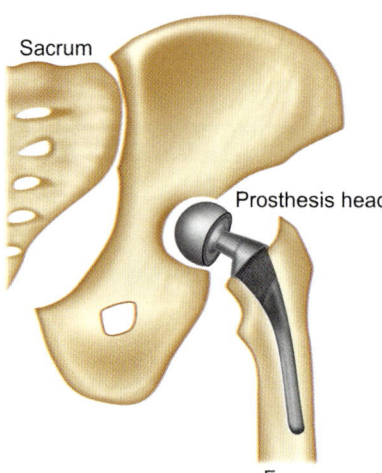

Fig. 27.14: Hemiarthroplasty of hip joint.

c. **Total replacement arthroplasty (Fig. 27.15):**
Here both the articular surfaces are excised and replaced with metal and high-density polyethylene. It is held in place using acrylic cement. It is commonly used in hip joint. Often used in knee and other joints. Absolute care should be taken against sepsis. Good asepsis, proper sterilization like autoclaving, proper preparation, hypersterile laminar OT is extremely important in preventing infection. If infection occurs, prosthesis has to be removed and problem will still persist. Deep vein thrombosis (DVT) is a common problem. It can be prevented by elevation, exercise, crepe bandaging the limbs, and anticoagulants.

OSTEOTOMY

It is therapeutic cutting of the bone to correct or stabilize the joint (Fig. 27.16).

Indications

- Correction of angulations, bowing, rotation deformity.
- Correction of discrepancies in the limbs.
- To correct or compensate malalignment of the joint.
- To correct instability of joint.
- To control and relieve pain.

It is useful in vagus or varus deformity, osteoarthritis of the joint.

Multiple drills are made in the cortex of the bone. Bone is divided and necessary corrections are made. Fragments are fixed using nail and plate. Patient should be immobilized in POP cast or splints for 6 weeks or until fracture are united.

Problems:
Improper correction, infection.

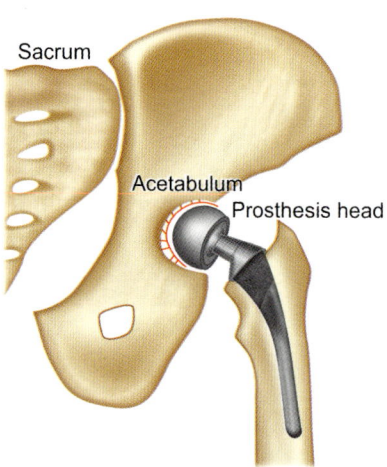

Fig. 27.15: Diagram showing total hip replacement arthroplasty (THRA).

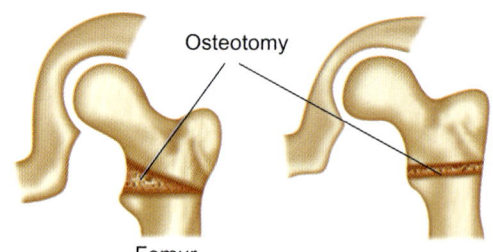

Fig. 27.16: Osteotomy of femur.

A bone to the dog is not charity. Charity is the bone shared with the dog, when you are just as hungry as the Dog

INFECTIONS OF THE BONE

- Bone gets infected by Gram-positive and Gram-negative bacteria, tuberculosis, brucellosis, typhoid, syphilis.
- Infection of the bone along with bone marrow is called as *osteomyelitis*. It can be acute or chronic.

ACUTE OSTEOMYELITIS

It is acute bacterial infection of the bone.

Causes

Gram-positive bacteria like staphylococci, streptococci, Gram-negative bacteria like *Klebsiella*, *Pseudomonas*.

Mode of Infection

- Direct—through the traumatic wounds.
- Hematogenous—from an infective focus from different parts of the body, like skin infections.

Mode of Spread

Bacteria spread through metaphyseal vessels into the metaphysis of the bone and multiply there releasing toxins and evoking inflammation. These vessels being end arteries get compressed by increased pressure in the metaphysis causing pus formation and suppuration. This pus can spread longitudinally into the diaphysis or across the joint capsule into the joint causing arthritis. It can spread outward into the soft tissues (muscles and fascia) and reach the subcutaneous plane causing a swelling. It eventually bursts through the skin forming discharging sinuses. Periosteum lays new bone eventually, as a reaction.

Features

- Common in young boys.
- Fever, toxicity.
- Pain in the bone. Tender swelling at the site.
- Effusion in adjacent joint.
- Inability to move the limb.

Investigations

- X-ray shows no changes for 2 weeks. Later it shows widening of cortical margin with new bone formation. Often joint effusion may be visualized.
- Total count and erythrocyte sedimentation rate (ESR) may be increased.
- Blood culture.
- MRI bone.

Treatment

- Antibiotics—Erythromycin, Cefotaxime, Cefadroxyl.
- Rest and immobilization.
- Often drainage of pus from the bone is required. Bone is drilled to reach the marrow with pus, which is drained and sent for culture and sensitivity.

Sequelae

- Septicemia can develop.
- Chronic osteomyelitis.
- Limb shortening, disability.
- Recurrent infection.
- Chronic discharging sinus formation.
- Malignancy—*squamous cell carcinoma from the skin*.

Nursing Care

- Adequate rest and maintenance of hygiene.
- Immobilization using proper splints.
- Observation of joint fullness and pain.
- Later physiotherapy and rehabilitation.

CHRONIC OSTEOMYELITIS

It is chronic, recurrent bacterial infection and inflammation of bone and bone marrow usually of long bones. There is new bone

*Smile, it is the key that fits the lock of everybody's heart—**Anthony J D'Angelo***

formation called as *involucrum* (like envelope) with discharging *sinus* with bone spicules in the sinus. It occurs either due to trauma or as sequelae of acute osteomyelitis. Dead part of the bone within the infected bone is separated by granulation tissue and is called as *sequestrum* (Dead bone in situ) (Fig. 27.17A).

Features

- Discharging sinus with swelling.
- Bone pain and tenderness. Thickening of the bone.
- Shortening, restricted mobility and deformity.

Investigations

- X-ray of the part shows sequestrum and new bone formation with sinus (Fig. 27.17B).
- Culture and sensitivity of discharge.
- MRI of bone.

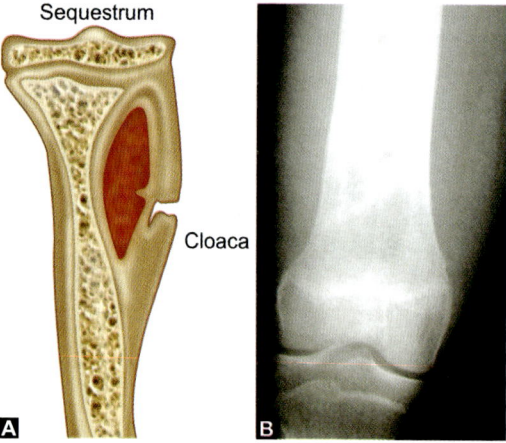

Figs. 27.17A and B: (A) Diagram showing osteomyelitis; (B) X-ray showing chronic osteomyelitis of femur.

Treatment

- Surgical exploration of the wound and removal of the sequestrum with laying open of the sinus cavity.
- Antibiotics—often are given for long duration of 3-6 weeks.

Problems

- Deformity.
- Malignant change—squamous cell carcinoma.
- Amyloid deposition.
- Recurrence.
- Pus can get localized in the metaphysis to form an abscess called as **Brodie's abscess**. It can cause pain, tenderness and swelling in the bone. It can lead to pathological fracture. It requires open drainage and curettage.

Nursing Care

- Care of the limb and regular physiotherapy and exercise.
- Care of the splint and plaster cast whenever used.
- Regular dressing of the wound.
- Psychotherapy and counseling to the patient.

PAGET'S DISEASE OF BONE

It is also called as *Osteitis deformans* wherein there is increased blood supply to the bone, causing bone to enlarge more than normal because of more vascularity and laying of coarse fibered abnormal bone. This is thick but not strong and is vulnerable for pathological fracture. Common bones involved are long bones like femur and tibia, spine, skull, also known to involve mandible. This bone is more prone to develop osteogenic sarcoma.

Features

- Common in elderly male.
- Thickening and increase in visible size of the bone like in skull causing requirement of larger sized caps.
- Dull continuous pain in the bone with often pathological fracture.
- Due to increased vascularity of bone there is hyperdynamic circulation leading to congestive cardiac failure.

To be effective means doing the right thing. To be efficient means doing the thing right

- Bending (bowing) of leg bones. Paraplegia due to vertebral involvement.
- Deafness due to middle ear sclerosis.
- The involved bone is more prone for osteosarcoma than normal bone.

Investigations

- Raised serum alkaline phosphatase.
- Elevated urinary excretion of hydroxyproline.
- X-ray shows dense sclerotic bone.
- Bone scan confirms the diagnosis.

Treatment

- Diphosphonates, Calcitonin.
- Correction of pathological fracture.

RICKETS

Formed bone matrix is not calcified leading to rickets. Bones contain uncalcified bone matrix called as *osteoid*.

Causes

- Dietary deficiency of vitamin D prevents calcium absorption from the gut.
- Excessive excretion of calcium in the kidney leading to less available calcium for bone calcification—*Renal rickets*.

Features

- Seen in infants.
- *Ricketic rossary* in costochondral junction.
- Bosselated frontal bone.
- Tri-radiate pelvis.
- Bowing of long bones.
- Stunted growth.
- X-ray confirms the disease.
- Serum calcium and serum phosphatase level estimation.

Treatment

- Vitamin D supplementation.
- Osteotomies to correct the bone deformity.

Note: **Osteomalacia** is vitamin D deficiency seen in adults (features are like rickets). Treatment is also same.

BONE DISEASE OF HYPERPARATHYROIDISM

Increased parathormone secretion by hyperfunctioning parathyroid glands or by parathyroid adenoma causes calcium resorption from the bone replacing the bone with fibrous tissue often with cystic spaces. It is called as **osteitis fibrosa cystica**. Bone becomes friable and leads to pathological fracture.

Features

- Common in phalanges, jaw bones and skull bones.
- Pathological fracture can occur.
- Serum calcium is high. Serum phosphorus is low. Serum alkaline phosphatase is raised.
- Serum PTH is raised. Thallium scan shows hyperfunctioning parathyroids. CT neck or MRI shows the nodule in parathyroid.
- X-ray of skull, hand, jaw shows salt and pepper lesion.

Treatment

- Correction of hypercalcemia by Calcitonin, Glucagon, Mithramycin, Diphosphonates.
- Surgical removal of parathyroids.
- Treatment for fracture.

OSTEOPOROSIS

It is reduction in total skeletal bone mass leading to thinning of the cortical margins, less dense cancellous bone.

Causes

- After menopause in women.
- In old age (elderly).
- Disused due to lesser activity.

*Learn not only to find what you like, learn to like what you find—**Anthony J D'Angelo***

Problems

These individuals are more prone for fracture by minor trauma, which is often unnoticed. Commonly observed fractures are Colle's fracture, fracture neck of femur, compression fracture of vertebrae, intertrochanteric fracture.

Treatment is of fractures wherever occurs.

SCURVY

Deficiency of vitamin C causes defective endochondral ossification with more unossified cartilages leading to hemorrhages and swelling in the epiphyseal region.

They present with hemorrhages, swelling, pathological fracture.

OSTEOGENESIS IMPERFECTA

It is a congenital inherited disease with defective collagen synthesis leading to brittle bones, which are prone for multiple fractures in multiple bones.

Features	
• Multiple fractures.	• Ligament laxity.
• Sclerosed ear (otosclerosis).	• Blood chemistry normal.
• Blue eyes (blue sclerotics).	• Bone histology normal.

ACHONDROPLASIA

It is a familial congenital disease where there is failure of normal ossification of long bones and skull bones.

Features
• Long large head, normal trunk.
• Short proximal part of the limb.
• Lumbar lordosis.
• Trident hand and wide pelvis side-by-side.
• Mental impairment is not present.

TENDINITIS

Inflammation of the tendon is called as tendinitis. It is commonly due to friction, trauma, and calcification. Common sites are supraspinatus tendon, patellar tendon, Achilles tendon in the foot, plantar fasciitis.

It causes painful movements of the tendon, with stiffness, and restricted function.

Supraspinatus tendinitis causes *painful arc syndrome* with restriction of mid 60° of abduction of the shoulder.

Treatment

- Powerful contraction of the muscle and tendon is avoided.
- Rest.
- Steroid injection locally.
- Analgesics and physiotherapy.
- Rarely surgical removal of calcification in the tendon and decompression is done. But results are not fully assured.

DIAPHYSEAL ACHALASIA (MULTIPLE EXOSTOSES)

It is a growth disorder due to defective endochondral ossification with failure of remodeling of bone ends.

Features

- It is commonly familial.
- Common in lower end of femur, upper end of tibia, humerus.
- Dwarfism is common.
- Exostosis is peduncle with cartilage as cap with a bursa in between. It grows away from the joint surface.

Complications

- Bursitis.
- Compression of neurovascular bundle and tendons.

The important thing is not to stop questioning. Curiosity has its own reasons for existing

- Restriction of joint movements.
- Turning into chondrosarcoma (5%).

Treatment
Usually excision is done once epiphysis fuses, not earlier. Cosmetic complications are indications for excision.

ENCHONDROMATOSIS (OLLIER'S DISEASE)

There is abnormal proliferation of cartilage cells of the growth plate into the metaphysis of long bones. It is commonly seen in bones of fingers, toes and other long bones. It also can turn into chondrosarcoma (5%).

ARTHRITIS

ACUTE PYOGENIC ARTHRITIS

It is acute infection of a joint caused by *Staphylococcus, Streptococcus, Pneumococcus* organisms either through hematogenous spread from distant focus or trauma. Exudates may be serous, serofibrinous or purulent depending on the severity of infection. Pus formation in the joint leads to destruction of articular cartilage; it may track through the soft tissues and skin causing abscess and sinus. Often severe virulent infection causes septicemia and if not treated properly death may ensue.

Features
- Pain and swelling in the joint.
- Restricted joint movement, tenderness, warmness, redness, and fullness over the joint.
- Joint is in maximum ease position.
- Spasm of the muscles adjacent to the joint.

Investigations
- Total count is increased.
- Pus aspirated is sent for culture and sensitivity.
- X-ray of joint shows widened joint space.

Treatment
- Broad-spectrum antibiotics.
- Immobilization of the joint.
- Analgesics.
- Aspiration of the pus and immobilization.
- Arthrotomy and drainage of pus with saline wash and later immobilization.
- Later physiotherapy.
- If there is destruction of joint surfaces, it leads to bony ankylosis (fusion of joint).

Arthritis can occur in infants, in patients with gonococcal infection and also syphilis.

CHRONIC PYOGENIC ARTHRITIS

It is due to chronic recurrent infection of the joint by Gram-positive or other bacteria. It causes deformity, disability and eventually bony ankylosis of the joint.

RHEUMATOID ARTHRITIS

It is an autoimmune connective tissue disorder involving many systems including skeletal system. In joints, it causes inflammation of the synovial membrane which gets thickened, edematous, and vascular. Eventually articular cartilage also gets involved in inflammatory process leading to formation of granulation tissue called *pannus*. *Pannus* eventually extends to capsule, periarticular tissue and deeper bone surfaces. Finally joint ankylosis, muscle atrophy occurs.

Features
- Common in women.
- It has got different phases with remissions and exacerbations.
- Small joints of hand and feet are involved first. Later proximal joints are involved.
- Morning stiffness and pain are typical.
- Restricted painful joint movements with effusion and swelling of the joint occur.

Don't reinvent the wheel, just realign it—**Anthony J D'Angelo**

- Flexion deformity of fingers and toes occurs often with buttonhole or swan neck deformity.
- In severe cases patient may be permanently crippled.
- Symmetrical joint involvement is seen.
- Patient may present with carpal tunnel syndrome, tennis elbow, plantar fasciitis, rheumatoid subcutaneous nodules, vasculitis with ischemia or gangrene of fingers or toes, pleural effusion, pericardial effusion, muscle wasting.

Investigations

- X-ray shows narrowed joint space with subchondral cystic areas.
- High ESR.
- IGM rheumatoid factor is positive.
- Synovial fluid shows high cell count (> 10,000) and high protein (>5 g%).
- Synovial biopsy is diagnostic.
- Arthroscopy is very useful.

Treatment

- Rest, analgesics (Aspirin, Indomethacin, Ibuprofen), Chloroquine, Prednisolone.
- D-penicillamine, gold therapy (sodium aurothiomalate).
- Splint and immobilization.
- Later physiotherapy.
- Intra-articular injection of hydrocortisone.
- Wax bath therapy.
- Cytotoxic drugs like Cyclophosphamide, Methotrexate, Azathioprine.
- Synovectomy, capsulotomy, osteotomy, arthrodesis, arthroplasty.

OSTEOARTHROSIS

It is a degenerative disease of the joint. There is degeneration of articular cartilage due to wear and tear. There is low grade or no inflammatory process. There is fragmentation and fibrillation. Cartilage once gets thinned out, bone surface is exposed. Reactive hypertrophy is observed in peripheral margins of the bone surfaces which forms osteophytes. Ankylosis of joint is not common. As there is not much of inflammatory reaction, it is better called as *osteoarthrosis* not as osteoarthritis.

Types

- *Primary osteoarthrosis* occurs in weight-bearing joints like knee, hip and spinal joints. It is common in old age, women, and obese individuals.
- *Secondary osteoarthrosis* is due to other diseases in the joint like avascular necrosis, trauma and so on. It is due to mechanical incongruity of the articular surfaces.
  Common joint involved is knee, then hip.

Features

- Pain, stiffness, difficulty in squatting.
- Muscle wasting, position of ease.
- Restricted movements, disability.
- Joint effusion and swelling.
- Crepitations over the joint.
  X-ray reveals narrowed joint space with subchondral sclerosis and osteophytes over the margins of the articular surfaces.

Treatment

- Rest, skin traction, analgesics, physiotherapy, exercise, weight reduction.
- In severe cases intra-articular hydrocortisone injections may be useful.
- Osteotomy, arthrodesis, arthroplasty are surgical treatment required.
- Osteoarthritis is a morbid condition.

Types of arthritis	
• Rheumatoid arthritis.	• Gouty arthritis.
	• Reactive arthritis.
• Osteoarthritis (osteoarthrosis).	• Tuberculous arthritis.
	• Psoriatic arthritis.
• Hemophilic arthritis.	

Never insult an alligator until after you have crossed the river.

ANKYLOSING SPONDYLITIS

- It is a chronic, progressive disease of spine and sacroiliac joints, which is genetically predisposed as **HLA-B-27**.
- There is progressive restriction of movements of all joints in the spine. Patient cannot bend with total stiffness and calcification of ligaments of the spine *(Bamboo spine)*.
- Costovertebral ankylosis causes *poor chest expansion* (<5 cm) leading to pulmonary complications.
- Eventually ankylosis of hip, knee, temporomandibular joints occur.
  Condition is diagnosed by clinical features, X-ray, ESR, positive HLA-B-27, negative rheumatoid factor.

Treatment

- Hard bed with a single pillow is used for sleeping.
- Correction of anemia.
- Chest and spine physiotherapy.
- Total hip/knee replacement.
- Lumbar spinal osteotomies.

KYPHOSIS

It means there is an exaggerated anterior curvature of thoracic spine with obliteration of lumbar lordosis.

Causes

- Tuberculosis of spine—angular—Gibbus type.
- Adolescent kyphosis.
- Trauma, osteoporosis.

Types

- Angular—only one or two vertebrae are involved.
- Rounded—many vertebrae are involved.

SCOLIOSIS

It is lateral curvature of the spine. It is common in thoracic spine.

Causes

- Idiopathic is the commonest. It is common in girls. Main primary convex curve is towards one side with secondary compensatory curves above and below towards opposite side.
- Postural in young people.
- Neuropathic like polio, cerebral palsy.
- Myopathic due to muscular dystrophies.
- Osteopathic due to hemivertebrae, fusion vertebrae.

Commonly patient presents with respiratory difficulties.

Scoliosis may be mobile or rigid.

X-ray is diagnostic.

Treatment

- Spinal exercises and breathing exercises.
- Heel and sole raise.
- Spinal braces.
- Spinal fusion using different types of rods and bone graft.

SPONDYLOLISTHESIS

It is defined as slipping forward of one vertebra over the next lower vertebra, usually seen in L_4-L_5 or L_5-S_1 junction. It causes sudden severe pain with lumbar lordosis and step like depression over the sacrum. X-ray is diagnostic. It is treated by exercises, physiotherapy, often by lumbosacral fusion.

INTERVERTEBRAL DISC PROLAPSE

Intervertebral disc prolapse (IVDP) is herniation of the nucleus pulposus of the disc through the nucleus fibrosus of the disc, commonly in posterolateral direction in one or both sides (Fig. 27.18).

It is better to conquer yourself than to win a thousand battles. Then the victory is yours. It cannot be taken from you, not by angels or by demons, heaven or hell—**Buddha**

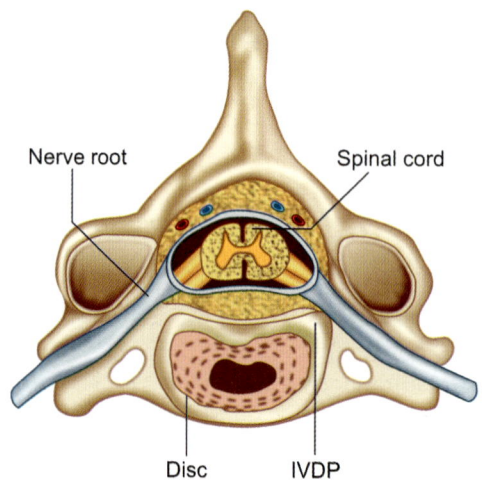

Fig. 27.18: Intervertebral disc prolapse (IVDP) posterolateral.

It is common in L_4-L_5 or L_5-S_1 region. Prolapse of L_4-L_5 disc compresses the lower nerve root –L_5. Prolapse of L_5-S_1 compresses the S_1 nerve root.

X-ray shows findings only at late stage. Myelogram, MRI are diagnostic (Fig. 27.19).

Features

* It is the commonest cause of back pain.
* Always possible neurological deficits should be looked for.
* SLR test will be positive.

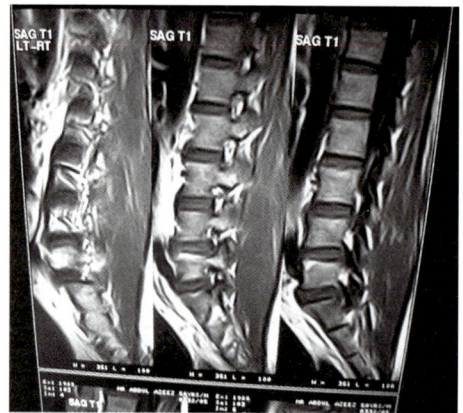

Fig. 27.19: MRI is the ideal investigation for IVDP.

Treatment

* Absolute bedrest, analgesics, pelvic traction, avoiding weight lifting for 6 months.
* Laminectomy and discectomy is the surgical procedure done.

BONE TUMORS

* It is either benign or malignant.
* Malignant can be either secondaries or primary.
* Secondaries are the commonest malignant bone tumor.
* Osteochondroma is the commonest benign bone tumor.

Benign Bone Tumors

* Osteoma.
* Osteochondroma.
* Chondroma.
* Osteoblastoma.

OSTEOMA

It is a benign tumor arising from the surface of a long/flat/skull bone (Fig. 27.20).

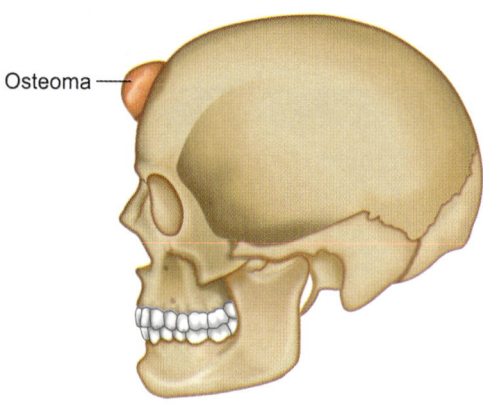

Fig. 27.20: Osteoma in the skull. Frontal bone is the common site.

Types (Fig. 27.21)

1. *Ivory osteoma* is hard compact. It usually occurs in skull bone like frontal bone/parietal bone. It presents like bony hard localized swelling which is nontender, nonmobile,

*Never complain and never explain—**Benjamin Disreali***

with free skin over the surface. It does not turn into malignancy. It can be left alone. Only if it is cosmetically troublesome it can be excised. But it should be differentiated from other swellings in the scalp like dermoid cysts or secondaries. Frontal bone osteoma may rarely extend into frontal sinus or orbital cavity and if it is so after doing CT scan it needs surgical excision.
2. *Cancellous osteoma* is usually arising from spongy bone with a localized swelling. Features are similar to ivory osteoma.

CHONDROMA

It is a tumor arising from cartilage.

Types (Fig. 27.21)

1. *Ecchondroma* grows outwards from the bone. It is common in flat bones like scapula/ilium or bones of hands and feet. In flat bones they often reach large size. It may turn into malignancy occasionally as chondrosarcoma.
2. *Enchondroma* is more common in bones of hands and feet. The affected bone expands from within leading to thinning of the bone cortex. Pathological fracture can occur. If this is not troublesome it can be left alone.
3. *Multiple chondromas* in major long bones is called as *dyschondroplasia/multiple chondromatosis or Ollier's disease*. It usually begins in childhood as enchondromatosis in the region of the growing epiphyseal cartilages of many bones. So, there will be interference of the growth of the epiphyseal plates, which causes shortening and deformity.

OSTEOCHONDROMA

❖ It is the commonest benign tumor of the bone.
❖ It begins in childhood from the growing epiphyseal cartilage plate. As the bone grows tumors is left behind and so appears like migrating towards the shaft of the bone. It grows outwards from the bone like a mushroom. Its stalk and proximal part is bony but distal part is cartilaginous like a cap often with a bursa in between (Fig. 27.22).
❖ Usually it is single but it can be familial. Multiple osteochondromas involving several long bones is called as diaphyseal, aclasis/multiple exostoses.
❖ Osteochondroma should be excised only after completion of the development of the bone.

Complications

❖ It often can compress neurovascular bundle. It presents with painless swelling.
❖ Only cartilaginous component turns into malignancy—chondrosarcoma. Osseous part will not turn into malignancy.

OSTEOCLASTOMA

❖ Osteoclastoma often termed as giant cell tumor. It occurs in ends of long bones

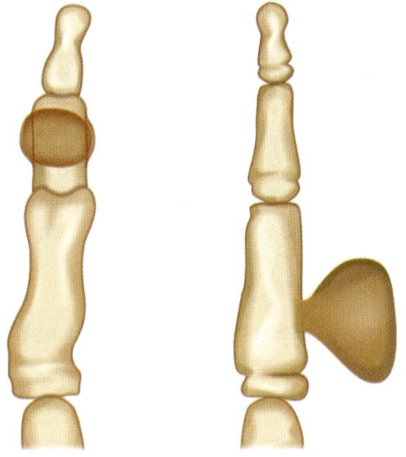

Enchondroma   Ecchondroma
Fig. 27.21: Chondroma types. Enchondroma grows from within. Ecchondroma grows outwards.

*Don't fear change - embrace It—**Anthony J D'Angelo***

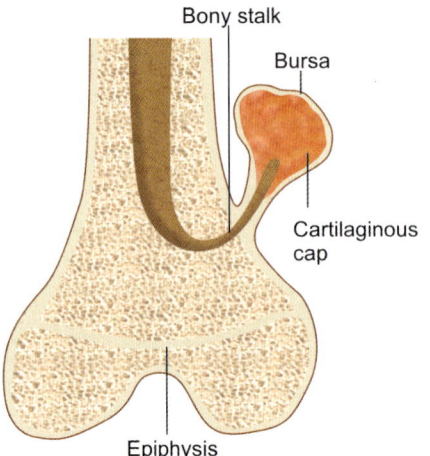

Fig. 27.22: Osteochondroma.

from epyphyses, often extends into the joint cavity. It also occurs in jaw either mandible or maxilla (Figs. 27.23A and B).
- It can be benign/intermediate or malignant (10%). Malignant osteoclastoma spreads into lungs through blood.
- It forms an expanding tumor with localized swelling, which is bony hard. It has got typical loculated appearance. Histologically, it contains spindle cells (typical) with osteoclastoma giant cells. It can cause pathological fracture.

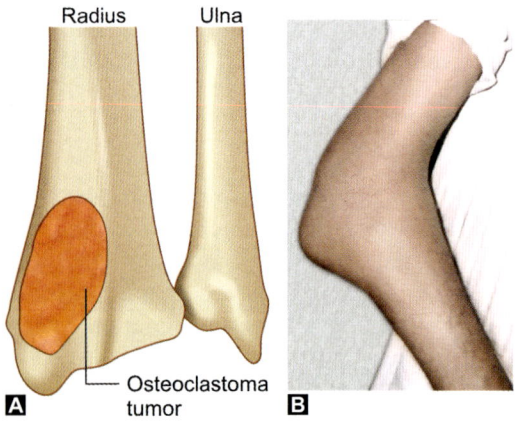

Figs. 27.23A and B: Osteoclastoma in elbow region.

- X-ray/incision biopsy and CT/MRI are the needed investigations.
- Treatment is wide excision/hemimandibulectomy. Partial removal/curettage is not advisable because recurrence is likely.

Malignant Bone Tumors

Secondaries is the *commonest* malignant tumor of the bone.

Primary malignant bone tumors	
• Osteosarcoma.	• Ewing's tumor.
• Chondrosarcoma.	• Multiple myeloma.
• Fibrosarcoma of bone.	

OSTEOSARCOMA

- It is common primary malignant tumor of the bone (Fig. 27.24A).
- It is common in children/adolescence.
- Common sites are lower end of femur/upper end of tibia/upper end of humerus.
- It arises from metaphysis.
- It expands outwards, extends into adjacent soft tissues.
- It spreads into lungs commonly through blood.
- It is very aggressive tumor.
- It causes extensive destruction of bone with rising of the periosteum with new bone formation.
- Pathological fracture is common.
- Localized pain, swelling which is warm, hard, and vascular are the features.

Investigations

- X-ray shows tumor in the end of the long bone with cortical destruction, Codman's triangle, *'sun-ray' appearance*, pathological fracture.
- Open incision biopsy.
- MRI of the lesion.
- CT chest to look for secondaries.

Start by doing what's necessary; then do what's possible; and suddenly you are doing the impossible—**Francis of Assisi**

Secondaries in bone tumors	
Common primaries causing secondaries in bone are: • All sarcomas. • Carcinoma kidney (RCC). • Carcinoma breast—70% cases in females. • Follicular carcinoma thyroid. • Carcinoma prostate. • Carcinoma lung.	**Common bones involved:** • Vertebral bodies. • Ribs and sternum. • Pelvis. • Upper end of femur and humerus. **Types** • Osteolytic—common. • Osteosclerotic—carcinoma prostate. • Combined osteosclerotic and osteolytic.

Treatment

- Amputation above the level of the lesion.
- Wide local excision if possible to salvage the limb.
- Radiotherapy/chemotherapy (Adriamycin, Cisplatin, Methotrexate) as sandwich therapy along with surgeries.
- Condition has got poor prognosis.

EWING'S SARCOMA

- It is highly malignant endothelial sarcoma of bone arising from bone marrow. It begins in diaphysis (Fig. 27.24B).
- It is soft, vascular tumor arising commonly from shafts of femur/tibia/humerus.
- It expands outwards with successive layer by layer formation of new bone.
- It commonly spreads through blood into lungs.
- It commonly occurs in children.
- Soft, vascular, firm, fusiform swelling in the shaft of long bones with warm skin over the tumor.
- X-ray has typical *'onion-peel'* appearance.
- Open biopsy, MRI bone, chest CT are the investigations needed.
- It should be differentiated from osteoid osteoma, osteomyelitis.
- Treatment is chemotherapy (Actinomycin D, Vincristine, Adriamycin, Cyclophosphamide), surgery (amputation) and radiotherapy (tumor is radiosensitive).

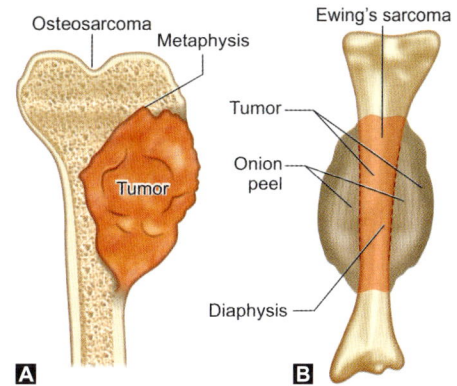

Figs. 27.24A and B: Osteosarcoma and Ewing's sarcoma.

MULTIPLE MYELOMA

- It is malignant aggressive tumor arising from plasma cells of the bone marrow.
- It mainly involves spine, skull, flat bones and ends of long bones.
- Generalized pain and illness, anemia, bone pain, pathological fracture, neurological deficits often with paraplegia are the features.
- X-ray shows multiple radiolucent areas in spine, pelvic bones, and skull bones.
- Blood smear shows *'cart-wheel shaped'* plasma cells.
- *Bence Jones proteins* are positive in urine of the patient.
- Specific immunoglobulin will be elevated and is diagnostic.
- Bone marrow biopsy is essential.
- Radioisotope study of bone is useful.
- Treatment is chemotherapy (Melphalan and Cyclophosphamide) and radiotherapy.
- It carries poor prognosis.

Hope puts our feet on the path when our eyes cannot see it

CHAPTER 28

Esophagus

Chapter Outline

- Anatomy
- Lower Esophageal Sphincter
- Dysphagia
- Achalasia Cardia
- Gastroesophageal Reflux Disease
- Barrett's Esophagus
- Hiatus Hernia
- Reflux Esophagitis
- Corrosive Stricture of Esophagus
- Plummer-Vinson Syndrome (Patterson-Kelly Syndrome)
- Mallory-Weiss Syndrome
- Boerhaave's Syndrome
- Tracheoesophageal Fistula
- Carcinoma Esophagus

ANATOMY

Esophagus begins at the lower edge of the cricoid cartilage (C_6 vertebra) and ends at esophagogastric junction (T_1 vertebra). Upper end is closed by cricopharyngeus muscle which is 18 cm from upper incisors. Lower end is 40 cm from the upper incisors (upper jaw is fixed and so is used as the landmark to measure, but not the lower jaw which is mobile) (Fig. 28.1).

It lies anterior to vertebral column and posterior to the trachea. It lacks serosal layer but is surrounded by a layer of loose fibroareolar adventitia.

Parts

1. **Cervical esophagus**:
   It extends from cricopharyngeus. It is part of inferior constrictor muscle, which is located as lower horizontal part. Upper oblique part is called as thyropharyngeus. Gap between two is called as *Killian's dehiscence*, which

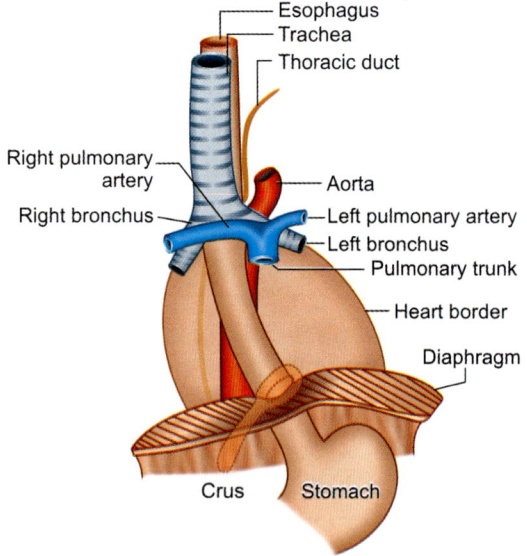

Fig. 28.1: Anatomical relations of esophagus.

An unspoken word never does harm

is a *site of occurrence of pharyngeal pouch*. Cervical esophagus is related to trachea and recurrent laryngeal nerve.
2. *Thoracic esophagus*:
   Lies initially towards the right side. In lower third it deviates towards the left and continues as abdominal esophagus. It is related to azygos vein, thoracic duct (which crosses the esophagus posteriorly from right to left), aorta, pleura and pericardium.
3. *Abdominal esophagus:*
   It is 2.5 cm long and grooves behind the left lobe of the liver.

Three areas of anatomic narrowing:
1. *Cervical constriction*—occur at the level of cricopharyngeal sphincter—narrowest point of gastrointestinal tract (GIT).
2. *Bronchoaortic constriction*—located at the level of T_4.
3. *Diaphragmatic constriction*—occurs where esophagus traverses the diaphragm.

Arterial supply of esophagus:
By inferior thyroid artery, esophageal branches of the aorta, gastric arteries and inferior phrenic arteries (Fig. 28.2A).

Venous drainage of esophagus:
By inferior thyroid veins, brachiocephalic vein, left hemiazygos vein, azygos vein, coronary vein, splenic vein and inferior phrenic vein. Veins are longitudinal and they lie in submucosal plane in lower third and in muscular plane above (Fig. 28.2B).

Lymphatic drainage:
Lymphatics in esophagus are longitudinal and so spread of carcinoma to distant lymph nodes occurs early.

Lymph nodes are:
- *Paraesophageal groups* in the wall of the esophagus—are cervical, thoracic, paraesophageal and paracardial nodes.
- *Periesophageal groups* located immediately adjacent to esophageal wall. They are deep cervical, scalene, paratracheal,

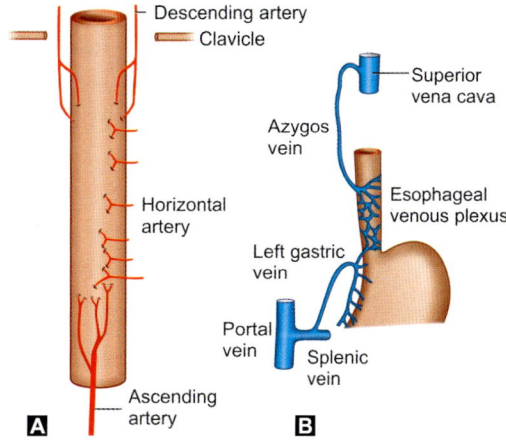

Figs. 28.2A and B: (A) Arterial supply and (B) Venous drainage of esophagus.

mediastinal, diaphragmatic, gastric and celiac lymph nodes.
- *Lateral esophageal groups* receive lymph from para- and peri-esophageal lymph nodes.

Nerve Supply

- Esophagus is innervated by vagus. There is both sympathetic and parasympathetic innervation.
- *Meissner's plexus* of nerves is located in the submucosa.
- *Auerbach's or myenteric plexus* lies between the longitudinal and circular layer of muscle.

Three types of contractions in the esophagus

1. *Primary*—progressive, triggered by swallowing.
2. *Secondary*—progressive, generated by distention or irritation.
3. *Tertiary*—nonprogressive.

LOWER ESOPHAGEAL SPHINCTER

- It is a high physiological pressure zone located in the lower end of the esophagus in terminal 4 cm region (4 cm in length), with a pressure of 10–25 mm Hg.

You may forget with whom you laughed, but you will never forget with whom you wept—Kalil Gibran

- Lower esophageal sphincter (LES) prevents reflux of gastric and duodenal contents.
- It is influenced by food, gastric distension, gastric pathology, smoking, GI hormones, alcohol.
- Normally there is a *transient relaxation period* wherein reflux (*physiological*) occurs but then immediately gets cleared by esophageal clearance mechanism.
- So *pathological reflux or gastroesophageal reflux disease (GERD)* can occur due to decreased LES tone, altered relaxation time, and reduced esophageal clearance mechanism, or other altered mechanical factors.
- Esophageal clearance mechanism is due to primary esophageal peristalsis which carries saliva with high bicarbonate content which neutralizes and clears the transient physiological reflux. Manometry with special microtransducers is used to measure the LES pressure.

DYSPHAGIA

It is difficulty/inability to swallow.

Causes for dysphagia

- Gastroesophageal reflux disease (GERD).
- Carcinoma esophagus.
- Achalasia cardia.
- Foreign body in esophagus.
- Plummer-Vinson syndrome.
- Hiatus hernia.
- Esophageal diverticula.
- Corrosive strictures.
- Esophageal candidial infection.
- Carcinoma post 1/3 of the tongue.
- Carcinoma pharynx.
- Diffuse esophageal spasm.
- Boerhaave's syndrome.
- Drug-induced dysphagia (KCl, Quinine, NSAID).
- Congenital anomalies of esophagus.

Investigations for dysphagia

- Barium swallow.
- Esophageal manometry.
- Ultrasound abdomen.
- Esophagoscopy.
- pH study of esophagus.
- MRI study.
- CT scan.
- Endosonography.

BARIUM SWALLOW X-RAY (FIG. 28.3)

It is done in cases of dysphagia, which may be due to carcinoma esophagus, achalasia cardia, stricture esophagus, hiatus hernia; to look for external compression, esophageal spasm, pharyngeal diverticula, esophageal webs. Varices can also be visualized. While screening motility of esophagus can be visualized.

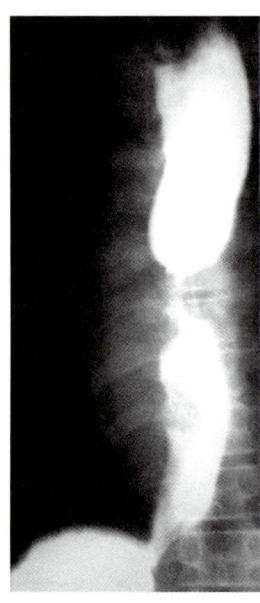

Fig. 28.3: Barium swallow showing irregular filling defect and *shouldering sign* in middle third esophagus.

ESOPHAGOSCOPY

Indications

- To identify the lesion (Fig. 28.4) and to take biopsy in carcinoma esophagus (Fig. 28.5).
- For diagnosing other esophageal conditions.
- To remove foreign body.
- To dilate stricture.
- To place endostents for inoperable carcinoma esophagus.
- To inject sclerosants for varices.

Self-respect—that a corner-stone of all virtue

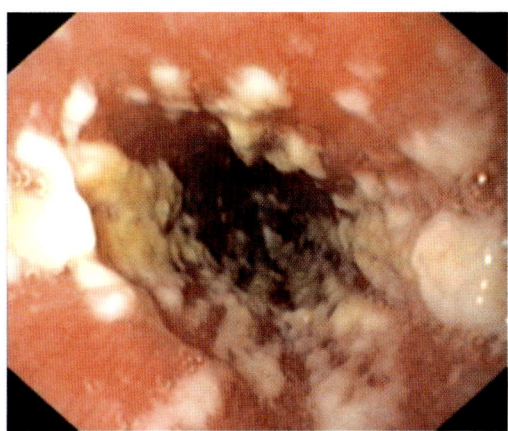

Fig. 28.4: Esophageal candidiasis—note the multiple lesions.

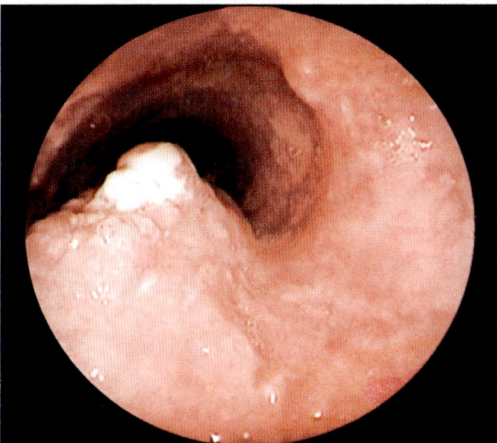

Fig. 28.5: Endoscopic view of carcinoma esophagus.

Types

1. **Rigid esophagoscope (Negus type):**
   - It is done under general anesthesia. Head is extended and head end of the table is tilted upwards, scope is passed behind the epiglottis and cricoid through the cricopharyngeal opening. This is the most difficult part in esophagoscopy. After that procedure, negotiation through the esophagus is easier. The lesion is identified and biopsy is taken if required.
   - **Complications** are perforation, bleeding.

2. **Fiberoptic flexible esophagoscope:**
   - It can be done under local anesthesia. Reflux and hiatus are well-identified. Stomach also can be visualized. Easier to pass and perforation is unlikely.
   - But tissue taken for biopsy is smaller and removal of foreign body is also difficult.

Esophageal endosonography
- It is a useful method of finding and assessing different layers of esophagus especially in carcinoma esophagus.
- It shows all layers clearly and distinctly and so invasion can be better made out and so operability can be decided.

ACHALASIA CARDIA

It is failure of relaxation of cardia (esophagogastric junction) due to disorganized esophageal peristalsis, as a result of integration of parasympathetic impulses causing *functional obstruction.*

Etiology
- Stress.
- Vitamin B_1 deficiency.
- Chaga's disease.
- There is pencil-shaped narrowing of cardia (O-G junction) with enormous dilatation of proximal esophagus, which contains foul smelling fluid and is more prone for aspiration pneumonia (Fig. 28.6).
- Achalasia cardia *is a precancerous* condition.

Clinical Features
- Common in females between 20–40 years age group.
- Present with progressive dysphagia, which is more for liquid than to solid food. Regurgitation and recurrent pneumonia are common.

Triad
• Dysphagia. • Regurgitation. • Weight loss.

Malnutrition and general ill health.

Don't judge each day by the harvest you reap but by the seeds that you plant—**Robert Louis Stevenson**

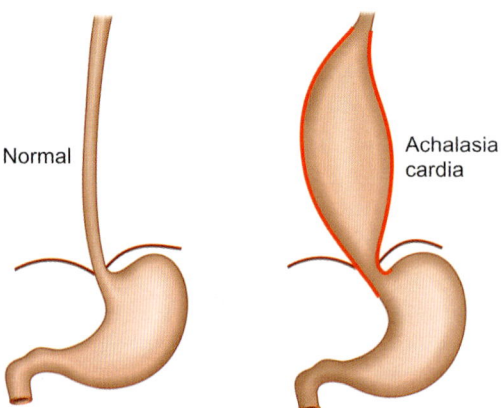

Fig. 28.6: Diagrammatic representation of achalasia cardia.

Investigations

- *Barium swallow is diagnostic*—shows (Fig. 28.7).
  - Pencil-like smooth narrowing of lower esophagus.
  - Dilatation of proximal esophagus.
  - Absence of fundic gas bubble.
- Chest X-ray shows patches of pneumonia.
- Esophageal manometry shows unrelaxed lower sphincter of esophageal sphincter.
- Esophagoscopy is done to confirm the diagnosis and to rule out carcinoma esophagus.

Differential Diagnosis

- Carcinoma esophagus.
- Stricture esophagus.

Treatment

1. *Modified Heller's operation—esophagocardiomyotomy* (Fig. 28.8).
   Either through thoracic or through abdominal approach, thickened circular muscle fibers are cut longitudinally for about 8–10 cm, 2 cm proximal to the thickened muscle to 1 cm distal to O-G junction. Care should be taken not to open the mucosa.
2. *Nissen's fundoplication* is done along with the above procedure to prevent reflux.
3. Rarely *Negus hydrostatic dilatation* is done to dilate O-G junction. It is not very well-accepted method as chances of perforation are high.

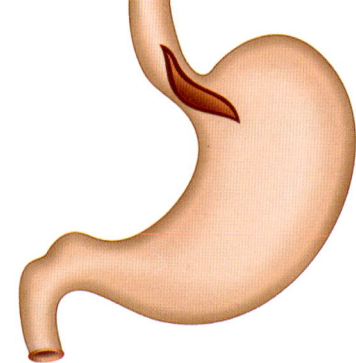

Fig. 28.8: Heller's cardiomyotomy for achalasia cardia. Only circular muscle layer is cut longitudinally in O-G junction until mucosa protrudes out without perforating the mucosa.

GASTROESOPHAGEAL REFLUX DISEASE

It is a pathological reflux from the stomach into the lower esophagus.

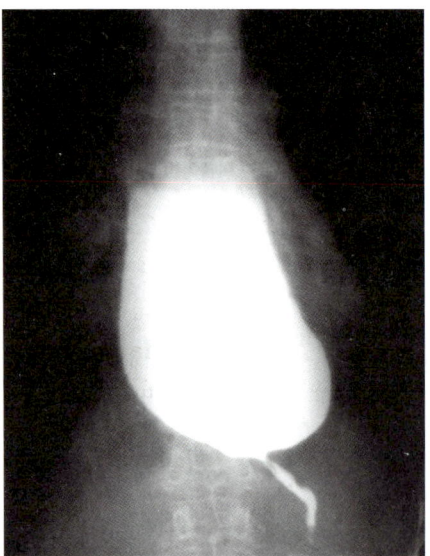

Fig. 28.7: X-ray picture of achalasia cardia.

God gives every bird its food, but He does not throw it into the nest

Anatomical Factors

- Obesity.
- Altered length of intra-abdominal esophagus.
- Altered obliquity of O-G junction.
- Reduced pinching action of crus of diaphragm.

Physiological Factors

- Reduced LES pressure.
- Altered transient relaxation period in LES.
- Reduced esophageal clearance mechanism.
- Delayed gastric emptying due to diabetes, neuromuscular block, gastroparesis, medications.
- Increased gastric distension and gastric acid hypersecretion.

Other Factors

Alcohol, smoking, stress, lifestyle.

Types
• Symptomatic uncomplicated GERD.
• Symptomatic, complicated GERD.

Features

- Fatty dyspepsia.
- Odynophagia.
- Appearance of symptoms within seconds of ingestion of food is typical.
- Chest pain and heartburn (*pyrosis*).
- Laryngeal symptoms.
- Dysphagia occurs once complications begin.
- Symptoms are more with change of position.
- Chronic cough, shortness of breath and hoarseness.

Complications	
• Reflux esophagitis.	• Esophageal shortening.
• Sliding hiatus hernia.	• Barrett's esophagus.
• Stricture lower end esophagus.	• Carcinoma (Adeno) esophagus.

Investigations

- Barium study in head down position.
- Endoscopy and biopsy.
- Esophageal manometry.
- 24-hour esophageal pH monitoring.

Differential Diagnosis

- Achalasia cardia.
- Carcinoma esophagus.
- Peptic ulcer.
- Gallstones.
- Pancreatic diseases.
- Gastritis.

Treatment of Uncomplicated GERD

- Control of obesity.
- Stop smoking and alcohol.
- Avoid tea, coffee.
- Propped up position.
- H_2 antagonists.
- *Proton pump inhibitors (PPI's)*:
  - Omeprazole 20 mg
  - Lansoprazole 30 mg
  - Pantoprazole 30 mg
  - Esomeprazole 20 mg.

Indications for Surgical Treatment

- Failure of drug treatment.
- Sliding hernia.
- Barrett's ulcer.

Surgeries

- *Total or partial Nissen's fundoplication* (Fig. 28.9) wherein after narrowing the crus of the diaphragm, mobilized fundus is wrapped around the O-G junction area either totally or partially.
- *Laparoscopic fundoplication* is safe and a popular alternate approach.
- *Belsey Mark-4* operation is plication of esophagus to the diaphragm through many sutures and so as to push the lower end of esophagus downwards and make it intra-abdominal.

Success is not how high you have climbed, but how you make a positive difference to the world—**Roy T Bennett**

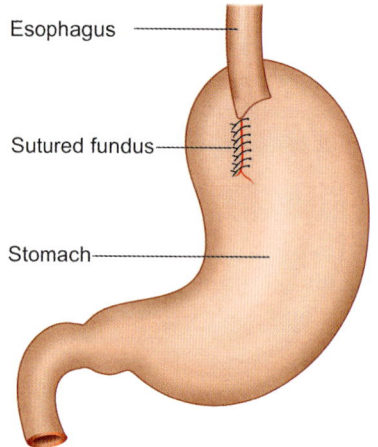

Fig. 28.9: Nissen's fundoplication.

- Placement of *Angelchik prosthesis* in lower end of esophagus, also prevents the reflux.
- *Collis' vertical gastroplasty* is done using fundus of stomach (by giving vertical cut and suturing fundus) for esophageal shortening (a complication of GERD).
- *Esophagogastrectomy* may be required in severe cases (lower end of esophagus and part of stomach).

BARRETT'S ESOPHAGUS

- It is metaplastic changes in the mucosa of the esophagus in response to GERD.
- Squamous epithelium of lower end of the esophagus is replaced by diseased columnar epithelium (columnar metaplasia).
- There is macroscopic visible length of columnar mucosa with microscopic features of intestinal metaplasia.
- If the length of metaplasia is more than 3 cm. it is called as *long segment Barrett's esophagus*.
- If the length is less than 3 cm, it is called as *short segment Barrett's esophagus*.
- This diseased columnar epithelium is more prone for malignant transformation, i.e. when there is intestinal metaplasia, the risk of malignant transformation increases that too when there is more amount of dysplasia.

Features

- Features of GERD.
- Hematemesis.

Management

- Regular endoscopic biopsy.
- Ablation of Barrett's esophagus by laser.
- Photodynamic therapy.
- Argon beam coagulation.
- Proton pump inhibitors.
- Antireflux treatment by surgery.
- Resection.

HIATUS HERNIA

It may be (Figs. 28.10 and 28.11):
- Sliding hernia (85%).
- Rolling hernia (10–12%).
- Combined.

Sliding hernia is commonly associated with GERD (should be discussed like GERD).

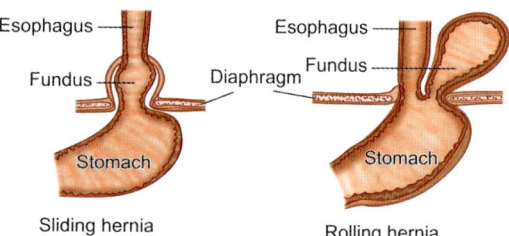

Fig. 28.10: Types of hiatus hernia.

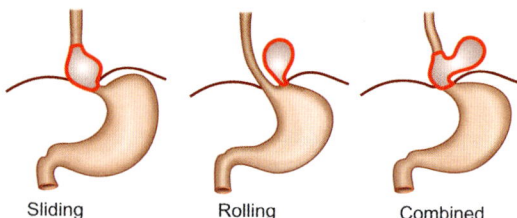

Fig. 28.11: Different types of hiatus hernia—sliding, rolling and combined.

Habit is either the best of servants or the worst of masters

ROLLING HERNIA (PARAESOPHAGEAL HERNIA)

* It is herniation of stomach or rarely other abdominal contents through a hiatus usually towards left side.

Clinical features	Complications
Pain	Gangrene of stomach.
Hiccough	Perforation into the mediastinum.
Regurgitation	Perforation into the peritoneum.
Cardiac abnormality	Gastric volvulus.

* **Investigations:** Plain X-ray; Barium meal study; electrocardiogram (ECG).
* **Treatment**
  - Treatment is always *surgical*.
  - Excision of sac and repair of the defect.
  - If it is gangrenous, gastrectomy is required.

REFLUX ESOPHAGITIS

Types

1. *Acute:* Following *burns, trauma, infection, peptic ulcer.*
2. *Chronic:*
   - Reflux of acid in sliding hernia, after gastric surgery.
   - Reflux is quiet common in pregnancy.
   - Site is always in lower esophagus.

Pathology

There is bleeding granulation tissue in lower esophageal mucosa with spasm of longitudinal muscle, which pulls the adjacent gastric area upwards into the esophagus causing sliding hernia.

Features

* It is a part of GERD, pain and burning sensation in retrosternal area often referred to shoulder, neck, arm, etc.
* Heartburn is common.
* Dysphagia, anemia.

Diagnosis

* Barium meal X-ray.
* Gastroscopy and biopsy.

Barrett's ulcer is an ulcer with gastric (columnar) metaplasia in lower esophagus.

Treatment

* H_2 *blockers*: Ranitidine, Famotidine, etc.
* *Proton pump inhibitors*:
  - Omeprazole 20 mg OD one hour before food (Morning).
  - Lanzoprazole 30 mg
  - Pantoprazole 40 mg
  - Esomeprazole 20 mg
  - Rabeprazole 20 mg
* *Treating GERD and associated causes.* By fundoplication and other surgeries.
* *Resection in severe cases.*

CORROSIVE STRICTURE OF ESOPHAGUS

* Mainly due to alkali sodium hydroxide, occasionally due to acid (sulfuric acid, nitric acid, etc.). Acid commonly damages the stomach.
* It causes extensive inflammation of the mucosa with periesophagitis, which if not treated leads to multiple strictures in esophagus.
* Sometimes, it causes severe life-threatening necrotizing lesion, which requires immediate surgical intervention.

Management

* Careful gentle endoscopy.
* Steroids for 3 weeks.
* Antibiotics.
* Later regular esophageal dilatation is done for stricture.

You cannot strengthen the weak by weakening the strong

In multiple strictures, treatment is esophageal resection with colonic transposition. Colonic transposition bypass without resection of esophagus can also be done.

PLUMMER-VINSON SYNDROME (PATTERSON-KELLY SYNDROME)

- *Esophageal webs* seen in uppermost portion of esophagus with spasm of circular muscle fibers. It is a premalignant condition.
- *Iron deficiency anemia.*
- *Superficial glossitis*, cheilitis, *kolionychia*.
- Splenomegaly.

In esophageal webs, mucosa is hyperkeratotic, friable, desquamated and causes severe dysphagia.

Esophagoscopy and biopsy is required to rule out malignancy.

Treatment

- Oral iron—ferrous sulfate 300 mg tid with vitamins.
- Blood transfusion is given when there is severe anemia (transfusion of packed cells).
- IV or IM iron therapy.
- Once anemia comes under control, webs will clear and patient can swallow. ***Follow-up endoscopy is a must***.

MALLORY-WEISS SYNDROME

- It is seen in adults with a severe prolonged vomiting causing longitudinal tear in the mucosa of stomach at and just below the cardia, *leading to severe hematemesis*.
- Violent vomiting often may be due to migraine or vertigo.
- Presents with severe *vomiting* and later *hematemesis*, with features of *shock*.
- **Investigations:** Gastroscopy, Hb%, PCV, blood grouping.

- **Differential diagnosis (Figs. 28.12A and B)**
  - Bleeding peptic ulcer.
  - Esophageal varices.
  - Erosive gastritis.
  - Carcinoma stomach.

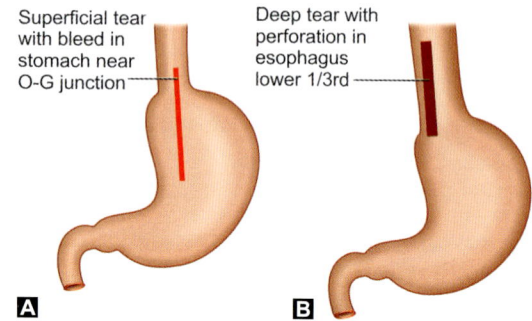

Figs. 28.12A and B: (A) Mallory-Weiss syndrome; (B) Boerhaave's syndrome.

- **Treatment**
  - Conservative, as tear is only mucosal.
  - Blood transfusion, IV fluids, sedation.
  - Hemostatic agents like vasopressin.
  - Endoscopic injection therapy if required.
  - Surgery is rarely required.

BOERHAAVE'S SYNDROME

- It is a tear in the lower third of the esophagus which occur when a person vomits *against a closed glottis*, causing leak into the mediastinum, pleural cavity and peritoneum.
- **Investigations:** Chest X-ray and MRI; total count.

Boerhaave's syndrome		
Presentations	Differential diagnosis	Complications
• Sudden onset of symptoms	• Myocardial infarction	• Mediastinitis
• Severe chest pain	• Pancreatitis	• Septicemia
• Pain abdomen		
• Shock		

Instead of worrying about what you cannot control, shift your energy to what you can create—**Roy T Bennett**

Treatment

- Nil by mouth; antibiotics.
- IV fluids; total parenteral nutrition (TPN).
- Feeding by jejunostomy.
- Often surgery with resection may be required.
- When severe mediastinitis occurs, condition has high mortality.

TRACHEOESOPHAGEAL FISTULA

Types (Figs. 28.13A to D)

In 85% cases, it is a blind upper end with lower end communicating with trachea.

It may be associated with **VACTER** anomalies.

- V—Vertebral defects.
- A—Anal atresia.
- C—Cardiac defect (PDA/VSD).
- TE—Tracheoesophageal fistula.
- R—Radial hypoplasia and renal agenesis.

Features

- Tracheoesophageal fistula (TEF) should be recognized within 24 hours of birth.
- Newborn baby regurgitates all feeds and there is continuous pouring of saliva from the mouth, which is a *diagnostic feature*.
- It is commonly associated with maternal *hydramnios*.

Investigations

- Obstruction while passing nasogastric tube.
- Contrast study reveals fistula and obstruction.
- Look for other anomalies.
- Chest X-ray.
- Echocardiography.

Treatment

Surgery

Through right sided thoracotomy (opposite to the side of aortic arch), fistula is identified and resected. Lower segment is anastomosed to the blind upper segment. If the length is inadequate then, colonic interposition has to be done.

Complications of surgery	
· Pneumonia.	· Reflux.
· Leak from anastomotic site.	· Dysphagia.

CARCINOMA ESOPHAGUS

Etiology

Diet, deficiencies	5% common
Mycotoxin	Common after 45 years
Alcohol and tobacco	Common in men
Achalasia cardia	Common in China– Henan province
Esophageal webs	

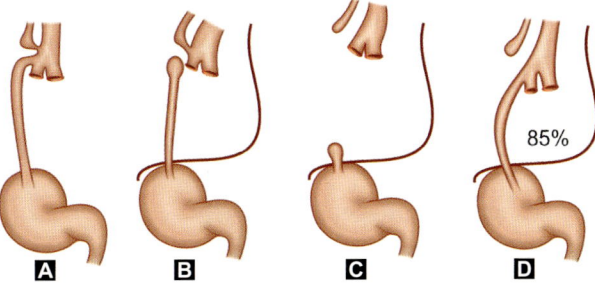

Figs. 28.13A to D: Types of tracheoesophageal fistula: (A) H type; (B) Lower end blind, upper end connected to trachea; (C) Both ends blind; (D) Upper end blind, lower end connected to stomach.

You cannot help men permanently by doing for them what they could and should do for themselves.

Pathology

Site	Incidence
• Middle third	• > 50% (common)
• Lower third	• 33%
• Upper third	• 17%

Type
- Squamous cell carcinoma—in proximal 2/3rd
- Adenocarcinoma and SCC—in lower 1/3rd
- Adenocarcinoma—in OG junction

Note:
Lower 3 cm of esophagus is lined by columnar epithelium, and so adenocarcinoma is common here. Barrett's columnar metaplasia which occurs in lower third esophagus is also more prone for adenocarcinoma.

Gross

- Annular.
- Ulcerative.
- Fungating—cauliflower-like.

Spread

Direct

- In upper third, it spreads through muscular layer and get adherent to left main bronchus, trachea, and left recurrent laryngeal nerve (causes hoarseness), aorta or its branches (causes fatal hemorrhage, but rare).
- It may perforate and cause mediastinitis.
- It may get adherent to pleura also.

Lymphatic Spread

- It spreads both by lymphatic permeation and lymphatic embolization.
- It can cause satellite nodules elsewhere in the esophagus away from the main tumor.
- Above in the neck it spreads to left supraclavicular lymph nodes.
- In the thorax it spreads to paraesophageal, tracheobronchial lymph nodes to subdiaphragmatic lymph nodes.
- In the abdomen it spreads to celiac lymph nodes.

Blood Spread

It occurs to *liver commonly;* occasionally to lungs and bones.

Clinical Features

- Recent onset of dysphagia is the commonest feature. For the dysphagia to develop two-third of the lumen should be occluded.
- Regurgitation.
- Anorexia and loss of weight (severe) (*cachexia*).
- Pain—substernal or in the abdomen.
- Liver secondaries.
- Bronchopneumonia.
- Features of bronchoesophageal fistula in carcinoma of upper third esophagus.
- Supraclavicular lymph nodes may be palpable.

Investigations

- *Barium swallow*: *Shouldering sign* and irregular filling defect (Fig. 28.14).
- Esophagoscopy to see the lesion, extent and type.

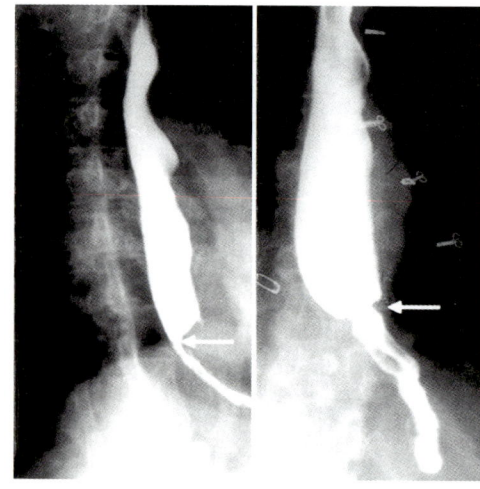

Fig. 28.14: Barium study showing shouldering sign and irregular filling defect—carcinoma lower esophagus.

Believe in your heart that you're meant to live a life full of passion, purpose, magic and miracles—**Roy T Bennett**

- Biopsy for histological type and confirmation.
- Chest X-ray to see pulmonary infection.
- Bronchoscopy, to see invasion in upper third growth.
- Esophageal endosonography to look for the involvement of layers of esophagus.
- CT scan to look for local extension and status of tracheobronchial tree in case of upper third growth.
- Ultrasound abdomen to look for liver and lymph nodes status in abdomen.
- Endoscopic esophageal staining with labeled iodine results in normal mucosa being stained brown, but mucosa remains pale in carcinoma (in carcinoma mucosa will not take up iodine).

Treatment

Curative treatment

Indications:
- Early growth, when patient is fit for surgery.
- When there is no involvement of lymph nodes, bronchus, and liver.

Postcricoid Tumor

- It is treated mainly by radiotherapy.
- Often *pharyngolaryngectomy is done along with gastric or colonic transposition*. But complications are more in this procedure.

Upper Third Growth

- Treated mainly by radiotherapy.
- Commonly it is advanced with left recurrent nerve palsy and bronchial invasion.

If it is early and operable, McKeown three staged esophagectomy and anastomosis is done in the neck.

Initially laparotomy is done to mobilize the stomach. Then thoracotomy through right 5th space is done and esophagus is mobilized. Through right side neck approach, esophagus with growth is removed. Anastomosis between pharynx and stomach is done in the neck.

Middle Third Growth

Ivor Lewis operation: After laparotomy stomach is mobilized. Pyloroplasty is done. Through right 5th space thoracotomy is done and growth with tumor is mobilized. Partial esophagectomy and esophagogastric anastomosis is done in the thorax. Intercostal tube drainage is placed during closure.

If growth is inoperable, palliative radiotherapy is given.

Lower Third Growth

Here through left thoracoabdominal approach, partial esophagogastrectomy is done with esophagogastric anastomosis. Often jejunal Roux-en-Y loop anastomosis is done.
- *Orrhinger and Orrhinger approach,* i.e. *trans-hiatal blind total esophagectomy* (Fig. 28.15) with anastomosis in the left side of the neck—through laparotomy, stomach and lower part of the esophagus are mobilized. Through left sided neck approach, upper part of the esophagus is mobilized using finger. Blind dissection is completed by meeting both fingers above and below in the thorax. Later esophagus is pulled up, out through the neck wound and removed. Continuity is maintained in the neck. It is a *palliative* surgery.
- *Thoracoscopic-laparoscopic esophagectomy* is practiced in a few centers.

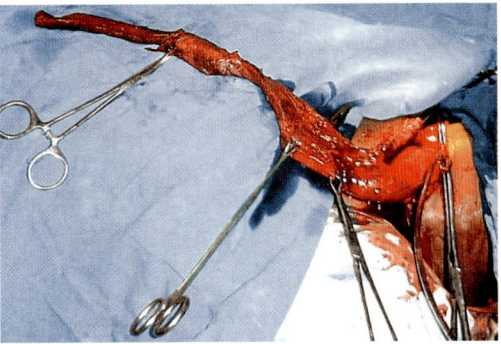

Fig. 28.15: Transhiatal blind esophagectomy on table surgical specimen.

You give but little when you give of your possessions. It is when you give of yourself that you truly give—**Kalil Gibran**

- When interposition is required, mobilized *stomach or jejunum or colon (left)* are used. Commonly it is placed in the thorax. Often it can be placed in substernal space or in front of the sternum in subcutaneous plane (especially colon).

Palliative Treatment

Gastrostomy should not be done as a palliative procedure.
- Palliative radiotherapy.
- Intraluminal brachytherapy (radiation intraluminally).

Chemotherapy:
Cisplatin, Methotrexate, 5-FU.

Intubation

- Atkinson tube.
- Celestin tube.
- Souttar tube.
- Mousseau-Barbin tube—cheaper, but requires laparotomy to pass.
  - *Expanding metal stents* are passed through endoscope under C-arm guidance.
  - *Endoscopic laser* is used to core a channel through the tumor to improve dysphagia.

Complications of major surgeries: Infection, leak, bleeding.

Terminal events in carcinoma esophagus

- Cancer cachexia; sepsis; immunosuppression.
- Malignant tracheoesophageal fistula (causes severe respiratory infection and death. Here expansile endoluminal stents are used at the site of fistula to have temporary benefit).

Prognosis

Not good because of early spread due to longitudinal lymphatics, aggressiveness, difficult approach, late presentation.

So long as enthusiasm lasts, so long is life still with us

CHAPTER 29

Neurosurgery

Chapter Outline

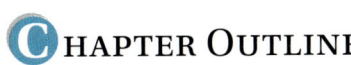

- Head Injuries
- Extradural Hematoma
- Subdural Hematoma
- Depressed Skull Fracture
- Subarachnoid Hemorrhage
- Intracranial Abscess
- Intracranial Aneurysm
- Hydrocephalus
- Intracranial Tumors
- Pituitary Tumors
- Spina Bifida

HEAD INJURIES

Mechanism

- *Distortion of the brain*: Brain is a soft structure, therefore has 'mobility' and readily distorts. This distortion and mobility is accentuated by cerebrospinal fluid (CSF) and vascular components. Any impact creates shearing forces in the brain causing damage to neurons, supporting tissues and blood vessels. This leads to loss of consciousness, focal neurological deficits. Such distortive damage may be temporary or permanent.
- *Mobility of the brain in relation to the skull and membranes* causes cerebral damage and bleeding in dural spaces from torn vessels in the dura, commonly the veins. In old age, the brain shrinks, as a result of which 'mobility' of brain increases favoring rupture of veins which cross the subdural space.
- *Configuration of interior of skull*: Damage is less severe over the smooth area but is more severe over the rough and sharp areas. So the damage is severe over the anterior cranial fossa, over the falx, and over the tentorium.
- *Deceleration and acceleration injuries*: *Deceleration injuries* occur when moving head strikes an immovable object (like in road traffic accidents). *Acceleration injuries* occur when stationary skull is struck by a moving object (like in assault).
- *Cerebral concussion* is slight distortion causing temporary physiological changes leading to transient loss of consciousness with complete recovery.
- *Cerebral contusion* is more severe degree of damage with bruising and cerebral edema leading to diffuse or localized changes.
- *Cerebral laceration* is tearing of brain surface with collection of blood in different spaces and with displacement of dural parts.

Effects of Brain Injuries

- *Brain edema* is accumulation of fluid both intracellular and extracellular. It is due to

Do whatever your enemies don't want you to do

Clinical types	Causative types	Primary lesions
• Open injury. • Closed injury.	• Blunt injury. • Sharp injury. • Missile injury.	• Diffuse axonal injury. • Shearing lesions. • Contusion. • Laceration.
Cerebral concussion	**Injuries**	**Secondary lesions**
• It is temporary physiological paralysis. • Transient loss of consciousness. • Transient amnesia. • Usually shows complete recovery. • Should be observed for any possible complications like extradural or subdural hematoma.	• Cerebral concussion. • Contusion, laceration. • Hemorrhages. • Midline shift, coning. • Brain edema. • Diffuse neuronal injury. • Intraventricular injury/hemorrhage. • Brainstem injury. • Coup and contre-coup injury.	• *Brain swelling* due to edema, hypoxia, congestion. • *Hemorrhages* like extradural, subdural, intracerebral. • *Infections* like meningitis, subdural empyema with pus collection as localized, encephalitis. • *Features due to increased intracranial pressure.* • *Electrolyte changes.*

congestion and dilatation of blood vessels. It may be diffuse or localized.
- *Brain necrosis* is of severe variety with destruction and is due to hemorrhagic infarction.
- *Extradural hematomas* occurs usually in temporoparietal region. It is commonly due to tear in middle meningeal veins and often middle meningeal artery. It causes intracranial hypertension, displacement, Kernohan's effect and often death.
- *Subdural hematoma* is due to tear of veins between cerebrum and dura due to shearing forces. It is diffuse and commonly associated with cerebral injury.
- *Intracerebral hematoma* can occur in different parts of cerebrum may be in frontal lobe, temporal lobe, etc.
- *Intraventricular hemorrhage* is very severe type of hemorrhage.
- *Brain ischemia* is due to increased pressure. This in turn leads to alteration in the perfusion of brain which itself aggravates the ischemia and this forms a vicious cycle, causing progressive diffuse ischemia of brain.
- *Coup injury* occurs on the side of the blow to the head. **Contre-coup** injury occurs on the side opposite to the blow on the head.

❖ Coning:
It is due to rise in intracranial pressure causing either:
i. Herniation of contents of supratentorial compartment through *the tentorial hiatus*
   or
ii. Herniation of the contents of infratentorial compartment through the *foramen magnum.*
In supratentorial herniation, there is compression of ipsilateral third cranial nerve and midbrain.
Midbrain is displaced away from the mass (hematoma) and midbrain is pressed by the sharp edge of tentorium cerebelli of opposite side leading to dysfunction of corticospinal fibers (which after decussation supplies on the opposite side in the body, i.e. same side of the injury). This leads to:
a. Deterioration in the level of consciousness.
b. Dilatation of pupil on the side of compressing mass (hematoma).
c. Hemiparesis on the same side of the mass lesion (hematoma) due to compression of the contralateral corticospinal tract. This effect is called as **Kernohan's notch effect (Fig. 29.1)**.

*Experience is a comb that nature gives man after he has gone bald—**Thai Saying***

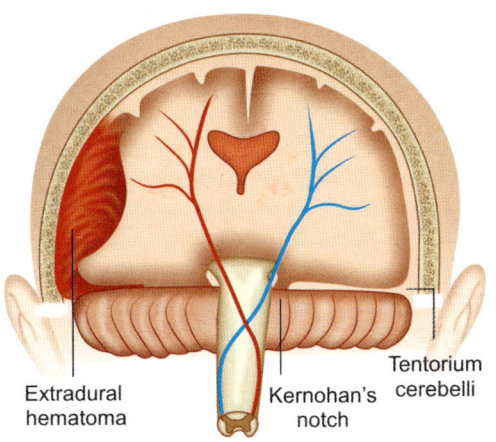

Fig. 29.1: Coning with Kernohan's notch.

Herniation of infratentorial contents through the foramen magnum causes obstruction of cerebral aqueduct which further damages the brain function.

* *Respiratory failure* altering PO_2 and PCO_2 levels.
* *Raised intracranial pressure* causing bradycardia, hypertension, vomiting. Raised intracranial pressure may precipitate coning and thus aggravates brain ischemia.
* Fluid and electrolyte imbalance.
* Hyperpyrexia.
* *Convulsions* due to irritation of gray matter.
* CSF rhinorrhea or CSF otorrhea.

Clinical Approach of a Patient with Head Injury

* Detail history of injury has to be taken and also the process of deterioration—rapid or gradual.
* History of alcohol intake: Alcohol intake mimics head injury and alcoholism itself may mask the features of head injury.
* *Neurological assessment*:
  By:
  – Level of consciousness.
  – Glasgow Coma Scale.
  – Pupillary reaction to light and size.
  – Pulse.
  – Temperature.
  – Blood pressure.
  – Respiratory rate.
  – Reflexes.
  – Limb movements—normal/mild weakness/severe weakness/spastic flexion/extension/no response.
* Status and protection of airway.
* General assessment and other injuries like fractures, abdominal organ injuries, and thoracic injuries are looked for.
* Presence of any scalp hematoma, fractures of skull bone which may be depressed has to be looked for Figure 29.2 shows a head injury patient having a black eye.
* Any blood from nose or ear, CSF rhinorrhea or CSF otorrhea has to be looked for.

Adelaide Coma Scale: It is used in children. Scores for eye opening and motor responses are same as Glasgow Coma Scale.

But *verbal response score differs*—Oriented-5. Words-4. Vocal sounds-3. Cries-2. Nil-1.

Orientation cannot be evaluated below 5 years. For first 6 months, the best verbal response is cry.

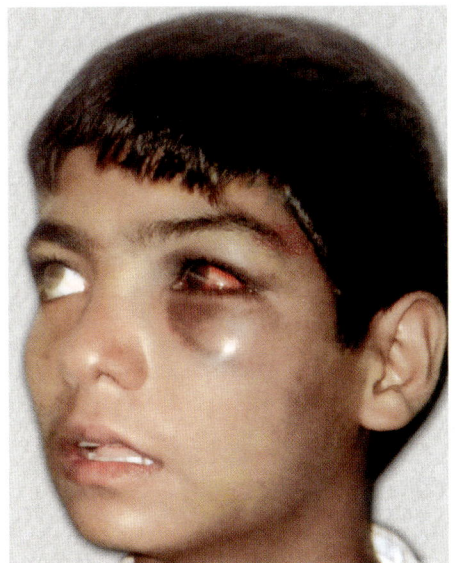

Fig. 29.2: Head injury patient having black eye.

Friends come and go, but enemies accumulate

Indications for hospitalization
• Any altered level of consciousness.
• Skull fracture.
• Focal neurological features.
• Persistent headache, vomiting, systolic hypertension, bradycardia.
• Alcohol intoxication.
• Bleeding from ear or nose.
• Associated injuries.

Investigations

- X-ray skull: To look for fracture, relative position of the calcified pineal gland, presence of intracranial air.
- Serum electrolyte measurement.
- Blood grouping and cross matching.
- CT scan—plain (not contrast) to look for cerebral edema, hematomas (Figs. 29.3 and 29.4), midline shift, fractures, ventricles, brainstem injury.
- Carotid arteriography.
- Investigations for other injuries like ultrasound of abdomen.
- Monitoring of intracranial pressure.

Treatment

General

- Protection of airway using mouth gag, endotracheal intubation or tracheostomy whenever required.
- Throat suction, bladder and bowel care, good nursing are very essential.

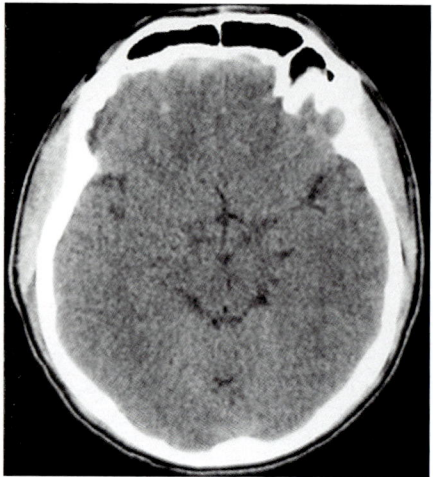

Fig. 29.3: CT scan head showing scalp hematoma both sides. There is no internal injury.

- Nasal oxygen or often ventilator support.
- IV fluids initially, later Ryle's tube feeding has to be done.
- Electrolyte maintenance.

Drugs

- *No sedation is given.*
- Analgesics and anticonvulsants like Phenytoin or Phenobarbitone is started.
- Diuretics are given to reduce cerebral edema—either mannitol 20%, 200 mL IV 8th hourly or Frusemide 40 mg IV 8th hourly. It should not be given in conditions like intracranial hematomas.

Glasgow coma scale						
Eye opening		*Verbal response*		*Motor response*		
Spontaneous.	4	Oriented.	5	Obeys commands.	6	
To speech.	3	Confused.	4	Localizes pain.	5	
To pain.	2	Inappropriate words.	3	Flexion to pain.	4	
None.	1	Incomprehensible words.	2	Abnormal flexion.	3	
		None.	1	Extension to pain.	2	
				None.	1	
Total score: 15.
Mild head injury—Score: 13–15.
Moderate head injury: 9–12.
Severe head injury—less than 8: (3–8).						
Score 1—dead or dying. Score 2—vegetative state. Score 3—severe disability.
Score 4—moderate disability. Score 5—good recovery.						

A sweet friendship refreshes the soul

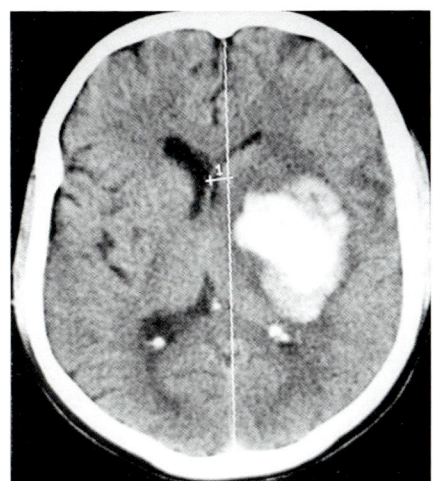

Fig. 29.4: CT scan head showing intracerebral hematoma.

- Antibiotics like penicillins, ampicillins are given to prevent the onset of meningitis.
- Corticosteroids either dexamethasone or betamethasone is used commonly but its beneficial effect is not confirmed.

Indications for Surgery

- Acute extradural hematoma.
- Acute subdural hematoma.
- Depressed skull fracture.

Procedure: Craniotomy is done and cranial flap is raised. After evacuating the clot *hitch stitches* are applied between dural layer and scalp. Postoperative antibiotics, analgesics, anticonvulsants are given.

Complications of Head Injuries

A. **Early**
  1. Brainstem injury—due to coning.
  2. Compression over cerebellum and medulla.
  3. CSF rhinorrhea.
  4. Meningitis—common.
  5. Pituitary damage and endocrine failure—requires high dose of hydrocortisone 200 mg 6th hourly.
  6. Aerocele.
  7. CSF otorrhea.
  8. Depressed fractures often causes injury to dural venous sinuses and may lead to torrential hemorrhage which may be life-threatening. So such depressed fractures should never be elevated.

B. **Late**
  1. Chronic subdural hematoma.
  2. Early post-traumatic epilepsy—they need anticonvulsants for 3 years.
  3. Late post-traumatic epilepsy is due to scarring and gliosis of cerebrum.
  4. Post-traumatic amnesia.
  5. Post-traumatic hydrocephalus.
  6. Post-traumatic headache.

CSF RHINORRHEA

It is due to communication between intracranial cavity and the nose. There is a tear in the dura following the fracture involving the sinuses—frontal, ethmoid, sphenoidal sinuses. Meningitis is the common complication of CSF rhinorrhea.

Treatment: Initial management is only conservative for 10 days—by antibiotics and observation.

Indications for surgical intervention:
- Fracture middle third face.
- CSF rhinorrhea persisting for more than 10 days.
- Fracture of sinuses.
- An aerocele.
- An attack of meningitis.

Surgeries:
- Reduction of middle third of face.
- Exploration of anterior cranial fossa.

EXTRADURAL HEMATOMA

It is collection of blood in the extradural space between the dura and skull. Commonest site is *temporoparietal* region. It can be *unilateral* or *bilateral*.

Vessels commonly involved:
- Middle meningeal veins.
- Anterior branch of middle meningeal artery.
- Posterior branch of middle meningeal artery.

The greatest truths are the simplest; and so are the greatest men

Usually is associated with fracture of temporoparietal region.

Immediately after injury, there will be transient loss of consciousness and the patient soon becomes normal. Later after 6–12 hours, he again falls ill and the condition deteriorates. This is the time taken to develop raised intracranial pressure, coning and its effects. This crucial time gap which is unnoticed and often missed is called as '**lucid interval**'.

Coning of the supratentorial content through sharp edge of the tentorial hiatus due to midline shift and injury to opposite midbrain occurs and is called as **Kernohan's notch effect *(refer Fig. 29.1)***.

Pathology

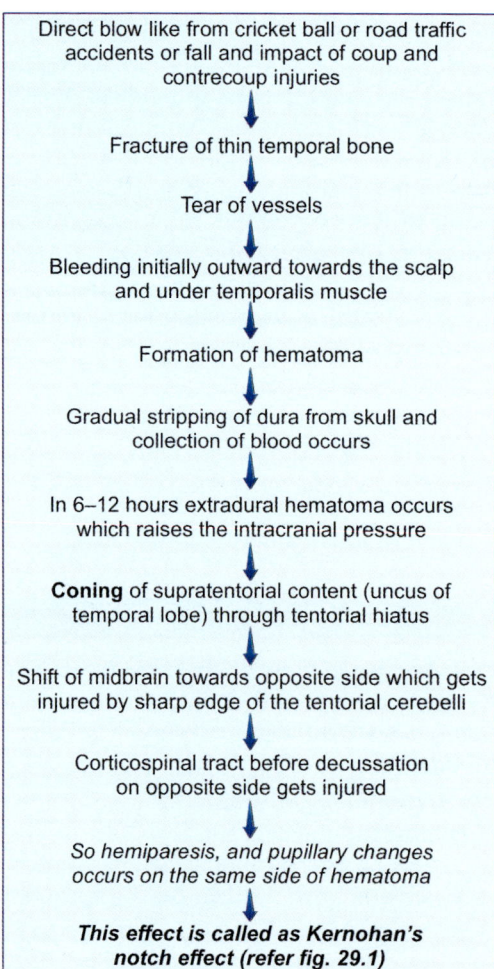

Features

History of transient loss of consciousness following a history of blow or fall. Patient soon regains consciousness and again after 6–12 hours starts deteriorating (***Lucid interval***).

Later the patient presents with confusion, irritability, drowsiness, and hemiparesis on same side of the injury. Initially pupillary constriction and later pupillary dilatation occurs on the same side, finally becomes totally unconscious.

Death can occur if immediate surgical intervention is not done.

Features of raised intracranial pressure like high blood pressure, bradycardia, vomiting is also seen. Occasionally *convulsions* may be present.

Wound and hematoma in the temporal region of scalp may be seen.

Investigations

- X-ray skull may show fracture of temporal bone.
- Electrolyte estimation.
- CT scan—head is diagnostic. Extradural hematoma shows *biconvex* lesion (Figs. 29.5 and 29.6).

Treatment

Immediate surgical intervention is essential to save the life of patient.

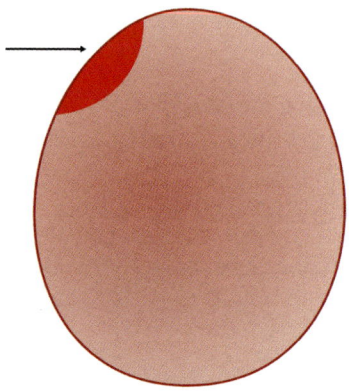

Fig. 29.5: Extradural hematoma. Note the biconvex configuration of the hematoma.

*It does not matter if you fall down as long as you pick up something while you get up—**Allen Smith***

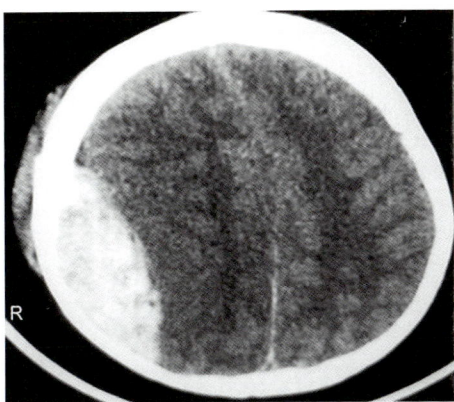

Fig. 29.6: CT scan head showing extradural hematoma with biconvex lesion.

Craniotomy is done and cranial flaps are raised. The dura is opened and the clot is evacuated. The dura is fixed to galea using interrupted sutures—*Hitch stitches*. Antibiotics and anticonvulsants are given postoperatively.

Recovery is good after surgery.

Complications

- Post-traumatic epilepsy.
- Meningitis.
- Post-traumatic amnesia.

SUBDURAL HEMATOMA

Types

Acute or Chronic

a. Acute subdural hematoma:
It is a collection of blood between the brain and dura. It is due to injury to the cortical veins and often due to laceration of cortex of brain which bleeds and blood gets collected in the subdural space forming a hematoma.

Here hematoma is extensive and diffuse. There is no lucid interval. There is a severe primary brain damage.

Hematoma may be coup and contrecoup type.

Loss of consciousness occurs immediately after trauma and is progressive.

Convulsion is common.

Features of raised intracranial pressure are obviously seen—high BP, bradycardia, vomiting.

Focal neurological deficits or hemiparesis can occur.

CT scan shows concavo-convex lesion.

Treatment: Antibiotics, anticonvulsants, etc. *Surgical decompression has to be done by craniotomy.*

b. Chronic subdural hematoma:
It is due to the rupture of veins between dura and brain (cerebral hemispheres), causing gradual collection of blood in subdural space. It is commonly seen in elderly people following any minor trauma like fall, slipping, etc. (which might have gone unnoticed). In elderly people, brain atrophies and even minor injuries can cause shearing and bleeding from these veins. Blood collects gradually over 2–6 weeks. Plasma and cellular components get separated. Eventually cellular part gets absorbed leaving only fluid component. It is called as **subdural hygroma**.

Usual hematoma collection is 60–120 mL. Often it is bilateral in 50% of cases.

This chronic hematoma may get infected, gets filled with localized pus and is called as **chronic subdural empyema**.

Features

- Common in old age, with history of minor trauma.
- Patient presents with confusion, disorientation, gradually with altered level of consciousness and drowsiness.
- Later convulsions, features of intracranial hypertension, features of coning develop.
- Extensor plantar response and pupillary changes develop eventually.

*We all have dreams. But in order to make dreams come into reality, it takes an awful lot of determination, dedication, self-discipline, and effort—**Jesse Owens***

Investigations (Figs. 29.7 and 29.8)

- CT scan (shows *concavo-convex* lesion).
- Serum electrolytes.
- Blood grouping and cross matching.

Differential Diagnosis

- Electrolyte imbalance.
- Intracranial space occupying lesion.

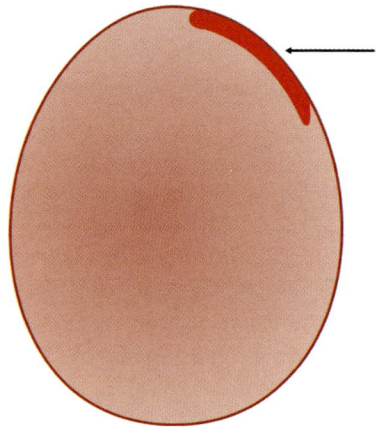

Fig. 29.7: Subdural hematoma. Note the concavo-convex configuration of the lesion (C/W EDH).

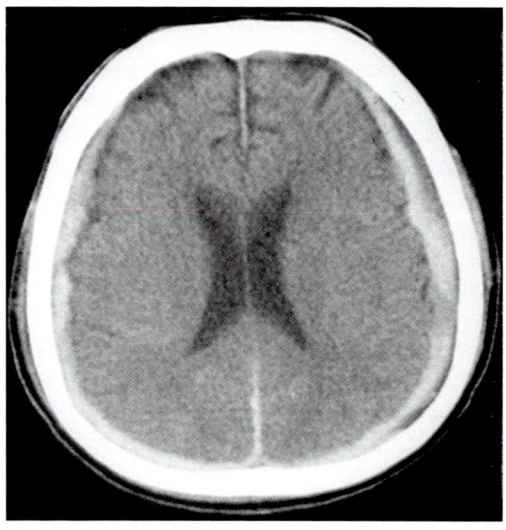

Fig. 29.8: CT scan head showing subdural hematoma with concavo-convex lesion.

Treatment

- Craniotomy and evacuation of clot has to be done when required on both sides.
- Antibiotics.
- Anticonvulsants for 3 years.

Complications

- Epilepsy; meningitis.
- Coning; neurological deficits.

DEPRESSED SKULL FRACTURE

It is a common neurosurgical problem among the head injuries.

It means fracture depression is more than the depth of the inner table of skull.

Problems in depressed fracture
• Tear in the dura beneath.
• Hematoma in the deeper plane.
• Injury to the cerebrum.
• Injury to the venous sinuses—may cause life-threatening hemorrhage. *Fracture should not be elevated* in such occasion as it itself can precipitate bleeding.
• Convulsions.
• Meningitis.

Investigations

CT scan.

Treatment

Antibiotics, anticonvulsants.
Elevation of the depressed fracture: Burr holes are made in the adjacent normal skull. Fracture is elevated. Bony fragments and necrotic materials are removed. Dural tear is closed with interrupted sutures.

SUBARACHNOID HEMORRHAGE

It is a type of intracranial hemorrhage into the subarachnoid space usually from basal cisterns. It is usually spontaneous.

You can muffle the drum, and you can loosen the strings of the lyre, but who shall command the skylark not to sing?—**Kahlil Gibran**

Causes

- Intracranial aneurysms. Commonest cause (50%).
- Hypertension.
- AV malformations.
- Blood dyscrasias.
- Anticoagulant drugs.
- Brain tumors (malignant).

Features

- Sudden onset of severe headache with vomiting.
- Features of raised intracranial pressure.
- Photophobia.
- Neck stiffness.
- Focal neurological deficits: Hemiplegia, dysphasia.
- Eye changes: Ptosis, dilated pupil, changes in the eyeball movements.
- Sudden loss of consciousness.
- Features of brain edema and cerebral ischemia.

In 40% of recovered patients, rebleeding occurs in 6-8 weeks which is commonly fatal.

Differential Diagnosis

- Meningitis.
- Coning due to any cause.

Investigations

- Lumbar puncture should be done to differentiate from meningitis.
  - It has to be done carefully as it may precipitate coning.
  - In subarachnoid hemorrhage blood stained CSF is collected.
- CT scan.
- Carotid and vertebral angiogram.

Treatment

- Clipping, or wrapping the aneurysm.
- Craniotomy and proceed.
- Ligation of common carotid artery—there is risk of hemiplegia.
- Therapeutic embolization.
- Excision of vascular malformations.

INTRACRANIAL ABSCESS

Types

1. ***Extradural abscess***: Caused by:
   - Osteomyelitis of skull.
   - Middle ear infection.
   - Frontal sinusitis.

   Pott's puffy tumor is infection and inflammation of the scalp. There is acute localized headache and tenderness in the skull, localized pitting edema of the scalp usually in the frontal region.

2. ***Subdural abscess*** is caused by septic thrombophlebitis from the frontal sinusitis or other infections. It is often very severe with extension into the venous sinuses.

3. ***Intracerebral abscess*** is caused by:
   a. Extension from middle ear or sinuses.
   b. Blood born infection.
   c. After intracranial injuries.

Common sites: Temporal lobe, cerebellum, frontal lobe. It can be:

a. *Acute:* There is acute septic encephalitis without pus formation. It may cause ventriculitis or localized abscess formation.
b. *Subacute:* Commences in 3 weeks, by the formation of a glial wall, i.e. thickness is more near the cortex and less towards ventricle.
c. *Chronic:* Occurs in 6 weeks with thick wall which may persist or may get enlarged behaving like a space occupying lesion.
d. *Metastatic:* Abscess in brain occurs either in cerebrum (parietal or temporal lobes) or in ventricles (ventriculitis is more dangerous and often fatal).

*Winning and losing isn't everything. Sometimes, the journey is just as important as the outcome—**Alex Morgan***

Features

- Evidence of focus of infections are seen, i.e. middle ear (CSOM), sinusitis.
- Focal neurological features are seen, depending on the location of abscess. In temporal lobe abscess they have dysphasia, contralateral hemiparesis; all cerebellar symptoms are seen in cerebellar abscess.
- Epilepsy.
- Features of raised intracranial pressure: (a) slow pulse, (b) rising BP, (c) headache and vomiting, (d) papilledema, (e) deterioration in level of consciousness, (f) visual disturbances.

Investigations

- CT scan; MRI; EEG.
- Carotid angiogram; ventriculography.
- Isotope brain scan.
- Total count, ESR.
- Investigation specific for focus of infection.

Lumbar puncture should be avoided in acute abscess as coning can occur.

Treatment

- Antibiotics—high dose Penicillins, Benzyl penicillins are given.
- Burr hole exploration is done and Dandy's brain cannula is placed. Pus is aspirated and sent for culture and cytology.
- In case of chronic abscess, exploration of cranial cavity and excision of brain abscess has to be done.

Complications

- Intracranial hypertension.
- Coning; neurological deficits.

INTRACRANIAL ANEURYSM

Types

1. **Subclinoid type** occurs in the internal carotid artery within the cavernous sinus. It causes ptosis, defective external ocular movements, 5th nerve palsy. It can cause carotid cavernous fistula.
2. **Supraclinoid type** is common type.
   a. *Berry's aneurysms*: *A congenital type* occurs in circle of Willis in relation to internal carotid artery [40% (most commonly at the origin of posterior communicating artery)], anterior communicating artery, middle cerebral artery, vertebrobasilar artery. It occurs due to weakness in the media of major arteries.
   b. *Acquired aneurysms* due to atheromas, hypertension.
   c. *Mycotic aneurysms* occur due to infection in the wall of cerebral vessels as a result of any bacteremia. Common sites are peripheral branches of middle cerebral artery.

Presentations

- Subarachnoid hemorrhage.
- Pressure effects.
- Convulsions.
- Eye and pupillary signs.
- **Investigations:** CT scan; carotid and vertebral angiogram.

Treatment

- Clipping or wrapping of aneurysms.
- Therapeutic embolization.
- Open neurosurgical approaches.

HYDROCEPHALUS

Dilatation of ventricles due to blockage of cerebrospinal flow (CSF).

Classification I

a. **Communicating type**:
   Ventricles communicate freely into the subarachnoid space.
   Here there is defective absorption of CSF following any inflammation, subarachnoid hemorrhage or trauma.

*The hard days are what make you stronger—**Aly Raisman***

b. *Noncommunicating type*:
      Obstruction is in the ventricle or its exit due to any tumors or any inflammatory process.

Classification II

Congenital
- Associated with spina bifida and myelomeningocele.
- Failure of formation of CSF pathways.
- Arnold-Chiari malformation.
- Congenital stenosis of aqueduct of Sylvius.

Features

Bulging of anterior fontanel (Fig. 29.9A), engorged scalp veins, separation of suture lines, '*sun-setting*' sign.

Acquired
- May be unilateral or bilateral (midline obstruction).
- Chronic meningitis.
- Trauma.
- Brain tumors.
- Colloid cyst of 3rd ventricle.
- Arachnoid cysts.

Features

- Presents with widening of sutures, tense fontanelles and decreased cortical thickness.
- Enlargement of head occurs, either prenatal (can cause obstructed labor) or postnatal.

Investigations

CT scan (Fig. 29.9B), ventriculography, air encephalography, MRI.

Treatment

- Tapping of lateral ventricles.
- Ventriculocysternostomy using polythene catheters—Torkildsen operation.
- Ventriculoatrial (VA) shunt.
- Ventriculoperitoneal (VP) shunt.

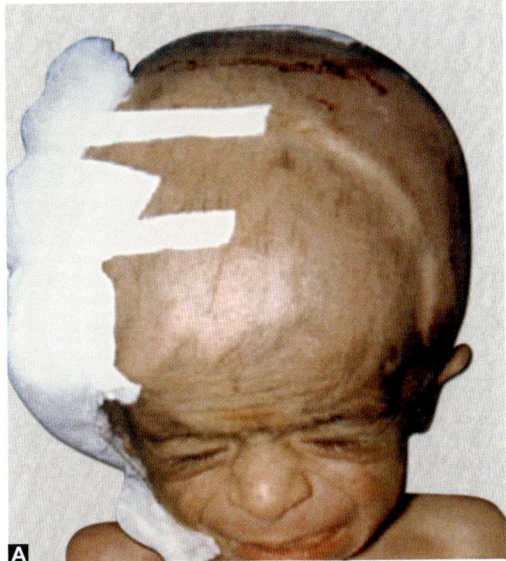
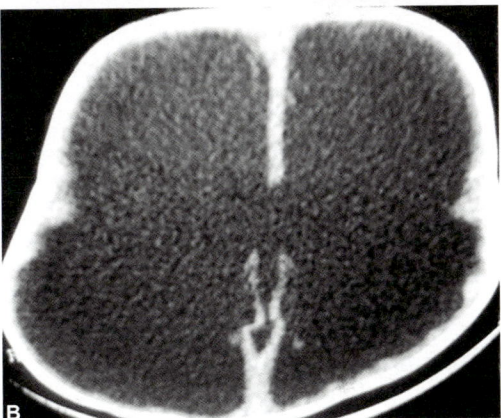

Figs. 29.9A and B: Hydrocephalus child. CT scan head picture in hydrocephalus.

INTRACRANIAL TUMORS

Secondaries are the commonest malignant tumor in the brain. Metastasis occurs usually from lung (commonest), nasopharynx or from any other organ in the body.

Primary Brain Tumors

1. ***Gliomas (43%) (Fig. 29.10).***
   a. ***Astrocytomas*** are the commonest type. They are usually malignant. They can

Anything good is either illegal, immoral, or fattening

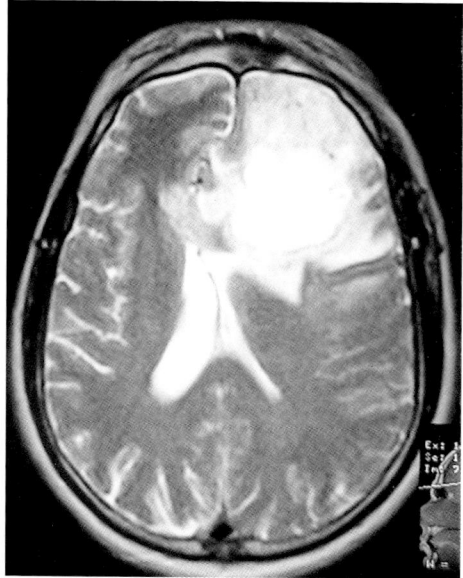

Fig. 29.10: MRI brain showing glioma brain.

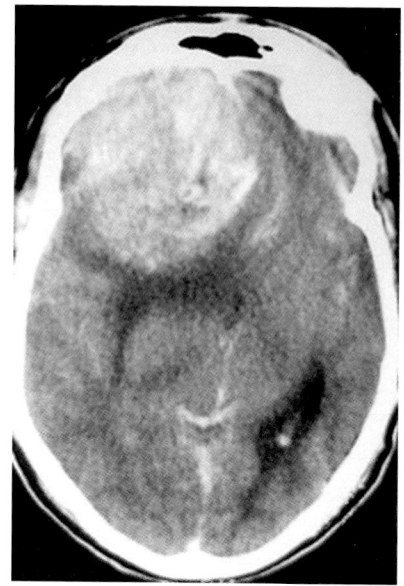

Fig. 29.11: CT scan head showing large meningioma in frontal region.

occur anywhere in the cerebral hemispheres, medulla, and brainstem. They can be *diffuse, solid,* or *cystic.* They contain star-shaped cells resembling adult neuroglial cells. Astrocytic gliomas are graded as *Grade I, II, III, IV as per the quantity of adult and primitive cells.*

b. *Oligodendrogliomas.*
c. *Spongioblastoma polare* arises from the primitive spongioblasts affects optic chiasma, third ventricle, hypothalamus, etc. They are irremovable but are radiosensitive.
d. *Medulloblastoma* occurs in children, affecting vermis of the cerebellum which grows rapidly with seedling elsewhere in the brain.
e. *Ependymomas*: Cells here resemble ependymal cells. It can occur throughout the cerebral hemispheres.

2. *Meningiomas (18%)*: They are usually globular, arising from the arachnoids. Tumor gets attached to the dura. It gets blood supply from dural arteries and veins, from emissary veins and veins of diploe and scalp. Along these veins tumor cells invade the bone, causing bone destruction and reactive hyperostosis. Meningiomas can be *calcified, fibroblastic, endothelial* and *angioblastic.*

Sites: (1) Parasagittal, (2) Frontobasal, (3) Posterior fossa, (4) Choroid plexus (Fig. 29.11).

Microscopic: It contains whorls of spindle cells, with central hyaline material, with Psammoma bodies.

3. *Schwannoma (8%)*: Common in auditory nerve also called as *acoustic neuroma.*

 Occurs in the internal auditory meatus which projects into the cerebellopontine angle (CP angle), compressing 5, 6, 7, 8th nerves. It presents with compressive features like unilateral deafness, trigeminal neuralgia, squint, cerebellar compression syndrome.

4. *Pituitary tumors (12%).*
5. *Craniopharyngiomas (5%).*
6. *Blood vessel tumors (2%).*

Future comes one day at a time

Features
- Initial period of silent growth.
- Focal syndromes with epilepsy.
- Raised intracranial pessure with headache, vomiting, deterioration of level of consciousness, altered vision slow pulse, high BP, papilledema.
- Brain displacement and stage of coning.

Specific Features
- Frontal lobe tumors: Personality and emotional changes, epilepsy of generalized type, contralateral facial weakness.
- Parietal lobe tumors: Jacksonian epilepsy, progressive hemiparesis, astereognosis, acalculia.
- Occipital lobe tumors: Aura of flashing of light in contralateral field, homonymous hemianopia.
- Temporal lobe tumors: Progressive aphasia, visual, auditory, smell and taste hallucinations, hemiparesis, superior quadrantic hemianopia.
- Midline tumors: Produces bilateral hydrocephalus.
- Tumors of the third ventricle (colloid cyst is common): Causes bilateral hydrocephalus, progressive cerebral atrophy, dementia, sexual precocity, endocrine disturbances.
- Pineal tumors: Causes precocious puberty.
- Cerebellar vermis tumors: Usually medulloblastomas, occur in young children, presents with progressive hydrocephalus and features of herniation of cerebellar tonsils through foramen magnum.
- Cerebellar hemisphere tumors: Commonly are astrocytomas, produce cerebellar syndromes, nystagmus.

Investigations
- X-ray skull
  - Calcifications like in meningiomas, craniopharyngiomas.
  - Separation of sutures.
  - A *beaten silver* appearance.
  - Lateral displacement of pineal body.
  - Hyperostosis, expansion, destruction in skull bones.
- Isotope scan.
- CT scan.
- MRI.
- Positron emission tomography (PET).
- Carotid angiogram (introduced by Egas Moniz).
- Ventriculography.
- EEG.

Treatment
- Relief of raised intracranial pressure:
  - Ventricular tap and drainage through a posterior parietal burr hole.
  - Tapping of cystic tumors and abscesses.
  - Administration of mannitol.
  - Emergency decompression by partial removal of tumor.
  - Steroid therapy—dexamethasone.
- Establishment of pathological diagnosis:
  - Burr hole and biopsy.
  - Craniotomy and biopsy using brain cannula.
  - Frozen section biopsy.
  - CT guided stereotactic biopsy.
- Removal of benign tumors—by different craniotomy approaches.
- Decompressive surgeries for malignant tumors.
- Shunt surgeries to drain CSF ventriculoperitoneal shunt or ventriculoatrial shunt.
- Radiotherapy—external radiotherapy is used as primary treatment or as an adjuvant therapy after surgery.
- Chemotherapy is occasionally used.

Prognosis
If tumor is benign and surgically accessible then has got better prognosis.

The pessimist complains about the wind; the optimist expects it to change; the realist adjusts the sails—**William Arthur Ward**

PITUITARY TUMORS

Classification

1. **Eosinophil (acidophil) adenomas**:
   - Tumor is usually small. Rarely it causes compressive features.
   - It secretes excess growth hormone causing acromegaly in adults and gigantism in children.
2. **Chromophobe adenomas**:
   - These are common in females and in the age group (20–50 years). Initially it is *intrasellar* and after sometime becomes *suprasellar*. Later it extends *intracranially* often massively, causing features of intracranial space occupying lesion.
   - It presents with myxedema, amenorrhea, infertility, headache, visual disturbances, bitemporal hemianopia, blindness, intracranial hypertension, epilepsy.
   - Differential diagnosis: Meningiomas, aneurysms.
   - CT scan, angiogram, X-ray skull are diagnostic.
   - Treatment is surgical decompression by craniotomy through subfrontal approach or transsphenoidal approach. Deep external radiotherapy and steroids are also used.
3. **Basophil adenomas**:
   - They are usually small. They secrete adrenocorticotropic hormone (ACTH) and presents as Cushing's disease with all its features.
4. **Prolactin secreting adenomas**:
   - Causes infertility, amenorrhea and galactorrhea.
   - It could be hypersecreting or hyposecreting by compression and atrophy.
   - It could be micronodular if tumor size is less than 10 mm.
   - It could be macronodular if tumor size is more than 10 mm.

Investigations

- X-ray skull: Shows calcifications, destruction of sella turcica, mass lesion, and enlarged pituitary fossa.
- CT scan.
- Magnetic resonance imaging (MRI).
- Hormone assay—like prolactin, growth hormone, ACTH, steroids, sex hormones, etc.

Treatment

- Surgery:
  - By subfrontal craniotomy approach or transsphenoidal approach. Care should be taken not to injure optic chiasma, arteries, cavernous sinus.
- External radiotherapy.

SPINA BIFIDA

- It is failure of enfolding of nerve elements within the spinal canal during developmental period.
- It is usually seen in lumbosacral region. There is failure of fusion of the one or more posterior vertebral arches.
- It is often associated with other anomalies.

Sites

- Lumbosacral.
- Thoracolumbar.

Types

Spina bifida occulta:
- There is dimpling of skin with dermoids, lipomas in the site. Impulse on coughing can be seen.
- Initially there is no neurological deficit but later due to tethering, traction on dura, and infection neurological deficits can occur.

*Promise yourself to live your life as a revolution and not just a process of evolution—**Anthony J D'Angelo***

Spina bifida aperta:
- Neurological deficit is present. It may be *myelomeningocele* wherein spinal cord and nerve roots are in the sac. It may be *meningocele* wherein sac consists of meninges and fluid only.
- Meningocele is brilliantly transilluminant. Myelomeningocele is not transilluminant.

Features (Figs. 29.12 to 29.14)
- Motor paralysis; sensory paralysis.
- Visceral paralysis with incontinence of urine and feces.
- Swelling in the spine at the site of the lesion, may be lipoma or dermoid with impulse on coughing.
- Bony defect at the site.
- Hydrocephalus.

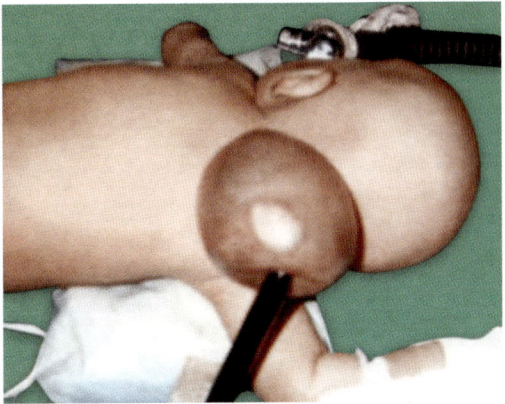

Fig. 29.13: Meningoencephalocele.

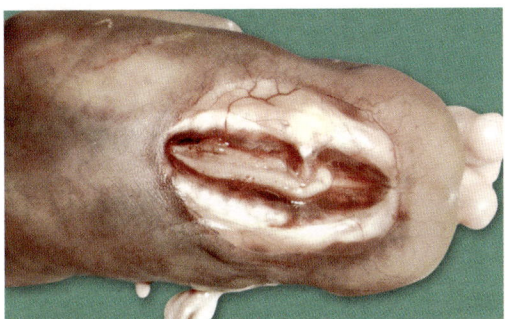

Fig. 29.14: Spina bifida in a newborn.

Investigations
- Plain X-ray of the spine.
- CT scan/MRI of spine and head.

Treatment
- Correction of deformity.
- Maintaining the visceral function.
- Development of limb function.
- Ventriculoperitoneal shunt or ventriculoatrial shunt surgery for hydrocephalus.

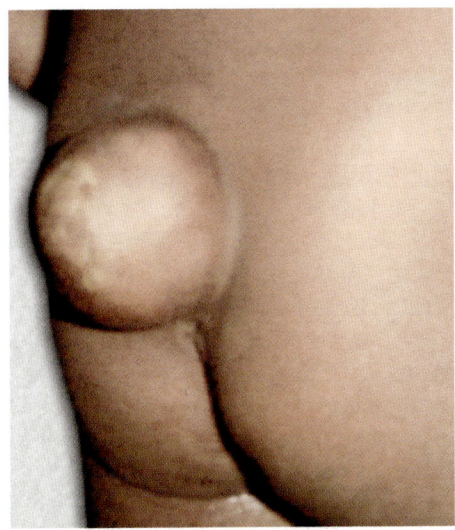

Fig. 29.12: Spina bifida with protruding dermoid through the defect.

Happiest people are not only happy in themselves; they are the cause of happiness to others

CHAPTER 30

Adjuvant Therapy

Chapter Outline

- Radiotherapy
- Chemotherapy
- Immunosuppression
- Hormone Therapy
- Immunotherapy
- Hybridoma
- Gene Therapy

RADIOTHERAPY

It is use of high energy ionizing radiation in the management of malignant tumors. It may be electromagnetic waves, X-rays, gamma rays, electrons, protons, neutrons or alpha particles.

It may be:
- External radiotherapy/brachytherapy/combined.
- Curative/palliative radiotherapy.
- Preoperative/postoperative/both pre- and postoperative radiotherapy.

Principle

Radiation is used to kill actively proliferating malignant cells at their mitotic level.

Common malignancies which are *Radiosensitive* are:
- Squamous cell carcinoma.
- Basal cell carcinoma.
- Bladder tumors.
- Carcinoma cervix.
- Seminoma testis.
- Hodgkin's lymphoma.

Other areas where radiotherapy is commonly used are:
- In carcinoma breast with secondaries in bone during postoperative period. Sometimes as preoperative radiotherapy, as part of *QUART Regime*.
- In follicular carcinoma of thyroid: For secondaries, radioactive I^{131} 5 m curies is given orally. External radiotherapy is also given for bone secondaries along with internal fixation if there is pathological fracture.
- Malignant brain tumors like astrocytomas.
- Many sarcomas.
- Carcinoma prostate.
- Carcinoma esophagus.
- Carcinoma lung.
- Fixed secondaries in neck as palliation to reduce pain, fungation and erosion into major vessels.
- Multiple myelomas.

Radioresistant tumors include:
- All gastrointestinal (GI) malignancies.
- Melanoma.
- Medullary carcinoma of the thyroid.

Reality doesn't bite, rather our perception of reality bites—Anthony J D'Angelo

Sources of radiotherapy	Classification	Efficacy depends on
• X-rays, electrons—from high energy X-ray machine, i.e. linear accelerator. • Gamma and beta rays from radioactive isotopes like cobalt-60, cesium 137, iridium 197. • Protons, neutrons and heavy ion nuclei from cyclotrons.	• *Low LET* (low energy transfer) radiation- X-rays, gamma rays, electrons. • *High LET* radiation—neutrons, protons, alpha particles and negative ions. It has heavier mass with dense localization and hence biologically more effective.	• Cell cycle phase. • Oxygen content of cells. ***Methods of delivery*** • External beam radiation (teletherapy). • Brachytherapy. • Systemic irradiation using radioisotopes like I^{131}.

Sources of Radiotherapy

- Cobalt 60 machine—most commonly used.
- Kilovoltage machines.
- Linear accelerator.
- Betatron/microton.
- Radioactive materials like cesium 137 (pellets), iridium 192 (wire), gold 198 (seeds), iodine 125 (seeds).

Measurement of Ionizing Radiation

Roentgen unit is a measure of ionizations produced per unit volume of air by X-rays and gamma rays but it is not used for photon energies above 3Mev. SI unit for exposure is coulomb per kg.

Radiation absorbed dose (RAD)
Absorbed dose is De/dm. It is mean energy imparted by the ionizing radiation to material of mass dm.

Old unit is *rad* which is equivalent to 100 ergs of energy per gram.
Newer international unit is presently used.
One Gray *(Gy)* is one joule of energy deposited per kilogram of material. One Gy = 100 rads = 100 cGy. 1 cGy = 1 rad.

Radiotherapy Plan

Type and doses of radiotherapy is decided by following factors:
- Site of tumor.
- Lymphatic field.
- Tumor size and extent.
- Histological type and grading.

BRACHYTHERAPY (*refer* Table on next page)

It is radiation given with source close to the tumor.
- It is given using iridium needles or moulds.
- It is curative radiotherapy.

Preoperative radiotherapy	Postoperative radiotherapy	Radiotherapy and chemotherapy combined
Advantages • Down-stage the tumor and reduces the tumor bulk. • No change in oxygenation of tissues. • Blockage of lymphatics by radiotherapy (RT) prevents tumor spread during surgical dissection. • Reduces the chances of microscopic spread. *Disadvantages* • Delayed healing due to reduced vascularity. • Flap necrosis, fistula formation. • Carotid blowout.	• More effective and extent of RT is well-defined. • Flap necrosis, fistula complications are less. *Indications* • When resected margin is positive for tumor. • When bone/cartilage are involved. • Extracapsular nodal spread. • Multiple neck nodes/node more than 3 cm in size in case of neck disease. • Poorly differentiated tumor.	• Commonly used before or during RT. • Chemotherapy after RT is not commonly followed. • Chemotherapy before RT is called *as induction chemotherapy* which reduces the bulk of tumor without altering the vascularity. • Chemotherapy with RT is called as *concomitant RT* which improves the effect of RT. Methotrexate and Bleomycin are radiosensitizers.

A fashion is nothing, but an induced epidemic—**Bernard Shaw**

Brachytherapy		
Types	Advantages	Disadvantages
• Intracavitary like in uterus, urinary bladder, maxillary antrum, bronchial or esophageal tree. • Interstitial wherein radioactive needles/wires/ribbons/seeds are inserted into the tumor area like in bladder or oral cavity. • Surface brachytherapy using moulds like in tumors of skin/eye/breast. Radionuclides used are caesium 137 (Cs^{137}), iridium 192 (Ir^{192}), gold 198 (Au^{198}) and iodine 125 (I^{125}). Brachytherapy is often combined with external beam radiotherapy.	• High, localized, single continuous dose of RT. • Deeper and adjacent tissues are spared. • High dose rate with short time. • Less side effects. • Curative and effective in early cancers. • After loading devices are available which reduces personal exposure. • Surgery is avoided and part is retained.	• Technically difficult. • Availability of the facility. • Local complications like displacement/erosion.

❖ It is used in carcinoma oral cavity, penis, breast, cervix and bladder.

Note: **Palliative radiotherapy** is always external teletherapy using cobalt 60.

Problems in Radiotherapy

❖ Loss of taste and sensations, loss of appetite.
❖ Infection, trismus, fibrosis, mucositis, dryness of mouth.
❖ Skin necrosis, sloughing, infection.
❖ Laryngeal edema, candida infection.
❖ Radiation-induced osteomyelitis commonly in mandible.
❖ Radiation-induced retinopathy and cataract.
❖ Endocrine deficit like of thyroid/pituitary.
❖ Radiation-induced nephritis and renal failure.
❖ Radiation-induced thimble bladder.
❖ Radiation oophoritis and infertility.
❖ Radiation-induced frozen pelvis.
❖ Radiation-induced malignancy.
❖ Hemopoietic suppression.
❖ Transverse myelitis.

Usual dose required depends on site, type of tumor, size of tumor and response of tumor. Usually 20–25 doses required. It is given 5 days a week. Two days gap is given so as to allow dormant cells to get activated because only active cells will be killed by radiotherapy.

Care of patients on radiotherapy

- Diet rich in proteins, vitamins and iron.
- All infected/problematic teeth should be extracted before RT.
- Care of skin by keeping area dry. Avoid washing with soap and water.
- Avoid exposure to sunlight and wet shaving.
- Adhesive plaster/dressings should be avoided.
- Soft silk cloth should be used to cover the RT area.
- Avoid alcohol, tobacco, spicy food.
- Milk of magnesia is used for mucositis. Xylocaine gel 10% is used to relieve pain.
- Prevention of infection especially candida by topical Nystatin/Clotrimazole.

CHEMOTHERAPY

❖ Today chemotherapy is an important modality of treatment in management of cancer.
❖ It is the main modality of treatment in most of the advanced malignancies.
❖ It is used preoperatively to downstage the tumor so as to increase the possibilities of surgical resection.
❖ When used postoperatively it reduces the rate of recurrence.
❖ It is the primary treatment for non-Hodgkin's lymphoma (NHL), leukemia.

Build your reputation by helping other people build theirs—**Anthony J D'Angelo**

- These drugs mainly act by blocking the mitotic activity in the nucleus in different phases of the cell cycle.
- It is given either orally, intravenously (systemic), intra-arterial, intrathecal and intravesical (regional) or as isolated limb perfusion.
- Intra-arterial chemotherapy is used in head and neck cancers and hepatic cancers.
- Isolated limb perfusion is used in melanoma.

ANTIMALIGNANCY DRUGS

Mode of action:
- They damage the active cells.
- They also affect hemopoiesis, cellular activity, epithelial tissues and gonads.
- They also suppress the immune system.

Side effects in general:
- Bone marrow suppression.
- Alopecia.
- Hepatotoxicity.
- Nephrotoxicity.

Mustine hydrochloride: Used in Hodgkin's lymphoma. It is Mechlorethamine.

Cyclophosphamide: It is used in ovarian carcinoma, lymphomas, colonic carcinoma, bronchogenic carcinoma.
Side effects: Alopecia, bone marrow suppression, cystitis (hemorrhagic).
Dose: 3 mg/kg IV daily for 5 days in dextrose, as monthly cycle for 6 months. Orally as 50 mg tablets.

Melphalan (Phenylalanine mustard): Used in multiple myeloma and melanoma.
Dose: 10 mg daily for 3 weeks. Available as 2 mg tablets.

Busulfan: 2 mg tablet. 10 mg for 3 weeks. Used in chronic myeloid leukemia.
Side effect: Pulmonary fibrosis.

Chlorambucil: 10 mg for 3 weeks. Used in chronic lymphatic leukemia.

Methotrexate: 10 mg orally. It competes with folic acid.
Side effects: Megaloblastic anemia, hepatic damage and dermatitis.

6-Mercaptopurine: It alters the purine metabolism. 50 mg tablets.
It is used in leukemias and choriocarcinoma.
Dose: 150 mg for 5 days monthly for 6 months. It causes hyperuricemia.

5-Fluorouracil: 15 mg/kg. It is given daily for 5 days in dextrose bottle for 6 months cycle.
Uses: Adenocarcinomas of GIT, breast cancers and cancer cervix.
Side effects: Neurotoxicity, stomatitis, bone marrow suppression.

Vinca alkaloids: It inhibits mitosis.

Vincristine: *Dose*: 1.4 mg/sq.m. It is neurotoxic.

Vinblastine: *Dose*: 0.1 kg body weight. It causes bone marrow toxicity.

Rubidomycin: 40 mg/m/day IV. Myocardial depressant.
Used in acute myeloblastic leukemia.

Adriamycin: It is commonly used in NHL, hepatoma, medullary carcinoma of thyroid, osteosarcoma and soft-tissue sarcomas. It is cardiotoxic. So should be infused with cardiac monitoring.
Dose: 30 mg/day for 3 days.

0'-p DDD (Mitotane): It destroys selectively adrenal cortex. It is used in carcinoma adrenal cortex.
Dose: 10 g orally for 8 weeks.

Bleomycin: 20 units IV or IM twice a week. It causes pulmonary fibrosis.
It is used in squamous cell carcinoma of skin and other regions and in lymphomas.

Cytosine arabinoside: 4 mg/kg IV for 2 days. Used in leukemias and lymphomas.

Lomustine (CCNU) and Carmustine (BCNU): It is used in brain tumors and lymphomas.

Procarbazine: 300 mg 3 times a day. Used in Hodgkin's lymphoma and oat cell carcinoma lung.

Never explain—your friends do not need it and your enemies will not believe it—**Elbert Hubbard**

Cisplatin: 30 mg daily. Used in testicular and ovarian tumors.

Etoposide: *Dose*: 100 mg/sq.m.
Uses: Testicular tumor, bladder tumor, lymphomas.

Hydroxyureas: 80 mg/kg.
Uses: Myeloma, leukemias.

IMMUNOSUPPRESSION

It is mainly used:
- In transplantation to prevent graft rejection.
- In transplantation of kidney, liver, heart, small bowel, pancreas.

Drugs used are:
- *Azathioprine* (Imuran, Purine analog).
- *Cyclosporine*: It is a very good immunosuppressant, derived from fungus. It causes inhibition of lymphocytic activity, delayed hypersensitivity, interleukins, memory cells, etc. It is initially given intravenously and later given orally. It is given usually for long duration for 12–24 months. It is *nephrotoxic* as well as *bone marrow suppressant*. So constant monitoring by blood urea, serum creatinine, blood count, Hb% at regular intervals is required. Dose should be adjusted depending on these parameters. Cyclosporine is very effective immunosuppressant in transplantation.
- Antilymphocytic globulin.
- Steroids.
- Cytosine arabinoside.

HORMONE THERAPY

Ablative procedures: Hormone therapy is often used as adjuvant therapy in certain malignancies. Examples are oophorectomy and adrenalectomy in carcinoma breast and orchidectomy in carcinoma prostate.

Added hormones in few malignancies like prednisolone, progestogens, estrogens and androgens.

Hormone Antagonists
- Tamoxifen is used as estrogen receptor antagonist in carcinoma breast.
- Cyproterone acetate competes for binding receptors.
- Luteinizing hormone-releasing hormone (LHRH) analog like goserelin in carcinoma breast.
- Phosphorylated diethyl stilbestrol in carcinoma prostate.

Drugs that Interfere with Hormone Synthesis
- Aminoglutethimide as adrenal inhibitor.
- L-thyroxine 0.3 mg daily as suppressor of thyroid stimulating hormone (TSH) in papillary carcinoma of thyroid.

IMMUNOTHERAPY

It is enhancing the host response of patient whenever required commonly against malignant cells. Often it is also used in conditions where there is severe immunosuppression due to any reason like bone marrow suppression, or in specific conditions like severe hepatitis.

Immunotherapy can be:	
• Active.	• Restorative.
• Passive.	• Adoptive.

Immunotherapy Agents
- Monoclonal antibodies.
- Bone marrow transplantation.
- Cell transfer.
- Lymphokines.
- Thymic hormones.
- Levamisole and BCG (as immunomodulators).
- Prostaglandins.
- Interferons, interleukins.
- Immunoglobulins.
- Antibody derived specific to certain tumor like melanoma.

Tumors where immunotherapy is used
- Melanoma.
- Bladder tumor.

You don't have to hold a position in order to be a leader—**Anthony J D'Angelo**

- Carcinoma colon.
- Renal cell carcinoma.
- In many tumors it is under trial.

Disadvantages
• Very costly. • Nonavailability. • Effect is not 100%.

HYBRIDOMA

- It is a biotechnological process wherein *multiplication* property of **Myeloma cells** is combined with *synthetic* property of some other required cells **to achieve** rapid and large quantity manufacturing of required chemical.
- Myeloma cells with only retained multiplication activity is fused with human cells or lymphocytes or other cells (nature to produce the required product) by **hybridization**. The resulting cell has got the capacity to multiply rapidly and to produce required product in large quantity. It is called as **hybridoma**.
- It is used to generate monoclonal antibodies, insulin and many other antibodies, immunoglobulins, etc.

Monoclonal antibodies are used for:
- Immunodiagnosis—for radioimmunoassay, radionuclide scan.
- Antibody for detection of tumor antigen
    - For cancer therapy,
    - For serotherapy,
    - As conjugates (with drugs, toxins, isotopes).
- Production of other chemicals and as a *research tool*.

GENE THERAPY

The ability to alter specific genes of interest is nowadays an exciting and powerful tool in the potential management of a wide range of diseases. Instead of giving a patient a drug to treat or control the symptoms of the genetic disorder, physicians may be capable of treating the basic problem by altering the genetic makeup of the patient's cell.

Typically two methods have been considered: Germ line and somatic cell gene therapy.
- *Germ cell therapy* involves insertion of a gene into fertilized egg for the correction of a genetic disease. Because these genes are dispersed throughout the tissues of the egg, they end up in the germ cells of the fetus, and hence are passed on to the future generations.
- *Somatic cell therapy* involves the insertion of genes or otherwise manipulating the gene machinery of a cell to treat a disease. In this case the cells are restricted to the population that has been treated and any genetic change remains restricted to these cells and is not passed to the germ cell line.

The goals of human somatic therapy are usually one of the following:
- To repair or compensate for a defective gene
- To enhance the immune response directed at a tumor or pathogen.
- To protect vulnerable cell populations against treatments such as chemotherapy.
- To kill tumor cells directly.

Several single gene disorders are candidates for gene therapy. Current thinking has expanded to include treatment of acquired immunodeficiency syndrome (AIDS) and atherosclerosis using gene therapy techniques.

Vectors used for gene therapy fall into two main classes—viral and nonviral.
- **Viral**:
    Initially retroviruses were used as vectors. Other potential vectors include adenovirus, herpes virus and vaccinia virus.
- **Nonviral systems:**
    - Liposome mediated DNA transfer.
    - DNA protein conjugates.

However, exciting and appealing the prospects of gene therapy may appear, this technique is still in the experimental stages.

---

*I never see what has been done; I only see what remains to be done—**Buddha***

CHAPTER 31

Instruments and Suture Materials

CHAPTER OUTLINE

- Instruments
- Suture Materials

INSTRUMENTS

CHEATLE'S FORCEPS (FIG. 31.1)

It is used to pick sterilized articles like instruments and drapes so that touching of the instruments can be avoided while transferring them. It is kept dipped in antiseptic solutions. It does not have lock.

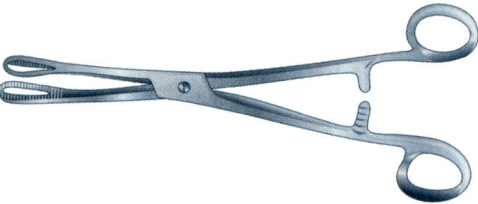

Fig. 31.2: Sponge holding forceps.

MAYO'S TOWEL CLIP (FIG. 31.3)

- ❖ It is used to fix drapes in operative field.
- ❖ It is used to fix suction tubes, diathermy wires, and laparoscopic cables in operative table.
- ❖ It is used to fix ribs in flail chest.

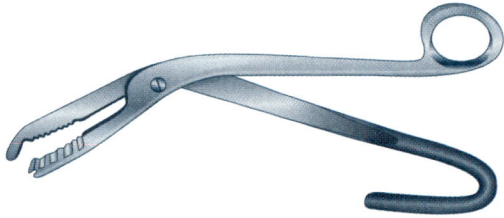

Fig. 31.1: Cheatle's forceps.

SPONGE HOLDING FORCEPS (RAMPLEY'S) (FIG. 31.2)

It has got fenestrated, serrated, flat distal end. It is used to clean the operative field, to swab the cavities, to mop the oozing area, to hold gallbladder and cervix during surgeries, for blunt dissections, and as ovum forceps.

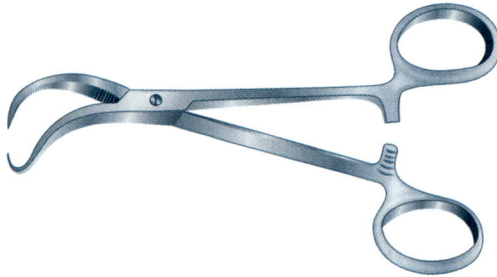

Fig. 31.3: Mayo's towel clip.

Many receive advice, only the wise profit by it

ARTERY FORCEPS (HEMOSTAT) (FIGS. 31.4A TO C)

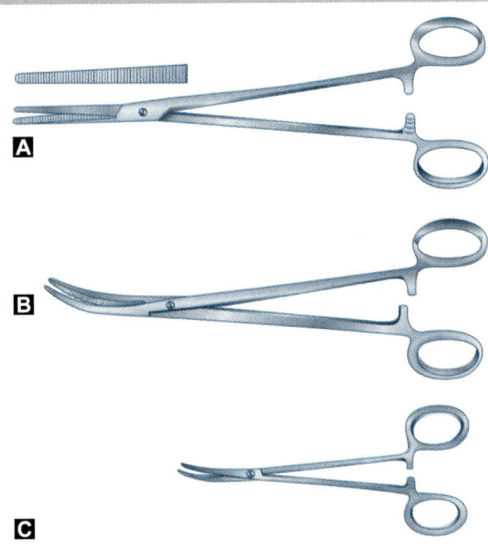

Figs. 31.4A to C: Artery forceps: (A) Straight; (B) Curved; (C) Mosquito.

Types

Based on size:
- Small or mosquito artery forceps.
- Medium-sized artery forceps.
- Large artery forceps.

Based on shape:
- Straight artery forceps.
- Curved artery forceps.

Features of artery forceps:
- Distal blades are having transverse serrations which are well apposed.
- Lock in the proximal part.

Uses

- To catch bleeding points.
- To open the facial planes in different surgeries.
- To pass a ligature.
- To hold fascia, peritoneum, aponeurosis.
- To hold sutures.
- To drain an abscess like a sinus forceps.
- To hold gauze as peanut.

RIGHT ANGLE FORCEPS (FIG. 31.5)

It is used to dissect pedicles and to pass ligatures. It is used in depth dissection. It is used in thyroidectomy, neck dissections and laparotomy procedures.

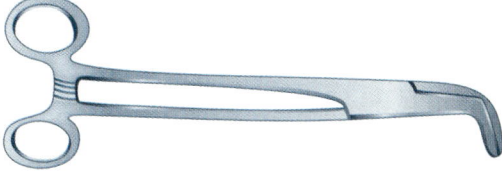

Fig. 31.5: Right angle forceps.

KOCHER'S FORCEPS (FIG. 31.6)

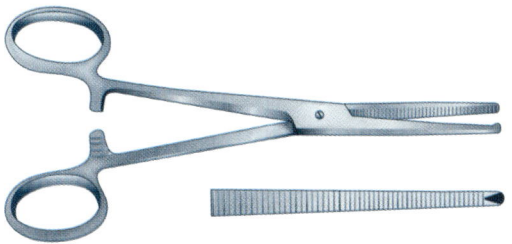

Fig. 31.6: Kocher's forceps.

It has got serrations in the distal blades and apposing tooth in the tip.

It is used to hold pedicles, tough structures, cut ends of the muscles.

It is used to hold gauze for blunt dissection, to hold resected bowel, to hold ribs during rib resection.

ALLIS TISSUE HOLDING FORCEPS (FIG. 31.7)

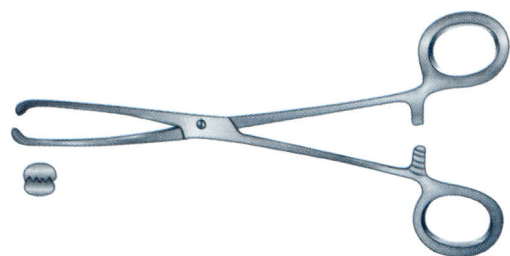

Fig. 31.7: Allis tissue holding forceps.

Here distal blades are not apposing each other.

Anger is short madness, so control your passion, or it will control you—Horace

Tip has got teeth in each blade which are apposing.

It has got lock.

It is used to hold skin flaps, fascias, aponeurosis, and bladder wall.

BABCOCK'S FORCEPS (FIG. 31.8)

Its distal part of blades is curved with triangular fenestra in it which allows soft tissues to bulge out. Tip is nontraumatic with transverse serrations on it. It has got a lock.

It is used to hold any part of the bowel, fallopian tubes, appendix, ureter, cord, etc.

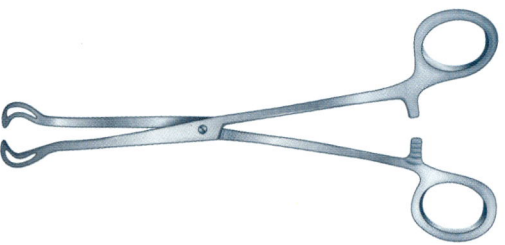

Fig. 31.8: Babcock's forceps.

LANE'S TISSUE HOLDING FORCEPS (FIG. 31.9)

It has got thick, stout distal blades with oval fenestra in each blade. It has got apposing tooth in the tip. It has got lock.

It is used to hold bulky and tough structures, to hold lymph nodes. It is also used as towel clip, as sponge holding forceps.

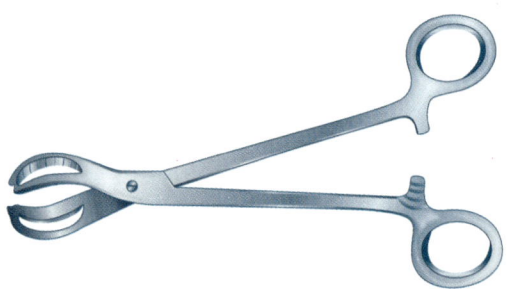

Fig. 31.9: Lane's tissue holding forceps.

SINGLE HOOK RETRACTOR (FIG. 31.10)

It is used to retract skin.

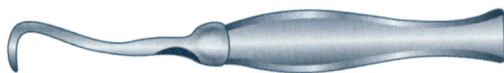

Fig. 31.10: Single hook retractor.

VOLKMANN'S RETRACTOR (FIG. 31.11)

It is used to retract fascias in soles and palms.

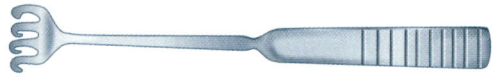

Fig. 31.11: Volkmann's retractor.

LANGENBECK'S RETRACTOR (FIG. 31.12)

It has got a long handle and a small solid blade. It is used in hernia surgery or any superficial surgeries to retract skin, fascia and aponeurosis, etc.

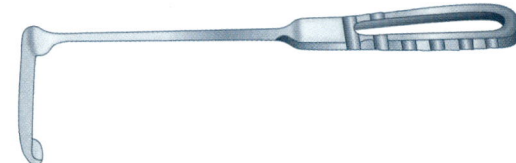

Fig. 31.12: Langenbeck's retractor.

CZERNEY'S RETRACTOR (FIG. 31.13) (HERNIA RETRACTOR)

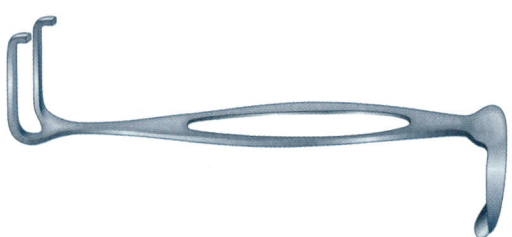

Fig. 31.13: Czerney's retractor.

The optimist sees the rose and not its thorns; the pessimist stares at the thorns, oblivious of the rose—**Khalil Gibran**

This retractor has got thick, small blade on one side and biflanged hook on the other side in opposite directions. It is used in surgeries like hernia, laparotomy especially during closure.

MORRIS' RETRACTOR (FIG. 31.14)

- It may be single blade type or double blade type.
- It is used to retract abdominal wall incisions.

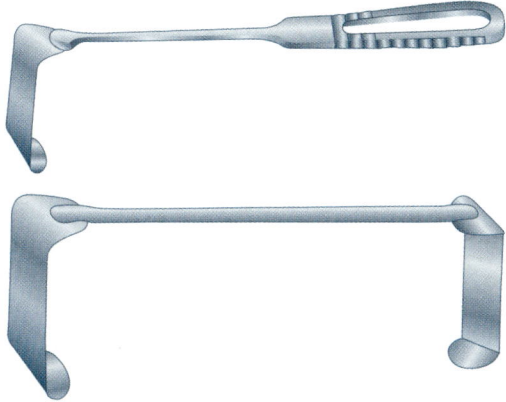

Fig. 31.14: Morris' retractor.

DEAVER'S RETRACTOR (FIG. 31.15)

- It is used to retract the abdominal wall.
- It is a retractor with a broad, gently curved blade.
- It is used to retract liver, spleen and other abdominal viscera.
- It is atraumatic and gives adequate exposure of the surgical field.

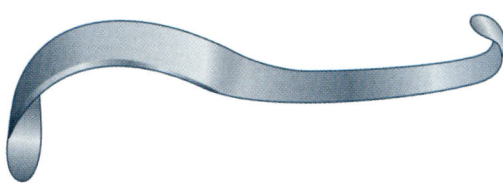

Fig. 31.15: Deaver's retractor.

DOYEN'S RETRACTOR (FIG. 31.16)

It is used in pelvic surgeries.

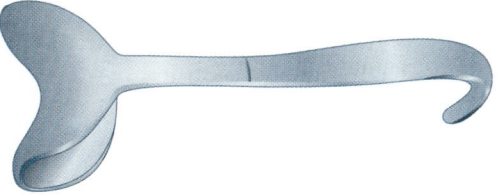

Fig. 31.16: Doyen's retractor.

SELF-RETAINING RETRACTOR (FIG. 31.17)

It has got different adjustable blades so as to retract abdominal wall and tissues during surgery.

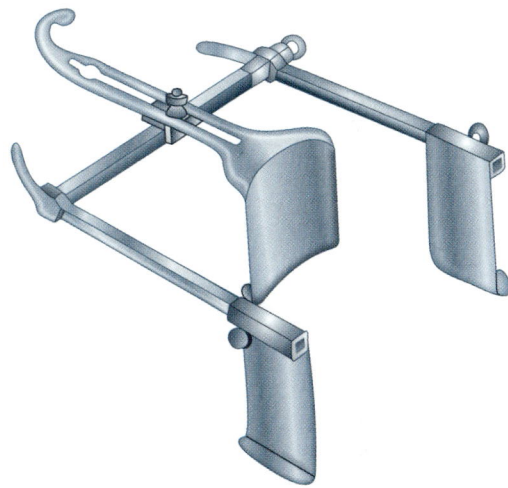

Fig. 31.17: Self-retaining retractor.

DISSECTING FORCEPS (FIGS. 31.18A AND B)

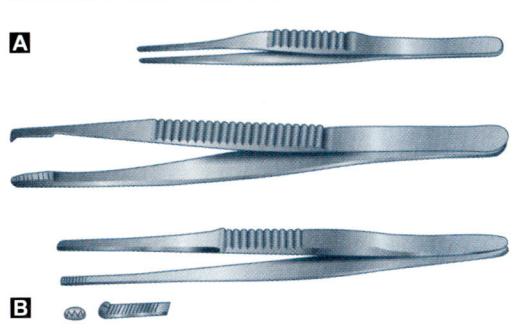

Figs. 31.18A and B: Dissecting forceps: (A) Nontoothed; (B) Toothed.

A child is God's opinion that the world should go on—***Carl Sandburg***

PLAIN NONTOOTHED DISSECTING FORCEPS

It is used to hold delicate structures like peritoneum, vessels, bowel, nerves, and tendons.

TOOTHED DISSECTING FORCEPS

It is used to hold skin and tough structures.

SURGICAL NEEDLES (FIG. 31.19)

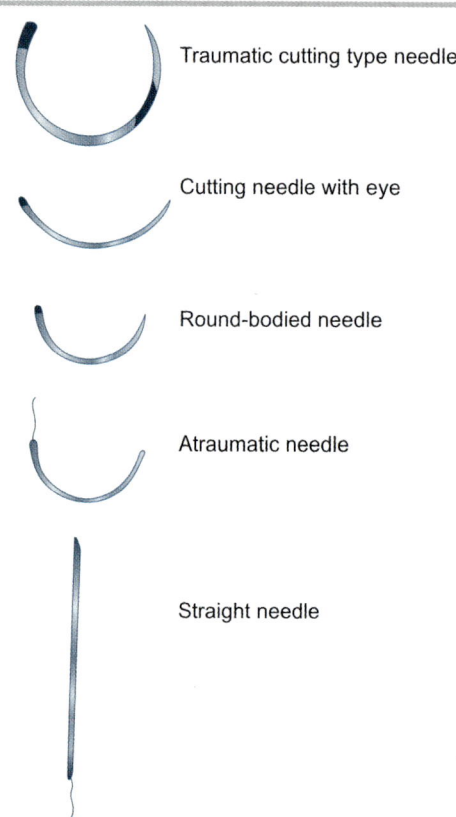

Fig. 31.19: Different types of needles.

Types

Based on the edge:
- Round body needle.
- Cutting needle.
- Reverse cutting needle.
- Taper cut needle.

Based on curvature:
- Straight needle.
- Curved needle. Half circle; 5/8th circle, etc.

Based on existence of the eye:
- **Atraumatic needle** is eyeless. Here suture material is attached to the needle by swaging. Size of the suture material and that of needle is same and so tissue trauma is less. Needle once used is disposed (not reusable).
- **Traumatic needle** is eyed needle. Needle in the eye area is wider than the body of the needle and so tissue trauma is more. These needles are reusable.

Round body needles are used in soft structures like peritoneum, muscle, vessel, nerves, tendons, bowel, and soft tissues.

Cutting needles are used to suture skin, aponeurosis and tough structures.

Reverse cutting needle is used to suture mucoperiosteum.

NEEDLE HOLDER (FIG. 31.20)

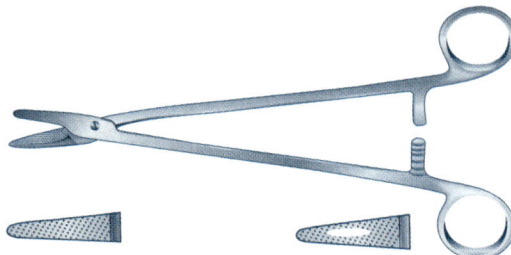

Fig. 31.20: Needle holder.

Smaller distal blades with criss-cross serrations often with a groove in the middle are the features of needle holder.

It may be straight or curved. It may be available in different sizes. While holding a needle in a needle holder one should get a good control and good grip. This is achieved by placing the needle at proximal 2/3rd and distal 1/3rd. Needle holder should be held between thumb and ring finger.

*Progress is impossible without change; and those who cannot change their minds cannot change anything—**George Bernard Shaw***

JOLL'S THYROID RETRACTOR (FIG. 31.21)

It is a self-retaining retractor specifically used for thyroid surgeries.

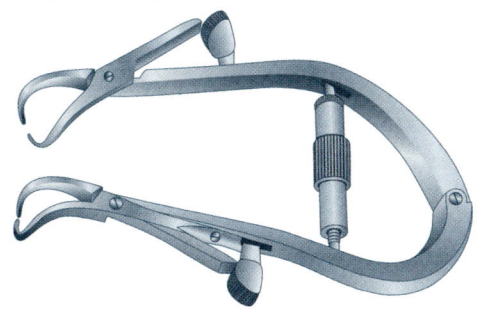

Fig. 31.21: Joll's thyroid retractor.

MOYNIHAN'S OCCLUSION CLAMP (FIG. 31.22)

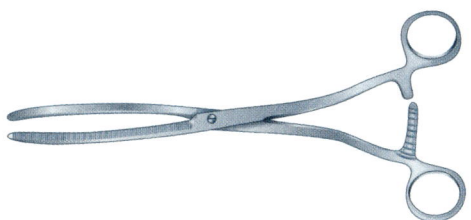

Fig. 31.22: Moynihan's occlusion clamp.

* It has got long distal blades with longitudinal serrations.
* It may be straight or curved.
* It is nontraumatic, noncrushing type.
* It occludes lumen of the bowel/stomach and so prevents spillage of the content of the bowel.
* It also occludes the vessels in the wall of the bowel and so prevents bleeding during surgery.
* It is used during anastomosis of the stomach and other parts of the bowel.

PAYR'S CRUSHING CLAMP (GASTRIC) (FIG. 31.23)

It is stout and heavy instrument with double lever in the handle.

It crushes the bowel once applied. So before applying it, line of resection of stomach/bowel should be assessed properly. It is applied to the part which is removed. Viability of the bowel is lost once it is applied.

It is used in gastrectomy and resection and anastomosis of the bowel.

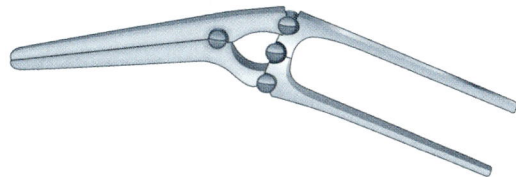

Fig. 31.23: Payr's crushing clamp.

DESJARDIN'S CHOLEDOCHOLITHOTOMY FORCEPS (FIG. 31.24)

It has got long distal blades with smooth serrations and fenestra in the tip. It does not have lock and so accidental damage of common bile duct (CBD) mucosa or crushing of the CBD stone are avoided.

It is used for choledocholithotomy (removal of CBD stones).

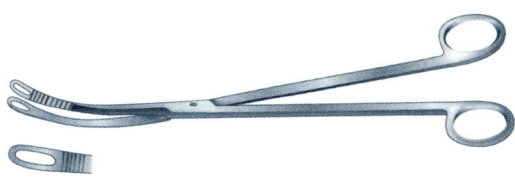

Fig. 31.24: Desjardin's choledocholithotomy forceps.

BAKE'S DILATOR (FIG. 31.25)

It is long malleable metallic instrument with olive tip at the terminal end.

It is used to assess the CBD, duodenal papilla for patency or block.

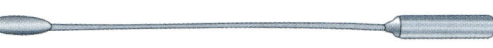

Fig. 31.25: Bake's dilator.

Many people will walk in and out of your life, but only true friends will leave footprints in your heart—**Eleanor Roosevelt**

SINUS FORCEPS (LISTER'S) (FIG. 31.26)

It has got straight, long blades with serrations in the tip. It does not have lock.

It is used to drain pus from abscess cavity (Hilton's method). It is called as sinus forceps because it is initially originated to pack the sinus cavities. It is less traumatic.

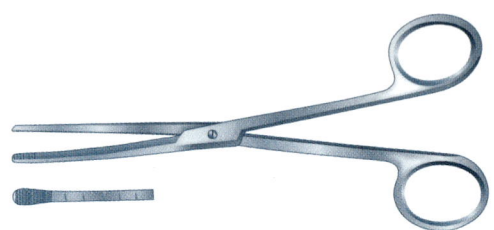

Fig. 31.26: Lister's sinus forceps.

TRACHEOSTOMY TUBE (FIGS. 31.27A AND B)

1. ***Fuller's bivalved tracheostomy tube***: It has got outer tube and inner tube. Outer tube is biflanged and so insertion is easier. Inner tube is longer with an opening on its posterior aspect. Inner tube can be removed and reinserted easily whenever required.
2. ***Jackson's tracheostomy tube***: It has got outer tube, inner tube and an obturator.
3. Red-rubber tracheostomy tube.
4. Polyvinyl chloride (PVC) tracheostomy tube.
   Modern tracheostomy tubes are made of plastic. They are soft, least irritant and disposable. They have inflatable cuff which makes it easier to give assisted ventilation. Cuff should be deflated at regular intervals to prevent pressure necrosis of trachea (For assisted ventilation endotracheal tube can be kept for 7 days. Beyond that period patient needs tracheostomy for further ventilation).

Indications for tracheostomy:
* In head, neck and facial injuries.
* Tetanus.
* Tracheomalacia after thyroidectomy.
* Laryngeal edema/spasm.
* Major head and neck surgeries like commando's operation, block dissection, etc.

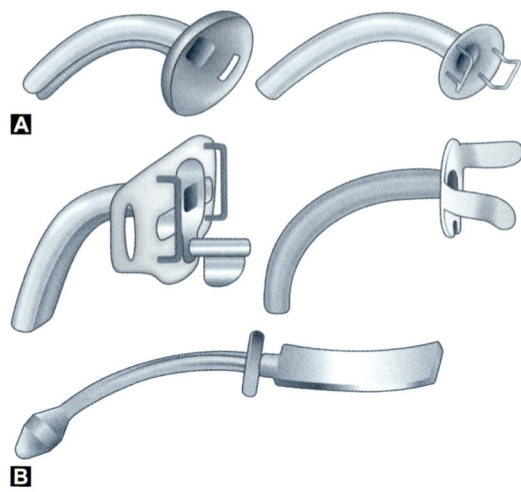

Figs. 31.27A and B: Tracheostomy tube: (A) Fuller's bivalved tracheostomy tube; (B) Jackson's tracheostomy tube.

DRAINS

A drain is a created channel which allows any fluid collected to come out after closure of the main wound.

Types

* ***Corrugated rubber drain (Fig. 31.28A)***: It drains by capillary action and gravity. It is cheaper and technically easier. But it allows soakage of dressings and causes discomfort to the patient.
* Tube drains (Fig. 31.28B):
  – Malecot catheter can be used as tube drain.
  – Penrose soft latex rubber tube.
  – Multiple perforated tubes (Fig. 31.28C).
* Closed suction tube drain system.
* ***Glove drain***.
* ***Wick drain*** is a gauze drain to drain pus, discharge, etc.

*Talent hits a target no one else can hit; Genius hits a target no one else can see—**Arthur Schopenhauer***

Chapter 31 : Instruments and Suture Materials

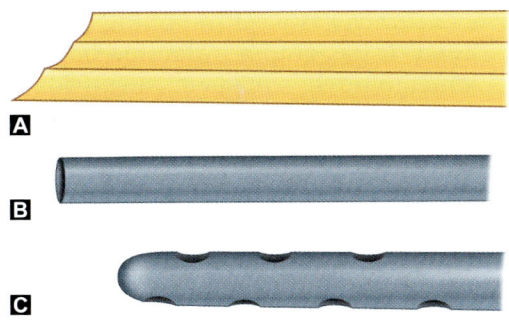

Figs. 31.28A to C: Drains: (A) Corrugated rubber drains; (B) Tube drain; (C) Multiple perforated drains.

❖ **Jackson-Pratt drain** *(JP drain, brain drain, 1972)* is a closed suction device consists of a perforated round or flat tube connected to a negative pressure collection device which is a bulb with a drainage port which can be opened to remove fluid or air. After compressing the bulb to remove fluid or air, negative pressure is created as the bulb returns to its normal shape. It is used in surgeries of abdomen, breast, brain, joints, etc. (Figs. 31.29A and B).

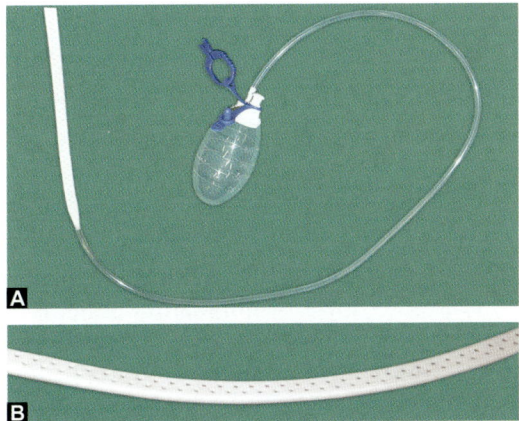

Figs. 31.29A and B: Jackson-Pratt suction drain.

❖ **Redivac drain:** Redivac drain is a close system drain with many holes at the end of a fine tube(s); it is connected to an evacuated glass bottle providing suction. It is used to drain blood beneath the skin, e.g. after mastectomy or thyroidectomy, or from deep spaces, e.g. around a vascular anastomosis (Fig. 31.30).

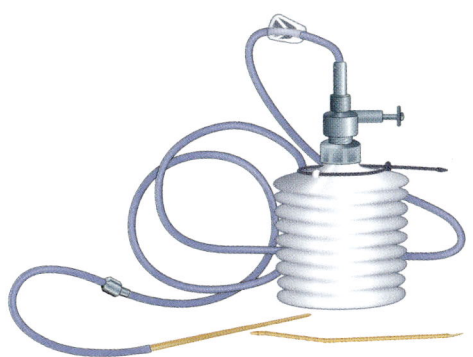

Fig. 31.30: Romovac suction drain. Here suction is created by pressing the suction corrugation. There is a sharp metallic introducer to pass the tube into the required area after puncturing the skin. It is used for thyroidectomy, mastectomy, radical dissection, wide excisions, flap surgeries, etc.

Advantages of Tube Drains

❖ Quantity of fluid like bile, pus can be measured.
❖ It can be kept for longer time.
❖ Skin excoriation will not occur.
❖ Patient will be more comfortable.
❖ Infection rate is less.
❖ Removal is easier.
Dye can be injected and cavity or communication can be assessed using 'C-arm'.

Classification of Drain Systems

1. **Open (static) drains**: Corrugated drain, Penrose drain. Infection rate is higher.
2. **Closed siphon drains**: Here drain is connected to a sterile bag with or without one-way valve. It reduces the infection.
3. **Closed suction drain**: Here negative pressure of –100 to –500 mm Hg is used to create vacuum to drain the secretions.
4. **Sump suction drain**: Here negative suction with a parallel air-vent is used to prevent the adjacent soft tissues being sucked into the lumen of the drain.

*Exaggeration is truth that has lost its temper—**Khalil Gibran***

5. **Under water seal drain** to drain pleural space.

Indications for Drains

- In drainage of an abscess.
- In bleeding surgical conditions like trauma, peroperative bleed.
- In hemo-, pyo- or pneumothorax.
- In acute abdominal conditions like peritonitis, hemoperitoneum.
- In major abdominal surgeries like of pancreas, biliary tree, stomach, etc.
- In thyroid surgery.
- In hydrocele surgery.

Problems in Drains

- Infection through the drain.
- Displacement.
- It may not drain adequately and can give a false information.
- It may interfere with healing process inside.

Presently keeping a drain itself a questioned debate and controversy all over.

Older dictum was 'when in doubt keep a drain and the surgeon can sleep happily'—is questioned at present.

Drains if not used properly may be counter-productive.

FOLEY'S CATHETER (FIG. 31.31)

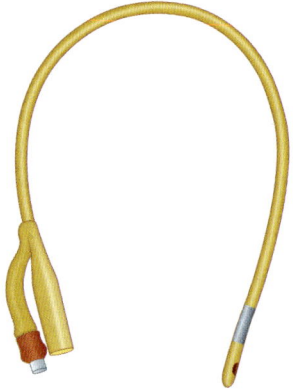

Fig. 31.31: Foley's catheter.

Foley's catheter is a self-retaining urinary catheter. It has got an inflatable balloon proximal to tip. It is inflated using distilled water (not with saline). It is made up of latex. After passing the catheter wih all aseptic precautions, it is inflated. Quantity of distilled water to be used is written in the catheter—usually 15–20 mL. It is kept for 1 week. If there is a need for longer duration of catheter then silicone coated Foley's catheter is used. While removing the catheter, same quantity of distilled water should be withdrawn prior to removal. It is very commonly used catheter in surgical practice.

MALECOT CATHETER (FIG. 31.32)

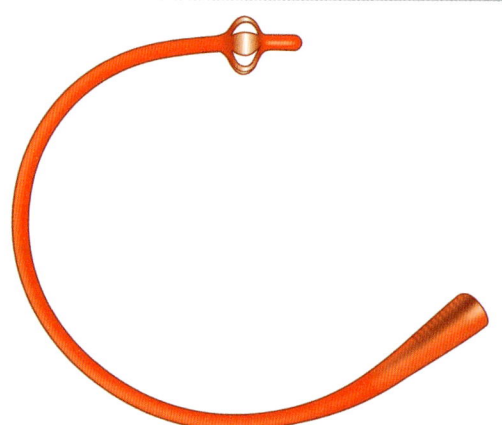

Fig. 31.32: Malecot catheter.

Malecot's catheter is also self-retaining one with flexible flower/umbrella in the tip. It is used for suprapubic cystostomy to drain urine, in draining pus or fluid or blood from cavities. It cannot be passed per urethrally. It is made up of red rubber. It is radiopaque. It is removed by gentle continuous pressure.

SIMPLE RED RUBBER TUBE (FIG. 31.33)

Simple red rubber catheter is non-self-retaining urinary catheter. It is made up of red rubber. It is blunt at tip with side opening. It is used to drain urine temporarily in retention of urine.

*One thorn of experience is worth a whole wilderness of warning—**Lowell***

It can also be used as tourniquet, for suction, to give nasal oxygen.

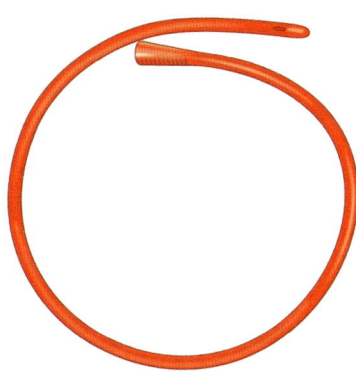

Fig. 31.33: Red rubber catheter.

LISTER'S URETHRAL DILATOR (FIG. 31.34)

It has got olive tip and it is used dilate stricture urethra.

Other dilators are Clutton's dilator and filiform bougies.

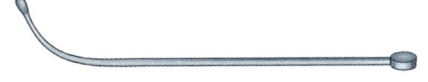

Fig. 31.34: Lister's urethral dilator.

RYLE'S TUBE (FIG. 31.35)

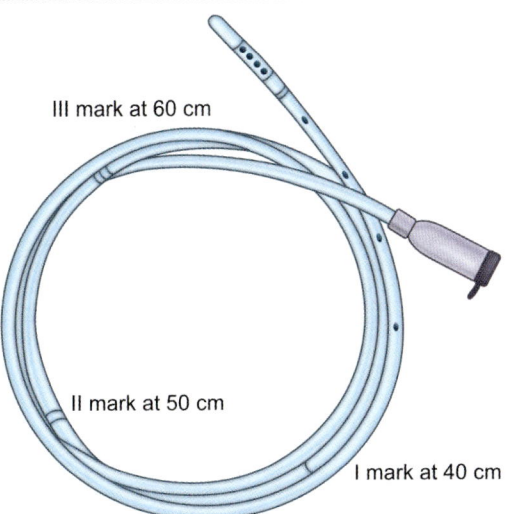

III mark at 60 cm

II mark at 50 cm

I mark at 40 cm

Fig. 31.35: Ryle's tube.

It is one meter long which is made up of red rubber or plastic.

It has got three lead shots in the tip which makes it radiopaque. It also facilitates easy passage of the tube through the esophagus.

It has got markings at different levels:
1. At 40 cm distance signifies the level of gastroesophageal junction.
2. At 50 cm distance signifies the level of body of the stomach.
3. At 60 cm distance, the level of the pylorus.
4. At 65 cm distance, the level of the duodenum.

Indications

Diagnostic:
- For gastric function tests. To assess free acid and total acid.
- Hollander's test for completion of vagotomy.
- To diagnose tracheoesophageal fistula.
- Baid test for pseudocyst of the pancreas.

Therapeutic:
- In acute abdominal conditions like peritonitis/intestinal obstruction, etc.
- In abdominal trauma.
- After abdominal surgeries.
- In pyloric stenosis.
- In upper GIT bleeding conditions.
- In paralytic ileus.
- For feeding purpose in cases like comatose patients, faciomaxillary injuries, major head and neck surgeries.

INFANT FEEDING TUBE (FIG. 31.36)

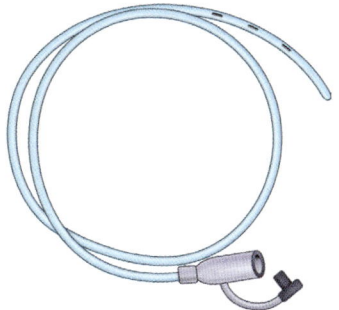

Fig. 31.36: Infant feeding tube. Lead shots are not present in the tip of infant feeding tube.

Good, to forgive; Best, to forget—Browning

Infant feeding tube is used in newborn babies and infants and children. Lead shots in the tip are not present in this tube unlike in nasogastric tube.

KEHR'S 'T' TUBE (FIG. 31.37)

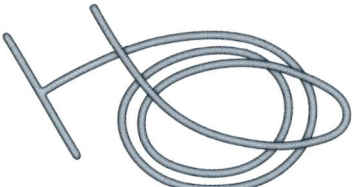

Fig. 31.37: Kehr's 'T' tube.

- It is used after opening of CBD (choledochotomy). CBD is closed with 'T' tube in the CBD.
- It is made up of latex or red rubber.
- 'T' tube has got horizontal part which is kept in the CBD and vertical part which is allowed to come out to drain bile. Amount of bile draining daily is measured out.

Before removal of 'T' tube, CBD patency should be confirmed.

It is done by following methods:
- Clamp the vertical limb (done in 12–14 days) and observe for development of pain, fever and jaundice in 24 hours. If normal then one can presume that there is no obstruction in the CBD.
- Water-soluble iodine dye is injected through the tube to visualize biliary tree and free flow of dye into the duodenum (postoperative 'T' tube cholangiogram). It is done in 14 days which is the time required to develop fibrous track. Once there is free flow, tube is removed and track gets closed on its own.

SCISSORS (FIG. 31.38)

Scissors do not have ratchets. Scissors can be Mayo's tissue scissors, straight cutting scissors, long scissors, fine scissors, stitch removal scissors. Scissors should not be sterilized in autoclave as its sharpness will alter. It is sterilized by immersing in glutaraldehyde solution.

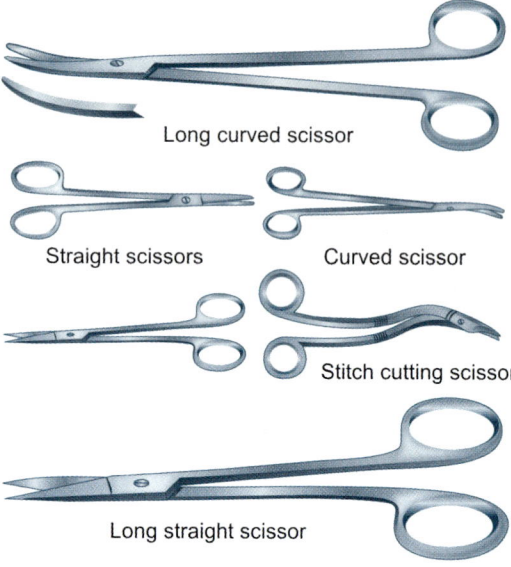

Fig. 31.38: Different types of scissors.

GIGLI'S WIRE/SAW (FIG. 31.39)

Gigli's wire is used to cut the bone like mandible. Pubis, ilium, ischium, etc. It has got fine sharp projections which makes it to cut the bone.

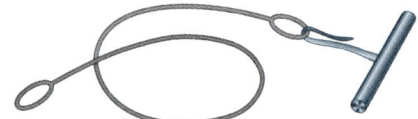

Fig. 31.39: Gigli's wire/saw.

MYER'S VEIN STRIPPER (FIG. 31.40)

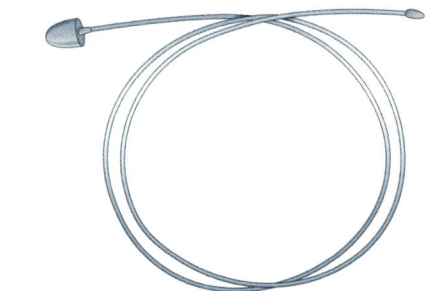

Fig. 31.40: Myer's varicose vein stripper.

Nature never deceives us. It is always we who deceive ourselves

It is a long metallic stripper used in stripping varicose veins. It has got a T shaped handle with blunt tip which is advancing. After passing through the vein tip is detached and specific required sized round knob is attached to the tip with screwing action. Vein is stripped by jerky movements over the T handle.

VOLKMANN'S SCOOP (FIG. 31.41)

Volkmann's scoop is used to scoop the granulation tissue, ulcer bed, sinus cavity. It has got a stiff handle.

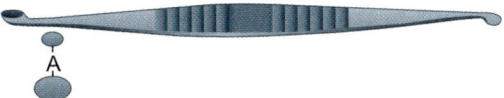

Fig. 31.41: Volkmann's scoop.

SCALPEL WITH BLADES (FIG. 31.42)

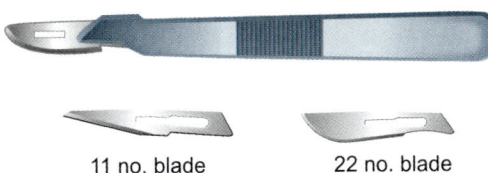

Fig. 31.42: Scalpel handle (knife) with different sized blades.

Scalpel handle (knife) is used to make incisions. Different types of handles are available. Different types of blades are available. No. 11 blade (sharp) is used for incision and drainage. No. 22 blade is used for making incision.

HUDSON BRACE WITH PERFORATOR AND BURR (FIG. 31.43)

Hudson's brace is used to do burr holes in skull bone. Using brace initially, perforator is used to reach and open the inner table. Perforator should be carefully used to avoid injury to deeper structures. Later burr is used to widen the hole made by perforator.

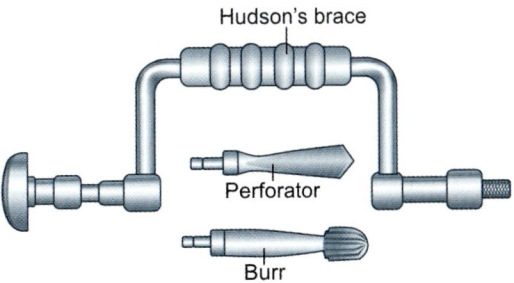

Fig. 31.43: Hudson's brace perforator and burr.

ANEURYSM NEEDLE (FIG. 31.44)

Aneurysm needle is stout instrument with a deep hook in one end with an eye opening in the tip. This facilitates the passage of the ligatures across the deeper plane.

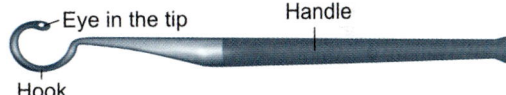

Fig. 31.44: Aneurysm needle.

PROCTOSCOPE (FIG. 31.45)

Proctoscope is used to visualize anal canal and only lower part of the rectum. It can be non-illuminating wherein torch from outside is used during proctoscopy or illuminating wherein tip of the proctoscope contains illuminating light. Proctoscope is used to see piles, to do procedures like banding, cryosurgery or to take biopsy.

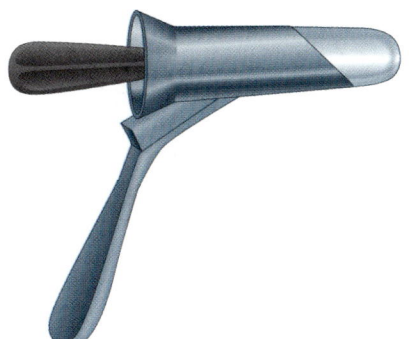

Fig. 31.45: Proctoscope.

*A little knowledge that acts is worth infinitely more than much knowledge that is idle—**Kalil Gibran***

SUTURE MATERIALS (FIG. 31.46)

Features of ideal suture material:
- Adequate tensile strength.
- Good knot holding property.
- Should be least reactive.
- Easy handling property.
- Should have *less memory*.
- Should be easily available and cost effective.

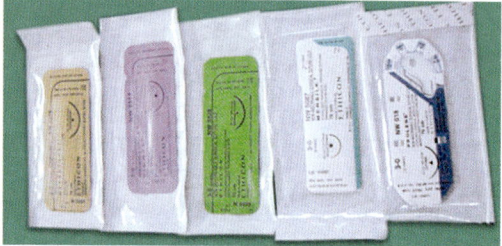

Fig. 31.46: Different types of suture materials (with pack).

CLASSIFICATION I

Absorbable Suture Materials

1. **Plain catgut** is derived from submucosa of jejunum of sheep.
   - It is yellowish white in color.
   - It is absorbed by inflammatory reaction and phagocytosis.
   - Absorption time is 7 days.
   - It is used for subcutaneous tissue, muscle, circumcision in children.
2. **Chromic** catgut is catgut with chromic acid salt.
   - It is brown in color.
   - Its absorption time is 21 days.
   - It is used in suturing muscle, fascia, external oblique aponeurosis, ligating pedicles, etc.
3. **Vicryl** (polyglactic acid):
   - It is synthetic absorbable suture material.
   - It gets absorbed in 90 days.
   - Absorption is by hydrolysis.
   - It is violet in color (braided).
   - It is multifilament and braided.
   - It is very good suture material for bowel anastomosis, suturing muscles-closure of peritoneum.
4. **Dexon** (polyglycolic acid) is synthetic absorbable suture material like vicryl. It is creamy yellow in color (braided).
5. **Maxon** (polyglyconate) monofilament.
6. **PDS** (poly dioxanone suture material) is absorbable suture material. It is creamy in color with properties like vicryl. It is costly but better suture material than vicryl.
7. **Monocryl** (polyglecaprone) monofilament.
8. **Biosyn** (glycomer) monofilament.

Uses of absorbable suture materials

1. In bowel anastomosis like gastrojejunostomy, resection and anastomosis vicryl is used.
2. In cholecystojejunostomy (CCJ), choledochojejunostomy (CDJ), pancreaticojejunostomy vicryl is used.
3. In suturing muscle, fascia, peritoneum, subcutaneous tissue, mucosa, etc.
4. In ligating pedicles. 1-zero chromic catgut or vicryl are used, e.g. ligation of pedicles during hysterectomy.
5. In circumcision usually 3-zero plain or chromic catgut are used.
6. In suturing tongue, inner aspect of lip, oral mucosa, etc.

Absorbable suture materials should not be used in suturing tendon, nerves, vessels (vascular anastomosis).

Nonabsorbable Suture Materials

1. *Silk* is natural multifilament braided nonabsorbable suture material derived from cocoon of silkworm larva. It is black in color. It is coated suture material to reduce capillary action.
2. *Polypropylene* (prolene) is synthetic monofilament suture material. It is blue in color. It has got high memory (*Memory of suture material* is recoiling tendency after removal from the packet. Ideally

There is no seven wonders of the world in the eyes of a child.
*There are seven million—***Walt Streightiff**

suture material should have low memory) (Prolene mesh used for hernioplasty is white in color).
3. *Polyethylene* (ethylene) is synthetic monofilament nonabsorbable suture material. It is black in color.
4. *Cotton* is twisted multifilament natural nonabsorbable suture material. It is white in color.
5. *Linen* is derived from bark of cotton tree.
6. *Steel, polyester, polyamide (sutupack), nylon* are other nonabsorbable suture materials.

Uses of nonabsorbable suture materials
1. In herniorrhaphy for repair.
2. For closure of abdomen after laparotomy.
3. For vascular anastomosis (6-zero), nerve suturing, tendon suturing.
4. For tension suturing in the abdomen.
5. For suturing the skin.

CLASSIFICATION II
Natural
1. Catgut.
2. Silk.
3. Cotton.
4. Linen.

Synthetic
1. Vicryl, dexon, polydiaxanone (PDS), maxon.
2. Polypropylene, polyethylene, polyester, polyamide.

CLASSIFICATION III
1. **Braided**: Polyester, polyamide, vicryl, dexon and silk.
2. **Twisted**: Cotton, linen.

CLASSIFICATION IV
1. **Monofilament**: Polypropylene, polyethylene, PDS, catgut, steel.
2. **Multifilament**: Polyester, polyamide, vicryl, dexon, silk, cotton.

CLASSIFICATION V
1. **Coated**: Polyamide, polypropylene, catgut, PDS.
2. **Uncoated**: Cotton, polyester.

Numbering of Suture Material

2—	Thick. For pedicle ligation.
1—	
1-zero	
2-zero.	For bowel suturing.
3-zero.	
4-zero.	
5-zero.	For vascular anastomosis.
6-zero.	
7-zero.	
8-zero.	
9-zero.	For ophthalmic surgery. Requires operating microscope.

TYPES OF SUTURING (FIG. 31.47)
1. Continuous suturing.
2. Interrupted simple suturing.
3. Interrupted mattress suturing.
4. Subcuticular suturing.
5. Horizontal tension suturing (Fig. 31.48).
6. Vertical tension suturing.

TYPES OF KNOTS (FIG. 31.49)
1. Reef knot.
2. Granny knot.
3. Surgeon's knot.

The greatest gift that you can give yourself is a little bit of your own attention—**Anthony J D'Angelo**

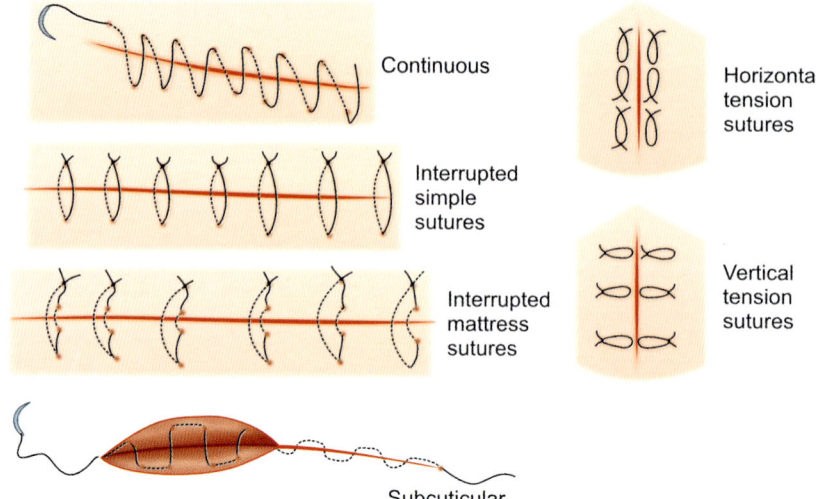

Fig. 31.47: Types of suturing.

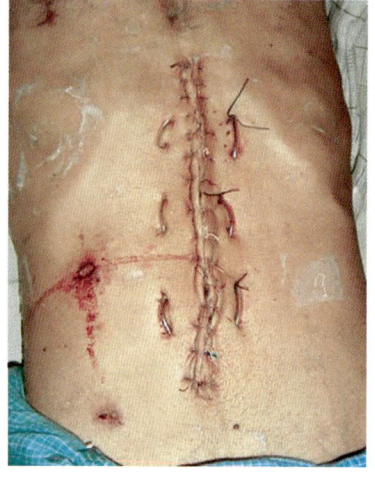

Fig. 31.48: Horizontal tension sutures.

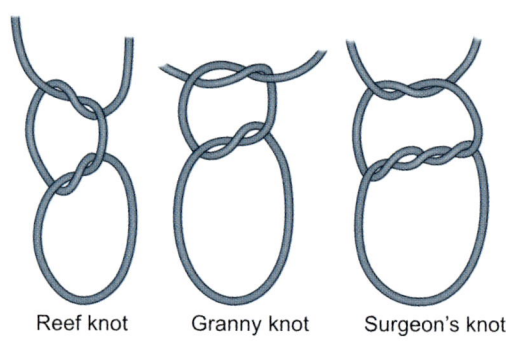

Fig. 31.49: Types of knots.

I don't know the key to success, but the key to failure is trying to please everybody—**Bill Cosby**

CHAPTER 32

Cautery, Laser, Cryosurgery and Day Care Surgery

Chapter Outline

- Diathermy (Electrocautery)
- Lasers in Surgery
- Cryosurgery
- Day Care Surgery

DIATHERMY (ELECTROCAUTERY)

It is the method to control bleeding or to cut the tissues during surgery (Fig. 32.1).

Types

Based on type of current
1. Unipolar cautery.
2. Bipolar cautery. It is safer because its effect is seen only in between electrode points. Adjacent tissues will never get damaged.

Based on type of action
1. **Coagulation cautery** which causes hemostasis by tissue coagulation. Here temperature is 100°C.
2. **Cutting cautery**: Here temperature is 1000°C which disintegrate the tissues. It is not hemostatic.
3. **Blended current** is combination of both coagulation and cutting.

Uses

- For coagulation of bleeders during surgery to achieve hemostasis.
- To cut muscles, fascia, etc.

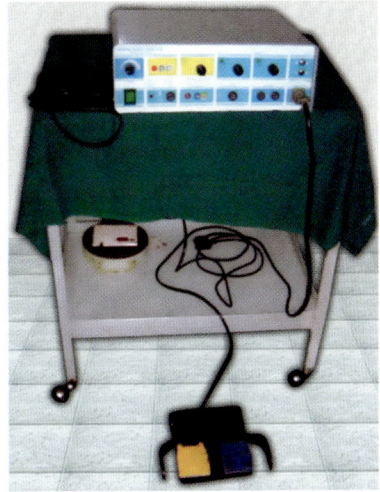

Fig. 32.1: Diathermy machine with plate, foot switch for use.

- It is essential for laparoscopic surgical procedures. Bipolar is commonly used.
- It is used to remove small cutaneous lesions, to control bleeding duodenal ulcer.
- *For dissection* it is used now most commonly especially in oncosurgery. Precise dissection using blended cautery becomes bloodless and perfect. But absolute con-

Your life is not a coincidence but it's a reflection of you

centration and care is needed to avoid injury due to lateral heat. Late tissue necrosis, infection and long time discharge—are the problems. One should be careful while using cautery close to the major vessels, nerves, vital tissues.

Disadvantages
- Infection.
- Cauterization of normal tissues.
- Explosive problems.
- Diathermy burn to the patient where diathermy plate is kept.
- Burn injury or electrical shock to surgeon and assisting personnel.

Precautions
- Proper earthing.
- Avoid loose contact of electrodes.
- It should be kept off when not in use during procedure.

LASERS IN SURGERY

(**L**ight **A**mplification **S**timulated **E**mission of **R**adiation).

Molecules are placed in a compact area and power is passed through this so as to activate the molecules. Molecules get activated at different periods and move in different directions, which they hit to each other releasing energy. This energy is allowed to act through optical system to the area wherever required.

Depending on the molecules used it is named:
- Argon laser.
- Yttrium-aluminum garnet laser (YAG laser).
- CO_2 laser.
- Neon laser.
- Holmium laser.
- Erbium laser.

Uses of Laser
- In *cranial surgery* in children.
- In *ENT to* treat vocal cord lesions, laryngeal lesions.
- In *ophthalmology* it is very useful in retinal surgery like for detachment:
  - Iridotomy.
  - Dacrocystitis.
  - Capsulotomy.
  - To liquefy human lens.
  - In glaucomas, etc.

In *general surgery:*
In bleeding duodenal ulcer
- For palliative decoring of tumors in carcinoma esophagus.
- In carcinoma rectum.
- In hemorrhoidal treatment (1st and 2nd degree).
- In bladder tumor resection.
- In cervical cancer.
- To achieve bloodless field.
- Often in making incisions in abdomen and other places.

Advantages of laser
- Blood less field; Faster.
- Small lesions can be removed easily and completely.

Precautions
- All reflecting instruments should be avoided otherwise laser will reflect and can injure normal tissues or the working team in the OT itself.
- All should wear protective spectacles to protect their eyes.

Disadvantage
Availability and cost factors.

CRYOSURGERY

It is the destruction of tissues by **controlled cooling**.

System contains an automatic defrosting device with a cryoprobe (Fig. 32.2).

Gases used are
1. Nitrous oxide—98°C temperature.
2. CO_2—60°C.

It is not how much we have, but how we enjoy, that makes us happy

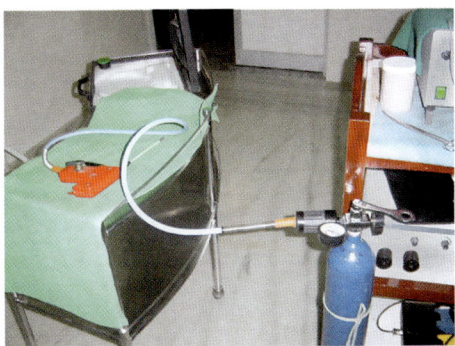

Fig. 32.2: Cryosurgery instrument kept ready for procedure.

3. Liquid N_2—180°C.
4. Freon—190°C.
❖ Commonly used is nitrous oxide as it is easily available, cheaper and achieves optimum temperature required for different procedures.

Mode of Action

❖ It produces intracellular crystallization, dehydration and denaturation of proteins and cell death.
❖ It causes the obliteration of microcirculation and so cell death.

Indications

❖ To remove warts and lesions in the skin.
❖ Cryotherapy for piles.
❖ For chronic cervicitis.

Advantages

❖ Relatively bloodless and painless.
❖ Adequate control of extent and depth in freezing.
❖ Equally effective.

Disadvantage

Infection; discharge from the site.

Procedures done in day care surgery

- Excision of cysts, lipomas, bursae, neurofibromas.
- Lymph node biopsy, hemorrhoid surgery, endoscopies, circumcision, hydrocele.
- Wound suturing, toe amputation.

DAY CARE SURGERY

Day care surgery is an upcoming field in surgical practice. It is an unique method wherein general practitioner, nurse at day care ward and theater, surgeon, anesthetist work in hand so that hospital stay and the cost is reduced. Patient comes to hospital in morning for surgery and leaves the hospital on same day evening.

Advantages

❖ Minimal hospital stay; patient's acceptance.
❖ Becomes cheaper.

Precautions

❖ Patient should be assessed properly before sending to day care surgery.
❖ The nurse should give proper instruction to the patient as patient stays in the hospital for a short period.
❖ Patient should be warned about possible problems like bleeding, vomiting, pain, discomfort, and sedation.
❖ Before discharging, patient should be seen by the doctor for the fitness.
❖ All records should be carefully documented.
❖ Patient should be advised to rush to hospital if any problems arise or to communicate immediately.

Nurses hold an important role in day care surgery.

---

*If you cannot work with love but only with distaste, it is better that you should leave your work—**Khalil Gibran***

CHAPTER 33

Advanced Imaging Methods

Chapter Outline

- Ultrasound
- Doppler
- CT Scan
- Magnetic Resonance Imaging

ULTRASOUND

Ultrasound contains waves with a frequency of more than 20,000 cycles/second which the human ears cannot hear.

In medical sonography frequencies used are commonly 2–10 MHz. The transducer or the probe works as both transmitter of **sound waves** and receiver of **echoes**. The piezoelectric crystal is the producer of ultrasound waves. Received signals from the patient are fed into the computer which forms the image.

There are three types of ultrasound image display.
1. **A-mode**: Only one-dimensional static display as spikes are obtained. It is used only in eye scan.
2. **B-mode**: Two-dimensional real time images in the form of grains. It is most widely used type. Using this mode *Transverse, Longitudinal* or *Oblique* sections can be taken.
3. **M-mode**: Images are recorded as dots. It is mainly used in moving parts like echocardiography. M-mode is also called as TM Mode, i.e. *Time Motion Mode*.

Uses

- All abdominal and pelvic conditions, often in thoracic conditions.
- **Ultrasound of thyroid** is very useful method to differentiate between solid and cystic lesions (Fig. 33.1).
- Ultrasound is used in testicular tumors, epididymo-orchitis, trauma to testis, erectile dysfunction, etc.
- Ultrasound breast to differentiate solid from cystic tumors.
- Soft tissue and musculoskeletal system ultrasound.
- Ocular ultrasound is ideal method to image eye and intraocular structures.

Advantages

- No radiation.
- Noninvasive.
- Effective with efficiency.
- Painless.
- Low cost.
- Availability even as portable machines.
- Stones are well-visualized with **acoustic shadow**.

You, yourself, as much as anybody in the entire universe, deserve your love and affection—**Buddha**

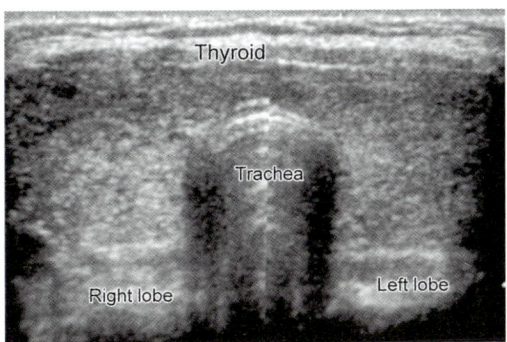

Fig. 33.1: Ultrasound thyroid showing thyroid both lobes.

Disadvantages

- Interpretation can be inadequate.
- *Bowel shadow may prevent proper visualization.*
- In obese patient image will be inadequate.
- **Interpretation** is based on echogenicity either *hyperechogenic* or *hypoechogenic*.

Advanced Ultrasound Techniques (Fig. 33.2)

- Endosonography (EUS) used in visualization of walls of esophagus or stomach through gastroscopy.
- Transvaginal ultrasound.
- Transrectal ultrasound to see prostate.
- Doppler ultrasound to study arterial and venous diseases.

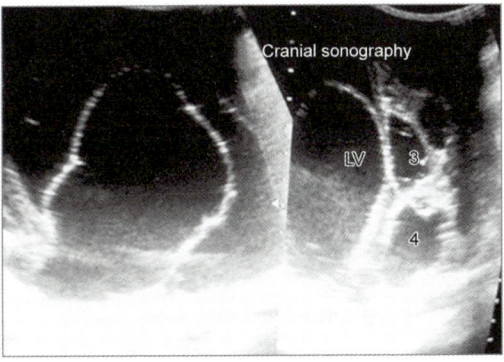

Fig. 33.2: Cranial sonography is done to see intracranial problems through suture lines—usually done in infants and children.

Ultrasound as Therapeutic Use

- To guide aspiration of amebic liver abscess, pericardial tap, abscess neck, abscess breast, etc.
- On table ultrasound to assess the operability of tumor (During laparoscopy to assess the extent of tumor, lymph node status, etc.).

DOPPLER

Doppler effect is a change in the perceived frequency of sound emitted by a ***moving source***. So it measures blood flow. Spectral Doppler wave form and ultrasound image are combined in **Duplex scanning**.

Types

1. Continuous waves.
2. Pulsed waves.
   Doppler will provide both audio and video signals.
   Color Doppler imaging displays flowing blood as **red** when direction of flow is towards the transducer. Image will be **blue** if flow is away from transducer.

Uses

- To study cardiovascular system.
- To study vascularity of tumors.
- To study blood flow and velocity in arterial diseases so as to assess stenosis (its extent, cause, etc.) like in atherosclerosis, thromboangiitis obliterans (TAO), cervical rib, aneurysm, atriovenous (AV) fistulas.
- To find out deep venous thrombosis (DVT), varicose veins, perforator incompetence.
- To study grade of varicocele in males.

Advantages

- It has replaced venogram and angiogram in many places as a diagnostic tool.
- It is reliable and noninvasive.

---

*Start by doing what's necessary, then do what's possible and suddenly you are doing the impossible—**Saint Francis of Assiss***

CT SCAN

Computerized tomography scan was invented by **Godfrey Hounsfield** in 1963. He was a Physicist. He received **Nobel Prize** (1972) for the same. The first CAT scan is in the London museum.

Narrow X-ray beams are passed from rotating X-ray generator through **the gantry** where patient is placed. When X-rays pass through the tissues, some of the X-rays get absorbed and some pass through, depending on the tissue density. The different grades of absorption in different tissues are detected through sensitive detectors which are translated to a Gray scale image by a computer.

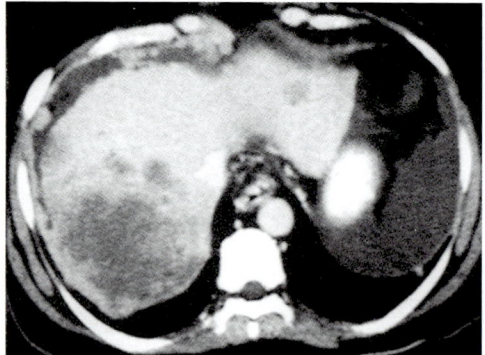

Fig. 33.3: CT scan picture showing liver secondaries.

Density of tissues is numbered as **Hounsfield Number (HN)**
- Water—Zero HN.
- Air— –1000.
- Bone— +1000.

Other tissues come in between air and bone with different HNs.

Presently spiral CT scan has become popular. They are faster and in a single breath-holding time, whole CT scan can be taken.

Both plain and contrast CTs are done whenever required.

Contrast Agents

- **Ionic**: Water-soluble iodide dyes like *sodium diatrizoate, meglumine iothalamate (Conray, Urograffin, Angiograffin)*. They are cheaper but often toxic and cause anaphylaxis.
- **Nonionic are** safer but expensive, like *IOHEXOL (Omnipaque), Iopamiro*.

In abdominal CT, contrast agents can be given orally to delineate bowel properly.

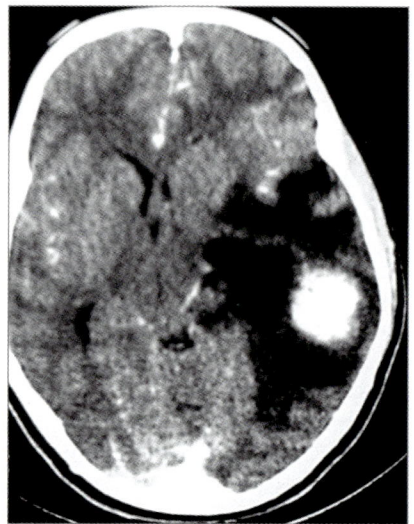

Fig. 33.4: CT picture showing astrocytoma.

(Fig. 33.3). For example, brain, abdominal, retroperitoneal, thoracic and spinal tumors (Fig. 33.4).
- **Inflammatory conditions** in various places also, e.g. psoas abscess, pseudocyst of pancreas (Fig. 33.5).

Indications

- **Trauma** like head injury, chest injury, abdomen trauma. In trauma **only plain CT scan** is taken.
- **Neoplasms**: To see the exact location, size, vascularity, extent and operability

Advantages of CT scan
• One to two mm sized sections are possible.
• Amount of X-ray exposure is less.
• More accurate, sensitive, and specific.
• Small lesions are also detected.
• CT-guided biopsies are done at present safely.

Set high standards and few limitations for yourself—Anthony J D'Angelo

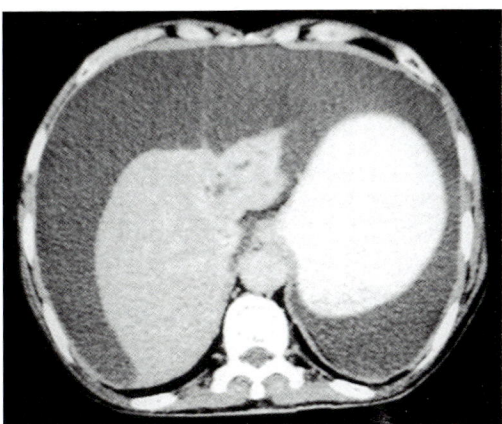

Fig. 33.5: CT scan showing ascites (gross).

Disadvantages
• **Interpretation** by an experienced radiologist is important. • **Artefacts** can be present. • **Cost factor** and **availability**.

Findings

* Extradural hematoma—***biconvex lesion.***
* **Subdural hematoma**—*concavo-convex lesion.*
* Smooth margin in benign condition.
* Irregular margin in malignant condition.

Advantages of spiral CT scan
• **Reduced** scan time. Useful in children and critically ill patients. • Imaging in both arterial and venous phases is possible. • Improved lesion detection. Missing a lesion is uncommon. • Multiplanar and 3-dimensional analysis like CT angiography, complex joint imaging, facial bone imaging is possible.

High resolution CT (HRCT) is a CT technique used in chest scan where thin sections are taken to have better quality images.

MAGNETIC RESONANCE IMAGING

Earlier named as *nuclear magnetic imaging (NMR)*, the term is not used now.

Principle

When patient is placed in an *external high magnetic field*, protons of hydrogen atoms rotate in phase with each other and gradually return to their original position releasing small amounts of energy which is detected by sensitive coils. Proton density and relaxation time are assessed by radiofrequency pulse and the computer generates a Gray scale image from this data.

T1 relaxation time is the time taken to return to original axis. **T1 images** are used to find out **normal anatomical detail**. It has got high soft tissue discrimination. Here fluid (CSF) looks black.

T2 relaxation time is the time taken by the proton to diphase. It is used to assess **pathological** processes. **In T2 images** fluid looks white.

In proton density images fluid looks in between black and white.

It can be **plain MRI** or **contrast MRI**. Contrast agent is *gadolinium* given intravenously.

Uses of MRI (Figs. 33.6 and 33.7)

* It is very useful in intracranial, spinal and musculoskeletal lesions including *joint pathologies.*
* It gives direct anatomical sections of the area with lesions at a high resolution.
* MR angiogram **is done without injecting IV contrast agents**.
* **Cardiac MRI** is very useful.
* **Breast MRI** is used in multifocal recurrent cancers.

The worth of your lives comes neither in what we do nor whom we know but by whom we are

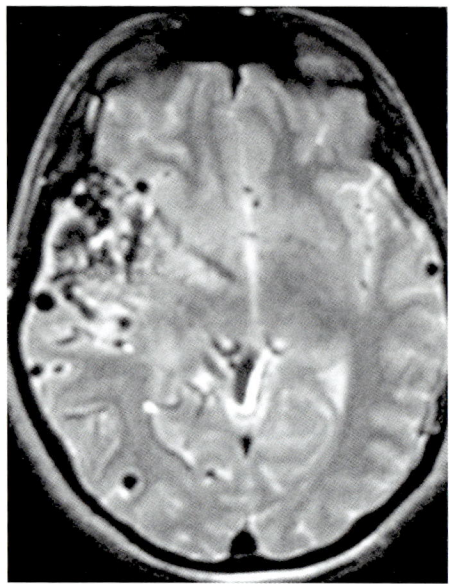

Fig. 33.6: MRI showing AV malformation.

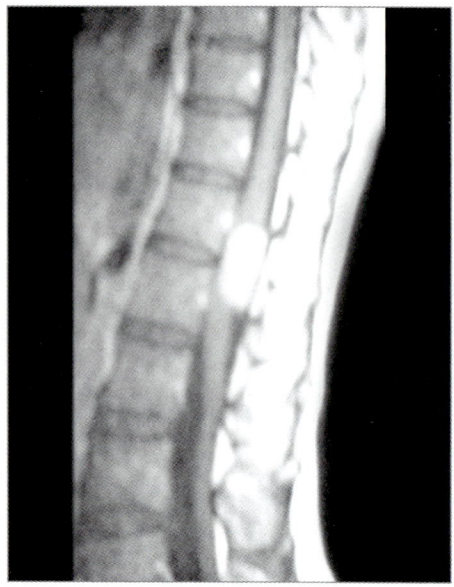

Fig. 33.7: MRI picture, which shows extradural schwannoma.

- **Magnetic resonance cholangiopancreatography** *(MRCP)* is a very useful non-contrast diagnostic tool which may replace diagnostic ERCP.
- **MR spectroscopy** is chemical analysis of elements in a tissue to differentiate between tumor, inflammation, and degeneration.

Advantages

- Artefacts are not common.
- More sensitive and specific than CT scan.

Contraindications
Patients with prosthesis in the body, metallic foreign bodies, pacemakers, cochlear implants, cranial aneurysm clips *should never* **undergo MRI**.

Precaution
Before entering the MRI room, the patient and other personnel should remove all magnetically attractive materials.

Disadvantages

- **Availability** and **cost factor**.
- It is time consuming.
- Patient compliance is poor.
- In is not feasible in patients suffering from *claustrophobia*.
- It is not ideal in emergencies and critically ill patients.
- It is not useful in lung pathology and subarachnoid hemorrhage.

*Good judgment comes from experience, and experience comes from bad judgment—**Barry LePatner***

CHAPTER 34

Anesthesia

Chapter Outline

- Preoperative Assessment
- General Anesthesia
- Muscle Relaxants
- Reversal Agents
- Instruments in Anesthesia
- Steps in General Anesthesia
- Complications in General Anesthesia
- Postoperative Care
- Regional Anesthesia
- Spinal Anesthesia
- Epidural Anesthesia
- Caudal Anesthesia

PREOPERATIVE ASSESSMENT

History

- Chronic cough, smoking, alcohol, drug intake, drug allergy.
- Any previous diseases like hypertension, diabetes mellitus, epilepsy, bronchial asthma tuberculosis, hepatitis, cardiac diseases.
- Drug therapy: Steroids, antihypertensives, sedatives, antibiotics, antiepileptics.

Examination

General: Posture, teeth, mouth opening, dilated veins, neck movements, tremor, airway. Anemia, edema, jaundice, cyanosis.

Respiratory system: To look for asthma, tuberculosis, emphysema, chronic obstructive pulmonary disease (COPD).

Airway: Mouth opening, Malampatti scoring, tyromental distance, temporomandibular joint assessment.

Cardiovascular system: Hypertension, ischemic heart disease, arrhythmias, cardiac failure, valvular diseases.

Spine: Curvature, intervertebral space, skin over the area for any infection.

Other systems: Abdomen, skeletal system.

Preoperative Investigations

Hematocrit, blood sugar, blood urea, serum creatinine, electrolytes, chest X-ray, electrocardiogram (ECG), blood grouping, blood-gas analysis, cardiac assessment.

Preoperative Treatment

- Control of respiratory and cardiac diseases.
- Improvement of Hb% status, if anemia is present.
- Preoperative antibiotics is given.
- Blood should be kept ready for major cases.
- *Starvation for 4 hours for liquids and 6 hours for solids.*

Hope puts a smile on our face when the heart cannot manage

- Bladder and bowel should be emptied to prevent soiling on the operation table. Urinary catheter may be passed and enema may be given.
- Dentures, contact lenses, jewellery must be removed.
- Surgical area should be cleaned and properly prepared.

Premedication

It is given one hour before surgery:
- *For sedation and relief of anxiety.* Pethidine 50 mg/Morphine 10 mg/Diazepam 10 mg. Midazolam 1–2.5 mg.
- *To suppress vagal activity.* Atropine 0.6 mg IM.
- *To reduce vomiting.* Promethazine (Phenergan) 12.5 mg.

GENERAL ANESTHESIA

It means abolition of all sensations, i.e. touch, pain, posture and temperature with a state of reversible loss of consciousness.

It has got three components:
(1) Analgesia, (2) Hypnosis and (3) Muscle relaxation.

Volatile anesthetics: They vaporize in room in air.

Agents used are: Ether, Trichloroethylene, Halothane, Enflurane, Isoflurane, Sevoflurane.

Ether which is irritant, unpleasant, flammable, is commonly used agent in developing countries.

Enflurane and Isoflurane are noninflammable, nonexplosive, nonirritant, stable. Here anesthesia is rapid with faster recovery.

Gaseous anesthetics

Nitrous oxide: It is noninflammable, nonirritant, good analgesics but weak anesthetic agent. It is given along with 30–50% oxygen for balanced anesthesia (blue-colored cylinder in India).

Cyclopropane is highly flammable.

Intravenous anesthetics

Thiopentone: It is ultrashort acting barbiturate which causes hypnosis during induction of anesthesia. It does not have analgesic effect. It causes hypotension, respiratory depression, laryngeal and bronchospasm. Recovery is rapid. Extravasation of drug can cause skin ulceration. Intra-arterial injection causes vasospasm and gangrene. *Dose:* 4–7 mg/kg.

Methohexitone sodium.

Propanidid. 4–7 mg/kg. It can cause anaphylaxis.

Ketamine: 2 mg/kg IV. It is a good analgesic. It causes dissociative anesthesia. It can lead to hypertension, apnea, laryngospasm. In children it can be given IM—5 mg/kg. It does not require intubation for small procedures.

Propofol: It is widely used induction agent which has got predictable onset and recovery. It has got least side effects on CVS and respiratory system. It is also used for total IV anesthesia. *Dose:* 1–2.5 mg/kg.

Fentanyl is neuroleptanalgesic. It causes sedation, catatonia, dissociation, hypotension and preferred in asthmatics.

Oxygen

- oxygen is given through Boyle's apparatus (33.3%).
- Oxygen in high concentration is respiratory depressant and also affects eyes.
- A 5% CO_2 mixture in oxygen is called as *carbogen*.
- Oxygen is available in black and white-colored cylinder.

MUSCLE RELAXANTS

Depolarizing muscle relaxants

They act on the acetylcholine receptors which widens the refractory period after depolarization causing paralysis. It is short-acting muscle relaxant.

a. *Suxamethonium chloride (scoline):*
   It lasts for 2–4 minutes.
   It causes muscle twitching—fasciculations—paralysis.

Become a student of change. It is the only thing that will remain constant—**Anthony J D'Angelo**

It is metabolized by plasma pseudocholinesterase. Atypical or deficiency of this enzyme prolongs the action of the scoline. *Side effects* are hyperkalemia, myotonia, apnea and cardiac arrest.
b. *Suxthonium bromide.*

Nondepolarizing Muscle Relaxants

They block the channels of entry of acetyl choline. They are long-acting relaxants.
1. *Tubocurarine*: It lasts for 45 minutes. 30 mg is the dose.
2. *Gallamine (Flaxedil)*: Dose is 1–2 mg/kg. It is cheaper. It is contraindicated in renal diseases.
3. *Pancuronium bromide (Pavulon)*: It is synthetic steroid muscle relaxant. It lasts for 45 minutes. Dose is 0.08–0.1 mg/kg.
4. *Vecuronium bromide*: It is a steroid muscle relaxant, given at a dose of 0.05–0.1 mg/kg.
5. *Rocuronium* is short-acting steroid muscle relaxant. It starts its action in one minute.
6. *Atracurium*: It lasts for 20–30 minutes. Dose is 0.6 mg/kg.
7. *Mivacurium*: Dose is 0.15–0.25 mg/kg.

REVERSAL AGENTS

They are anticholinesterase drugs which increase the acetylcholine and thus act as antagonizing agents for nondepolarizing muscle relaxants. They cause bradycardia.

Neostigmine (2.5 mg) is used commonly along with atropine (1.2 mg).

Endrophonium (short-acting) and pyridostigmine (long-acting) are other drugs.

INSTRUMENTS IN ANESTHESIA

1. ***Boyle's apparatus (Fig. 34.1)***
   It consists of:
   a. Cylinders for N_2O and O_2.
   b. Pressure guage—to know the amount of gas remaining.

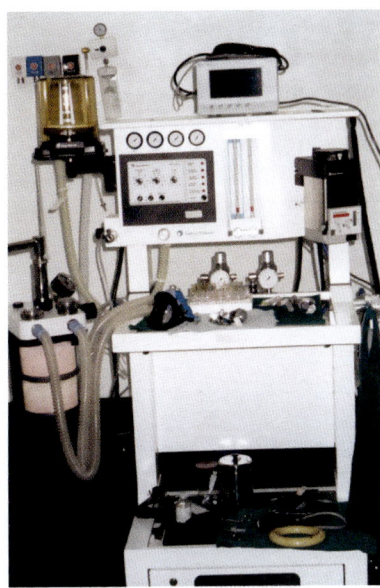

Fig. 34.1: Boyle's apparatus.

   c. Pressure regulator—to regulate the pressure of gas used.
   d. Rotameter—to know the flow of gas.
   e. Vaporizer.
2. **Endotracheal tube:** These are tubes inserted into the trachea and is used to conduct gases and vapors to and from the lungs. Depending on the diameter, it is available in various sizes. It has a cuff at one end which when inflated stabilizes the tube in position and also prevents aspiration. Noncuffed tubes are also available. The other end near the mouth is connected to the breathing circuit through which anesthetic gases are delivered. The tube is inserted using a direct laryngoscope. The proper placement in the airway is confirmed by auscultating for the breath sounds over the chest when the gases are delivered.

Complication
❖ Postoperative sore throat.
❖ Hoarseness after intubation.
❖ Upper airway edema.

No good deed goes unpunished!—CB Luce

- *Magill's forceps (Fig. 34.2).*
- Mouth gag.
- Laryngoscope.
- Connectors.
- Laryngeal mask airway (LMA).

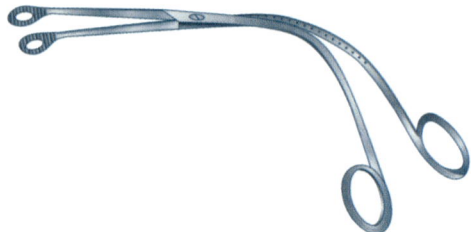

Fig. 34.2: Magill's forceps.

STEPS IN GENERAL ANESTHESIA

Components of general anesthesia
- Premedication.
- Induction.
- Maintenance.
- Recovery.

- **Premedication** is given one hour before surgery with Pethidine 50 mg/Diazepam 10 mg, Atropine 0.6 mg IM and Promethazine (Phenergan) 12.5 mg.
- **Induction:** Patient is preoxygenated with 100% oxygen for 3 minutes then induced with IV Thiopentone given 4–5 mg/kg. Patient *loses consciousness*. Induction is maintained by 67% nitrous oxide and 33% oxygen.
- Scoline is given IV to relax muscles so as to facilitate *endotracheal intubation*.
- Once intubated *ventilation* can be either *controlled* using muscle relaxants or spontaneous using a volatile anesthetic agent.
- **Reversal** is done using Neostigmine and Atropine or Glycopyrrolate.

COMPLICATIONS IN GENERAL ANESTHESIA

- Intraarterial injection of the drug.
- Myocardial depression and cardiac arrest.
- Hypertension.
- Laryngeal and bronchial spasm.
- Cardiac arrhythmias.
- Respiratory failure.
- Acute respiratory distress syndrome (ARDS).
- **Mendelson's syndrome**: It is due to regurgitation of the acid from the stomach causing aspiration of acid leading into bronchospasm, pulmonary edema and circulatory failure. This is treated with oxygen, suction, hydrocortisone, aminophylline, antibiotics, Ryle's tube aspiration and ventilator support.
- Hypoxia.
- Pneumothorax.
- Anaphylaxis.
- **Malignant hyperthermia**: It is an inherited myopathic disorder occurs under anesthesia due to drugs like halothane, scoline. There is marked increase in metabolic rate with rise of temperature. There is high levels of creatinine phosphokinase (CPK) enzyme. Condition will cause metabolic acidosis and hyperkalemia. It has got high mortality. Treatment is IV Dantrolene, cooling, oxygen and cold IV fluids.
- Hypothermia.

POSTOPERATIVE CARE

Immediate postoperative period is important and critical because patient may not be fully conscious. Patient should be kept in recovery room until he/she recovers from anesthesia.

- Care of respiratory system: Adequate breathing is important otherwise hypoxia sets in which gradually lead to cardiac arrest. Respiratory problems may be:
  - Laryngeal spasm.
  - Falling of tongue backwards blocking the airway.
  - Aspiration.
  - Bronchospasm.
  - ARDS.
  - Respiratory failure.

Oxygen supplement through mask, observation, proper positioning are the treatment.

*It's not that I'm so smart, it's just that I stay with problems longer—**Albert Einstein***

- Hypercarbia.
- Circulatory problems:
  - Hypotension.
  - Arrhythmias.
  - Hypertension.
  - Cardiac arrest.
- Gastrointestinal tract (GIT):
  - Vomiting.
  - Regurgitation.
  - Mendelson's syndrome.
- Renal problems:
  - Oliguria, i.e. urine output is less than 30 mL/hour. It may be due to hypovolemia, hypotension, acidosis, sepsis, transfusion reaction, toxins.
  - The ratio of urine/plasma osmolality of 2:1 signifies prerenal failure. Ratio of 1.7:1 indicates renal failure.
  - Blood urea and serum creatinine is done at regular intervals.
  - Fluid and electrolyte imbalance if any is corrected.
  - 100 mL 20% mannitol or frusemide 40–80 mg are often required.
  - Other problems:
  - Restlessness, shivering, pain.

MONITORING THE POSTOPERATIVE PATIENT

- Pulse, temperature BP chart.
- Breathing type.
- Level of consciousness.
- Urine output.
- Oxygen saturation and heart rate using pulse oximeter.
- Checking and encouraging limb movements.
- Skin color, tongue color for adequacy of oxygenation.
- Tongue for hydration.
- Cardiac monitor.
- Blood gas analysis in case of patient on ventilator.
- Serum electrolyte assessment.

REGIONAL ANESTHESIA

Carl Koller, an ophthalmologist introduced cocaine as local anesthetic in ophthalmic practice.

Mode of action: It causes temporary conduction block of the nerve, thus preventing the propagation of nerve impulse.

Advantages of local anesthetic agent:
- Technically simpler.
- General anesthesia is avoided.
- Consciousness is retained.
- Patient can have food earlier after surgery.

Drugs used: Cocaine, Procaine, Cinchocaine—amino esters. Lignocaine, Prilocaine, Bupivacaine, Ropivacaine amino amides.

Lignocaine/Lidocaine/Xylocaine: It is the commonest local anesthetic agent used. It is available as 0.25–5% concentrations.

It is metabolized in the liver and excreted in the kidney as xylidines. It is also an antiarrhythmic drug and so commonly used in cardiology and cardiac surgery.

Side effects: Giddiness, headache, postural hypotension, tinnitus, circumoral anesthesia.

Dose: 4 mg/kg. Effect lasts for 90 minutes.

Uses:
- Topical—4%.
- Infiltration block—0.25%.
- Field block—0.5%.
- Nerve block—1.0%.
- Epidural—1.5–2.0%.
- Spinal—5%.

It can be used with or without adrenaline.

Xylocaine with adrenaline has got longer duration of action. It creates relatively bloodless field.

But it should not be used in places where end arteries are present like glans penis, ear lobule, tip of the nose, lip, fingers and toes.

Bupivacaine (Marcaine): It has got prolonged action. It is a vasodilator also.
- Dose: 3 mg/kg.
- Epidural block: 0.5%
- Spinal 0.5% 3 mL.

*Our friends show us what we can do. Our enemies teach us what we must do—**Goethe***

TOPICAL ANESTHESIA

It is used for minor surgeries of eye, laryngoscopy, bronchoscopy, cystoscopy, gastroscopy, submucus injection.

It is available as instillation, spray, viscous, ointment, gel, EMLA (eutectic mixture of local anesthetic).

INFILTRATION BLOCK

Direct injection of local anesthetic under the skin for small procedures.

FIELD BLOCK

It is achieved by blocking the entire field of excision where lesion is located.

NERVE BLOCK

- Block of inferior dental nerve and lingual nerves in the region of the mental foramen for extraction of teeth.
- Finger block of digital nerves. Here plain xylocaine is used (without adrenaline).
- Intercostal block.
- Ankle block.
- Median and ulnar nerve block.
- Brachial plexus block (Winnie's block)
  It can be given through
   - Interscalene,
   - Axillary,
   - Supraclavicular approaches.

Supraclavicular approach is commonly used. 1 cm above the mipoint of the clavicle, needle is passed downwards, backwards and medially towards first rib. Once needle hits the first rib, 15–20 mL of 1.5% xylocaine is injected (with walking or stepping over the first rib). Complications are pneumothorax and injury to the great vessels.

Other blocks:
- Cervical plexus block.
- Sciatic nerve block.
- Femoral nerve block.

INTRAVENOUS REGIONAL ANESTHESIA (BIER'S BLOCK)

Limb is exsanguinated and occluded with tourniquet. Pressure in the tourniquet must be 30 mm Hg more than the systolic pressure of the patient. Needle is placed in the selected vein. 40 mL of 0.5% xylocaine for upper limb and 80 mL of 0.25% of xylocaine for lower limb is injected into the vein. *Xylocaine with Adrenaline should not be used.* It gives very good analgesia for 2 hours.

Side effects: Sudden release of drug into the circulation can cause hypotension, convulsions and often death.

Bupivacaine should not be used.

Indications: For upper and lower limb surgeries it can be used without general anesthesia (GA) or spinal anesthesia (SA).

SPINAL ANESTHESIA

It is the injection of local anesthetic into the subarachnoid space causing loss of sympathetic tone, sensation and motor function. The sympathetic block is 3 segments higher than sensory block, motor block is 3 segments lower than sensory block.

Position: Lateral decubitus position with head, hips and knees being fully flexed so as to open the interlaminar spaces. Highest point of iliac crest corresponds to 4th lumbar vertebra.

Drugs used:
- Lignocaine 5% in 6% dextrose 2 mL.
- Bupivacaine 0.5% in 5% dextrose 3 mL.
- Cinchocaine 0.5% in 6% dextrose 2 mL.

Technique

24–26 gauge needle with stilette is used. Needle is passed through the interspinous space and ligamentum flavum to reach the subarachnoid space to get clear fluid (0.5 mL/sec). Needle is rotated 360° and drug is

We must teach our children to dream with their eyes open—Harry Edwards

injected slowly. Patient is repositioned to supine. Drug takes 15 minutes to act.

Types

1. Caudal (up to L_5).
2. Low spinal (up to L_1).
3. Midspinal (up to T_{10}).
4. High spinal (up to T_6).
5. Unilateral spinal.

Advantages

- Economical.
- Hypotension reduces the bleeding.
- Adequate relaxation is achieved.
- Respiratory complications are less.

Disadvantages and Complications

- Cerebrospinal fluid (CSF) leak and aseptic inflammation of meninges causing headache.
- Meningism.
- Infection.
- Paraplegia. It is very rare.
- Occasionally it can become total spinal which requires intubation and ventilator support.

Contraindications

- Allergy.
- Increased intracranial pressure. It may precipitate coning.
- Sepsis.
- Spinal tumors.
- Back pain and spinal diseases.
- Neurological conditions like syringomyelia.

SADDLE BLOCK

- It is used for surgeries in perineal and anorectal region.
- It is spinal anesthesia using Xylocaine or Bupivacaine given in sitting position.

EPIDURAL ANESTHESIA

It is a potential space between dura anteriorly and ligamentum flavum posteriorly which has got negative pressure inside. It extends from foramen magnum to sacral hiatus.

Touhy needle is used for epidural anesthesia. Once the needle is in the space there will be sudden indrawing of air or saline drop. An epidural catheter is placed in the space and fixed. 2% Xylocaine with Adrenaline or 0.5% Bupivacaine is injected into the space to achieve anesthesia up to the desired level.

Advantages

- It can be used for continuous repeated prolonged anesthesia.
- It can be used for postoperative analgesia.
- It can be kept for several days.

CAUDAL ANESTHESIA

Caudal space is the sacral component of epidural space and access is through the sacral hiatus.

Indications

- Hemorrhoidal surgery.
- Circumcision.
- Small procedures in the perineum like cystoscopy.

Procedure

It is given in lateral position. Needle is inserted through the sacral hiatus to enter the caudal epidural space. Drug is then injected into the space.

Complications

- Trauma to anal canal.
- Intravascular injection.
- Failure of caudal block.

Keep your face to the sunshine and you cannot see the shadows

CHAPTER 35A

Clinical Methods in Surgery for Dental Students

Chapter Outline

- Clinical Examination of Sinus or Fistula
- Examination of an Ulcer
- Examination of a Swelling/Lump
- Examination in Arterial Disease (Arterial System)
- Examination of Varicose Veins
- Examination of Thyroid Gland
- Examination of Oral Cavity
- Examination of Jaw and Temporomandibular Joint
- Examination Salivary Gland
- Examination of Inguinoscrotal Swellings
- Definition of Hernia
- Examination of Hydrocele

Study of basic clinical skill in surgery is very essential for dental graduates alike MBBS students.

Even with the availability of modern day technologies like 3D/4D ultrasonography (USG), CT scan, magnetic resonance imaging (MRI), clinical methods still has its role in evaluating and treating a patient. First of all it builds a bridge of confidence, rapport and mutual respect between the surgeon and the patient which is getting weakened by the advent of modern day technologies. Secondly, it improves the communication skills, interpretation skills and treating skills of the surgeon. Finally, whatever may be the modern technologies they are only supplementary to a clinical methodology but not a substitute.

Even for their clinical examination in 'surgery' subject this is essential. Hence, precisely clinical methods of different conditions which will be kept as cases for dental students are discussed here.

Common conditions students has to learn for clinical examinations are:

- Examination of swelling.
- Examination of ulcer.
- Arterial diseases—thromboangiitis obliterans (TAO), atherosclerosis.
- Varicose veins.
- Examination of lymphatics.
- Examination of thyroid swelling.
- Oral carcinoma.
- Neck swellings—secondaries/tuberculosis in lymph node/lymphoma.
- Parotid swelling.
- Hernia and hydrocele.

Without a sense of caring, there can be no sense of community—**Anthony J D'Angelo**

History Taking in a Surgical Case

Basic outline of history taking is discussed here. For detailed description please refer 'SRB's Clinical Methods in Surgery.'

'History taking' is nothing but taking a detailed account of patient's illness and noting it down methodically in a case sheet in the following order. Conversation with the patient is done in the language well known to the patient; if not possible then it is wise to take the help of an interpreter usually the ward nurse.

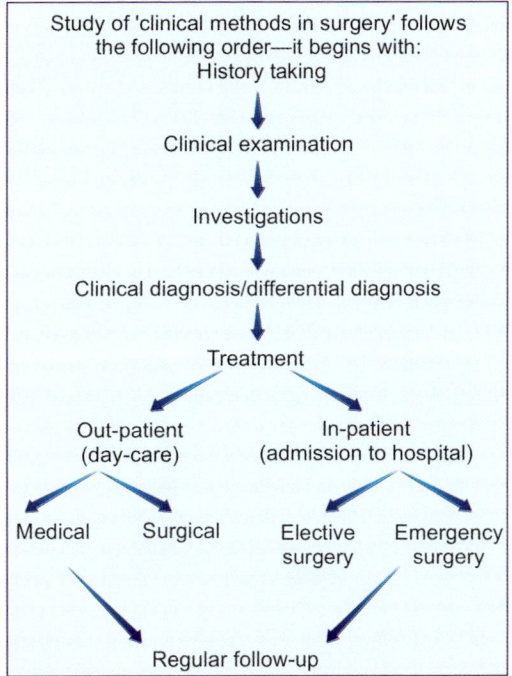

Name:
Addressing the patient by his name is very important as it helps in building up a rapport with the patient.

Age:
Noting the correct age of the patient is important as some conditions are age related, e.g. cleft lip/palate is seen in newborns; Wilm's tumor, cystic hygroma in children; oral malignancies are common above 40 years.

Sex:
Certain conditions are more common in one particular sex, e.g. gallstones, goiter, mobile kidneys are common in females.

Peptic ulcer, GI malignancies, carcinoma lip, cheek are more common in men.

Occupation:
People with certain occupation are more prone to certain diseases, e.g. varicose ulcer/veins are common in policemen, nurses, surgeon who stand for long hours, laryngocele common in trumpet blowers.

Place/address:
Certain conditions are found to be endemic to certain areas. Chronic pancreatitis is common in Kerala, gallstones/cholecystitis common in Bihar, thyroid swellings in hilly areas, Madura foot in Madurai, peptic diseases in south India.

Socioeconomic status:
Certain diseases like tuberculous lymphadenitis are common in lower socioeconomic status.

Chief complaints:
Should be noted in chronological order of occurrence. For example,
- Lump—1 month duration.
- Pain—1 week duration.
- Fever—2 days duration.

(*Symptoms*—are what patients complain; *Signs*—what the clinician elicits.)

History of present illness
- Mode of onset—gradual/sudden in onset. Swelling of gradual onset are benign/congenital; whereas those of sudden in onset are inflammatory/neoplastic.
- Progression of symptoms—slow (benign, chronic condition)/rapid (acute, malignant condition).
- Duration of illness—long (chronic conditions)/short (acute)
- History of pain—presence of pain suggests inflammatory process (boil, carbuncle). Painless swellings becoming painful

You can never get enough of what you don't really need—Eric Hoffer

suggest secondary infection, malignant transformation, infiltration of malignancy into underlying nerves.
- Factors aggravating/relieving the complaints, e.g. pain in gastric ulcer is aggravated by food whereas pain in duodenal ulcer is relieved by food.
- Associated constitutional symptoms like fever (low grade/high grade suggestive of inflammatory condition); vomiting; decreased appetite, altered bowel habits, loss of weight, anorexia, diarrhea.

Past history:
History of illness in the past like diabetes, tuberculosis, syphilis and treatment received for it. They may or may not be related to the current illness.

Personal history:
It includes detail history of personal habbits like cigarette smoking with its duration, number of packs smoked per day, as smoking is one of the important etiological factors for various carcinomas. History of tobacco chewing/paan chewing is important in oral carcinoma. History of alcohol is also very important. Enquiry about diet has to be done whether vegetarian/non-vegetarian. History of sleep disturbances is also important.

Menstrual history:
Should be noted in detail in all women which includes age of menarche, menstrual irregularities, vaginal discharge, postmenopausal bleeding, etc.

Family history:
Certain conditions like diabetes, atherosclerosis, hypertension, are familial. Certain malignancies like medullary carcinoma thyroid, colonic and breast malignancies are familial.

Treatment history:
Drugs taken for diabetes, hypertension, bronchial asthma, epilepsy, tuberculosis, oral anticoagulants should be noted. Any surgery in the past, hospitalization and blood transfusion should be noted.

General Physical Examination

- *General appearance:* Level of consciousness, cooperation, and comfortness is noted (Fig. 35.1).
- *Attitude:* It is the special posture of the body in lying/sitting position, e.g. patient with tuberculous cervical spine is found sitting with his hand supporting the chin; rigid neck in meningitis.
- *Build:* Normal/poor/well built based on height and weight of the patient. Built is poor in chronic malnutrition, uncontrolled diabetes, malignancies (Fig. 35.1).
- *Nourishment:* Normal/poor/well or over nourished based triceps skin fold thickness, subcutaneous fat, skin texture, muscle mass. Patients are poorly nourished in advanced malignancies (Figs. 35.2 and 35.3).
- *Gums:* Gums should be examined for epulis, nutritional deficiencies, ulcers, etc. (Fig. 35.4).
- *Anemia:* It is decrease in Hb%, manifests as pallor, looked in palpebral conjunctiva, nail beds, and tongue (Figs. 35.5A and B).

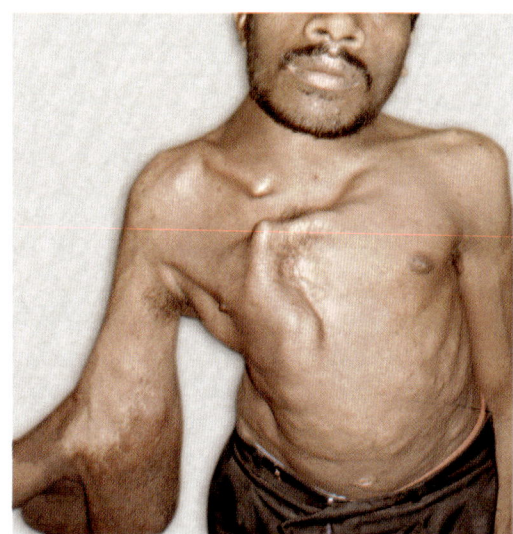

Fig. 35.1: Built, deformity should be looked for. Sternal deformity and plexiform neurofibroma over right forearm in this patient is obvious.

*I hear: I forget/I see: I remember/I do: I understand—***Chinese Proverb**

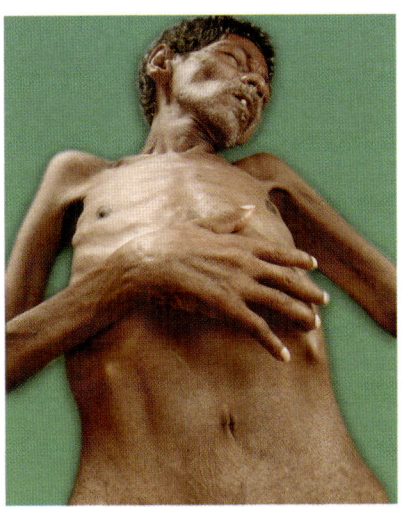

Fig. 35.2: Emaciated terminally ill patient.

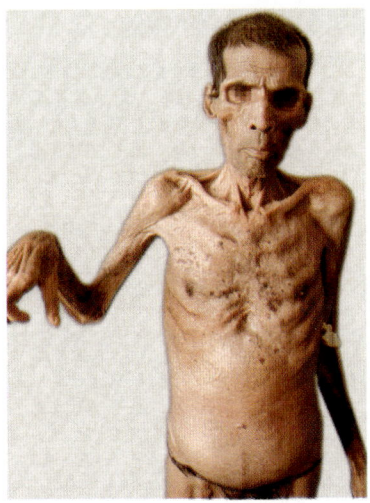

Fig. 35.3: Malignant cachexia.

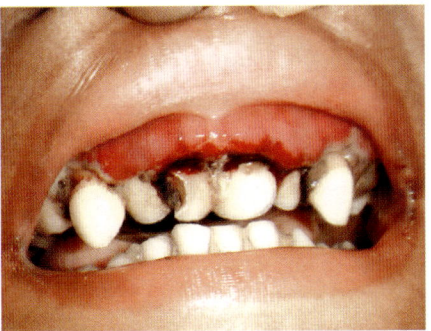

Fig. 35.4: Gum should be examined for epulis/nutritional deficiencies/ulcer/tumor.

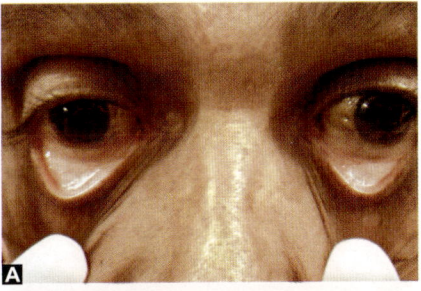

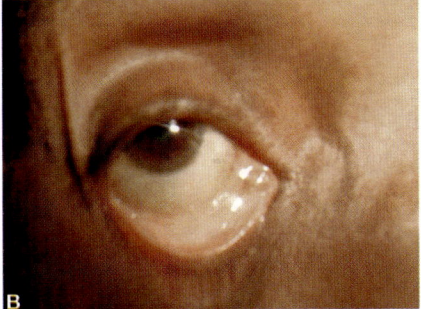

Figs 35.5A and B: Lower conjunctiva should be examined to check for anemia.

- *Icterus/jaundice:* Yellowish discoloration of skin and mucous membrane due to increase bilirubin level in blood (normal value is <1.2 mg %). It is looked for in upper sclera, nail bed, undersurface of tongue and palmar creases as bilirubin has high affinity for connective tissues which are abundant in these areas (Fig. 35.6).
- *Cyanosis:* It is bluish discoloration of skin and mucus membrane due to increased deoxyhemoglobin concentration in blood. It is looked for in fingers and nasal tips (peripheral cyanosis), tongue and lips (central cyanosis). It is due to circulatory/ventilator problem.
- *Clubbing:* It is bulbous enlargement of terminal phalanges of fingers and toes seen in cyanotic congenital heart disease, bronchiectasis, lung abscess, empyema, bronchogenic carcinoma, alcohol liver disease (Fig. 35.7).

*Never argue with a fool, onlookers may not be able to tell the difference—**Mark Twain***

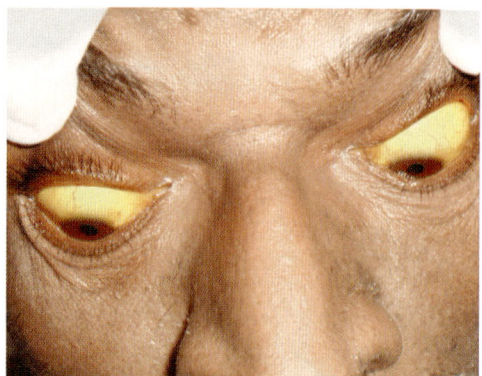

Fig. 35.6: Jaundice—severe probably obstructive in this patient.

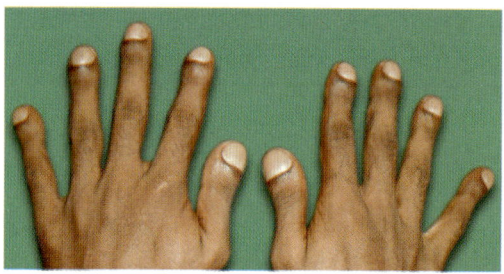

Fig. 35.7: Clubbing.

- *Edema:*
  - *Pedal edema:* It is checked by applying pressure with thumb over shin of the patient for 10–15 sec. Appearance of depression lasting for more than 30 sec is significant. Pedal edema is seen in cardiac failure, cirrhosis, nephrotic syndrome, protein-energy malnutrition, filariasis/lymphangitis (Figs. 35.8A to D).
  - *Upprt limb edema:* It can occur in filariasis, after modified radical mastectomy, axillary vein thrombosis (Fig. 35.9).
- *Pulse*—good indicator of cardiovascular system. Usually radial pulse is checked and counted for full 1 minute. The rate (normal 72/mt), rhythm (regular/irregular), volume, character are noted. Rate is increased in fever, thyrotoxicosis, exercise, shock, hemorrhage. Bilateral pulses are checked and peripheral pulses are also checked in vascular diseases.

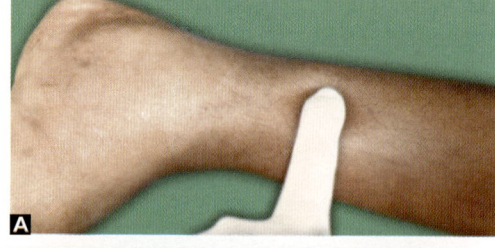
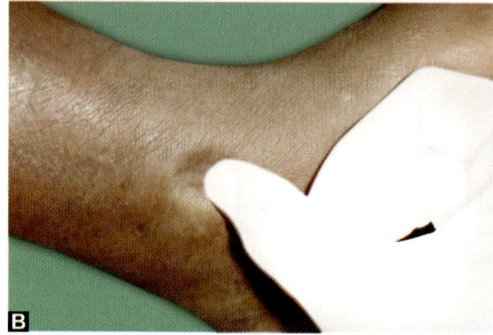
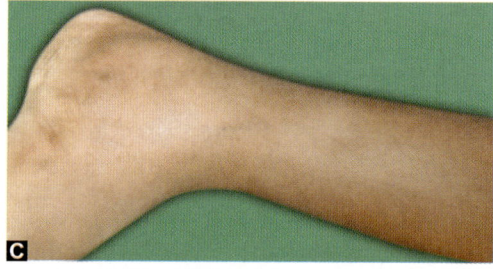
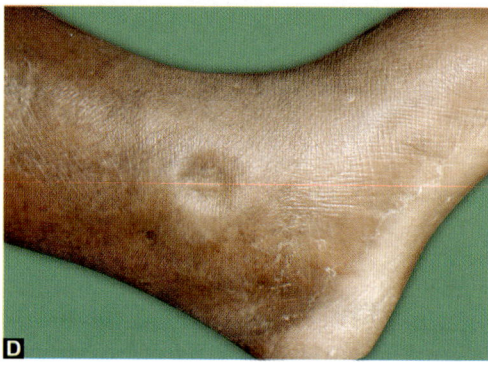

Figs. 35.8A to D: Edema foot—checked by pitting using finger over ankle region. Lymphedema is nonpitting.

- *Blood pressure*—normally checked on the left arm (normal—120/80 mm Hg). Hypertensive patients have to be identified, evaluated and treated.

*Logic will get you from A to B. Imagination will take you everywhere—**Albert Einstein***

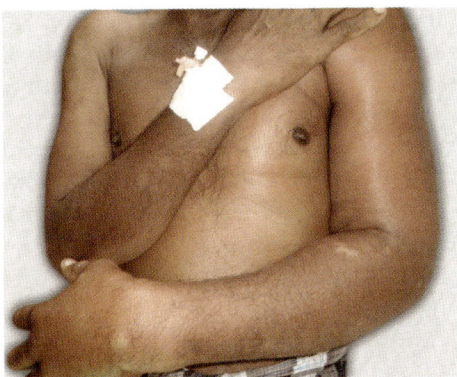

Fig. 35.9: Edema upper limb—could be lymphedema.

- *Temperature*—has to be recorded in the mouth or in the axilla (normal 37°C; raised in fever, thyotoxicosis). Fever may be low grade/high grade, continous/intermittent.
- *Respiration*—rate (normal 16–20/mt), type (abdominothoracic/thoracoabdominal) has to be noted. Rate is increased (tachypnea) fever, shock, hemorrhage etc. *Chynes-Stokes* breathing—alternating gradual overventilation and short periods of apnea.
- *Lymphadenopathy*—lymph nodes of neck, groin, axilla may be enlarged in inflammatory, tuberculous, neoplastic condition. Its number, consistency, tenderness, fixity are noted. They are soft, tender in inflammatory conditions; matted and firm in tuberculous; hard and fixed in malignant secondaries.
- *Skin* to be examined for purpura/rashes, etc. (Fig. 35.10).

Local Examination

- It is the examination of the affected area which has to be done in a quite closed room always in a presence of a nurse.
- The position of the patient for examination depends on the site of the pathology—standing position for varicose veins, inguinoscrotal swellings; sitting for thyroid, breast, head and neck swellings, oral cavity; supine for abdominal pathology, prone for pathology in the back.

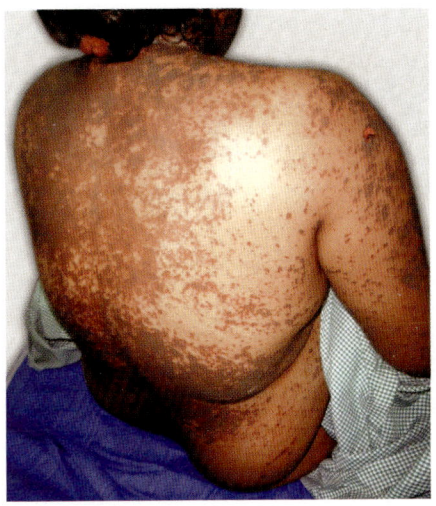

Fig. 35.10: Purpuric rashes all over the body.

The local examination follows the following order:

Inspection → palpation → percussion → auscultation.

- **Inspection:**
  With proper exposure and good light the diseased part is looked properly for the exact site, size, side, number of lesions, discharge if any, redness, visible pulsation, prominent veins, simultaneously comparing with the normal side.
- **Palpation:**
  All inspectory findings are confirmed by the palpation, which has to be gentle, done with the palmar aspect of the examiners hand giving reassurance to the patient. Sizes, surface, consistency, mobility, raised temperature, tenderness are some of the clinical aspects well appreciated with palpation.
- **Percussion:**
  It is carried out in inguinoscrotal lesions, abdominal conditions, neck and thyroid lesions; helps to differentiate gas containing organs (intestines, lungs) and collected free gas and free fluid (ascites, pleural effusion); to detect free fluid in the abdominal cavity (Figs. 35.11 and 35.12).

*Judge your success by what you had to give up in order getting it—**Dalai Lama***

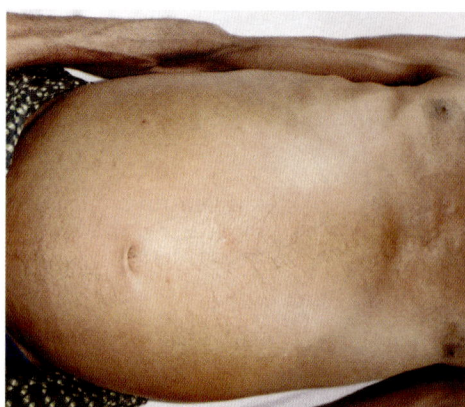

Fig. 35.11: Ascites. It could be due to hepatic, nutritional, renal or neoplastic causes.

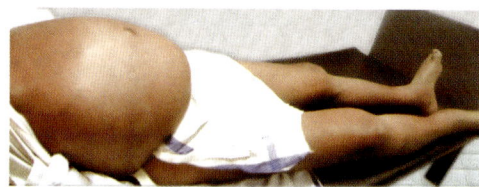

Fig. 35.12: Anasarca.

- ❖ **Auscultation:**
  With the stethoscope auscultate for the bruit (over the thyroid swelling) which is suggestive of increased vascularity, intestinal movement sound in inguinoscrotal lesions; over the trachea for air entry.
- ❖ **Measurements:**
  Measurements of the extremities (both length and girth) to identify wasting.
- ❖ **Movements:**
  Movements (active/passive) of limbs are checked in lesions over the limbs.
- ❖ **Examination of relevant parts:**
  Oral cavity— neck; chest—axilla and neck; abdomen—groin, scrotum perineum, lower chest, spine; hand and foot—groin and axilla.

Systemic Examination

- ❖ **Cardiovascular system**—for heart sounds, murmurs (due to anemia, valvular diseases, thyotoxicosis).
- ❖ **Respiratory system**—air entry in all lung fields, for adventitious sounds like rhonchi (bronchial asthma), crepitation (bronciectasis, lung abscess).
- ❖ **Abdominal examination**—for organomegaly (liver, spleen enlargement seen in malignancies, infections), for free fluid (ascites/hemorrhage).
- ❖ **Skeletal system** (for congenital deformities, pathological fractures).
- ❖ **Genitourinary system**.
- ❖ **CNS** (cranial nerves, muscle power).
- ❖ **Spine**—tenderness, deformity (kyphosis/gibbus).

Clinical Diagnosis

- ❖ After all these laborious procedure, it is essential to come to a clinical diagnosis which will help in going into further line of management.
- ❖ In order to come to a clinical diagnosis first ascertain the tissue of origin (anatomical)—lymph nodes, salivary glands, etc.
- ❖ Next, type of pathological process—congenital, inflammatory (acute/chronic), neoplastic (benign/malignant), traumatic, degenerative, metabolic, endocrinal.
- ❖ Pathological process may be in single or multiple sites—multiple matted lymph nodes in the neck suggests tuberculous lymphadenitis; nonhealing ulcer in the mouth with firm to hard lymph node swellings suggests oral cancer with lymph node secondaries.
- ❖ Based on all the clinical findings the most commonly occurring condition is thought of as the *provisional diagnosis*. If there is any confusion or doubt then other probable diagnosis are thought of (*differential diagnosis*).

Investigations

It is done to ascertain the diagnosis; to know the extent of pathological process; to know the fitness of the patient for surgery if needed.

*Choose a job you love and you'll never have to work a day in your life—***Confucius**

- *Blood*—Hb% (to look for anemia), total leukocyte count (raised in infection), erythrocyte sedimentation rate (ESR) (raised in tuberculosis, malignancy), blood urea and serum creatinine (renal function), liver function test (LFT) (bilirubin, liver enzymes), bleeding time and clotting time, platelet count and prothrombin time (PT-INR) (to rule out bleeding diathesis), blood sugar (fasting and post-prandial), thyroid function test.
- *Urine*—routine analysis and microscopy.
- *Stool*—ova cyst and occult blood.
- *Imaging*:
  - Chest X-ray—consolidation, opacity, effusion.
  - Bone X-ray—fracture, deformity.
  - Doppler imaging—blood flow.
  - Ultrasound—thyroid and neck swelling, abdomen.
  - CT scan.
  - MRI—joints and spine.
- Cytological/tissue diagnosis: Fine needle aspiration cytology (FNAC)/excision/incision biopsy/USG-CT guided biopsy.

With the help of all the above investigations along with the clinical findings we will be able to come to a *clinical diagnosis* of the disease.

CLINICAL EXAMINATION OF SINUS OR FISTULA

History of Present Illness

Mode of onset—congenital, present since birth (pre-auricular sinus) or later in life; history of fever, swelling following discharging sinus in osteomyelitis of mandible.

History of pain, fever, redness—suggest inflammatory origin.

Past History

History of tuberculous lymphadenitis, oral carcinoma being treated or on treatment.

Local Examination

Inspection

Site:
Helps in clinching the diagnosis.
- Branchial fistulae—anterior border of lower 1/3rd of sternomastoid.
- Parotid fistula—in parotid region.
- Thyroglossal fistulae—midline of neck below hyoid bone.
- Pre-auricular sinus—directed upwards and backwards, situated at the root of the helix.
- Median mental sinus—symphysis menti.
- Tuberculous sinus—neck.

Number:
It may be single or multiple (actinomycosis).

Opening:
- Wide and thin blue undermined margin—tuberculous.
- Sprouting granulation tissue—suggests foreign body underneath (sequestrum, foreign body).

Discharge:
- Tuberculous—serosanguinous/white thin caseous.
- Osteomyelitis—purulent pus.
- Actinomycosis—yellow sulphur granules.
- Branchial fistula—thin mucus discharge.
- Fecal fistula—fecal discharge (Fig. 35.13).
- Parotid fistula—thin watery.

Surrounding skin (Figs. 35.14 and 35.15):
- Red inflamed—in acute osteomyelitis.
- Scarred with pigmentation—tuberculous, chronic osteomyelitis, actinomycosis.

Palpation
- *Temperature* is raised and *tenderness* is seen in sinuses of acute osteomyelitis.
- *Discharge* if not seen can be pressed out by palpation and the nature should be noted.
- *Wall of the sinus* is palpated for thickening suggestive of chronic infection.
- *Mobility* is checked, in chronic osteomyelitis sinus is fixed to the bone.

You can learn a lot from people who view the world differently than you do—**Anthony J D'Angelo**

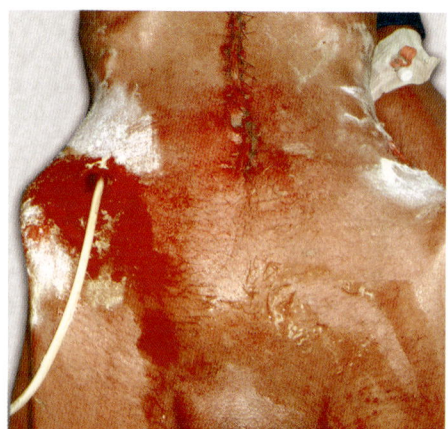

Fig. 35.13: Fecal fistula.

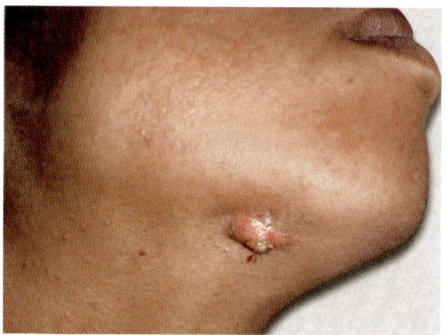

Fig. 35.14: Discharging sinus in the neck; could be nonspecific due to dental sepsis or tuberculosis.

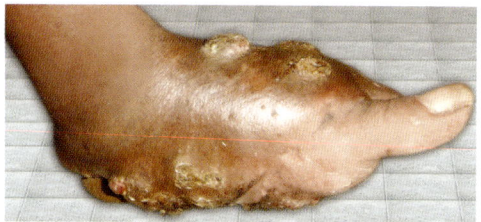

Fig. 35.15: Madura foot showing multiple discharging sinus foot.

* *Palpation of the underlying tissue*—thickening in chronic osteomyelitis; matted, enlarged lymph nodes in tuberculous lymphadenitis.
* *Palpation of regional lymph nodes*—firm and mobile—chronic infection; matted—tuberculous; hard and fixed in malignancy.

Other Relevant Local Examination
* Oral cavity—submental sinus, oral malignancy.
* Adjoining bone—osteomyelitis.
* Submandibular gland—bidigital examination.

Systemic Examination
Respiratory system; abdomen; spine.

Specific Investigation
* Fistulography/sinusography (injecting radiopaque fluid—lipiodol, hypaque)—helps to know the direction of the tract.
* X-ray of the adjoining bone for osteomyelitis.
* Biopsy from the edge of the sinus—for malignancy, tuberculosis.
* Discharge study—cytology, microscopy (Ziehl-Neelsen for acid-fast bacilli (AFB) and Gram staining).

EXAMINATION OF AN ULCER

HISTORY

Name:

Sex:

Age:
Certain diseases or ulcers may more common in certain age groups.

Occupation:
Venous ulcers are more common in individuals whose occupation requires long hours of standing like nurses, surgeons, traffic policemen, watchmen and bus conductors.

Place:

Chief complaints:
History of ulcer and its duration should be mentioned. History of specific condition related also should be mentioned.

History of Present Illness

Mode of onset and progression:
It is the initial way of formation of an ulcer. It may be after an attack of cellulitis of the part, or

You must first get along with yourself before you can get along with others—**Anthony J D'Angelo**

after trauma which breaks the continuity or due to any cause. Common cause of ulcer is trauma. Traumatic ulcer may heal fast or may progress to chronicity if it lies on a joint or due to improper rest to the part or if patient is diabetic or due to any other precipitating causes. Even minor trauma can cause extensive necrotizing fasciitis and ulcer later. Often patient will be having the idea of the cause of ulcer.

Tuberculous lymphadenitis leading into collar stud abscess eventually may form a fistula or an ulcer.

Ulcerative lesion may be rodent ulcer, carcinomatous ulcer or melanotic ulcer originating spontaneously.

Syphilis may lead into gummatous ulcer.

Venous ulcer may occur as a result of varicose veins; ischemic ulcer due to arterial insufficiency.

Regression or progression of an ulcer formed in specific method is important. Ulcer may often heal spontaneously and reform later repeatedly in the same site, e.g. formation of an ulcer in a pre-existing burn scar or formation of venous ulcer repetitively around ankle. Here ulcer heals by rest and reforms by trauma or other precipitating causes.

Duration:
Ulcer may be of long duration like in chronic venous ulcer or of short duration like in acute ulcer after trauma or cellulitis.

Pain:
Ulcer may be painful or painless. Often malignant ulcers are painless to begin with but may eventually become painful due to secondary bacterial infection or infiltration to deeper plane or nerve ending. Painful acute ulcer becomes painless once it turns to chronicity. Its time of onset, progress, and severity should be asked. Trophic ulcers, syphilitic ulcer, ulcers of neurological diseases like spinal injury/spinal diseases/peripheral neuropathy/tabes dorsalis are painless. Pain may interfere with patient's daily routine activities like walking, eating, bathing, defecation, etc. Tuberculous ulcer is usually painful.

History of fever:
Presence of fever signifies existing acute inflammation in an ulcer or in surrounding area.

Discharge from ulcer:
Presence and type of discharge is significant. Discharge can be assessed by looking at dressing pads also. Discharge may be profuse, scanty or absent. Color and smell of discharge, whether discharge is serous or purulent and if greenish it may be due to *Pseudomonas* bacterial infection.

Number of ulcers:
Often ulcers are multiple. If it is so, which ulcer developed first and which one later should be asked.

Associated symptoms:
History of presence of varicose veins; claudication, rest pain of arterial insufficiency should be asked for.

Past History

Past history of ulcer treated by dressing/drugs/skin grafting/hospital stay should be asked in detail. Number of days hospitalized, time taken up for healing of the ulcer should be noted. Previous history of treatment for tuberculosis, syphilis, diabetes or any other illness is important.

History suggestive of associated disease/treatment history like tuberculosis, tabes dorsalis, spinal diseases or diabetes mellitus. If patient is on treatment for any of such ailment, type of drugs taken, dose and method of intake should be asked.

Personal History

History of alcohol consumption/smoking/tobacco chewing/history of sexual contact/dietary habits are also important. Duration of such habits, quantity are also important. It has got direct relation to ulcer formation or ulcer healing or treatment strategy. *Altered appetite or weight loss* can also be mentioned under personal history—may be due to advanced malignancy or tuberculosis.

The weak can never forgive. Forgiveness is an attribute of the strong

Family History

Family history of any specific disease should be asked.

LOCAL EXAMINATION OF AN ULCER

Inspection (Fig. 35.16)

Inspection of an ulcer is done after taking and documenting detailed history. Lesion is inspected after proper exposing the area.

Site

If ulcer is on the toes, fingers or distal aspect of the foot, it could be ischemic or diabetic ulcer.

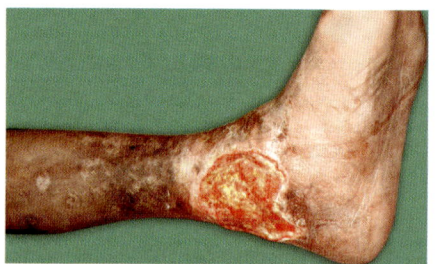

Fig. 35.16: Ulcer should be inspected for all features—location, edge, margin, and surrounding area.

If the ulcer is over medial malleolus, it is venous ulcer due to long saphenous vein varicosity. If it is over lateral malleolus, it is venous ulcer due to short saphenous vein varicosity.

Floor (Fig. 35.17)

Inspect the floor of an ulcer. Floor of an ulcer is the part, which is seen. Floor may contain *discharge* which may be blood, serous fluid, pus, and caseation material. It may be covered with slough, pale granulation tissue or healthy pink granulation tissue. It may be pigmented like in melanoma or covered with *wash-leather slough* like in syphilitic ulcer.

Margin

It is at the junction of edge and normal skin or mucosa. It may be well or ill defined or may be regular or irregular.

Edge

Edge is between floor and the margin. Sloping edge is seen in healing ulcer; undermined in tuberculous ulcer; raised and everted in squamous cell carcinomatous ulcer (epithelioma); punched out edge in trophic ulcer; raised and beaded in rodent ulcer (basal cell carcinoma).

Surrounding Area

Surrounding area should be inspected for redness, edema, pigmentation, ischemic features and for scars.

Palpation

Temperature

It may be warm or cold over the lesion. Surrounding area should be checked using back of the hand and should be compared to normal area.

Tenderness (Fig. 35.18)

Its location, severity and extent should be assessed.

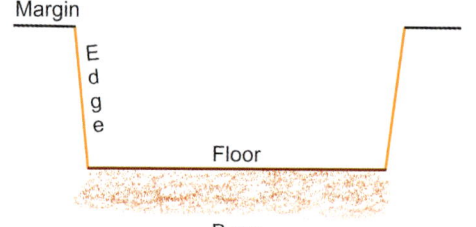

Fig. 35.17: Pathological anatomy of an ulcer—floor; edge; margin; base.

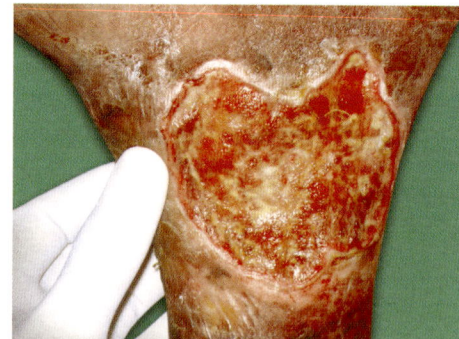

Fig. 35.18: Tenderness should be checked for in the edge and surrounding area.

*Children must be taught how to think, not what to think—**Margaret Mead***

Mobility of the Ulcer (Fig. 35.19)

It should be checked in two directions. If mobile, then it is superficial or easy to treat. If nonmobile base is formed by bone and it is difficult to treat.

Edge of the Ulcer (Fig. 35.20)

It is tender or not/*indurated* or not/friable or not. Induration is seen in epithelioma ulcer (squamous cell carcinoma). Friability is observed in malignancy or in acute inflammation.

Base of the Ulcer

It is one where ulcer rests on. Base may be bone, muscles or soft tissues. It is checked by mobility of the ulcer and also by contracting the muscle/tendon underneath. Base is also palpated for *induration*.

Bleeding on Palpation

It signifies either carcinoma or healthy granulation tissue.

Surrounding Area (Fig. 35.21)

Induration and tenderness in surrounding area should be checked for.

Bone thickening is looked for by running finger over the bone. It is an evidence of periostitis.

Palpation of Peripheral Pulses

Palpation of peripheral pulses like dorsalis pedis artery, posterior tibial artery should be done which gives the idea about the wound healing.

Sensation of the Part

Sensation of the part like vibration, sense of position, touch should be checked in order.

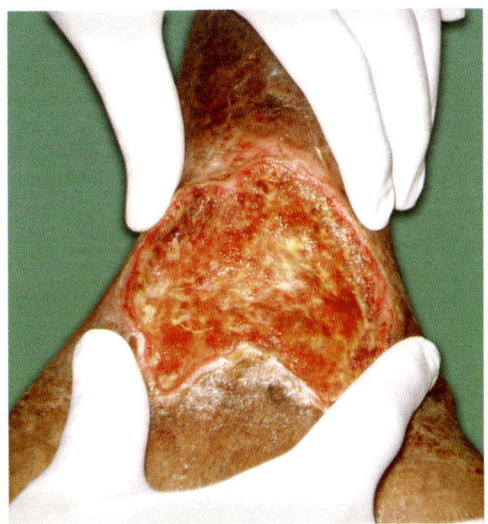

Fig. 35.19: Ulcer mobility should be checked—to find out base and fixity.

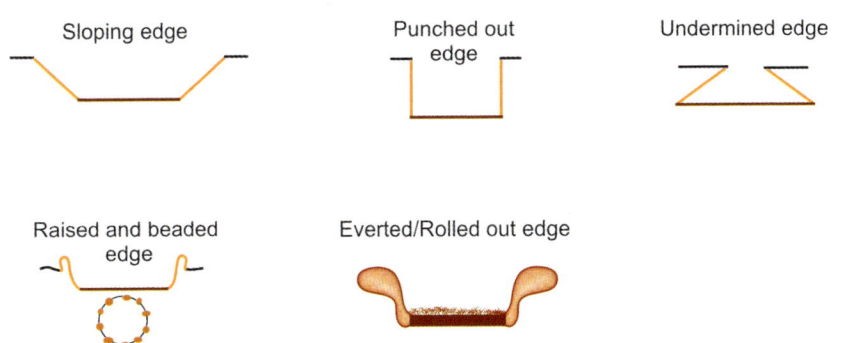

Fig. 35.20: Different edges observed in ulcers due to different conditions.

---

*Life is like riding a bicycle. In order to keep your balance, you must keep moving—***Albert Einstein**

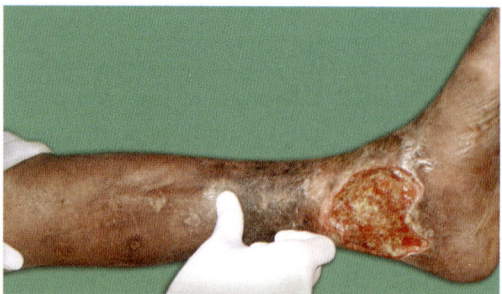

Fig. 35.21: Bone thickening should be checked—as evidence of periostitis.

Joint Movements (Fig. 35.22)

Joint movements are assessed. Plantar and dorsiflexion for ankle joint, inversion and eversion for subtalar joint is checked.

Regional Lymph Nodes (Fig. 35.23)

Regional lymph nodes like in groin (inguinal node vertical/horizontal group), axilla or neck depending on the location of primary lesion should be examined. Tender node is observed in inflammatory condition, nontender hard node in malignancy, and matted nodes in tuberculosis.

Other Examinations

Look for varicose veins or other relevant findings in relation to the ulcer.

Relevant Systemic Examinations

Systemic examinations like of abdomen, respiratory system or cardiovascular system should be done.

EXAMINATION OF A SWELLING/LUMP

Swelling/lump denotes enlargement or protuberance in the any part of the body due to congenital/inflammatory/traumatic or neoplastic causes.

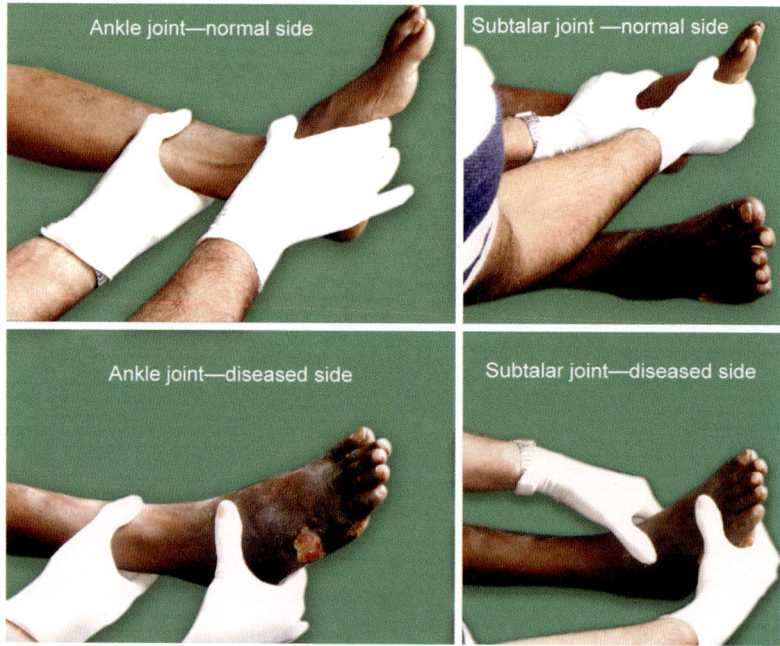

Fig. 35.22: Joints adjacent to the ulcer should be examined for both active and passive movements. Ankle and subtalar joints are examined in this patient.

*In the end, it's not the years in your life that count. It's the life in your years—**Abraham Lincoln***

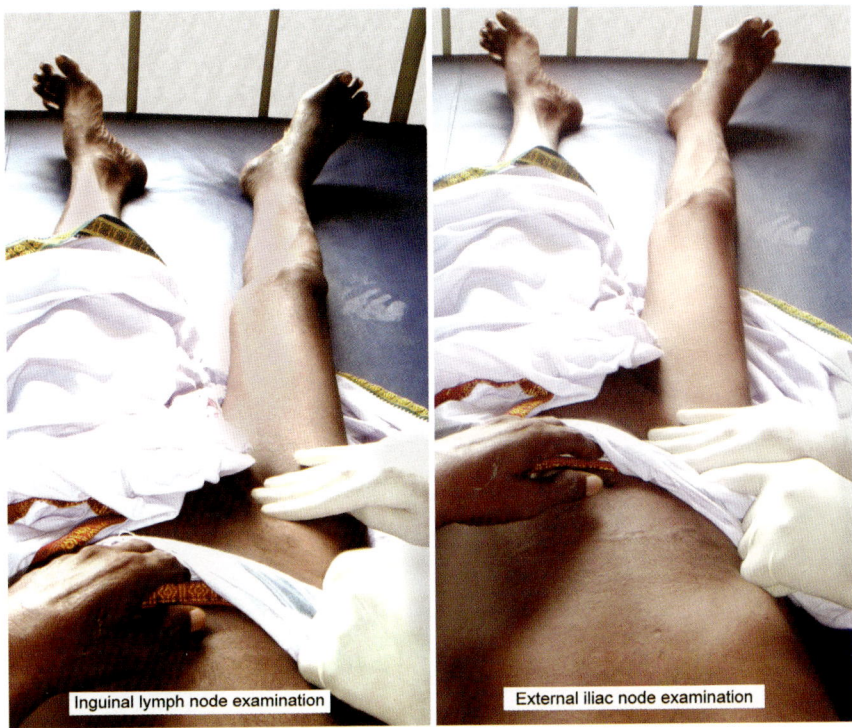

Fig. 35.23: Regional nodes should be examined in an ulcer patient.

HISTORY

History of Present Illness

* **Duration:**
  – Duration of swelling is important in all swellings. Swelling which is present since birth could be congenital like meningocele.
  – Swelling of short duration with pain may be inflammatory. Benign tumors are usually painless of long duration swelling.
  – Malignant tumors are of short duration, rapidly enlarging, initially painless (but can be painful later).
* **Mode of onset:**
  – Swelling whether started after trauma or spontaneously.
  – *Rapid progress or slow in progress*— malignant swelling progresses rapidly whereas benign swellings progress slowly.
  – Whether painful or not.
* *Pain:*
  – When pain started? Location of pain/ type of pain/severity/whether it interferes with work or not.
  – Inflammatory conditions are painful whereas malignant conditions are painless to begin with but later it becomes painful.
* *Presence of fever:*
  – Fever may be present in inflammatory conditions. Certain malignancies also can present with fever at later stage like in Hodgkin's lymphoma or renal cell carcinoma.
* *Presence of other lumps:*
  – Presence of other lumps/secondary changes in the swelling like ulceration/ fungation.
* History of previous surgery.
* Loss of function of part or as a whole.

*Children are the living messages we send to a time we will not see—**John F Kennedy***

Personal History

- *Loss of weight and decreased appetite:* It may signify that swelling is related to malignant condition and also probably advanced.
- History of alcohol consumption/smoking/tobacco chewing/history of sexual contact/dietary habits are also important.

Family History

Family history suggestive of similar swellings is important. Neurofibromatosis is often familial.

GENERAL EXAMINATION

Detailed general examination is a must. Anemia/edema/jaundice/clubbing/lymphadenopathy/radial pulse/blood pressure/raise in temperature/attitude of the patient/nutritional assessment by skin texture, subcutaneous fat, weight, body mass index/any other relevant findings should be mentioned.

LOCAL EXAMINATION

Inspection (Fig. 35.24)

- Location of the swelling
  - Exact anatomical location of the swelling/its size/shape should be noted—globular or hemispherical or oval or pear-shaped or irregular or kidney shaped/diffuse or well localized.
  - Vertical and horizontal dimension should be assessed and should be measured using a measuring tape.
  - Dermoid cysts occur in midline/outer canthus of eye/or along any line of embryonic fusion. Lipoma can occur anywhere in the body.
- Color of the swelling
  - Blue color of hemangioma/black color of nevus or melanoma/blue color of ranula are often diagnostic.
  - Redness over the swelling suggests inflammation.

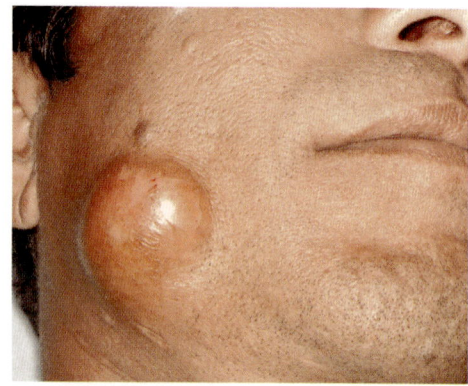

Fig. 35.24: Sebaceous cyst face.

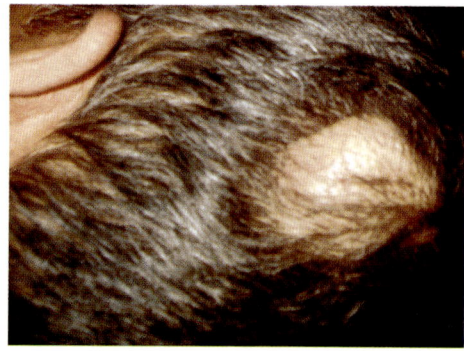

Fig. 35.25: Sebaceous cyst scalp. Note the loss of hair over the swelling.

- Surface over swelling (Fig. 35.25)
  - Smooth/irregular/nodular/cauliflower like.
- Number of the swellings
  - Neurofibromas and sebaceous cysts can be multiple. Dermoid cyst is usually single.
- Edge of the swelling
  - It may be well-defined or ill-defined/pedunculated or sessile should be looked for.
- Pulsation over the swelling
  - Arterial swelling has got *expansile pulsation*. It is checked by keeping two fingers over the swelling.
  - Swelling which is very close to artery or adherent to it also can show pulsation but it is transmitted pulsation.

Children find everything in nothing; men find nothing in everything—**Giacomo Leopardi**

- Reducibility
  - Whether swelling gets reduced while pressing and disappears. Hernia is reducible.
- Presence of expansile impulse
  - Presence of expansile impulse on coughing signifies hernia or communication into the deeper cavity like abdomen or thorax or cranium.
- Skin over the swelling should be inspected.
  - Skin over the swelling may be tense, glossy with prominent veins in sarcoma and malignancy.
  - It is red edematous in inflammatory swellings.
  - Pigmentation, ulceration/fungation/discharge from ulcer/bleeding from the fungation should be inspected.
  - Scar—its size, features whether healed by primary intention or secondary intention should be mentioned. Linear and regular/broad, puckered and irregular.
- Inspect the area and distally
  - Inspect the local area and distally especially when swelling is in the limbs for pressure effects and wasting.
  - Wasting should be confirmed by proper measurement of the part comparing with the corresponding part of the opposite limb, from equal distance from a bony point.

Palpation

- Local raise of temperature
  - It is checked using back of fingers. It may be due to inflammation (infection) or due to tumors.
- Tenderness
  - It is checked while palpating the swelling by observing the face of the patient.
  - Patient expresses the tenderness. Inflammatory conditions are tender.
  - Neoplastic conditions are initially nontender but later can become tender.
- Size
  - It is measured using tape (vertical × horizontal in cm); shape is confirmed and extent of the entire swelling and its anatomical location should be mentioned properly.
- Edge or margin of the swelling
  - It can be well-defined (distinct) or ill-defined (indistinct). In acute conditions and deep swellings it is ill-defined.
  - In superficial swellings it is well-defined. Margin may be irregular in malignancy and may be regular in benign swellings.
  - Edge of the swelling is examined using pulp of the index finger.
  - Erosion of the margin into the deeper plane like bone is also should be checked. Dermoid cyst commonly shows erosion into the underlying bone.
  - In lipoma margin slips away from the finger—*slip sign*.
  - In sebaceous cyst margin gets yielded by the finger.
- Surface of the swelling
  - It is done using palmar surface of the fingers.
  - It may be smooth like in a cyst/nodular in lymph nodes/lobular in lipoma/matted in tuberculous nodes/irregular in carcinoma.
  - It may be variable and if so should be mentioned *which part is smooth and which part is nodular*.
- Consistency
  - It may be soft (like consistency of lip)/may be firm (like consistency of nose)/may be hard (like consistency of forehead).
  - Lipoma, cystic swellings, abscess are soft.
  - Fibromas, neurofibromas, certain nodal enlargements are firm.
  - Chondroma, osteomas are bony hard. Malignant swellings are stony hard.
  - Variable consistency in one swelling may be observed. In such occasion

*Anything is possible when you have the right people there to support you—**Misty Copeland***

which area is soft, which area is firm or hard should be confirmed properly. Variability may be due to tumor necrosis/inflammation.
  – Swelling like sebaceous cyst or dermoid cyst which contains pultaceous material or putty like material gets *moulded by the palpating fingers.*
❖ Fluctuation
  – Swelling is fixed usually by holding both thumbs and middle fingers. With the index finger of one hand one side of the swelling is pressed and the index finger of other hand placed diagonally on the opposite side feels fluid movement and also a raise. Procedure should be done in perpendicular direction to confirm fluctuation (two right angle planes). This is **standard fluctuation**. Positive fluctuation signifies presence of fluid. Examples are hydrocele, cysts, etc. (*Note:* Often muscle gives fluctuation like feeling when elicited in one direction but not in two perpendicular directions).
  – In a swelling which cannot accommodate two fingers to do standard fluctuation test, margin of the swelling is fixed using two fingers (index and ring) and using middle finger summit/center of the swelling is pressed/indented to feel displacement of the fluid/yielding sensation. This test is called as **Paget's test** of fluctuation (Figs. 35.26A and B).
  – Fluctuation may be present in a cystic swelling which contains fluid with two components on either sides of an anatomical barrier (across an anatomical barrier). It is called as **cross fluctuation**. Ranula (across mylohyoid muscle), psoas abscess (across inguinal ligament), compound palmar ganglion (across flexor retinaculum), bilocular hydrocele (across a band or superficial inguinal ring) are cross-fluctuant.

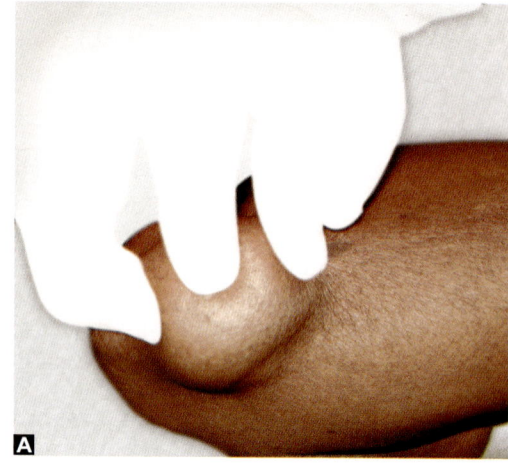
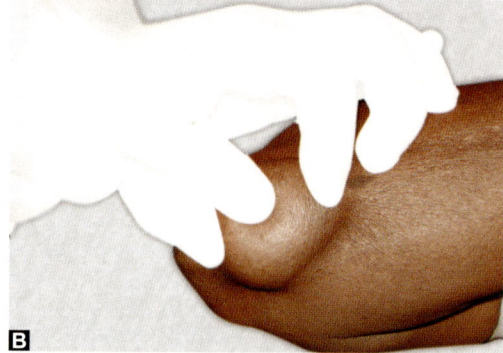

Figs. 35.26A and B: Paget's test is done for a small swelling to elicit fluctuation.

  – False fluctuation may be elicited in lipoma, myxoma and vascular swellings.
❖ Transillumination test
  – When light is illuminated over the swelling it transmits light through it. It is called as *transillumination/translucency*. It is positive means swelling illuminates to light. It means it contains clear fluid. It is negative when it contains blood, pus, pultaceous material. Torch light is placed on one side of the swelling and illumination is observed on the diagonally opposite side using a rolled paper or rolled X-ray sheath.
  – Lymph cyst, cystic hygroma, ranula, meningocele, hydrocele are transilluminant.

*Share your smile with the world. It's a symbol of friendship and peace—****Christie Brinkley***

- Reducibility
  - Swelling is pressed to get reduced completely and disappears. Hernia is a reducible swelling.
- Compressibility
  - Swelling on pressure reduces in size *only partially and will not disappear completely* and on releasing the pressure swelling again *comes back to its original size and shape immediately*. Usually vascular and lymphatic swellings are compressible. Example—hemangioma, lymphangioma.
- Pulsatility
  - Two fingers are placed over the swelling with adequate gap between two fingers. If fingers over the swelling are raised and separated with each beat of the artery it means pulsation is *expansile*.
  - If fingers are only raised but not separated from each other then pulsation of the swelling is *transmitted*.
  - Pure arterial swelling like aneurysm shows expansile pulsation. Swelling which is close to the artery because of its close proximity may show pulsation and it is only transmitted pulsation.
- Fixity to the skin (Fig. 35.27)
  - Mobility of the skin over the swelling is checked or skin over the swelling is pinched to confirm whether skin is free or attached to swelling underneath.
  - Sebaceous cyst is having adherent skin over the summit with a punctum which (70%) often may be present.
  - In dermoid cyst skin is always free. In lipoma usually skin is free. In neurofibromas skin may be adherent, depends on from which nerves the neurofibroma arises whether from deeper plane or from cutaneous nerves.
- Fixity to deeper structures (Fig. 35.28)
  - If swelling is freely mobile it could be in subcutaneous plane. Lipoma, sebaceous cyst, often neurofibroma are subcutaneous.

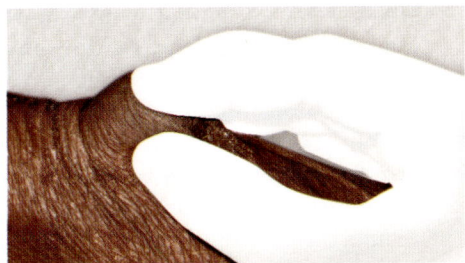
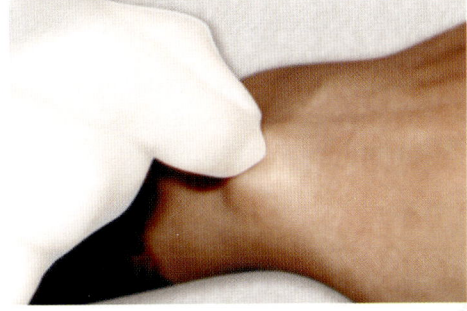

Fig. 35.27: Skin over the swelling should be pinched/held to check swelling is adherent to skin or not.

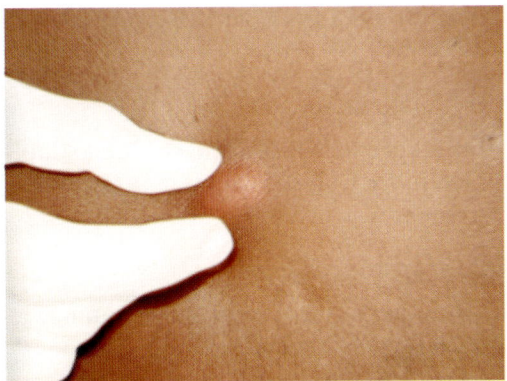

Fig. 35.28: Mobility of swelling should be checked to find out the plane of the swelling.

  - If swelling is adherent to the muscle underneath, its mobility is restricted when muscle is contracted against resistance but becomes more prominent. While muscle is relaxed swelling will be mobile.
  - If swelling is arising from the muscle or deep to muscle then size of the swelling decreases (less prominent) when muscle is contracted. Again mobility

A friend is one who overlooks your broken fence and admires the flowers in your garden

which is present initially will disappear completely during contraction of the muscle. Disappearance occurs much more significantly in swelling which is deeper to the muscle.
- Swellings arising from vessels or nerves will move only horizontally; in perpendicular direction to the line of nerve but will not show any mobility in longitudinal direction. Example—neurofibroma, aneurysm.
- Swelling arising from the bone is hard and absolutely fixed and cannot be moved separately from the bone.

Percussion

Percussion over the swelling in relevant area like hernia should be done.

Auscultation

It is done to look for bruit over the swelling like in AV malformation, arterial stenosis, aneurysms.

Joint Examination

Joints above and below the swelling should be examined both for active and passive movements.

Regional Lymph Nodes

Regional lymph nodes should be examined for significant enlargement.

Relevant Systemic Examination

Relevant systemic examination is very essential like respiratory, cardiac, skeletal and abdominal systems.
Proper diagnosis of the swelling should be given.

Relevant Investigations

FNAC, US of part, CT scan, MRI for bony and joint swellings, angiography and Doppler in vascular swellings, biopsy in soft tissue sarcomas.

Note:
- Swelling may be congenital/traumatic/inflammatory/neoplastic.
- It may be benign or malignant.
- In malignancy it may be early or advanced.

EXAMINATION IN ARTERIAL DISEASE (ARTERIAL SYSTEM)

Arterial diseases occur commonly in lower limb also occasionally in upper limb. Often both lower and upper limbs may get involved.

It is often classified as lower limb ischemia and upper limb ischemia. But wherever is the disease detailed examination of both lower limb and upper limb vessels is required in all patients.

Name:
Age:
Sex:
Occupation:
Address:

Atherosclerosis occurs in old age usually. Thromboangiitis obliterans (Buerger's disease) occurs in young males. Raynaud's disease is common in young/middle aged females.

Chief Complaints

- Pain in the limb right/left/both—its duration.
- Intermittent claudication—its duration.
- Blackish discoloration/ulceration.

HISTORY

History of Present Illness

- Pain
  - Site of pain, type of pain—severe burning/aching/deep persisting.
  - Whether pain radiates or not.
  - Presence of rest pain—its location/severity/whether patient has to hold the limb/foot/leg/toes to relieve pain little bit (probably by transmission of

*Try to be a rainbow in someone's cloud—***Maya Angelou**

temperature from holding hand into the part) or to hang the leg down to relieve the pain or by applying warmth. Pain, discomfort, color changes when exposed to cold.
- Intermittent claudication
  - Its duration, grade/distance how much patient can walk/whether pain subsides after stopping walk or after continuous walk/whether patient is able to walk in spite of pain/change in the claudication distance eventually/site of claudication—foot/leg/thigh/buttock.
- Ulceration
  - Whether precipitated by trauma/spontaneous onset.
  - Pain in the ulcer/type/duration/aggravating or relieving factors.
  - Discharge—type-serous-purulent-bloody.
  - Progression.
- Gangrene
  - Site of gangrene/its onset/progression/duration/pain.
- History of difficulty in walking/altered gait.
- Mode of onset
  - In atherosclerosis/Buerger's disease process is spontaneous and gradual.
  - Gangrene due to embolism is sudden in onset, rapidly progressive.
- History of fever.
- History of impotence—its duration.
- History of tingling/numbness/weakness in the limbs.
- History of syncope/blackouts/loss of consciousness/blurred vision.
- History of chest pain/cough or cardiac related symptoms.
- History of abdominal pain/bloody diarrhea/abdominal angina.
- History of paresthesia over the skin.
- History suggestive of superficial thrombophlebitis like swelling/redness/pain along the line of superficial vein.

Past History and Treatment History
- Similar history earlier.
- History of drug intake earlier for similar conditions like vasodilators/drugs to increase the perfusion.
- History of earlier surgery like/sympathectomy/omentoplasty/their results or effects.

Personal History

History of smoking—beedi or cigarettes/duration/number per day/stopped now or continuing/since when stopped smoking.

Family History

Any family history suggestive of atherosclerosis or vascular diseases.

GENERAL EXAMINATION

- Pulse—rate/rhythm/character/condition of vessel wall.
- Blood pressure of both arms and if possible of both lower limbs.
- Attitude of the limbs.

LOCAL EXAMINATION

Inspection (Fig. 35.29)
- Inspect both lower limbs
  - Inspect both lower limbs keeping side by side as comparison is needed during clinical examination.
  - Inspect for any deformity of limbs.
- Change in color
  - It is very important sign of ischemia.
  - Color proximal to gangrene area/ischemic area (usually ischemic area is palor) is checked carefully.
  - It is black in established gangrene; pale and dry in ischemia, red and cyanosed in pregangrene.
- Gangrene
  - Gangrene of toe/toes/foot/leg—its extent, discharge from area, type of gangrene—

*Education is what remains after one has forgotten what one has learned in school—**Albert Einstein***

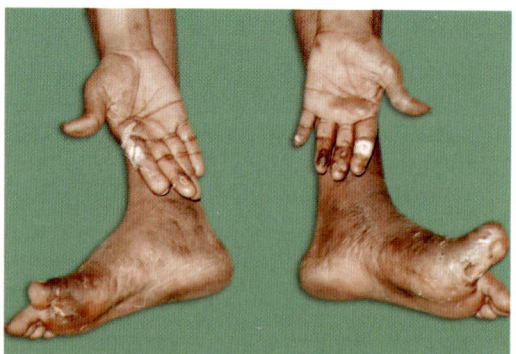

Fig. 35.29: Ischemia of all four limbs. Note the ischemic ulcers in fingers and toes.

dry or wet, line of demarcation—type/level/depth, color of gangrenous area—black/purple/greenish black (in gas gangrene) has to be checked.
- ❖ Ulceration
  - Ulceration when present—its extent/discharge/size/shape/floor/surrounding area is looked for.
  - Patchy ulcers proximal to gangrenous area—*skip lesions* which are usually black patchy lesions.
- ❖ Muscle wasting
  - Muscle wasting in the foot/leg/thigh should be observed.
  - It should be compared and also should be measured using a tape from a fixed bony point keeping equal distance in both limbs.
- ❖ Features of ischemia
  - Shiny thin skin/loss of subcutaneous fat/hair loss—its extent/nail changes—brittle nail/transverse ridges in the nail.
- ❖ Plantar aspect of the foot
  - Plantar aspect of the foot for infective focus/abscess/callosities/skin changes/superficial ulcers in heel/malleoli/toes.
- ❖ *Buerger's postural test*
  - Patient in supine position is asked to raise his legs one after other with knee kept straight. In normal limb, even after elevation to 90° limb remains pink without any pallor. Diseased limb after elevation shows marked pallor (over foot) with empty-guttered veins. The angle at which pallor develops (between limb and ground) is called as *Buerger's vascular angle of insufficiency.* In severe ischemia this angle will be less than 30°. If foot does not show pallor or when doubtful, then repeated ankle flexion and extension is done until pallor becomes evident with empty-guttered veins on the dorsum of foot. After lowering the foot cyanotic congestion appears in the foot.
- ❖ Edema in the foot/feet/legs.
- ❖ Status of the superficial veins
  - Normally filled veins or pale/discolored/guttered veins as seen in ischemic limb.
- ❖ *Capillary filling time*
  - Initially elevated limbs are made to hang down the bed. Limb will remain normal pink in elevated as well as in depressed position because of rapid capillary filling time. In ischemia, limb becomes pale on elevation and gradually becomes purple—red and then pink in more than 20 seconds. Purple pink color is due to deoxygenated blood. Prolonged capillary time signifies severe ischemia.
- ❖ *Venous refilling time*
  - Elevated limb when laid horizontal on the bed the normal venous refilling occurs within 5 seconds. It is delayed in ischemic limb.

Palpation
- ❖ Temperature of the skin
  - It is important factor in ischemic limb. Extent of cooling and proximally where exactly the limb/part become warmer also should be assessed.
- ❖ Tenderness
  - Site/extent/severity should be assessed.
- ❖ Gangrenous area
  - Gangrenous area is palpated for extent/whether it is dry and shriveled or whether it is wet and edematous.

Good friends are like stars. You don't always see them, but you know they're always there

- Presence or absence of crepitus in gangrenous should be checked.
- Limb above the gangrenous area should be palpated.
- *Capillary filling*
  - Tip of the nail or pulp of the finger or toe is pressed to blanch it and pressure is released to make it to become pink. Time taken for blanched area to turn pink is capillary filling time. It is prolonged in ischemic limb.
- *Harvey's venous refilling test*
  - Two fingers are placed over the vein. Pressure is elicited over the vein. Proximal finger is moved proximally for about 5 cm without releasing the pressure. Vein between the fingers gets emptied completely and becomes flat. Distal finger is released now to see the flow of the blood and its refilling is observed whether it is good or poor. It is poor in ischemic limb.
- *Elevated arm stress test (EAST)*
  - Both shoulders are abducted 90 degrees with arms fully externally rotated. Patient will open and close the hands rapidly for 5 minutes. Normal individual can do this without any discomfort and pain. Patient with thoracic outlet syndrome develops pain, fatigue, paresthesia of forearm with tingling and numbness of fingers. Patient will not be able to complete the test for 5 minutes. This test can also differentiate thoracic outlet syndrome from cervical disc prolapse disease.
- *Roos test*
  - Patient is asked to elevate and abduct the shoulders 90 degrees with external rotation of arms and keep it for 5 minutes. Patient feels fatigue in the diseased side.
- *Costoclavicular compression maneuver*
  - While feeling radial pulse of the patient he is asked to draw his shoulder backwards and downwards (exaggerated military position) causing absence/feeble radial pulse and a bruit may be heard while auscultating the supraclavicular region. This is due to compression of subclavian artery between clavicle and first rib.
- *Hyperabduction maneuver (Halsted test)*
  - While palpating the radial pulse, arm on the diseased side is passively hyperabducted causing feeble or absence of radial pulse. This is due to compression of artery by pectoralis minor tendon (*pectoralis minor syndrome*). An *axillary bruit* may be heard on auscultation.
- *Adson's test*
  - While feeling the radial pulse of the affected side of the patient, patient is asked to take deep breath and to turn his neck/head towards the same side so as to compress the thoracoaxillary channel. Pulse becomes feeble or absent (positive Adson's test) in thoracic outlet syndrome/scalenus anticus syndrome. While taking deep breath thoracic cage moves upwards and narrows the space causing aggravation of compression of subclavian artery by scalenus anterior muscle. Contraction of scalenus anterior further aggravates the feature (by turning neck towards same side).
- *Branham's/Nicoladoni's sign*
  - In arteriovenous fistula—pressure applied over the artery proximal to fistula will cause reduction in pulse rate and size of the swelling with pulse pressure becoming normal along with disappearance of bruit.
- *Allen's test*
  - It is used in hand to find out the patency of radial and ulnar arteries. Both radial and ulnar arteries of the patient is felt and pressed firmly at the wrist. Patient clinches his hand firmly (often repeated clinching) and holds it tightly. After 1 minute clinch is released to open the palm of the hand which looks pale.

I would rather walk with a friend in the dark, than alone in the light—**Helen Keller**

Pressure on the radial artery in wrist is released to see area of distribution of the radial artery. Normally it becomes flushed with pink color. If there is block in radial artery that area will remain white. Test is repeated again. This time pressure on the ulnar artery is released to check the patency of ulnar artery. Area will be pale and blanched after releasing in case of ulnar artery block. Otherwise in normal individual it becomes pink soon after release.

- ❖ Cold and warm water test
  - It is commonly done to confirm Raynaud's phenomena. Patient is asked to dip hands in cold water to precipitate the vasospasm and Raynaud's syndrome.
- ❖ Crossed leg test (Fuchsig's test) (Fig. 35.30)
  - Patient is asked to sit with the legs crossed one over the other so that the popliteal fossa of one leg will lie against the knee of other leg. Oscillatory movements of foot can be observed synchronous with the popliteal artery pulsation. If the popliteal artery is blocked oscillatory movements will be absent.
- ❖ Disappearing pulse syndrome:
  - Exercise the limb after feeling the pulse. Pulse will disappear once patient develops claudication. Due to exercise vasodilatation and increased vascular space occurs wherein arterial tension cannot be kept adequately and so pulse will disappear (unmasking the arterial obstruction).
- ❖ **Palpation of blood vessels (Figs. 35.31A to D)**
  - *Dorsalis pedis artery* is felt just lateral to the extensor hallucis longus tendon at the proximal end of first web space, felt against the navicular and middle cuneiform bones. It is absent in 10% cases.
  - *Posterior tibial artery* is felt against the calcaneus just behind the medial malleolus midway between it and tendo-Achilles.
  - *Anterior tibial artery* is felt in the midway anteriorly between the two malleoli against the lower end of tibia just above the ankle joint lateral to extensor hallucis longus tendon.

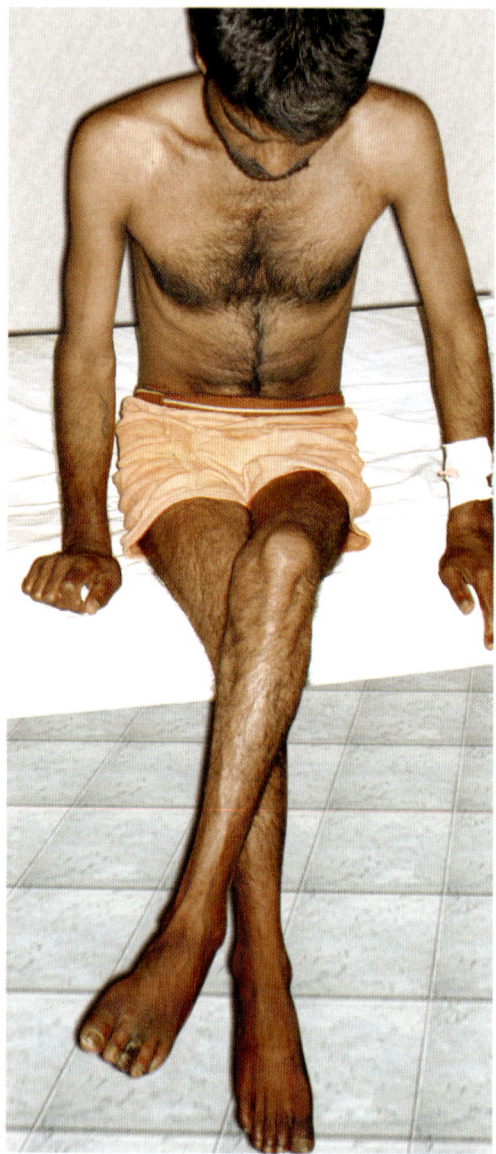

Fig. 35.30: Cross leg (Fuchsig's test) test to see oscillations.

Awards become corroded. Friends gather no dust—**Jesse Owens**

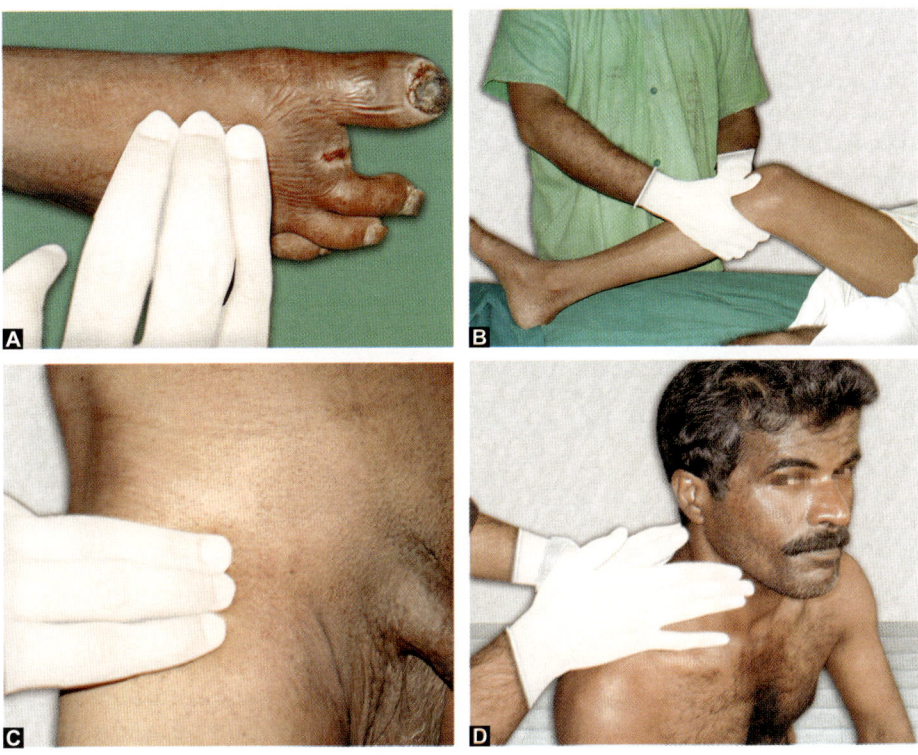

Figs. 35.31A to D: Methods of palpation of dorsalis pedis, popliteal, femoral and carotid artery pulsations.

- *Popliteal artery* is difficult to feel. It is palpated better in prone position with knee flexed about 40–90 degrees to relax popliteal fascia. It is felt in the lower part of the fossa over the flat posterior surface of upper end of tibia. Artery is not felt in upper end of the fossa, as there is no bony area in the intercondylar region. It can also be felt in supine position with knee flexed 45 degrees so as to relax the popliteal fossa and feel the pulsation over the upper part against tibial condyles.
- *Femoral artery* in the groin is felt just below the inguinal ligament midway between anterosuperior iliac spine and pubic symphysis (mid-inguinal point). Often hip has to be flexed for about 10–15 degree to feel it properly.
- *Radial artery* is felt at the wrist on the lateral aspect against lower end of the front of radius.
- *Ulnar artery* is felt at the wrist on the medial end against lower end of the front of ulna.
- *Brachial artery* is felt in front of the elbow just medial to biceps brachii tendon.
- *Axillary artery is felt on lateral aspect of the axilla* against upper end of the shaft of the humerus with raised and elevated arm.
- *Subclavian artery* is felt against first rib just above the middle of the clavicle in supraclavicular fossa while patient is lifting the shoulder to relax deep fascia.
- *Facial artery* is felt against body of mandible at the insertion of masseter.

A good friend is like a four-leaf clover: hard to find and lucky to have

- *Common carotid artery* is felt medial to sternomastoid muscle at the level of thyroid cartilage against carotid tubercle (Chaissagne tubercle) of transverse process of 6th cervical vertebra (in carotid triangle).
- *Superficial temporal artery* is felt just in front of the tragus of the ear against zygomatic bone.

All pulsations should be recorded in a table form mentioning right and left side

Pulse	Right	Left
Dorsalis pedis Posterior tibial Anterior tibial Popliteal Femoral Radial Ulnar Brachial Axillary Subclavian Carotid Superficial temporal	Should be mentioned as present/absent/feeble	Should be mentioned as present/absent/feeble

- *Condition of the vessel wall*, thrill and any tenderness on the artery should be mentioned.
- *Ulcer if present* should be examined for different features like tenderness/mobility/fixity/base/induration.

Auscultation (Fig. 35.32)

- Auscultation over the artery for *bruit* is done using bell of the stethoscope placing gently over the artery. It signifies localized stenosis causing turbulence flow.
- Machinery bruit/murmur also heard in AV malformations/fistulas.

Regional Lymph Node Examination

- It is important in case of infection.
- Tender lymph nodes in inguinal region may be present in lower limb ischemia.
- In upper limb ischemia axillary nodes are palpated.

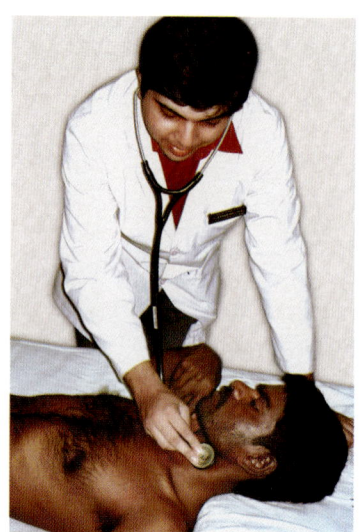

Fig. 35.32: Auscultation of carotid artery for bruit.

Systemic Examination

- Abdomen
  - Abdomen should be examined for the presence of abdominal *aortic aneurysms*. It presents as pulsatile mass above the umbilicus, vertically placed, smooth, soft, nonmobile, not moving with respiration, resonant on percussion. Expansile pulsation is confirmed by placing the patient in knee-elbow position.
- Cardiovascular system
  - CVS examination is an essential part of the arterial system to look for any associated or causative causes. There may be embolic focus in heart like fibrillation/endocarditis, etc.
- Neurological examination
  - Muscle tone/power at ankle, knee and hip; sensory examination for touch, pain and temperature; reflexes at ankle and knee; and plantar response should be checked for any associated neurological conditions (like tabes dorsalis, syringomyelia, hemiplegia, transverse myelitis).

It's not what we have in life, but who we have in our life that matters

- Other systems
  - Skeletal and respiratory systems should be examined in detail.

EXAMINATION OF VARICOSE VEINS

Chief Complaints

- Pain in the leg/thigh/foot with the side and duration of pain.
- Swelling/dilated veins in the leg and its duration.
- Pigmentation/ulceration in the leg with duration.

HISTORY

History of Present Illness

Pain
- Pain in the leg/foot/or thigh with duration. Origin of pain, its severity, onset whether acute or insidious has to be asked.
- Character of pain which may be dull aching or cramping. Whether pain gets aggravated by walking/standing. Dull aching pain along the line of the vein is typical; feeling of tightness in the calf as well as tiredness after activity and is usually more towards evening and gets relieved by lying down.
- Severe bursting pain in calf on walk of short duration may be due to associated deep vein thrombosis (DVT).
- Pain also can be due to ulcer/periostitis/infection.

Pigmentation
- It is due to stasis and release of chemicals and usually occurs around ankle region.
- It is associated with itching and often ulceration.

Ulcer
- History regarding mode of onset, duration, site of onset. Ulcer on the medial side of the ankle occurs in long saphenous vein varicosity. On the lateral aspect it is due to short saphenous vein varicosity.
- Discharge from ulcer its type, smell, quantity signifies the severity of the infection.
- Itching and bleeding in the ulcer bed are also important.

History of trauma. Often minor trauma precipitates ulcer formation in varicose vein patients.

History of swelling around the ankle.

History of pain/lump in the abdomen.

History of urinary/bowel symptoms.

History of similar complaints on the other leg.

Varicose veins are often bilateral.

Past History
- History suggestive of deep vein thrombosis earlier like pain, calf swelling and fever.
- History of immobilization, hospitalization.
- History of surgery earlier.

Treatment History

History of earlier varicose vein surgery, drug like warfarin intake for DVT, injection-sclerotherapy, wearing stockings/crepe bandages.

Personal History
- In females history of pregnancy, delivery and post-delivery period, oral contraceptive intake.
- Smoking/alcohol/working pattern.

Family History

Often varicose veins are familial, which are bilateral severe and observed in young individuals. There are absence/defective valves in these patients.

LOCAL EXAMINATION

- *Examination of both lower limbs—***standing** and on lying down.
- *Symptomatic limb should be examined first.*

True friends are never apart, maybe in distance but never in heart

Inspection (Figs. 35.33A and B)

Examination of veins in standing position is the first method in varicose veins.

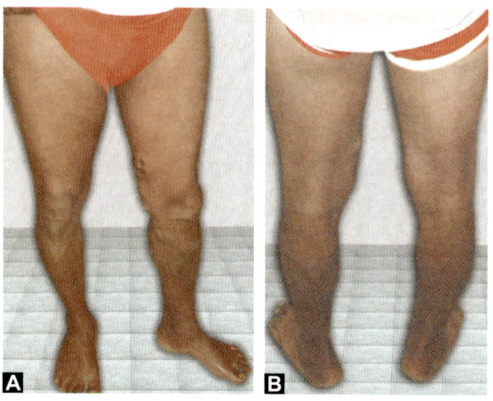

Figs. 35.33A and B: Inspection of varicose veins should be done on standing. Long saphenous veins on both sides should be inspected from medial aspect in standing position. Short saphenous vein should also be inspected from behind.

* Limb is looked for dilated veins both on the medial side for long saphenous vein and from behind and lateral side for short saphenous vein. Other communicating veins are also looked for.
* Beginning of the varicosity in the foot, later its extent above also should be seen. Great saphenous vein tortuosity often extends into the thigh whereas short saphenous vein varicosity ends at popliteal region.
* Always limb is looked for skin changes, pigmentation, edema, ankle flare, and ulcer. Cough impulse at saphenous opening (Morrisey's) may be significant.
* Extent, size, shape, margin, edge and discharge in an ulcer should be noted.

Palpation

* Ulcer if present should be described with tenderness, induration, warmness, mobility, fixity, etc.
* *Brodie-Trendelenburg test (Figs. 35.34 and 35.35):*
  - Vein is emptied by elevating the limb and milking the vein in lying down

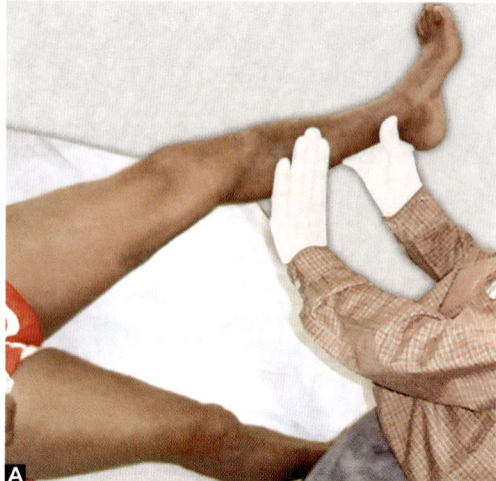

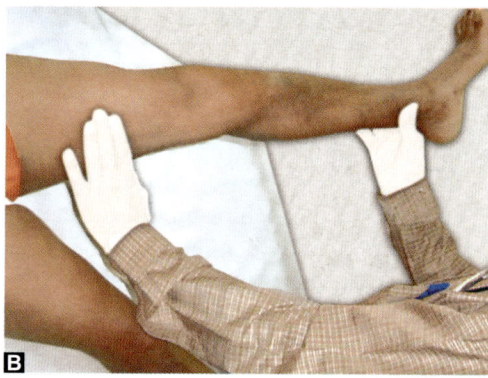

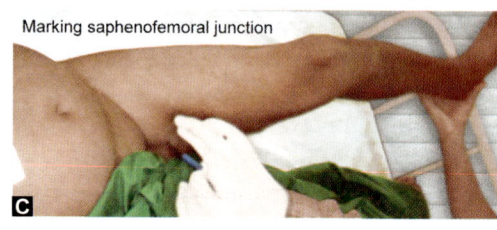

Marking saphenofemoral junction

Figs. 35.34A to C: Emptying of the superficial varicose vein is important in all tourniquet tests for varicose veins. It is done in lying down position with elevating and milking the vein. Emptying is not done in modified Perthe's test. Note the marking of the saphenofemoral junction before applying the tourniquet.

position and a tourniquet is tied just below the saphenofemoral junction (or saphenofemoral junction is occluded using thumb). Saphenous opening is located 3.5 cm below and lateral to

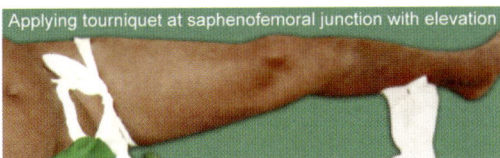

Fig. 35.35: Note the site of applying the tourniquet at saphenofemoral junction. It is 3.5 cm below and lateral to pubic tubercle.

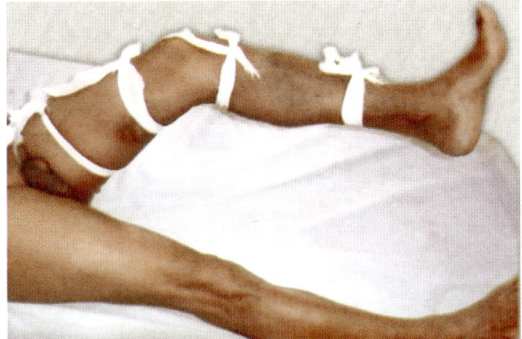

Fig. 35.36: Note the placement of tourniquets in multiple tourniquet tests.

the pubic tubercle. Pubic tubercle is palpated along the adductor longus tendon which is identified by adducting the thigh against resistance. Patient is asked to stand quickly. When tourniquet or thumb is released, rapid filling from above signifies saphenofemoral incompetence. *This is Trendelenburg test I.*

❖ In *Trendelenburg test II*, vein is emptied again in lying down position and tourniquet is applied at saphenofemoral junction. On standing limb is observed without releasing the tourniquet. Filling of blood from below upwards rapidly can be observed within 30–60 seconds. It signifies perforator incompetence.

❖ *Three/multiple (Oschner's Mahoner's test) tourniquet test (Fig. 35.36):*
  – It is to find out the site of incompetent perforator. Three tourniquets are tied after emptying the vein:
    - At saphenofemoral junction.
    - Above knee level.
    - Another below-knee level.
    - Additional tourniquets often may be applied at below-knee and above-ankle level.
  – Patient is asked to stand and limb is looked for filling of veins and site of filling. Then tourniquets are released from below upwards to look for incompetent perforators. Individual perforators may be tested by repeating the procedure.

❖ *Schwartz test*:
  – In standing position, when lower part of the vein in leg is tapped, impulse is felt at the saphenous junction or at the upper end of the visible part of the vein. It signifies continuous column of blood due to valvular incompetence.
  – It signifies continuous column of blood and also signifies that valves between two fingers are incompetent.
  – Positive test is usually found in gross venous varicosity.

❖ *Pratt's test:*
  – Esmarch bandage is applied to the leg from below upwards with a tourniquet at saphenofemoral junction.
  – After that the bandage is released to see the '*blowouts*' of perforators.

❖ *Fegan's test*:
  – Line of varicose vein is marked out. On standing, the site where the perforators enter the deep fascia bulges and these points are marked. Then on lying down, button like depressions (crescent like gaps) in the deep fascia are felt at the marked out points which confirms the perforator site.

❖ *Ian-Aird test:*
  – On standing, proximal segment of long saphenous vein is emptied with two fingers. Pressure from proximal finger is released to see the rapid filling from above which confirms saphenofemoral incompetence.

A friend knows the song in my heart and sings it to me when my memory fails—**Donna Roberts**

- *Perthes test*:
  - The affected lower limb is wrapped with elastic bandage and the patient is asked to walk around and exercise for 3–5 minutes. Development of severe cramp like pain in the calf signifies DVT.
- *Modified Perthe's test:* Tourniquet is tied just below the saphenofemoral junction without emptying the vein. Patient is allowed to have a *brisk* walk which precipitates *bursting pain* in the calf and also makes superficial veins more prominent. It signifies DVT.

> **Note:**
> - DVT is contraindicated for any surgical intervention of superficial varicose veins.
> - It is also contraindicated for sclerosant therapy.
> - Point to be remembered is that in case of acute DVT, Homan's/Mose's tests should not be done as it will precipitate the dislodgement of the clot and embolism.

- *Homan's test and Mose's sign*
  - *Homan's test* is dorsiflexion of the foot to elicit pain in the calf.
  - *Mose's sign* is squeezing the relaxed calf muscles sideward to elicit pain.
  - Both tests signify deep vein thrombosis (DVT).
- *Bone thickening*
  - *Bone thickening* in the shin (tibia and in ankle) is important which signifies periostitis.
- *Measurements*
  - Measurement of limb length and girth is needed especially in arteriovenous malformation with varicose veins and also to find out deformities.

Auscultation

It is done on the femoral/popliteal vein for venous hum or bruit of AV fistula.

Examination of Peripheral Pulses

It is important (dorsalis pedis/anterior tibial/posterior tibial/popliteal/femoral) as venous disease may be associated with arterial disease (ischemia).

Regional Lymph Nodes

Regional lymph nodes [(vertical inguinal nodes and external iliac nodes (above and medial aspect of the inguinal ligament)], ankle joint movements (plantar and dorsiflexion) are important.

Examination of the Other Limb

Examination of the other limb both in standing and in lying down position should not be forgotten.

Examination of Abdomen

- Abdomen should be examined for any mass which might be compressing the inferior vena cava (IVC) or iliac veins causing varicose veins.
- Per-rectal and per-vaginal examination should be done to rule out pelvic masses that would exert pressure over the iliac veins.
- Examination of external genitals should be done to exclude malignancies with secondaries in the para-aortic nodes.

Examination of Other Systems

Cardiovascular system (CVS), respiratory systems should be examined.

EXAMINATION OF THYROID GLAND

Name:

Address (Fig. 35.37):
Knowing the residential place may be important in certain types of goiters—endemic goiter due to iodine deficiency is common in interior areas, mountainous areas like Vindhyas, Himalayas. Goiter is more common in south India than in north India. It is also common in Middle East and European countries, North America, Bulgaria near river Struma which eventually

---

*A real friend is one who walks in when the rest of the world walks out—**Walter Winchell***

reaches Aegean Sea. Follicular and anaplastic carcinoma may be more common in areas of iodine deficiency but papillary carcinoma is not related to iodine deficiency. Chalk or limestone producing areas like Southern Ireland and Derbyshire are goitrogenic areas as calcium is goitrogenic.

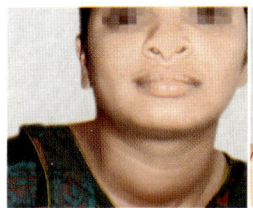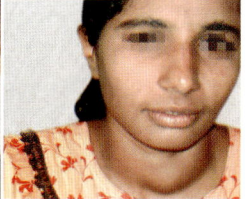

Fig. 35.37: Goiter may occur in many family members. Two siblings presented with goiter.

Occupation:

Age:

Simple goiter is often seen in girls during puberty. Goiter due to dyshormonogenesis occurs in younger age group. Physiological goiter occurs when there is increased metabolic demand of the hormone like in puberty, pregnancy. Solitary nodule, colloid goiter, papillary carcinoma and primary thyrotoxicosis are seen between 20–40 years. Multinodular goiter, follicular carcinoma and Hashimoto's thyroiditis are seen in middle aged women.

Sex

Most of the thyroid diseases like hyperthyroidism (8:1), hypothyroidism, goiters, neoplasms (3:1) are commonly seen in *females*.

Chief Complaints

- Swelling in front of the neck and its duration.
- Pain in the swelling and its duration.
- Hoarseness of voice due to recurrent laryngeal nerve palsy.
- Difficulty in swallowing or breathing.
- Tremor in the hands.
- Generalized weakness.
- Palpitation.
- Significant loss of weight.

HISTORY

History of Present Illness

- Swelling:
  - Its duration, onset—sudden or insidious. Origin of the swelling, its progress—gradual (benign), rapidly progressive (malignancy) or in an existing swelling rapid increase recently (benign turning into malignancy) or sudden rapid increase in size of swelling may be seen in hemorrhage.
- Pain:
  - Its duration, character like dull aching/pricking, site of pain, radiation, factors which alters the pain.
- Pressure symptoms:
  - Dysphagia, dyspnea, hoarseness of voice. Their duration, onset and progression.
- Features of toxicity:
  - Increased appetite/loss of weight/diarrhea/chest pain aggravated by exercise/palpitation/amenorrhea/irritability/nervousness/sleeplessness (insomnia)/hand tremors/increased sweating/heat intolerance/proximal muscle weakness in the thigh or arm like difficult in getting down steps or lifting weight using arms (myopathy)—due to difficulty in isometric contraction and increased muscle metabolism/wasting of muscles/visual disturbances with bulging of the eyes.
- Features of myxedema:
  - Weakness/lethargy/weight gain/facial puffiness/cold intolerance/menorrhagia/constipation/superciliary madarosis in lateral half of the eyebrows (loss of hairs)/change in voice.

Past History

- History of irradiation for carcinoma thyroid is important. Irradiation to head and neck region for benign lesions like adenoids, tonsillitis, thymus, acne vulgaris or hemangiomas or malignancy in younger age groups like for lymphomas.

*It's never too late to change old habits—**Florence Griffith Joyner***

- Chernobyl nuclear disaster in Ukraine in 1986 caused increased incidence of papillary carcinoma of thyroid in children.

Personal History
- Smoking, alcohol intake or any drugs which may cause alteration in thyroid function.
- Patient may be on thyroxine or on antithyroid drugs or beta blockers or other drugs like lithium, periodic acid-Schiff (PAS) or sulphonylureas which alter the thyroid function.
- Dietary habits should be asked. Brassica family of vegetables like cabbage, kale and rape are goitrogens. Type of salt used in the family iodized/home rock salt is also important.

Family History
- Dyshormonogenesis, medullary carcinoma of thyroid can be familial (MEN syndrome).
- Endemic goiter and Grave's disease can occur in families.
- Altered thyroid function may be cause for infertility.

Menstrual History
Hypothyroidism causes menorrhagia; hyperthyroidism causes amenorrhea or oligomenorrhea.

Treatment History
History of undergoing investigations or treatment relevant to thyroid disease.

GENERAL EXAMINATION
- Like any other long case.
- Exophthalmos should be seen.
- Myxedema face is typical.
- Pulse (Figs. 35.38A and B):
  - Its character, whether tachycardia, collapsing or pulsus paradoxus or ectopic or fibrillation has to be looked for.

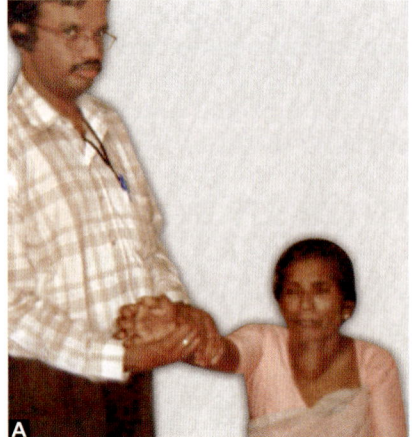
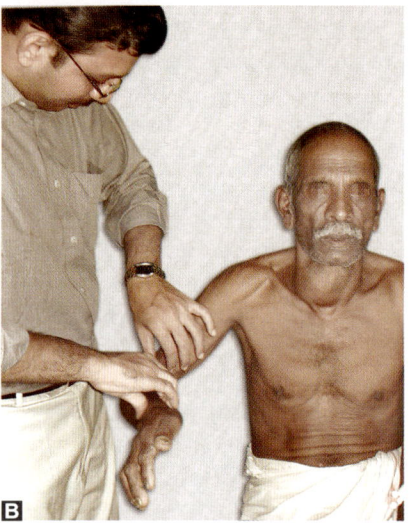

Figs. 35.38A and B: Checking radial pulse is essential in thyroid enlargement.

- *Sleeping pulse rate* is checked at late night or early morning for three consecutive nights and average is taken. Sedation like diazepam or phenobarbitone to be given to check sleeping pulse rate prior to sleep is controversial. Sleeping pulse rate is graded as Crile's grading.

Crile's grading	Sleeping pulse rate/minute
I	90–100
II	100–110
III	>110

Its okay to struggle, but it's not okay to give up on yourself or your dreams—Gabe Grunewald

- Blood pressure may be high in toxic thyroid.
- Toxic thyroid patient will be thin and underweight. In hypothyroidism, patient will be obese and overweight. In metastatic thyroid cancer, patient is cachexic.
- Agitated stressful facial expression is observed in toxic thyroid. Puffy, expressionless, dull and mask-like face is seen in myxedema.
- Rapid aggressive gait is seen in toxicity but lethargic and slow gait is observed in hypothyroidism.
- Skin is wet and warm in hyperthyroidism (moist palm while shaking hands).
- Ankle (Achilles tendon) reflex is prolonged with delayed relaxation in hypothyroidism and it is shortened and brisk in hyperthyroidism.
- Tremor of the hands and tongue (Figs. 35.39A and B).

LOCAL EXAMINATION

Inspection

- Swelling:
  - Its location/size (both vertical and horizontal dimensions of each lobe and isthmus or if it is one mass dimensions as a single swelling)/shape (butterfly shape if both lobes are involved)/extent (from posterior border of sternomastoid laterally to midline in one sided gland enlargement or from one side to opposite sternomastoid if both lobes are enlarged)/upper extent is usually up to thyroid cartilage/*lower margin is clearly visible or not* or visible during deglutition/**movement of swelling upwards with deglutition** (thyroid moves upwards during deglutition due to attachment of the condensed vascular pretracheal fascia *(Berry's ligament)* which is attached above, medially and behind to cricoid cartilage and also *pretracheal fascia* is attached to larynx, trachea and *inferior constrictor muscle which moves upwards during deglutition*)/scar or dilated veins

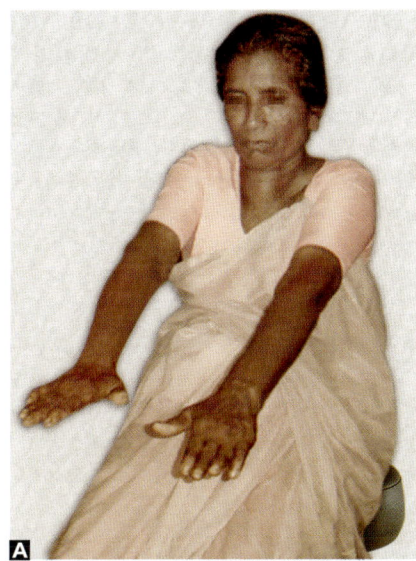

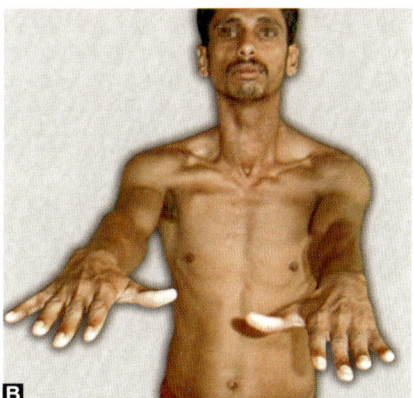

Figs. 35.39A and B: Method of looking for tremor of hands in thyrotoxicosis.

(in toxic goiter, carcinoma thyroid, venous compression, retrosternal goiter) or pigmentation on the skin over the swelling/pulsation over the swelling (toxicity, malignancy)/surface on inspection (smooth or nodular).

Swellings which move upwards with deglutition

- Thyroid swelling.
- Subhyoid bursa.
- Thyroglossal cyst.
- Pretracheal/prelaryngeal lymph nodes.
- Swelling from larynx/trachea.

Faith is knowledge within the heart, beyond the reach of proof— **KhalilGibran**

- In some occasions swelling whether moves upwards while protruding the tongue out or not should be looked for. Thyroglossal cyst moves upwards with protrusion of tongue. Patient is asked to open the mouth and then swelling/cyst is held firmly. Now patient is asked to protrude the tongue out to feel a upward movement of the swelling with a typical '*tug*' like feel.
- Any other swelling in the neck should be seen like for lymph nodes. Lymph nodes can be involved commonly in papillary carcinoma of thyroid and occasionally in follicular carcinoma of thyroid.

Palpation

- *Swelling (Figs. 35.40A and B):*
  - Temperature over swelling (swelling may be warm in toxic thyroid, malignancy, thyroiditis)/tenderness (hemorrhage, thyroiditis, tumor necrosis can cause tenderness)/extent/position/shape/size (should be measured in centimeter both vertically and horizontally)/movement of the swelling upwards with deglutition/surface (smooth or nodular)/consistency (soft or firm or hard or variable and if so different locations of different consistencies should be mentioned)/margin (well defined or diffuse, lower margin which is most important)/independent mobility of the swelling/plane of the swelling (it is checked by contracting the sternomastoid muscles by placing examiner's hand under the chin of patient and patient has to flex the neck against resisting hand) (single side gland relation to sternomastoid muscle is checked by contracting the muscle by turning the chin against resistance of the examiner's hand)/skin is free or not.
- *Thrill:*
  - Thrill is checked in the upper pole of the gland as superior thyroid artery is superficial and enters the gland in front upper pole. Thrill signifies toxicity or increased vascularity.
- *Methods of palpation of thyroid gland:*
  - Thyroid gland is palpated from behind with patient is sitting in a stool with neck partially flexed. Both thumbs of the examiner are kept over the occiput and fingers will be in front to feel the gland—both lateral lobes and isthmus for all features.
  - *Crile's method of palpation of gland:* It is the palpation of the nodule/swelling in front using the pulp of the thumb.
  - *Pizzillo's method of palpation (Fig. 35.41):* It is the method of palpation of thyroid gland in short neck and obese individuals. Patient is asked to keep her/his both hands over the occiput and gland becomes prominent which will be palpated from front or behind.
  - *Lahey's method of examination (Figs. 35.42A and B):*
    - It is the method used to palpate any nodules in posterior part of the gland. It is mainly useful in solitary nodule of thyroid. Examiner should stand in front of the patient. If right lobe is needed to palpate, left lateral lobe is pushed towards right to make posterior aspect

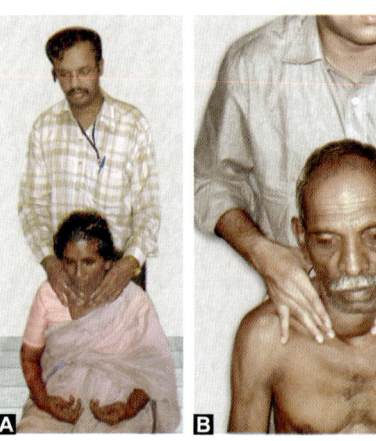

Figs. 35.40A and B: Method of palpation of thyroid gland from behind.

God made Truth with many doors to welcome every believer who knocks on them—KhalilGibran

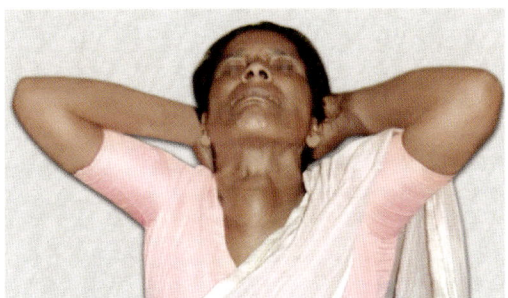

Fig. 35.41: Pizzillo's method of examination of thyroid gland.

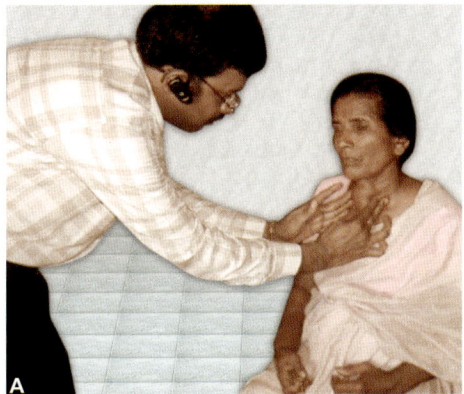

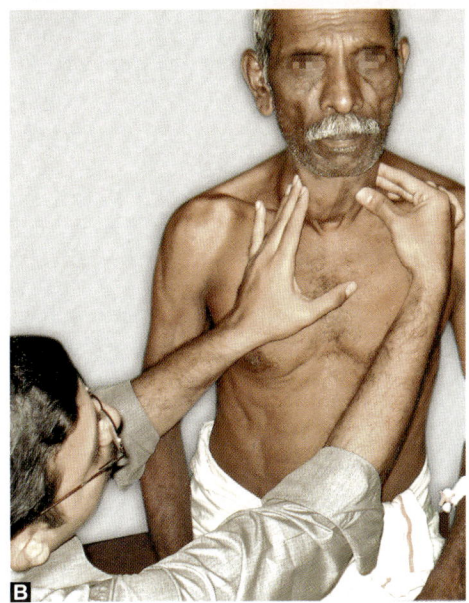

Figs. 35.42A and B: Lahey's method of palpating thyroid gland.

of the right gland more prominent as gland gets pushed and rotated towards right side. Posterior becomes posterolateral or lateral which is felt for any nodules. Posterior aspect of left lobe is palpated by pushing the right lobe towards left side.

- *Kocher's test:*
  - It is the test for *tracheal compression*. Patient is asked to see straight. Both lateral lobes of the thyroid gland are gently compressed with fingers and thumb directing posteromedially. If patient develops stridor—*Kocher's test is positive*. If there is no stridor means it is negative.
  - In a long standing goiter and large goiter, because of constant pressure tracheal rings get weakened which get narrowed/collapsed during compression. Goiter itself because of forward traction keeps trachea patent. But after thyroidectomy as there is no support to trachea causes tracheomalacia—weakening of the tracheal rings. Such patients need tracheostomy after thyroidectomy. It is usually temporary tracheostomy for 2–3 weeks by then tracheal rings regain their strength to maintain the patency of the trachea.

❖ **Confirmation of retrosternal extension:**
  - Lower margin of the swelling/goiter is not visible—even on deglutition.
  - Lower margin is not palpable on deglutition.
  - Dilated veins over neck or chest wall may be visible.
  - Normal resonant note becomes dull over the sternum on percussion.
  - *Pemberton's sign*—patient is asked to raise the both arms above the shoulder so as to touch the ears and made to keep like that for 3 minutes. Patient will develop dilated veins and cyanosis in the neck and upper chest

Your friend is your needs answered—**KhalilGibran**

wall, puffiness in face and respiratory distress and rarely dysphagia. It means sign is positive signifying retrosternal extension of goiter.

- Position of trachea:
  - It is checked by palpation using three fingers from below. Middle finger is kept just above the suprasternal space and index and ring fingers are placed over sternal heads of the sternomastoid muscles on each side. Middle finger is run upwards along the trachea to feel the position—central or deviated. In solitary nodule or disease of only one lateral lobe trachea will be usually deviated towards opposite side. In both lobes enlargement trachea will be usually central.
  - Other clinical features of tracheal deviation are—absence of hollowness on the side of the deviation *(trail sign)*, on auscultation hearing of breath sounds on the side of the deviation.
- Carotid pulsation:
  - Carotid pulsation should be checked. It is normally felt at the level of the upper border of thyroid cartilage over medial aspect of the sternomastoid muscle on the Chaissagne tubercle (carotid tubercle) on the transverse process of C6 vertebra.
  - It may be deviated posteriorly/laterally in a large goiter.
  - It may be absent in advanced carcinoma thyroid due to infiltration of the carotid sheath by the tumor/carcinoma (Berry's sign).
- **In primary thyrotoxicosis *exophthalmos* and all eye signs are looked for (Fig. 35.43):**
  - Both the eyelids cover the bulbar sclera partially in normal individual.
  - Upper sclera is visible in only lid retraction—due to spasm of involuntary levator palpebrae superioris muscle. Here lower eyelid is in normal position. It does not indicate exophthalmos.

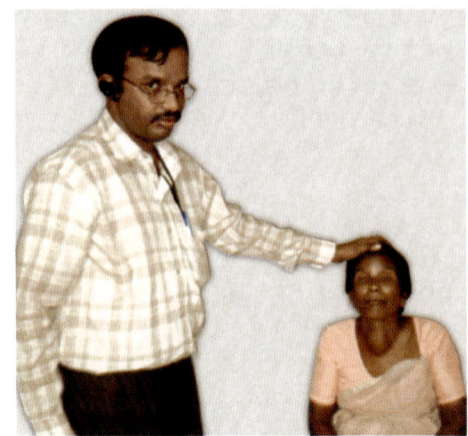

Fig. 35.43: Looking for eye signs is very important in thyroid swelling.

- In exophthalmos lower bulbar sclera is clearly visible and lower eyelid is below and will not cover the bulbar sclera. In severe exophthalmos sclera all over both above and below will be visible.
- Exophthalmos is measured using exophthalmometer.
- **Other eye signs**
  - *Eye signs are common in primary thyrotoxicosis. Lid lag, lid spasm can occur in secondary thyrotoxicosis also.*
    1. *Von Graefe's sign*: Lid lag sign—*is visible white sclera above the corneal margin during lid lag.*
    2. *Naffziger's sign:* While examiner standing behind the patient, patient's neck is extended and examiner looks from behind along the superior orbital margin of the patient. Eyeball is seen beyond the superior orbital margin in exophthalmos.
    3. *Dalrymple's sign*: Upper eye lid retraction, so visibility of upper sclera.
    4. *Stellwag's sign*: Absence of normal blinking—so *starring look*. First sign to appear.
    5. *Joffroy's sign*: Absence of wrinkling on forehead when patient looks up (frowns).

If your heart is a volcano, how shall you expect flowers to bloom?—**Kalil Gibran**

6. *Moebius sign*: Lack of convergence of eye ball. Defective convergence is due to lymphocytic infiltration of inferior oblique and inferior rectus muscles in case of primary thyrotoxicosis. There will be diplopia. It may be an early sign of eventual ophthalmoplegia.

Order of appearance of signs
- Stellwags sign—Mild. First sign to appear.
- Von Graefes sign—Mild.
- Joffroys sign—Moderate.
- Moebius sign—Severe.

Important signs to be remembered
- *Visible **lower sclera**—sign of exophthalmos.*
- Naffziger's sign.
- Von Graefes sign—upper lid lag-spasm of levator muscle.
- Joffroy's sign.
- Moebius sign—*most important—early sign of ophthalmoplegia.*

Examination of Neck Lymph Nodes for Secondaries

It is common in papillary carcinoma of thyroid. It is usually in level III and IV nodes. It could be firm, hard or cystic. It is usually brownish black in color often with papillary projections. Lymph nodes often can get enlarged in follicular carcinoma thyroid and lymphoma. *Lateral aberrant thyroid* is earlier thought as aberrant thyroid in lateral part of the neck but actually it is not so but it is secondary in lymph node with primary being papillary carcinoma of thyroid.

Percussion Over the Manubrium

- Percussion over the manubrium sterni is important. Usually direct method is used.
- Dullness signifies retrosternal extension.
- Tenderness may signify the secondaries in sternum from follicular carcinoma of thyroid.

Auscultation (Figs. 35.44A and B)

Auscultation over the upper pole of the gland for bruit—in toxic thyroid severe cases and very vascular tumors.

SYSTEMIC EXAMINATION

Cardiovascular System Examination

- It is important in thyrotoxicosis—commonly secondary type.

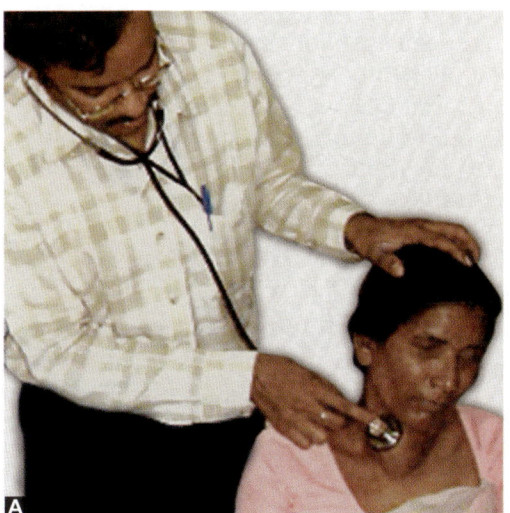
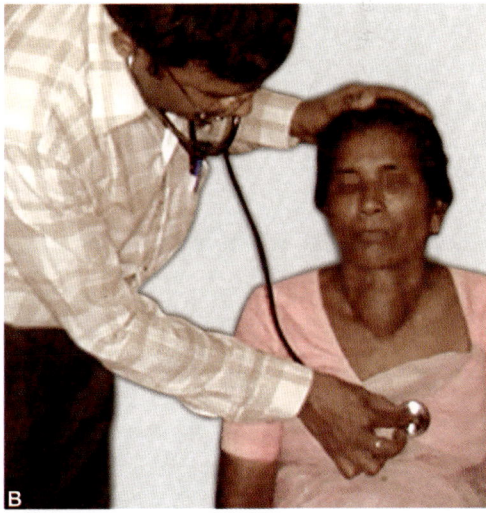

Figs. 35.44A and B: Auscultation over superior pole of thyroid to hear bruit in toxic thyroid and over cardiac region for any cardiac changes is needed.

Doubt is a pain too lonely to know that faith is his twin brother—**Kalil Gibran**

❖ Tachycardia, ectopic, pulsus paradoxus, extrasystoles, atrial fibrillation are the cardiac presentations.

Respiratory System Examination

Secondaries and pleural effusion can occur in follicular carcinoma of thyroid.

Abdomen Examination

❖ Hepatomegaly as secondaries in liver is known to occur in follicular carcinoma of thyroid.
❖ Hepatosplenomegaly can occur as part of Grave's disease or Hashimoto's disease.

Examination of Skull and Spine

Localized, warm, vascular, pulsatile secondaries can occur in skull commonly, rib and other bones occasionally as a spread from follicular carcinoma of thyroid.

Thyroid swelling which does not move with respiration

- Carcinoma thyroid with infiltration.
- Riedel's thyroiditis.
- Anaplastic carcinoma thyroid.

Causes of dyspnea/stridor in thyroid diseases

- Carcinoma thyroid causing infiltration of recurrent laryngeal nerve/trachea.
- Large, long standing goiter causing tracheomalacia.
- Retrosternal goiter.
- Congestive cardiac failure in thyrotoxicosis.

In a case of thyroid disease following things should be made very clear

- Functional status—hyperthyroid/euthyroid/hypothyroid.
- Compression to trachea/recurrent nerve.
- Neck lymph nodal status.
- Tracheal deviation.
- Carotid infiltration.
- Retrosternal extension.
- Systemic features like toxicity or malignant spread to different organs like bone/liver/lungs.

Recent rapid increase in thyroid swelling is due to:

- Previous MNG—malignant transformation.
- Hemorrhage into a nodule.
- Anaplastic carcinoma of thyroid.

Investigations for Thyroid Diseases

❖ T3, T4, TSH, free T3, free T4.
❖ US neck for thyroid and neck nodes.
❖ FNAC thyroid and lymph node.
❖ Radioisotope study to see the function of the thyroid.
❖ CT neck in malignancies or large goiter.
❖ Trucut biopsy if two trials of FNAC are inconclusive. But its use is questionable due to lack of its safety. It can injure deeper structures and also can cause hemorrhage.
❖ Frozen section biopsy on table and proceed may be needed.
❖ Serum calcitonin, serum thyroglobulin estimation in neoplasms of thyroid.
❖ US abdomen; CT chest; radioisotope bone scan to work up for metastases.

EXAMINATION OF ORAL CAVITY

History

❖ Carcinoma in oral cavity is common above 50 years, whereas cleft lip and palate are seen in childhood.
❖ Retention cyst occurs in any age.
❖ Cleft palate is common in females.
❖ Carcinoma lip is more common in men involved with outdoor activities (country man's lip).

Complaints and Other History

❖ Swelling or ulcer over the lip, cheek, tongue, floor of the mouth—in detail history regarding its mode of onset, duration, progress, etc. is asked. Retention cyst is of longer duration whereas carcinoma tongue has a short history.
❖ Pain:
  – Complains of pain in inflammatory conditions (aphthous ulcer), traumatic

---

Forgetfulness is a form of freedom—**Kalil Gibran**

ulcer, and tuberculous ulcer of tongue. It is late presentation in advanced carcinoma tongue. Pain is absent in leukoplakia, primary chancre, early carcinoma tongue. It may be at the diseased site or referred pain in the external ear (as the sensory center of the mandibular nerve receives signals from both lingual and auriculotemporal nerve).
- Redness of mucus membrane—in glossitis.
- Fever.
- Halitosis in advanced oral malignancies.
- Specific complaints:
  - Difficulty in chewing and swallowing (acute stomatitis, tonsillitis).
  - Difficulty in speech (cleft lip, palate and carcinoma tongue); alteration in voice (carcinoma posterior 1/3rd of tongue).
  - Inability to protrude the tongue or deviation of the tip of tongue (carcinoma tongue infiltrating the floor of the mouth).
  - Regurgitation of fluid and food—cleft palate; excessive salivation (commonest presentation in carcinoma tongue).

Past History

Past history of oral disease (carcinoma/leukoplakia), treatment histories like radiotherapy or chemotherapy or surgery for oral diseases.

Personal History

History of pan chewing, alcohol, smoking, betel nut chewing is common in oral malignancies.

Local Examination

- It has to be done in a good light. Head light or focusing light can be used.
- Examiner should wear gloves in order to protect his hands from contact with patient's saliva.
- Tongue depressor is used for proper exposure.
- Trismus should be assessed by placing fingers across the mouth opening.

Oral cavity should be properly exposed for examination (Figs. 35.45A to C):

- The lips are retracted to expose the buccal mucosa.
- The cheek is pushed outwards to examine labial aspect of gums.
- The tongue is pushed away from the floor of the mouth to examine the floor of the mouth, ventral aspect of the tongue, lingual side of the gum.
- The lateral aspect of the posterior third of the tongue is examined by pushing the tongue to one side.
- The tongue can be depressed for proper examining the tonsil and pharynx.

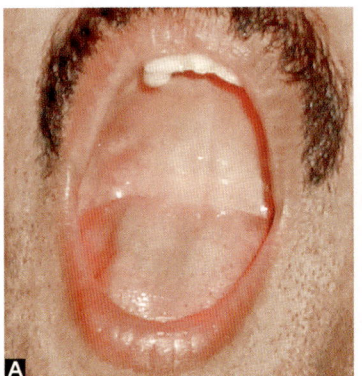 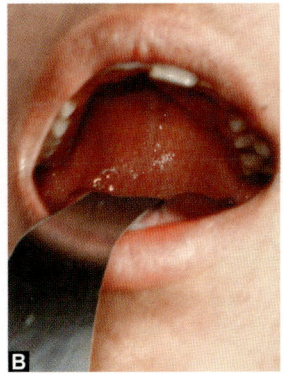 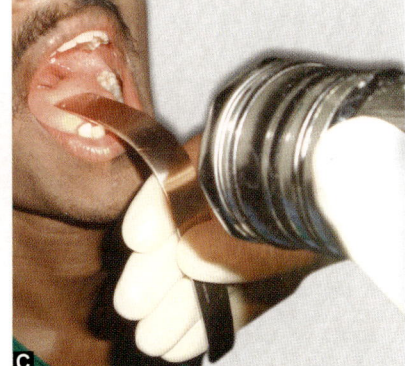

Figs. 35.45A to C: Proper inspection of the oral cavity is essential part of the examination. Often spatula/tongue depressor and a good light source should be used to inspect the oral cavity.

To be able to look back upon one's life in satisfaction, is to live twice—**Kalil Gibran**

Inspection

Ask the patient to open the mouth and look for any trismus (Fig. 35.46).

Lips:
- The mucous linings of the lips and cheek are examined by everting the upper and lower lip.
- Ulcer, swelling, leukoplakia, pigmentation, *macrochelia* (thickening of the lip commonly upper), *microchelia*, are looked for and their site, size, extent are noted (Fig. 35.47). Cleft lips are obviously visible.
- Cracked lips are indolent cracks in the midline of lower lip as a result of exposure to cold weather.

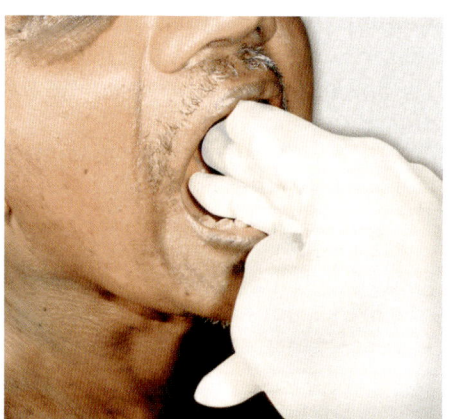

Fig. 35.46: Trismus in carcinoma cheek suggests pterygoids and soft tissue involvement. It is checked by placing fingers (of patient ideally) perpendicularly between opened jaws.

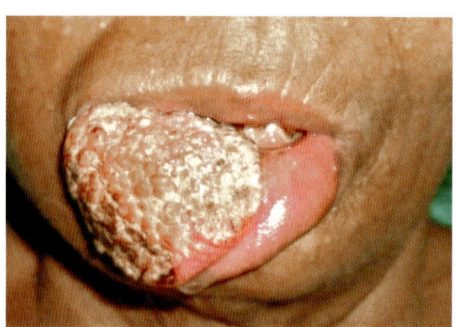

Fig. 35.47: Carcinoma lip. SCC is common in lower lip.

- Ectopic salivary gland tumors may present as slow growing lobulated tumors whereas carcinoma lip present as ulcerative lesions with everted edges.

Tongue:
- Examine the tongue for its *size* (massive tongue—*macroglossia*—hemangioma, lymphangiomas, muscular macroglossia, neurofibromas); *color* (leukoplakia—white colored patches in the tongue seen in chronic superficial glossitis, blue colored—venous hemangiomas, reddish glazes—when leukoplakic patches are shed away, pale—in anemia, black hairy tongue (in *Aspergillus* infection and chronic smokers); *cracks and fissure* (longitudinal in syphilis, horizontal in congenital); *ulcer and swelling* noting its site, size, number, etc.
- Swelling at the foramen cecum may be lingual thyroid.
- The site of the tongue ulcer is characteristic, sides of the tongue in dental, in dorsum in syphilitic, tuberculous on tip and sides, carcinomatous along the margin.
- *Movements of the tongue are checked* by asking the patient to protrude the tongue out, sideways, upwards, downwards.
- Presence of a short frenulum linguae will not allow the tongue to be protruded out (tongue tie); deviation of tongue to one side may be due to impairment of hypoglossal nerve supply to that half or carcinomatous infiltration of the nerve of that half of the tongue.

Palate:
- As cleft, ulcer, swelling, perforation in the palate is noted. In case of cleft palate note its extent, involvement of soft palate, whether nasal septum is attached or hangs free.
- Swelling and ulcer are examined in usual way as in any other case. Perforation may be due to syphilis or following any surgery for palate.

Love and doubt have never been on speaking terms—**Kalil Gibran**

Gums and teeth:
Gums are visualized by everting the lips and cheek; a spatula and a dental mirror can be used for proper visibility.
- Color of the gums (normal pink), any swelling (dental abscess), and ulcer are noted. Normally gums are bright pink with sharply defined, crenated edges, closely adherent to the teeth. Blue black line on the gum margins is seen in chronic lead poisoning.
- Deep red line along the free margin along with inflammation and swelling is seen in *pyorrhea alveolaris*.
- *Cancrum oris* is an ulcerative lesion associated with foul smell, begins at the premolar-molar region, progresses rapidly to expose the bone underneath. Gums are hypertrophied and teeth are buried in generalized hyperplastic gingivitis (idiopathic/hydantoin therapy), whereas localized hypertrophy of gums can occur by ill-fitting dentures.
- Teeth are counted; their color and any abnormal features are noted. Teeth may be congenitally absent or extracted. Staining of teeth may be due to tetracycline therapy in infancy, chronic smoking (yellowish brown staining), drinking water with excess fluorides (brown/black spots). Watch for syphilitic markers (*Hutchinson' teeth*—upper incisor teeth is small, notched, broad peg shaped, *Moon's molar*—doom-shaped first molar tooth).

Floor of the mouth (Fig. 35.48):
- It is exposed by asking the patient to fold the tongue upwards so as to touch the palate.
- Any swelling (ranula—bluish swelling; sublingual dermoid lies in the midline) or ulcer are noted along with its features.
- Congenitally short frenulum linguae causing tongue tie can also be seen on the floor of the mouth.
- Ulcerative/proliferative growth can be seen. Its extent, crossing midline or not should be looked for.

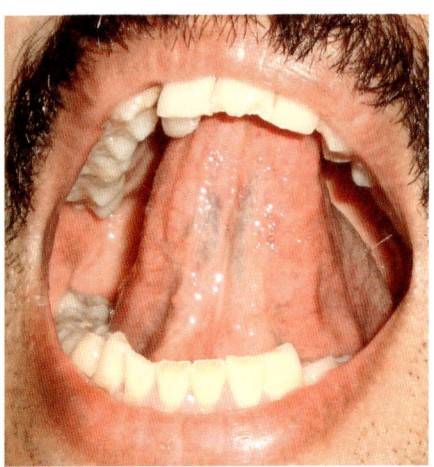

Fig. 35.48: Inspection of the floor of the mouth. Tip of the tongue should be kept upwards to touch the palate to inspect the floor of the mouth.

Cheek (Fig. 35.49):
- By retracting, the cheek is examined on its inner aspect for any swelling, ulcer, leukoplakia, cyst, carcinoma, and their respective features are noted in detail.

Fauces and tonsils:
Fauces and tonsils should be inspected (Fig. 35.50).

Palpation
Lips and cheek (Figs. 35.51 and 35.52):
- The mucus linings of the lips and cheek are examined by everting the upper and lower lip.
- Lip may contain ulcer (carcinoma, Hunterian chancre), swelling (carcinoma or retention cyst). In case of ulcerative lesion its mobility with respect to lip has to be checked.
- The lip is held and fixed with one hand and with index and thumb of the other the ulcer is moved against the lip.
- In carcinomatous lesion, it is always fixed.
- Mucus cyst is smooth surfaced, fluctuant swelling whereas papilloma is irregular surfaced, mobile swelling.
- Mucus retention cyst (normally present on the inner aspect of lower lip) can show

*You can do anything, but not everything—**David Allen***

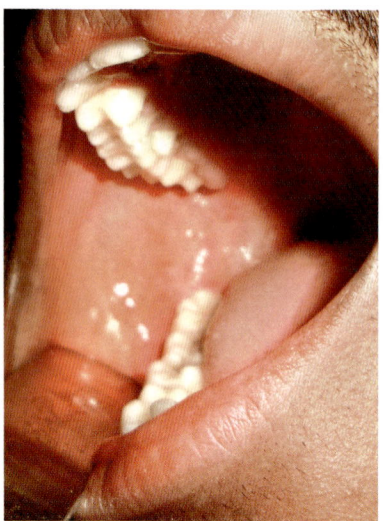

Fig. 35.49: Cheek is inspected using a spatula/depressor.

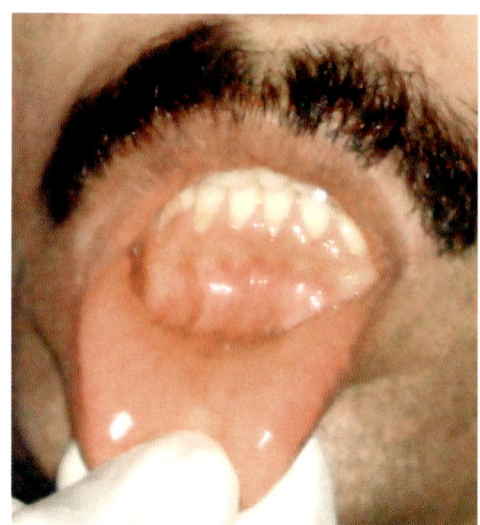

Fig. 35.51: Examination/palpation of lip should be done properly methodically.

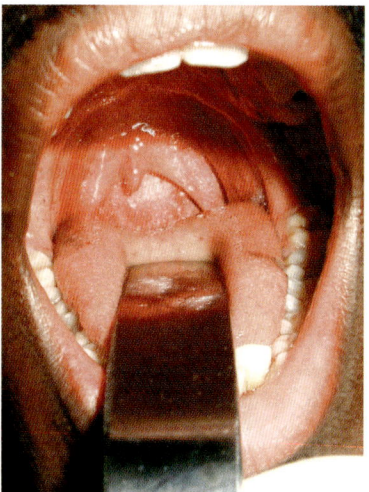

Fig. 35.50: Inspection of fauces is done using tongue depressor.

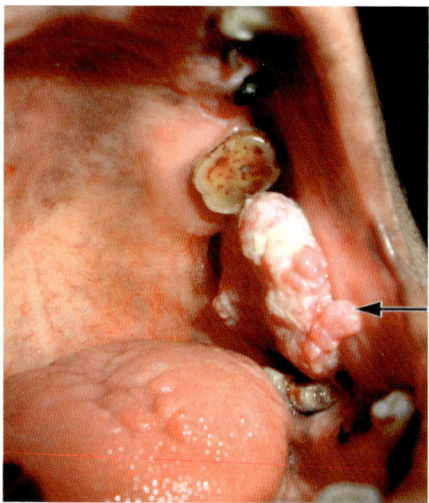

Fig. 35.52: Carcinoma cheek. Note the proliferative lesion.

  transillumination and fluctuation test positive when are sufficiently big in size.
- Buccal mucosa is palpated carefully for the extent of induration in case of carcinoma.

Gums and teeth:
- Gums are palpated to detect any localized swellings, tenderness (*pyorrhea alveolaris*), pus discharge (pyorrhea alveolaris, alveolar abscess, *Vincent's stomatitis*), bleeding on touch (pyorrhea, scurvy, uremia, blood dyscrasias).
- Teeth are palpated to detect any loose tooth. Erosion into the enamel can be detected by palpating with a probe. Pedunculated pink mass is seen in *epulis*.
- Tenderness over the teeth with apical abscess is seen in *median mental sinus*.

The richest man is not he who has the most, but he who needs the least

Tongue:

- In ulcerative lesions of the tongue it is necessary to note the induration due to infiltration. Induration is seen in carcinomatous/gummatous ulcer but not in tuberculous ulcer. To check for the induration, the tongue is placed inside the mouth in order to prevent the false sense of induration due to muscle contraction.
- Whether the ulcer bleeds on touch is noted. Any sharp tooth or dentures near the ulcer is noted. It is essential to palpate the back of the tongue for any ulcer or swelling. Patient is made to sit on a stool.
- Examiner stands on the right and with the left hand. The patient's head is supported against him. The index finger of the right hand is inserted in between the two jaws, passed along the cheek and behind the soft palate. Back of tongue, soft palate, tonsils and pharynx are palpated. Local anesthetic spray is used. Before palpation of these areas in order to prevent gag reflex (Fig. 35.53).

Palate:

Any ulcer or swelling is noted. Swelling, may be due to alveolar abscess (tender, red, fluctuant swelling from the alveolus) gumma (soft swelling in the middle of the hard palate), carcinoma of maxillary antrum (the palate is pushed downwards), rarely mixed salivary tumor from ectopic salivary gland.

Floor of the mouth:

- This is tested bimanually with finger of one hand in the mouth and the other in the sublingual region.
- Transillumination test is done for cystic swelling which is positive in ranula, negative in dermoid cyst.
- Carcinoma in floor of the mouth reveals indurated base and fixed to underlying tissues.
- Enlarged submandibular gland or stone in Wharton's duct may be felt on bidigital palpation.

Examination of Regional Lymph Nodes (Fig. 35.54)

Submental, submandibular, jugulodigastric, jugulo-omohyoid groups of cervical lymph

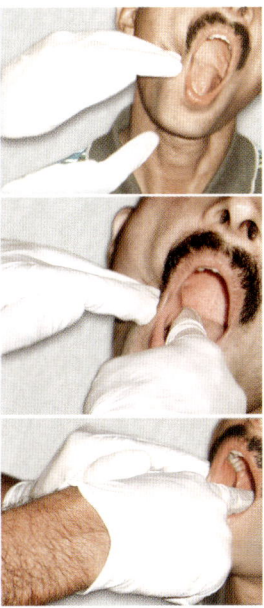

Fig. 35.53: Examination of posterior part of the tongue needs special method (see text).

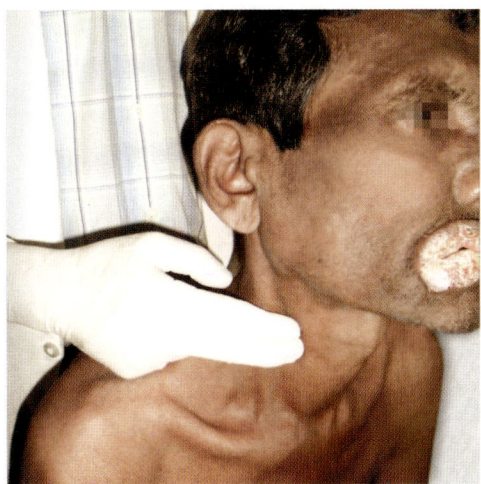

Fig. 35.54: Neck lymph nodes should be examined on both sides in oral cavity lesions.

*You miss 100 percent of the shots you never take—**Wayne Gretzky***

nodes on both sides of the neck are examined for enlargement, consistency, mobility, tenderness.

Systemic Examination

Respiratory system examination is done in carcinoma for secondaries, tuberculosis for primary focus.

Examination of oral cavity (Fig. 35.55)

History
- Swelling—in detail.
- Ulcer—detail.
- Pain.
- Type of pain, radiation to ear (through lingual and auriculotemporal nerves) or other places, severity.
- Fever.
- Excessive salivation is common in carcinomas.
- Difficulty in speech.
- Voice change.
- *Halitosis*—foul smelling breath.

Personal History
Smoking history, chewing pan and keeping pan/quid in the cheek, alcohol intake, spicy diet, trauma by teeth.

Contd...

Contd...

Examination
Inspection
- Site of lesion/type/extent/edge/margin/floor/ mouth opening (trismus) is adequate or not/ gums/dentition/floor of mouth/tongue/palate/ tonsils/lips/leukoplakia present or not.
- Skin over the cheek also should be inspected for swelling/edema/ulceration/discoloration.
- Tongue depressor is needed for proper inspection of the oral cavity.

Palpation
- Lesion is palpated after wearing a glove—for tenderness/extent/induration/mobility/fixity/ bleeding on touch/palpation of different parts of the oral cavity.
- Bone thickening is checked using two fingers— thickening/tenderness/irregularity/evidence of fracture site (pathological).
- All parts of the oral cavity should be palpated properly.

Neck is examined for significant lymph nodes of different groups and levels. Submandibular nodes are checked with neck flexed and tilted towards same side. It should be differentiated from submandibular salivary gland by bidigital palpation. Lymph gland is not bidigitally palpable whereas salivary gland is bidigitally palpable.

Relevant systemic examinations should be done.

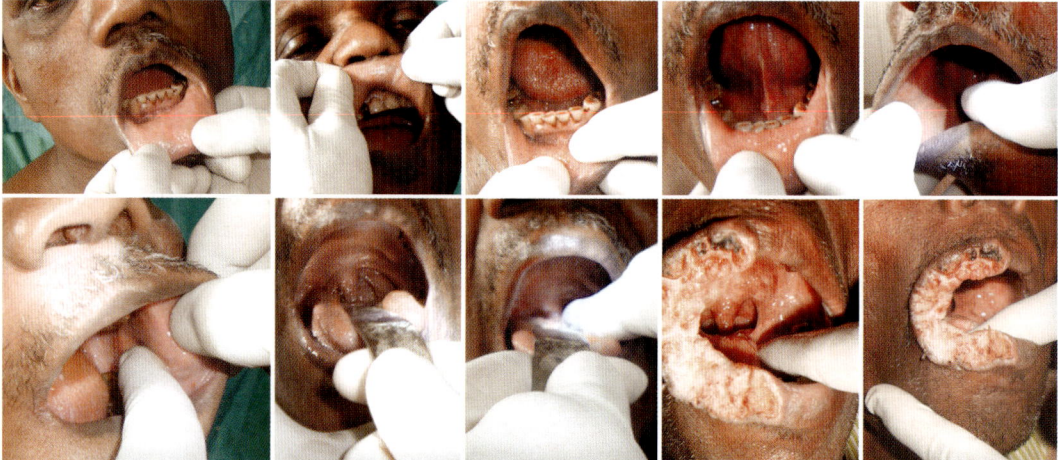

Fig. 35.55: Examination of oral cavity should be methodical—lips; gums; cheeks, tongue; floor of the mouth; palate; posterior aspect of the oral cavity.

*You must be the change you wish to see in the world—***Gandhi**

EXAMINATION OF JAW AND TEMPOROMANDIBULAR JOINT

Anatomy of Maxilla

It is pyramidal in shape. Any swelling or ulcer may be present in any of these surfaces which have to be thoroughly examined.

- *Superior surface* (orbital surface): This forms the floor of the orbit. The inferior orbital margins are palpated on both side, any differences in the margin (projections) are noted. Upward bulging of this surface will cause *proptosis* (forward pushing of the eyeball).
- *Inferior surface (palatine surface)*: The patient is asked to open the mouth, any swelling over the palate is noted. Also the teeth in the upper jaw are examined, note any missing tooth.
- *Medial surface* (*nasal surface*): This surface forms the lateral wall of the nostril and can be seen with the help of nasal speculum. Patient is asked to blow the nose occluding the nares at a time. The medial wall of the maxilla does not bulge if there is no obstruction. If there is obstruction, patient may give history of nasal discharge which may be purulent or serosanguinous.
- *Superficial surface:* The skin over the cheek is examined for any ulcer, pigmentation. If there is obstruction to the nasolacrimal duct, the patient gives history of constant flow of tears from that side. Any swelling/bulge may be obviously seen, and has to be felt by everting the upper lip.

HISTORY

- *History of trauma*, blood stained saliva, pain, swelling, nasal discharge, epistaxis, diplopia, headache, referred pain, ulcer, swelling in gums and antrum, caries teeth—should be asked for.
- *Past history* of any maxillary/mandibular disease or surgery should be asked for.
- *Personal history*—alcohol, smoking, pan chewing should be detailed.

Examination of Maxilla

Inspection (Figs. 35.56A and B)

- For swelling, nostrils, palate, alveolus, maxillary surface, ear, eye should be done.
- Oral cavity should be examined using good light source.
- Teeth should be examined for loosening, alignment.
- Trismus should be assessed.

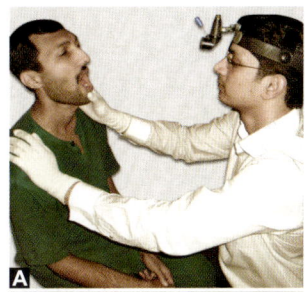
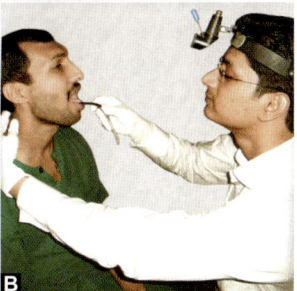

Figs. 35.56A and B: Inspect the oral cavity and palate carefully. Use a spatula and light source.

Palpation

- Tenderness on the surface.
- Swelling and its features in detail.
- Palpation of oral cavity is a must.
- Bidigital palpation of bone for thickening, tenderness, swelling, discrepancies.
- Any solid mass (sessile/pedunculated) arising from the mucoperiosteum must be noted which may be *epulis*. Note its consistency (firm/soft), may or may not bleed on palpation.

*We are what we repeatedly do; excellence, then, is not an act but a habit—***Aristotle**

- Teeth have to be counted. Dental cyst may be associated with caries tooth whereas dentigerous cyst may be associated with unerrupted permanent tooth.

Maxillary Antrum

- Maxillary antrum is palpated for tenderness. Tender antrum without any bulge and purulent discharge from that side suggest empyema (Figs. 35.57 and 35.58).
- *Transillumination test* is done for the maxillary antrum either by placing an illuminated torch over the maxilla in a dark room or by keeping the illuminated torch inside the mouth and closing the lip, transillumination is looked for which is absent in presence of pus or tumor.

Lymph Node Examination

Cervical lymph nodes must be looked for enlargement (submandibular) which can occur in tuberculous or carcinomatous lesions. Lymph nodes are not enlarged in sarcoma of upper jaw.

Examination of Mandible

- Any deformity/swelling/sinus in the mandible are looked for.
- History of trauma/fall should be asked in case of deformity. Patient may have blood stained saliva as most of the fracture mandible is a compound one, communicating with the oral cavity. There may also be difficulty in articulating the words. Patient is usually seen supporting the fragments with the hand.
- Slow growing large tumor usually suggests adamantinoma.
- Mandible is palpated bimanually keeping one hand in the mouth and other externally over the jaw (Figs. 35.59A to C).
- The hand is run along the lower border of the mandible externally and alveolus internally. Any swelling with tenderness, loss of continuity of the lower border and alignment of the teeth, crepitus always suggests fracture mandible. Fracture mandible is more common at the region of the canine teeth due to deep canine socket.

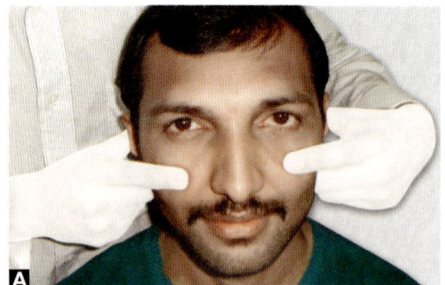
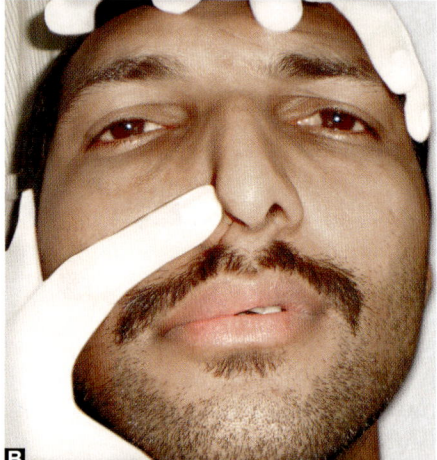
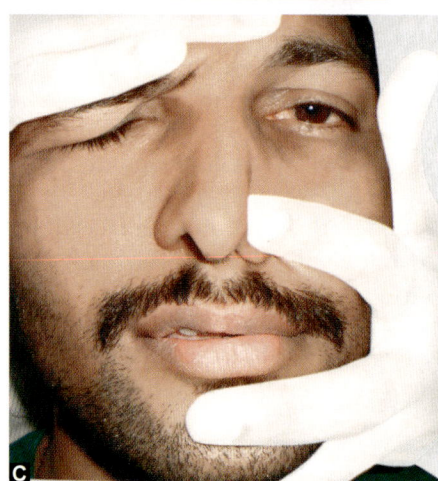

Figs. 35.57A to C: Eliciting the tenderness in maxilla and also checking the nasal blockage.

A wise man gets more use from his enemies than a fool from his friends—**Baltasar Gracian**

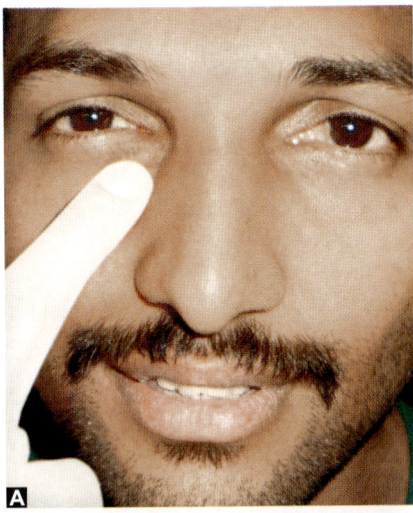

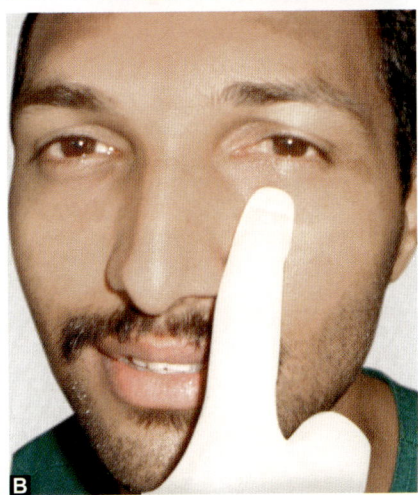

Figs. 35.58A and B: Palpating inferior orbital margin for tenderness or disruption.

- Any swelling if present is noted for its size, shape, consistency (uniform/variable), pulsation, egg-shell crackling, fluctuation, mobility, etc.
- Look for number and alignment of teeth in lower jaw.
- Look for any discharging sinus, if present, its location, number, discharge and granulation tissue.
- Discharging sinus in the symphysis menti is usually associated with sepsis of the lower teeth.

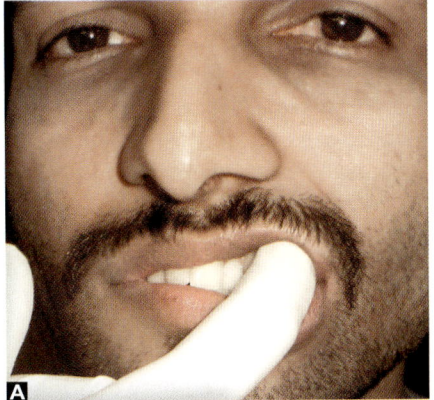

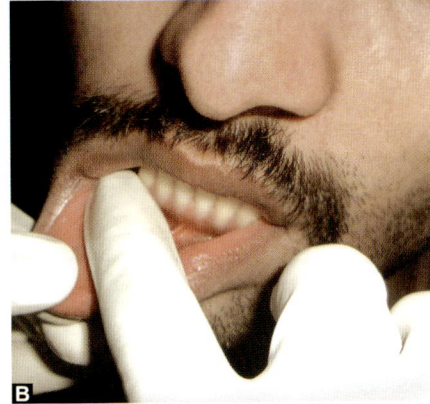

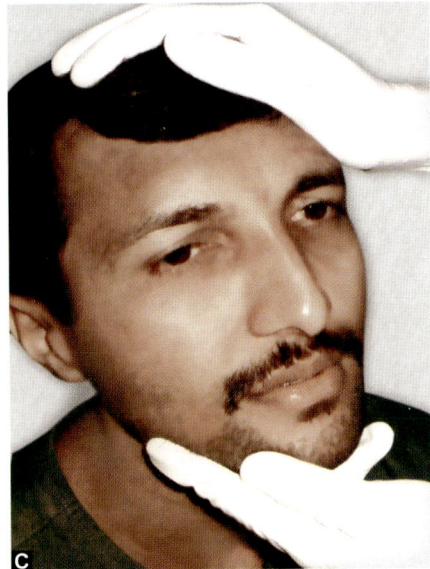

Figs. 35.59A to C: Palpating the alveolar margins of the jaw and lower margin of the mandible.

*But man is not made for defeat. A man can be destroyed but not defeated—***Ernest Hemingway**

* Tender, thickened mandible with discharging sinus suggests chronic osteomyelitis. Multiple discharging sinuses with sulfur granules are seen in actinomycosis of lower jaw.
* Cervical lymph nodes should be examined for enlargement.

Examination of Temporomandibular Joint (Figs. 35.60A to C)

* Patient is asked to open and close the mouth. The distance between the lower jaw and the upper is usually 2–5 cm. Patient sometimes cannot open the mouth due to muscular spasm around the joint (*trismus*); commonly seen when there is inflammatory process in the neighborhood, like dental abscess and parotitis.
* The movement of the condyle is appreciated by placing the fingers in front and just below the tragus. Any crepitus (seen in osteoarthritis), click in the joint is felt. It can also be well appreciated by placing a stethoscope in front of the joint.
* Dislocation of the joint has to be looked for. In bilateral dislocation, the mouth is open and fixed (prognathous deformity). In unilateral dislocation, the jaw is partially opened and deviated to the opposite side with a small hollow, felt just behind the condyle. The movement of the condyle can be felt by inserting the little finger into the external ear directed forwards, which is not felt in case of displaced condyles.

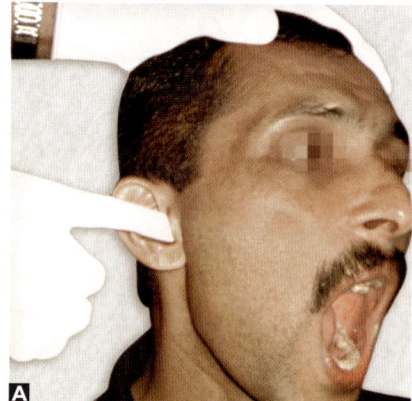
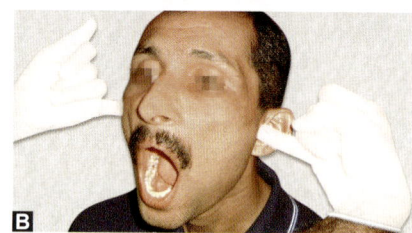
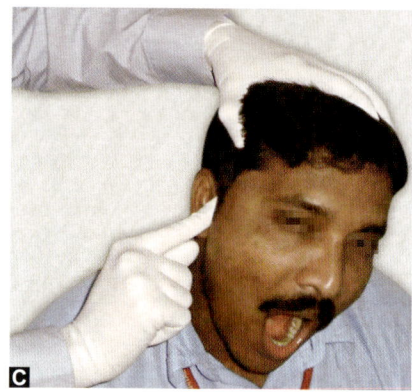

Figs. 35.60A to C: Temporomandibular joint movements should be checked both by placing little finger inside and from outside the ear.

Movements of Temporomandibular Joint

* It is checked by placing the little finger on the external auditory canal on both sides and patient is asked to open the jaw repeatedly. Joints also can be examined by placing the finger in front and above the tragus on the joint surface while opening the jaw.
* Forward, backward, gliding movements can be appreciated (Figs. 35.59A to C).

Examination of Nerves

* Maxillary division of trigeminal nerve is tested for integrity.
* Inferior alveolar nerve may be involved in mandibular trauma or tumor.

Investigations for Jaw Diseases

* Orthopantomogram to see the jaw bones.
* CT scan of jaw diseases.

A good teacher can inspire hope, ignite the imagination, and instill a love of learning—**Brad Henry**

- Biopsy of the lesion when suspecting for malignancy.
- FNAC of lymph node.

EXAMINATION SALIVARY GLAND

HISTORY

Swelling (Fig. 35.61)

- History of duration, mode of onset, site of onset, progress, recent increase in size, pain, whether initially painless, now becomes painful is asked. History of the swelling becoming tense and tender during meals is asked. Swelling of short duration with pain, trismus could be due to acute parotitis. Often it is bilateral in children due to viral cause (mumps). Bilateral enlargement of parotid along with other salivary glands and lacrimal gland is called as *Mikulicz syndrome*.

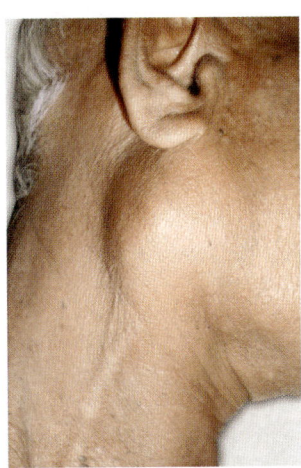

Fig. 35.61: Parotid gland enlargement. Note the location and ear lobule raise.

- Excessive salivation, joint pain along with enlargement of all salivary glandular is called as *Sjogren syndrome*.
- Pleomorphic adenoma is slowly growing tumor of long duration. Recent increase in size of swelling is important which suggests malignant transformation probably from a pre-existing pleomorphic adenoma. Adenolymphoma is slow growing tumor from lower pole of the parotid.

Pain

- History of duration/type/severity/radiation is asked. Sudden onset of severe pain is a feature of acute parotitis.
- Throbbing excruciating pain may be a feature of parotid abscess.
- Colicky pain during meals is a feature of salivary calculus with sialadenitis. Stone is more common in submandibular salivary gland but can also occur in parotid gland.

Fever

- It is a feature of acute sialadenitis or abscess.
- Acute sialadenitis with suppuration is common in parotid. Parotid abscess is usually unilateral. Mumps in children is bilateral.
- Neoplastic condition once necrosed can cause fever.

Difficulty in opening of mouth

It can occur in acute parotitis, submandibular sialadenitis, and malignancy extending into the soft tissues.

History of excess salivation

- Excessive salivation during meals/more pain during meals/swelling becoming more prominent during meals should be asked. It is a feature of stone in the salivary duct.
- Presence of sinus, its formation, discharge, etc. should be asked.

Discharge

- Discharge from sinus/fistula is usually saliva.
- Its quantity, duration, color whether increases while taking food should be clarified.

Recent increase in size

It suggests malignant transformation.

History of impairment of function

Drooling of saliva, inability to close eyes, tears in the eye, asymmetry of face, difficulty in opening of the mouth should be asked for.

When hungry, eat your rice; when tired, close your eyes. Fools may laugh at me, but wise men will know what I mean—**Lin-Chi**

History suggestive of metastases
In case of malignant salivary tumors like of lungs, bone and brain.

Past History
- Past history of surgery for parotid or submandibular swellings should be asked.
- Recurrent parotid tumors are known to occur in pleomorphic adenoma and malignancies.
- Detailed history of surgery, its nature of biopsy, postoperative management should be taken.
- Past history of radiotherapy in head and neck region; past history of other malignancy in the body.

Personal History
Personal history of alcohol intake is relevant in bilateral parotid enlargement.

LOCAL EXAMINATION

Inspection

Swelling
- Swelling is examined in detail. Position of the swelling is noted. Parotid swelling is below, behind and in front of the ear lobule. Parotid enlargement shows typical raise in ear lobule. Normal hollow/depression just below the ear lobule is obliterated.
- Size, shape, extent, skin over the swelling should be inspected. Skin is red and edematous in parotid abscess or inflammatory conditions. In inflammatory and mixed parotid tumor it assumes the shape of parotid, though it is much bigger in latter.
- Surface is bosselated and with well-defined margins in mixed parotid tumor; whereas it is smooth surfaced and with ill-defined margins in parotitis. In salivary calculus (submandibular calculus), swelling immediately becomes more prominent when lemon juice or chocolates are given to the patient to drink or eat.

Deep lobe (Fig. 35.62)
- Deep lobe of parotid enlargement is checked by inspecting the oral cavity for any bulge in the tonsil and lateral wall of pharynx.
- Floor of the mouth should be inspected for enlargement of deep lobe of the submandibular salivary gland.

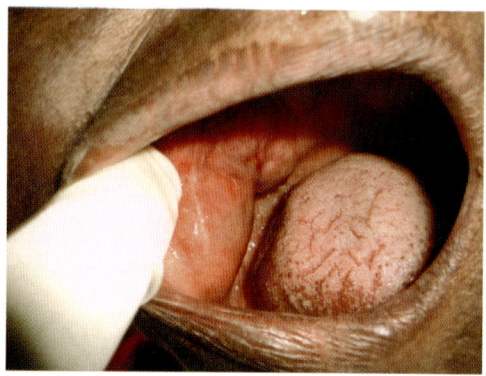

Fig. 35.62: Deep lobe of the parotid should be inspected from inside.

Stenson's and Wharton's duct examination
- *Stenson's parotid duct* is looked for on opposite to 2nd upper molar tooth (Fig. 35.63). Cheek should be retraced using spatula and with the help of good light source the duct is inspected properly. In suppurative parotitis, pus may be seen gushing out of the duct orifice after gentle

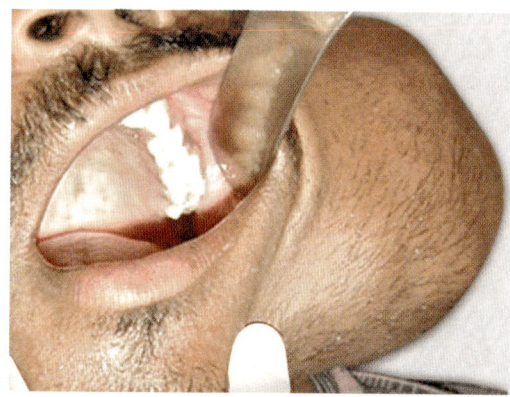

Fig. 35.63: Stenson's parotid duct should be examined opposite to 2nd upper molar.

Perfection is achieved, not when there is nothing more to add, but when there is nothing left to take away—**Antoine de Saint-Exupéry**

pressure over the parotid gland. Blood in the duct orifice (ampulla of duct) may be due to malignant parotid tumor.
* Opening and course of the *submandibular salivary duct (Wharton's)* should be inspected by asking the patient to fold the tongue upwards so that the tip of the tongue touches the palate. Duct orifice may be inflamed and edematous with pus discharging from it. Often stone may be visible near the duct orifice. Orifice is situated on either side of the frenulum linguae. Duct with impacted stone blocks the salivary flow and hence orifice on that side looks dry whereas orifice on normal side looks wet due to normal salivary flow. Two small dry swabs are placed over the orifices on each side and patient is asked to take stimulant like lemon juice; after a minute swabs are taken out and inspected; swab on the side with blocked orifice will be dry; swab over normal orifice will be wet.

Skin over the swelling
* Skin over the swelling should be inspected. Redness suggests sialadenitis. Sialadenitis is inflammation of the salivary gland.
* Ulceration or fungation may develop in advanced carcinoma parotid. Sinus or salivary *fistula* should be inspected for discharge and location.
* If parotid fistula is in relation with masseter then it is from the gland; but if it is premasseteric then it is from the duct.

Inspection of neck region
Neck is inspected for enlarged cervical nodes.

Movements of the jaw
Movements of the jaw may be restricted in malignant growth, infiltrating the jaw joint.

Palpation

Parotid swelling
Swelling (Fig. 35.64)
* Swelling should be palpated like for any other swelling—local rise of temperature,

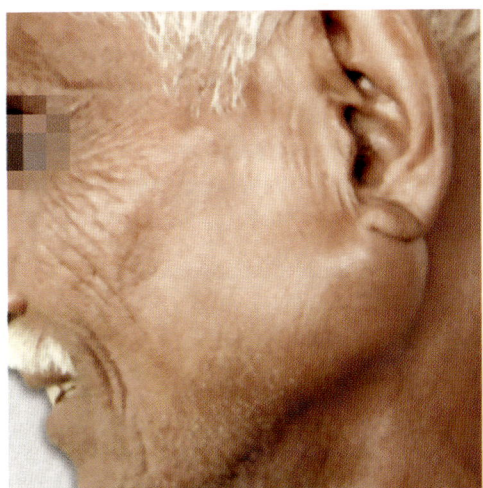

Fig. 35.64: Typical parotid swelling with ear lobe raised. Facial nerve should be tested by clenching the teeth.

tenderness, surface, consistency, mobility, *curtain sign,* whether skin is free or not, extension to deeper plane, relation to masseter and mandible.
* *Tenderness* suggests that it could be abscess, necrosis in a tumor or deeper infiltration.
* *Curtain sign*—deep fascia/parotid sheath is attached above to the zygomatic bone and so swelling arising from parotid gland cannot be moved up beyond zygomatic bone wherein deep fascia acts like a curtain preventing its further mobility. Swelling superficial to deep fascia can be moved beyond the level of the zygomatic bone above. Initially mobility of the swelling is checked in both directions; then patient is asked to clinch the teeth so that *masseter gets contracted* and mobility is checked again. If mobility is restricted then swelling is adherent to masseter muscle. Non-mobile swelling means it is adherent to bone beneath.
* Whether skin is adherent to swelling or not should be checked.
* *Consistency* is variable in different conditions—pleomorphic adenoma is firm but

Courage is not the absence of fear, but rather the judgement that something else is more important than fear—Ambrose Redmoon

can be hard with smooth surface. Malignant swellings often have nodular surface and of hard consistency; adenolymphoma (Warthin's) is smooth, soft often fluctuant and usually not transilluminant.

* Scar, fistula on the surface should be palpated.

Features of parotid swelling

- Ear lobule raise.
- Swelling in parotid region.
- Swelling occupying the groove between posterior part of the mandible and mastoid process.
- Moves upwards up to zygomatic bone—*curtain sign*.

Palpation

- Tenderness/temperature/extent/size/surface/consistency/mobility/fixity/plane of the swelling/masseter involvement/facial nerve involvement/skin over the swelling.
- Parotid duct palpation—by rolling the finger across the masseter muscle while patient is clinching the teeth to make masseter taut. Terminal part of the duct is palpated bidigitally using index finger inside and thumb outside.
- Palpation of oral cavity/bidigital examination for deep lobe is done with one finger inside the mouth behind the tonsillar fossa and the other outside in parotid region.
- All features of facial nerve palsy—inability to close eye/difficulty in blowing/altered nasolabial groove/clinching of teeth.
- Neck nodes should be examined.
- Examination of other salivary glands should be done.
- Relevant findings should be elicited in case of submandibular salivary gland enlargement.

Submandibular salivary gland swelling (Fig. 35.65)

It is also examined similar to any other swelling. Its medial, posterior extension, relation of the swelling to the lower margin of the body of the mandible should be checked. Enlargement of submandibular salivary gland occurs as a result of chronic sialadenitis or

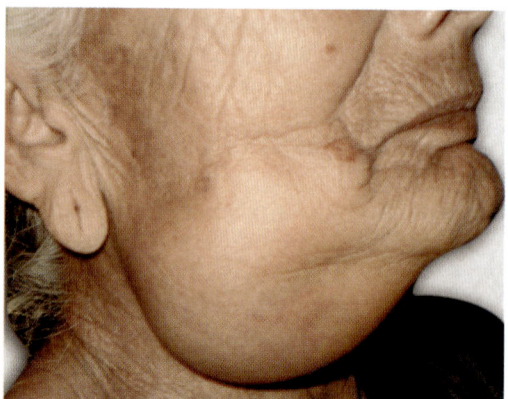

Fig. 35.65: Submandibular salivary gland tumor. Here oral cavity should be examined for deep lobe (bidigitally with one finger in the floor of the mouth); Wharton's duct (on either side of the frenulum of tongue); mandibular bone for thickening; hypoglossal nerve and lingual nerve palsy; neck nodes for spread.

neoplastic conditions. Its surface is usually smooth whereas in submandibular lymph node enlargement is usually nodular.

The *submandibular salivary gland* is best-palpated *bidigitally*. It confirms that swelling is submandibular salivary gland and also the deep lobe and duct can be palpated. Duct is palpated from behind forwards. First, dentures if present should be removed. Index finger of one hand is placed over the floor of the mouth medial to alveolus and lateral to tongue pushing the finger as deep as possible; fingers of the other hand are placed outside and medial to the mandibular margin, pushed the swelling upwards. By this way the finger inside the oral cavity not only helps to feel the deep lobe of the salivary gland which is deep to mylohyoid muscle but also the superficial lobe and often duct can be better assessed by this method. *Submandibular lymph node is not bidigitally palpable* as it is outside the mylohyoid muscle, superficial to the gland. Stone in the Wharton's duct also can be palpated by this method. Shape, size and consistency can be assessed by this method (Figs. 35.66 and 35.67).

It is well to give when asked but it is better to give unasked, through understanding—**KhalilGibran**

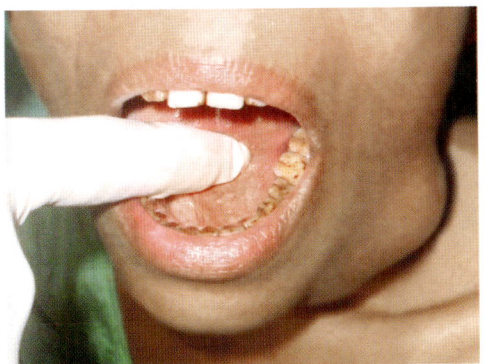

Fig. 35.66: Submandibular salivary gland duct should be palpated per orally.

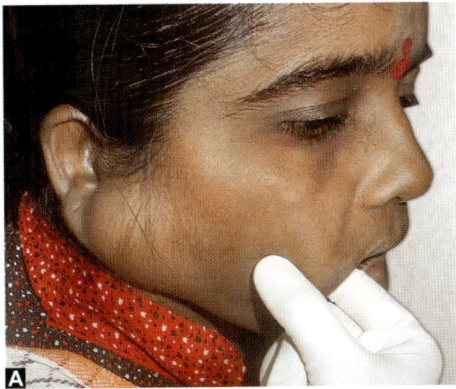

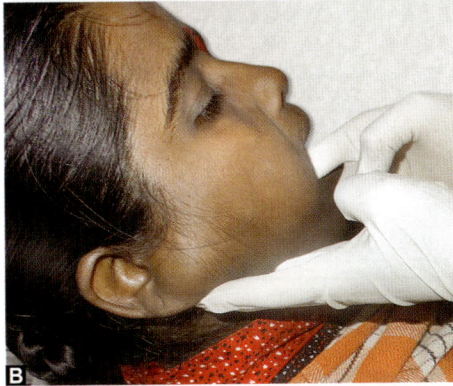

Figs. 35.68A and B: (A) Palpation of the parotid duct—bidigitally; (B) Palpation of the deep lobe of the parotid bidigitally.

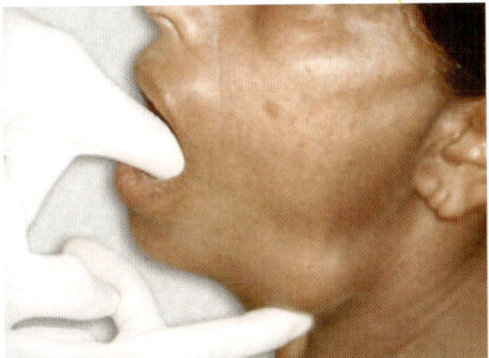

Fig. 35.67: Submandibular salivary gland bidigital palpation.

Intraoral Examination

- Parotid duct should be palpated using one finger inside the cheek and thumb outside the cheek. Duct can be better felt when masseter is taut. Only anterior part of the duct is felt.
- Enlarged *deep lobe of the parotid* can be felt by *bidigital palpation* with index finger of one hand placed inside the mouth in front of the tonsil and behind the 3rd molar tooth and fingers of the other hand placed outside and behind the ramus of the mandible (Figs. 35.68A and B).

Cranial Nerve Examination

- Involvement of *facial nerve* in parotid swelling should be checked for.

Features of facial nerve palsy (Figs. 35.69 to 35.71)

- Difficulty in chewing food as food accumulates in vestibule due to buccinator weakness.
- Deviation of angle of mouth while talking, laughing, blowing, whistling due to paralysis of orbicularis oris.
- Failure of closure of eyelids or easily opening of the eyelids after closure—paralysis of orbicularis oculi.
- Absence of furrows while looking upwards—paralysis of frontal belly of occipitofrontalis.
- Absence of corrugation in the forehead during frowning—paralysis of corrugator supercilii.
- Deviation of angle of mouth towards opposite side—paralysis of levator anguli oris.
- Loss of contraction of platysma in the neck while stretching the neck—paralysis of platysma.
- Inability to blow the air by the check and on palpation reduced tone of buccinator—paralysis of buccinator.
- Inability to whistle—paralysis of orbicularis oris.

To the man who only has a hammer, everything he encounters begins to look like a nail—Abraham Maslow

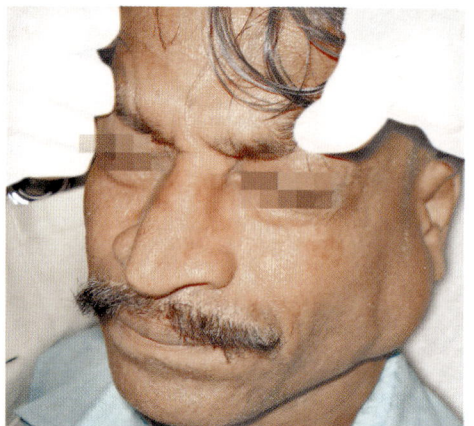

Fig. 35.69: Failure of closure of eyelids or easily opening of the eyelids after closure—paralysis of orbicularis oculi.

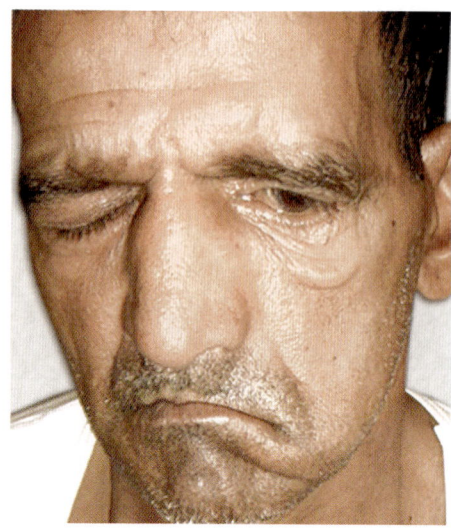

Fig. 35.71: Facial nerve palsy—typical look.

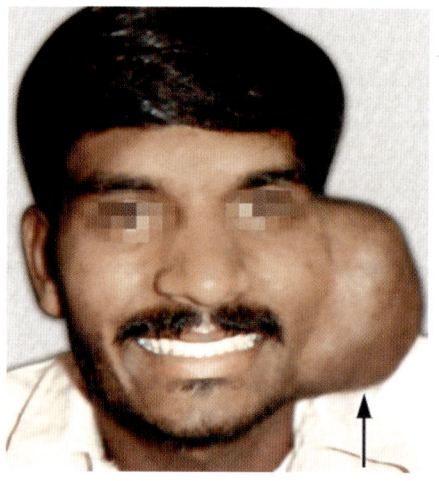

Fig. 35.70: Deviation of angle of mouth towards opposite side while clenching the teeth—paralysis of levator anguli oris.

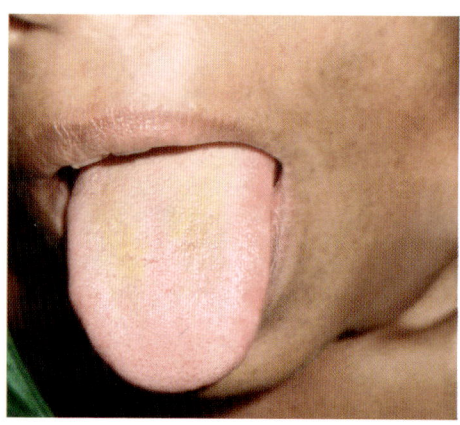

Fig. 35.72: Hypoglossal nerve should be assessed in submandibular salivary gland enlargement.

- *Hypoglossal nerve palsy* with tongue deviating towards same side while protruding should be checked for (Fig. 35.72).
- *Glossopharyngeal nerve palsy* should be checked for.

Differential Diagnosis for Parotid Enlargement

- *Idiopathic hypertrophy of masseter muscle*: It is a rare entity but presents like a swelling. When teeth are clenched, entire swelling hardens; but when relaxed swelling softens. It often can be bilateral.
- *Preauricular lymph node enlargement*: Swelling lies in front of the tragus; normal depression below and in front of the ear lobule is not obliterated; it may be suppuration, adenitis, tuberculosis or lymphoma. It feels more superficial.
- *Rarely parotid and paraparotid/subparotid lymph nodes* may be enlarged as secondaries from primary from oral mucosa and skin malignancies of head and neck

*The real voyage of discovery consists not in seeking new lands but seeing with new eyes—**Marcel Proust***

region (but these things are very rare and so students should not consider in usual clinical practice unless it is relevant). Still rarely parotid gland may be enlarged as nonmetastatic obstruction of the duct by carcinoma cheek.

Differential Diagnosis for Submandibular Salivary Gland Enlargement

- *Enlarged submandibular lymph nodes*: Bidigital palpation helps to confirm it. Lymph nodes are not bidigitally palpable.
- *Enlarged facial lymph node* lies adjacent to facial artery at the lower margin of the mandible which can be moved above the level of margin of the mandible into the face.

Examination of salivary gland

History
- Swelling—duration—progress.
- Pain—duration/type/severity/radiation.
- Fever.
- Difficulty in opening mouth.
- Excess salivation during meals/more pain during meals/swelling become more prominent during meals.

Examination

Inspection
- Swelling in detail.
- Deep lobe of parotid enlargement is checked by inspecting the oral cavity for any bulge in the tonsil and lateral wall of pharynx.
- Stenson's parotid duct should be inspected.
- Skin over the swelling should be inspected.

Palpation
- Tenderness/temperature/extent/size/surface/ consistency/mobility/fixity/plane of the swelling/ masseter involvement/facial nerve involvement/ skin over the swelling.
- Parotid duct palpation.
- Palpation of oral cavity/bidigital examination for deep lobe.
- All features of facial nerve palsy—inability to close eye/difficulty in blowing/altered nasolabial groove/clinching of teeth.
- Neck nodes should be examined.
- Examination of other neck nodes should be done.
- Relevant findings should be elicited in case of submandibular salivary gland enlargement.

EXAMINATION OF INGUINOSCROTAL SWELLINGS

- Elderly people are more prone for hernia. Men with strainfull occupation like manual laborers, sportsmen, weight lifters etc. are more prone for hernia. Indirect hernia occurs in young; direct hernia occurs in old. Strenuous workers; gymnastics; sportsmen; weight lifters may develop hernia due to straining.
- Funiculitis occurs in young age. Testicular tumor occurs in early adult age (seminoma) but can occur in young (teratoma). Varicocele presents in adolescents and young. Filarial funiculitis, orchitis and lymph varix are common in Orissa, West Bengal, coastal regions. Carcinoma of scrotal skin is seen in elderly. Torsion testis is seen in adolescents. Hydrocele is common in adult. Epididymal cyst, spermatocele are seen in adult. Tuberculous orchitis is seen in young individuals. Carcinoma of scrotal skin is often occupation related—those who come in contact with soot (Chimney sweep's cancer); tar or oil (Mule spinner's disease). Prolonged standing may cause varicocele.

Chief Complaints

- Swelling in the groin/inguinoscrotal region right or left or both side; durations of the swelling.
- Pain over the swelling—durations.

History

History of Present Illness

Swelling
- Duration of the swelling.
- Mode of onset of the swelling—spontaneously or on straining.
- Site of the first appearance of the swelling—in the groin or in the scrotum. Inguinal hernia begins in groin; hydrocele, testicular tumor begins in scrotum; varicocele begins

*Even if you're on the right track, you'll get run over if you just sit there—***Will Rogers**

- in root of the scrotum. Lipoma of cord, encysted hydrocele of the cord appears in groin or near root of the scrotum. Undescended testis presents with swelling in the groin with empty scrotum.
- Unilateral or bilateral. In bilateral swellings the side on which it appeared first and after how long has it appeared on opposite side should be asked. Hydrocele and inguinal hernia can be bilateral; varicocele is more common on left side but can be bilateral; bilateral impalpable undescended testes are called as *cryptorchidism*.
- Progress and extent of the swelling whether only limits to the groin or extends to the scrotum (complete inguinal hernia).
- Any changes in the size and extent of the swelling on standing/walking/straining/lying down.
- Whether swelling is reducible on lying down (reducible hernia will disappear on lying down, hydrocele will not disappear)/partially reducible or irreducible on lying down or needs any maneuver to reduce it—reducible hernias. History of gurgling sound in the scrotum signifies enterocele.
- If swelling is irreducible then whether it is painful or there is abdominal distension/vomiting—should be asked.
- History of trauma; trauma may precipitate hematocele or hydrocele. Trauma on bulb of urethra may cause urinary extravasation and swelling in the scrotum.
- History of rapid increase in size occurs in testicular tumors.
- Sudden pain and swelling in scrotum is probably due to acute epididymo-orchitis or pyocele.
- Other swellings in epigastric region in the abdomen (due to palpable enlarged para-aortic lymph nodes)/in the supraclavicular region due to enlarged lymph nodes may be elicited in history often.
- Scrotal edema may be due to filariasis or part of generalized anasarca.
- Gonococcal urethritis with stricture also can cause extravasation and scrotal swelling—*watering can perineum*.
- Swelling with heaviness in the scrotum may be initial presentation of testicular tumor.

Pain

- Site of pain—whether it is in the groin or in the scrotum.
- Duration of pain.
- Severity of the pain, type of pain—dull aching or severe pricking type, whether initially painless later become painful (in testicular tumor) should be asked.
- Aggravating or relieving factors: Aggravated by straining/walking/weight lifting; relieved by lying down.
- Epididymo-orchitis, funiculitis presents with pain, redness, swelling and often fever. Hematocele, pyocele can be severely painful. Torsion testis presents with severe pain often precipitated by straining due to sudden violent contraction of the cremaster. Periodic mild fever with pain, discomfort and swelling in the scrotum and spermatic cord are the features of filarial epididymo-orchitis.

History relevant to precipitating factors

Condition increasing the intra-abdominal pressure precipitating hernia are:
- Respiratory diseases like chronic cough, tuberculosis, bronchial asthma.
- Constipation, altered bowel habits, tenesmus, bloody stool—in relation to anorectal stricture/carcinoma.
- Dysuria/urgency/hesitancy/altered stream/night frequency/retention of urine/burning urine/hematuria—in relation to benign prostatic hyperplasia/urethral stricture.

Past History

- Past history of surgery (hernia/hydrocele)—same side/opposite side. Type of surgery

---

What we think, or what we know, or what we believe is, in the end, of little consequence. The only consequence is what we do—**John Ruskin**

done (whether mesh used or repair for hernia).
- History of appendicectomy earlier and if so detail about the surgery. Open appendicectomy can cause right inguinal hernia by injuring ilioinguinal nerve.
- Past history suggestive of irreducibility/ obstruction and treatment for that conservative/surgical.
- History of tuberculosis, venereal diseases.

Personal History

- Smoking—duration, number per day, whether beedi or cigarette. Pan chewing/ alcohol intake.
- Appetite and altered weight.
- History of infertility in case of varicocele.

General Examination

General built and nutritional status, pallor, clubbing, cyanosis, jaundice, lymphadenopathy, edema feet, pulse and blood pressure are noted.

Local Examination

Inguinoscrotal region should be examined in standing position as swelling commonly gets reduced and disappears in lying down position.

Inspection

Inspection in standing position (Fig. 35.73):
- Mention the side of the swelling, shape (globular in inguinal), margin—well defined/ill-defined.
- Site and extent of the swelling is important. Incomplete indirect inguinal hernia and usually direct inguinal hernias are in inguinal region. Complete indirect inguinal hernia (rarely complete direct inguinal hernia) is *inguinoscrotal*. Swelling extends from the proximal part of the inguinal canal towards the scrotum below.

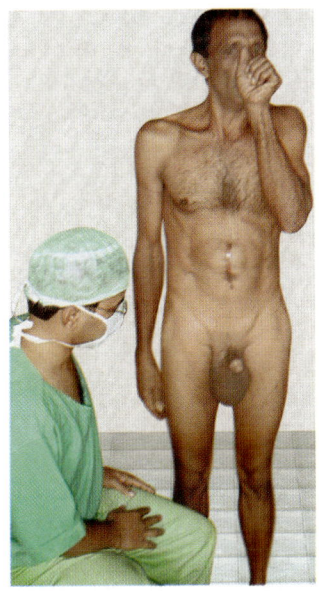

Fig. 35.73: Expansile impulse on coughing is better seen than felt. It should be inspected with patient standing and examiner sitting beside the patient

Swelling confined only to scrotum is due to hydrocele, epididymal cyst, spermatocele, scrotal edema, and varicocele. Hydrocele causes obvious large swelling. In encysted hydrocele of the cord, lipoma of the cord swelling may be in the groin or root of the scrotum. Swelling in the groin or superficial inguinal pouch may be due to undescended testis or ectopic testis. Here empty scrotum is obvious on inspection. Scrotal edema may be due to scrotal cellulitis, cardiac/ renal/hepatic causes, filariasis, advanced secondaries in the inguinal lymph nodes blocking cutaneous lymphatic drainage, extravasation of urine and often associated with penile edema. Penis may be buried in large hydrocele, large inguinoscrotal hernia, and scrotal edema.
- Skin over the scrotum/swelling/groin should be inspected. Surface smooth/ uneven in iguinal hernias:
  - It is red and edematous in funiculitis, and orchitis. Acutely inflamed skin with redness is often also a feature of torsion

Work like you don't need money, love like you've never been hurt, and dance like no one's watching

testis. Strangulated hernia also shows signs of inflammation over the skin which extends from scrotum to groin.
- Loss of rugosity of scrotal skin occurs in long standing hydrocele, syphilitic orchitis, tuberculous epididymitis and testicular tumors. Skin may be stretched in scrotal edema.
- Scrotal edema of filarial origin is non-pitting whereas due to other causes is pitting in nature. One has to remember that common cause of hydrocele is filarial. Clinician should be able to differentiate hydrocele from scrotal edema.
  - Ulcer in the scrotal skin may be due to **scrotal carcinoma** which will be having, raised and everted edge, slough in the floor. All features of an ulcer explained in chapter 'examination of an ulcer' should be mentioned.
  - **Testicular tumor** occasionally can fungate through scrotal skin (can be anywhere but *usually anterolateral*) and present as an ulcer.
  - Syphilitic **gummatous ulcer** is located always *on front (anterior)* of the scrotum which is adherent to testis due to syphilitic orchitis. It is punched out with wash leather slough.
  - **Tuberculous epididymitis** causes ulceration on the *posterior aspect* of the scrotum with an undermined edge. Only in anteverted testis positions are reversed.
  - Scrotal skin gangrene is a feature of **Fournier's gangrene**.
  - Multiple discharging sinuses in the scrotal skin are the features of the gonococcal urethritis with discharging urine—*watering can perineum*.
  - **Multiple sebaceous cysts** are common in scrotum. Scrotum may show whitish vesicle containing lymph due to filariasis **(lymph scrotum)** which may rupture causing **lymphorrhagia**.

- Both transverse and vertical dimensions of the size should be mentioned.
- *Expansile impulse on coughing over the swelling is diagnostic of inguinal hernia. It is better seen than felt.* Varicocele and lymph varix also show impulse on coughing but with fluid thrill.
- Groin should be inspected for swelling (inguinal nodes), ulceration, and fungation. Ulceration can occur in groin due to secondaries in the lymph nodes, bubo, tuberculosis, etc.
- Visible peristalsis over the inguinal swelling should be noted if present. It means it could be enterocele.
- Scar/dilated veins/discoloration.

Palpation

- **Position and extent**:
  Exact location of swelling on inspection is important whether it is in the inguinal/inguinoscrotal/scrotal region. Hernia is inguinal or inguinoscrotal. Encysted hydrocele of the cord is located usually in the middle of the cord near the root of the scrotum occasionally in the groin. It will not extend proximally above. Lipoma of the cord, funiculitis (inflammation of vas deferens), (filarial—common), ectopic testis in superficial inguinal pouch are other groin swellings to be considered. Skin should be held to see the fixity.
- **Get above the swelling (Fig. 35.74):**
  In standing position cord is palpated for structures by placing thumb in front and fingers behind on the root of the scrotum. Purely scrotal swellings like in hydrocele one can get above the swelling—means only cord structures are felt and nothing else. In inguinoscrotal hernia, one cannot get above the swelling. Cord with additional structures are also felt. This is important test to confirm scrotal swelling.
- Like any other swelling, *size* (in vertical and transverse directions), *shape,* margin (well

Try a thing you haven't done three times. Once, to get over the fear of doing it. Twice, to learn how to do it. And a third time, to figure out whether you like it or not—Virgil Garnett Thomson

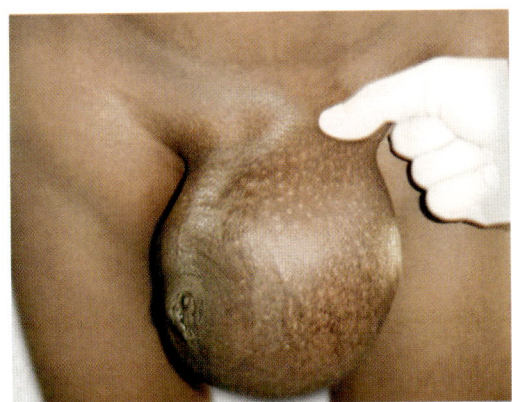

Fig. 35.74: One can get above the swelling in hydrocele. In inguinoscrotal swelling getting above the swelling is not possible.

defined or ill defined), **surface** smooth/lobular/tense), **warmness, tenderness,** should be checked.

* **Consistency** is soft and elastic in enterocele; doughy in omentocele. Encysted hydrocele is fluctuant, cystic (Paget's test is positive), transilluminant. Lymph varix is soft, cystic and doughy. Varicocele is soft, with typical feel of 'bag of worms'. Hydrocele is smooth and soft (firm if it is tensely cystic).
* **Location of the swelling:**
  Swelling is above and medial to pubic tubercle in inguinal hernia and below and lateral to pubic tubercle in femoral hernia.
* **Reducibility:**
  Inguinal and inguinoscrotal hernia is reducible. Reducibility of the swelling is checked by different methods. Whether swelling reduces spontaneously while lying down or needs any manipulation like *taxis* to get reduced. *Taxis* method is, after flexion and rotation of hip joint, contents of the scrotum is gradually and gently reduced into the abdominal cavity. Hernia gets reduced abruptly and rapidly. Whether it is reduced completely or partially is noted. In enterocele first part is difficult to be reduced but last part gets reduced easily whereas in omentocele, it is difficult to reduce the last part but first part gets reduced easily. Hydrocele is not reducible. *Exception*—congenital hydrocele, as it communicates with abdominal cavity is reducible. Varicocele and lymph varix also gets reduced while lying down but slowly and gradually.
* **Impulse on coughing:**
  - Hernia shows expansile impulse on coughing. Varicocele and lymph varix also show impulse on coughing like a fluid thrill but it is not expansile.
  - *Zieman's test* is done to find out over which finger impulse is felt and so which type of hernia it could be whether femoral/direct inguinal or indirect inguinal.
  - *Deep ring occlusion test (Fig. 35.75):* Once deep ring is occluded, if impulse on coughing becomes absent, it means it is indirect inguinal hernia. If impulse on coughing is still present then it is direct inguinal hernia.
  - *Finger invagination test*—size of the superficial ring and site on the finger where the impulse is felt, whether it is in the tip of the finger or pulp is noted.
* **Fluctuation:**
  This test is essential test for hydrocele. Upper part of the scrotum is held between thumb and fingers of one hand to steady

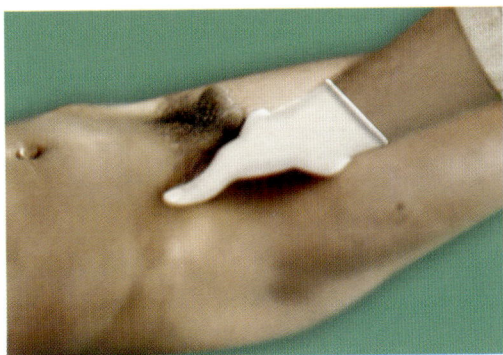

Fig. 35.75: Ring occlusion test is done to find out whether hernia is direct or indirect. If after occluding the ring swelling appears on the medial side, it is direct hernia. If swelling does not appear on occlusion and coughing it is indirect hernia.

Failure is simply the opportunity to begin again, this time more intelligently—Henry Ford

the swelling; thumb and fingers of other hand are held at lower pole. Intermittent pressure from lower fingers will push apart the fingers over upper part and vice versa. Test is repeated in opposite direction. It is important to elicit fluctuation in two directions. It is also important to fix the swelling prior to eliciting the fluctuation. In a small swelling Paget's test is used. In bilocular hydrocele, i.e. swelling in the groin and hydrocele with band like narrowing near external ring, fluctuation can be elicited across external ring above and below—*cross fluctuation* (other swellings which are cross fluctuant are—psoas abscess, ranula, and compound palmar ganglion). Hydrocele, encysted hydrocele, epididymal cyst, spermatocele, abscess are fluctuant swellings in the scrotum.

- **Transillumination/translucency (Fig. 35.76)**:
It is done in a dark room using a pen torch. Pen torch is placed laterally in the anterior part of the scrotum. It is never placed posteriorly as testis will interfere with proper illumination. Red glow of translucency is seen in the scrotum which is better appreciated using a roll of thick paper or X-ray sheet placed on the opposite side (medially) especially with day light. Hydrocele becomes non-transilluminant due to thick dartos, thick unclear fluid, thick sac, hematocele, chylocele, pyocele. Epididymal cyst is *brilliantly* transilluminant.

- **Traction test:**
It is the test for encysted hydrocele of the cord. Mobile swelling located above the testis becomes immobile once testis is pulled down from the swelling. It is used to differentiate it from epididymal cyst.

- Palpation of testis:
  - **Position:** Testis may be in normal position with testis in front, epididymis behind and globus major upwards. In *anteverted testis,* epididymis lies anteriorly and body posteriorly. In *inverted testis*, testis lies upside down with globus major inferiorly. In *incompletely inverted testis*, testis lies horizontally. Inverted or incompletely inverted testis precipitates torsion testis.
  - *Weight of the organ* in relation to size should be assessed. It is done by balancing the testis on the palm of the hand. Testis is *heavier in testicular tumor and hematocele*. It is lighter in gummatous testis even though size is large. Relation of swelling to testis also should be noted.
  - **Testicular sensation:** It is sickening sensation felt by the patient when a mild pressure is applied on the testis. It is absent in testicular tumor, syphilis (Gumma), leprosy, chronic hematocele. Both side testes should be palpated.

- Palpation of epididymis:
Epididymis will be enlarged, *craggy,* firm in tuberculosis. Firm, irregular enlarged epididymis is common in filariasis whereas in **acute epididymo-orchitis** it is smooth, soft, tender swelling posteriorly.

- Palpation of spermatic cord:
Cord is palpated for vas deferens. Vas deferens is palpated at the root of the scrotum between thumb and index finger *together on both sides*. Normally, it slips between fingers like whipcord. Vas is

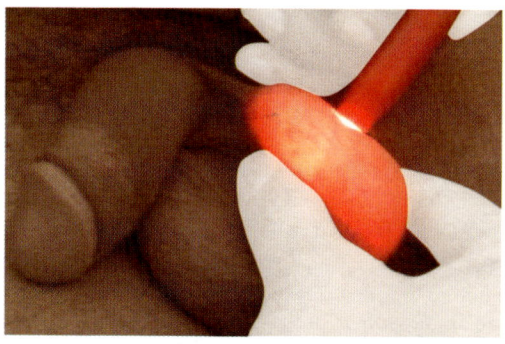

Fig. 35.76: Hydrocele which is transilluminant.

A little more persistence, a little more effort, and what seemed hopeless failure may turn to glorious success—**Elbert Hubbard**

thickened and tender in epididymo-orchitis—acute or chronic due to funiculitis. It is thickened and beaded in tuberculosis of vas. It is thickened and tender in filariasis. Soft, doughy feeling is felt in lymph varix; like 'bag of worms' in varicocele of spermatic cord. Rarely testicular tumor spreads along the spermatic cord making it nodular and hard.

- Palpation of bulbar urethra by lifting the scrotum and feeling in the midline for any thickening and button like depression—suggestive of stricture urethra.
- Opposite inguinal region, opposite testis, epididymis and spermatic cord should be examined. Impulse on coughing on opposite side is present or absent should be mentioned.

Percussion

In case of inguinal hernia, without reducing the contents of the swelling, percussion is done over the surface. If it is resonant, it is enterocele. If it is dull on percussion then it is omentocele.

Auscultation

Bowel sounds may be heard over the swelling if it is enterocele.

Systemic Examination

Per Abdomen Examination

- Abdomen muscle tone should be checked by head raising test, leg raising test and Valsalva maneuver. It should be inspected for Malgaigne bulging and should be palpated to check whether tone is adequate (firm) or inadequate (supple).
- Any scar in the abdomen (appendicectomy scar may cause right sided direct inguinal hernia), ascites or mass per abdomen should be mentioned.

Respiratory System Examination

It is important as secondaries can occur in testicular tumors; primary focus may be in lungs in tuberculosis and also to look for altered breath sounds (rhonchi, bronchial breathing), effusion, etc. to find out the precipitating causes of hernia.

Cardiovascular system, nervous system, spine and cranium for any neurological problems are examined for management of hernia.

Palpation of lymph nodes:
Scrotal skin drains into inguinal lymph nodes; testis and epididymis drains into pre- and para-aortic lymph nodes at the level of origin of testicular artery—transpyloric nodes. Inguinal and iliac nodes may be enlarged in scrotal skin conditions and also testicular tumor infiltrating the tunica and scrotal skin. Testicular tumor spreads to para-aortic nodes and then to left-sided supraclavicular nodes.

Digital Examination of the Rectum (P/R)

Rectal examination should be done in all hernia cases to look for prostate enlargement in elderly and rectal/anorectal strictures.

DEFINITION OF HERNIA

- Hernia means—*'To bud' or 'to protrude.' 'off shoot' (Greek). 'rupture' (Latin).*
- Hernia is defined an abnormal protrusion of a viscous or a part of a viscous through an opening, artificial or natural with a sac covering it.
- *Inguinal hernia is the commonest hernia (73%) because the muscular anatomy in the inguinal region is weak and also due to the presence of natural weakness like deep ring and cord structures.*
- *Femoral is 17%; umbilical is 8.5%; others are 1.5%.*

When solving problems, dig at the roots instead of just hacking at the leaves.—**Anthony J D'Angelo**

Etiology

* Straining.
* Lifting of heavy weight.
* Chronic cough (tuberculosis, chronic bronchitis, bronchial asthma, emphysema).
* Chronic constipation (habitual, rectal stricture).
* *Urinary causes:*
  – Old age: Benign prostatic hyperplasia (BPH), carcinoma prostate
  – Young age: Stricture urethra
  – Very young age: Phimosis, meatal stenosis.
* Obesity.
* Pregnancy and pelvic anatomy (especially in femoral hernia in females).
* Smoking.
* Ascites.
* Appendicectomy through McBurney's incision may injure the ilioinguinal nerve causing right sided *direct* inguinal hernia.
* An indirect inguinal hernia occurs in a congenital, preformed sac, i.e. the remains of processus vaginalis. Chances of presence of bilateral preformed sac are 60%.
* Familial—collagen disorder—Prune Belly syndrome.

Pathology of Hernia

Hernia comprises of:
* *Covering.*
* *Sac.*
* *Content.*

Sac

* Sac is a diverticulum of peritoneum with mouth, neck, body and fundus.
* Neck is *narrow in indirect sac but wide in direct sac*. Body of the sac is thin in infants, children and in indirect sac but is thick in direct and long-standing sac.
* Hernia without neck: Those hernias with larger mouth lacks neck, e.g. direct hernia, incisional hernia.
* Hernia without sac: Epigastric hernia—it is protrusion of extraperitoneal pad of fat.

Coverings of the sac are the layers of the abdominal wall through which the sac passes.

Contents of Sac

* Omentum—*Omentocele* (Epiplocele). Difficult to reduce the sac at the end.
* Intestine—*Enterocele*—commonly small bowel, but sometimes even large bowel. Difficult to reduce the sac initially.
* *Richter's hernia*—a portion of circumference of bowel is the content.
* Urinary bladder may be the content or part of the posterial wall of the sac.
* Ovary, often with fallopian tube.
* Meckel's diverticulum—*Littre's hernia*.
* *Fluid:* Fluid secreted from congested bowel or omentum. It may be a infected fluid or ascitic fluid or blood from the strangulated sac.

General Classification of Hernia

Classification I *(clinical):*
1. **Reducible hernia :** Hernia get reduced on its own or by the patient or by the surgeon. Intestine reduces with gurgling and first portion is difficult to reduce. Omentum is doughy and last portion is difficult to reduce. Expansile impulse on coughing present.
2. **Irreducible hernia**: Here contents cannot be returned to the abdomen due to narrow neck, adhesions, overcrowding, etc. Irreducibility predisposes to strangulation.
3. **Obstructed hernia**: It is an irreducible hernia with obstruction but blood supply to the bowel is not interfered. It eventually leads to strangulation.
4. **Inflamed hernia**: It is due to inflammation of the contents of the sac, e.g. appendicitis, salpingitis. Here hernia is tender but not tense; overlying skin is red and edematous.

Don't reinvent the wheel, just realign it—**Anthony J D'Angelo**

5. **Strangulated hernia**: It is due to obstruction causing blockage of blood supply leading into gangrene of the content. It is a surgical emergency. Patient will be toxic, with irreducibility and pain and tenderness. Emergency surgery, resection of the bowel and anastomosis should be done.

Classification II:
Anatomical classification in inguinal hernia:
- **Indirect hernia:** It arises through internal ring along with the cord. It is lateral to the inferior epigastric artery.
- **Direct hernia:** It occurs through the posterior wall of the inguinal canal. Sac is medial to the inferior epigastric artery (Fig. 35.77).

Classification III: According to the extent
- **Incomplete:**
  - **Bubonocele:** Here sac is confined to the inguinal canal.
  - **Funicular:** Here sac crosses the superficial inguinal ring but does not reach the bottom of the scrotum.
- **Complete:** Here sac descends to the bottom of the scrotum (Fig. 35.78).

Classification IV:
- Congenital.
- Acquired.

Classification V: According to the contents
- Omentocele—omemtum.
- Enterocele—intestine.
- Cystocele—urinary bladder.
- Litter's hernia—Meckel's diverticulum.

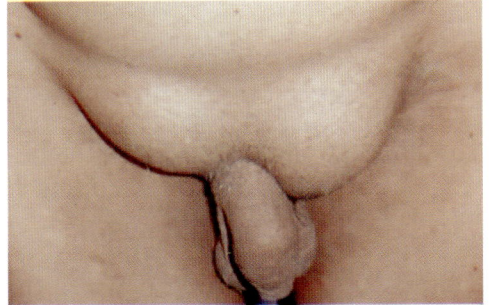

Fig. 35.77: Bilateral direct inguinal hernia. Note medial location of the hernia. It is always acquired.

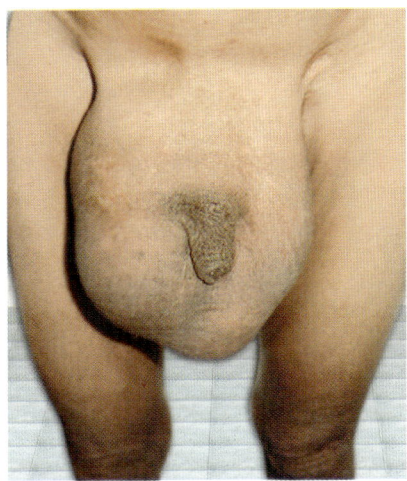

Fig. 35.78: Bilateral complete inguinal hernia. Here hernia descends into scrotum. Usually indirect inguinal hernia becomes complete.

- Maydl's hernia.
- Sliding hernia.
- Richter's hernia—part of the bowel wall.

Surgical Anatomy of Inguinal Canal (Figs. 35.79 and 35.80)

Superficial inguinal ring is a triangular opening in the external oblique aponeurosis and is 1.25 cm above the pubic tubercle. The ring is bounded by a superomedial and inferolateral crus. Normally the ring does not admit the tip of little finger.

Deep inguinal ring is a U-shaped condensation of the transversalis fascia, lies 1.25 cm above the inguinal ligament midway between the symphysis pubis and the anterosuperior iliac spine.

Inguinal canal—in infants both superficial and deep rings are superimposed without any obliquity of the inguinal canal. In adults it is 3.75 cm long, directed downwards and medially from the deep to superficial ring.

In males inguinal canal transmits the spermatic cord, ilioinguinal nerve and genital branch of the genitofemoral nerve. In females, its content is the round ligament.

Become a student of change. It is the only thing that will remain constant—**Anthony J D'Angelo**

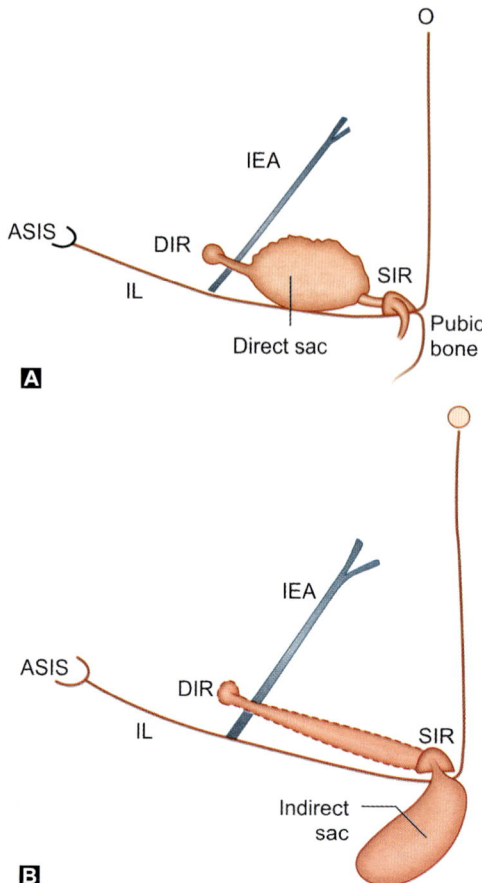

Figs. 35.79A and B: Diagrammatic representation of anatomical location of direct and indirect inguinal hernia.

Inguinal canal in female is called as canal of Nuck.

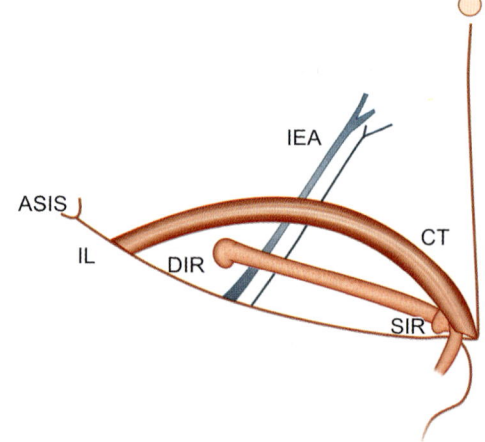

Fig. 35.80: Surgical anatomy of inguinal canal. (ASIS: anterosuperior iliac spine; DIR: deep inguinal ring; IEA: inferior epigastric artery; IL: inguinal ligament; SIR: superficial inguinal ring)

aspect of the spermatic cord, whereas the direct hernia pops out directly forward through the posterior wall of the inguinal canal.
- Neck of the indirect sac is lateral to inferior epigastric vessels but direct sac emerges medial to the inferior epigastric vessels with a wide neck.
- Saddle-bag or pantaloon hernial sac has got both medial and lateral component.
- Inguinal hernia is above and medial to the pubic tubercle. Femoral hernia is below and lateral to pubic tubercle.

Boundaries

- *In front:* External oblique aponeurosis and conjoined muscle laterally.
- *Behind:* Inferior epigastric artery, fascia transversalis and conjoined tendon medially.
- *Above:* Conjoined muscle (arched fibers of internal oblique).
- *Below:* Inguinal ligament.
   - An indirect inguinal hernia travels down the canal on the lateral and anterior

Hernioplasty

It is strengthening of posterior inguinal wall in case of indirect hernia or in any large hernia with weak abdominal wall using a supportive material. This allows and supports good fibroblast proliferation which in turn strengthens the weak posterior wall of inguinal canal or abdominal wall.

Material Used

- *Synthetic:* Prolene mesh (white in color)—Dacron mesh.

*You don't have to hold a position in order to be a leader—***Anthony J D'Angelo**

- *Biological:* Tensor fascia lata, temporal fascia and skin (presently biological materials are not well accepted as infection is common and its efficacy is not proved). *Prolene mesh* is commonly used at present. *Hernioplasty is ideal procedure for inguinal hernia.*

EXAMINATION OF HYDROCELE

- Hydrocele is collection of fluid in the scrotum between two layers of the tunica vaginalis testis. It can be primary idiopathic, or secondary due to filarial infection, trauma, tuberculosis, syphilis or malignancy.
- Hydrocele fluid is amber colored which contains water, salt, albumin and fibrinogen. Fluid per se does not clot but if comes in contact with the blood it gets clotted.
- Primary vaginal hydrocele occurs in middle age.
- Hydrocele is smooth, soft, fluctuant and often transilluminant (Fig. 35.81). When holding root of the scrotum only cord structures are felt not something else (Fig. 35.82). There is no impulse on coughing. It is by this method hydrocele is differentiated from inguinal hernia. In hernia one cannot get above the swelling and there is impulse on coughing.

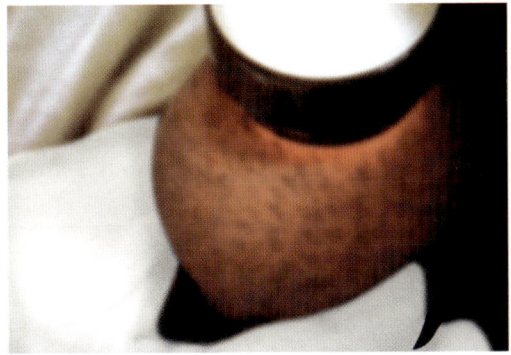

Fig. 35.81: Hydrocele is usually transilluminant. Thickened dartos, thick sac, infected fluid makes it non-transilluminant.

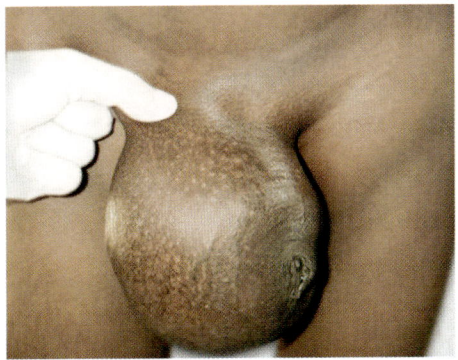

Fig. 35.82: Hydrocele is scrotal swelling. Get above the swelling is the clinical method used to differentiate from hernia.

Types

- **Vaginal hydrocele** limits to only scrotum.
- **Congenital hydrocele** communicates to peritoneal cavity.
- **Infantile hydrocele:** Here tunica and processus vaginalis (hydrocele) are distended up to internal ring, but sac has no connection with the general peritoneal cavity.
- **Encysted hydrocele of the cord:** It is a smooth, oval, and swelling associated with the spermatic cord. On gentle traction to the testis, the swelling becomes less mobile (traction test).
- **Hydrocele en bisac** (bilocular hydrocele).
- Hydrocele has got two intercommunicating sacs, one above and one below the neck of the scrotum.

Secondary Hydrocele

Causes

Infection: Filariasis
Tuberculosis of epididymis
Syphilis.

Injury: Trauma, post-herniorrhaphy hydrocele.

Tumor: Malignancy.

It is usually small, lax and testis is usually palpable (unlike primary hydrocele). Exception is secondary hydrocele due to filariasis.

Set high standards and few limitations for yourself—Anthony J D'Angelo

Filarial Hydrocele and Chylocele

- Occurs commonly in coastal region and in and around the equator.
- Usually occurs after repeated attacks of filarial epididymitis.
- Hydrocele is usually of large size and the sac is thickened.
- Fluid contains fat, rich in cholesterol, derived from ruptured lymph varix into the tunica.
- It is often difficult to differentiate from primary hydrocele.

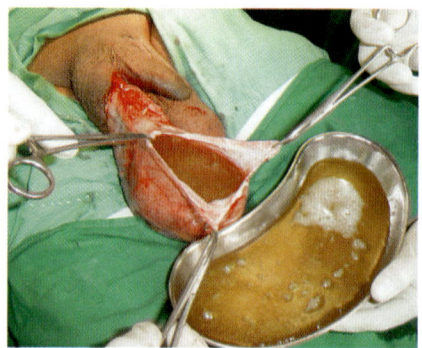

Fig. 35.83: Amber colored hydrocele fluid on table.

Complications of hydrocele
• Infection.
• Pyocele.
• Hematocele.
• Atrophy of testis.
• Infertility.

Treatment for Hydrocele

Surgery

- Subtotal excision. Radical cure—hydrocelectomy.
- Partial excision and eversion.
- Evacuation and eversion.
- Lord's plication.

Procedure (Fig. 35.83)

- Under general anesthesia or spinal or local anesthesia, after cleaning and draping, vertical incision of about 6–8 cm in length is made over the scrotum, anteriorly 1 cm lateral to the median raphe.
- Skin, dartos, external spermatic fascia, internal spermatic fascia are incised. *Bluish* hydrocele sac is identified (i.e. parietal layer of the tunica vaginalis of the testis). Fluid is evacuated using trocar and cannula. Sac is opened.
  - *If the sac is small, thin and contains clear fluid*, either *Lord's plication* (i.e. tunica is bunched into a 'ruff' by placing series of multiple interrupted chromic catgut sutures so as to make the sac to form fibrous tissue) (it is relatively avasular and so hematoma will not occur).
  - *Or evacuation and eversion* of the sac behind the testis (after eversion, everted sac is sutured with chromic catgut by continuous sutures) is done.
  - *If the sac is thick, in large hydrocele and chylocele, subtotal excision of the sac* is done (as tunica vaginalis is reflected on to the cord structures and epididymis posteriorly, total excision leads to orchidectomy with division of cord).
  - *Aspiration must be avoided as much as possible* as it is only a temporary measure (recurrence occurs very early) and chances of hematocele, infection are higher.
  - A drain is placed near the root of the scrotum on the lateral aspect because it becomes the most dependent portion once scrotal support is given. Scrotal support is given to reduce the scrotal edema for 10 days.
  - Wound is closed in layers.
  - Drain is removed in 48 hours.

Complications of surgery
• Reactionary hemorrhage.
• Hematocele.
• Infection.
• Pyocele.
• Sinus formation.
• Recurrent hydrocele.

Don't fear change - embrace It—Anthony J D'Angelo

CHAPTER 35B

Laboratory Values

CHAPTER OUTLINE

- Urine
- Blood
- Stool Examination

URINE

Specific gravity:
  Normal: 1.010 to 1.025. Low: less than 1.000. High: more than 1.025
  Fixed: 1.010 to 1.014
Reaction: Acidic with a pH of 6.0
Color: Clear and amber colored

Parameter	Values
Aldosterone	2–10 μg/day
Nitrogen	0.4–1.0 g/day
Amylase	30–250 somogyi units/hour
Calcium	<3.8 mmol/day
Catecholamines	<100 unit/day
Copper	<25 μg/day
Creatinine	1.0–1.6 g/day
Creatinine clearance	140–150 mL/min in males
	105–130 mL/min in females
Estrogens	4–25 μg/day (in males)
	5–100 μg/day (in females). Very high in pregnancy
17-hydroxycorticosteroids	2–10 mg/day
5-HIAA	2–9 mg/day
17-ketosteroids	7–25 mg/day in men
	4–15 mg/day in women
Magnesium	6.0–8.5 mEq/24 hours
Metanephrines	1.3 mg/day

Without a sense of caring, there can be no sense of community—**Anthony J D'Angelo**

Urine osmolarity	38–1400 mOsm/kg water
Phosphorus	0.9–1.3/day
Porphyrins	
Coproporphyrin	50–250 μg/day
Uroporphyrin	10–30 μg/day
Potassium	25–100 mmols/day
Protein	<150 mg/day
Sodium	100–250 mEq/day
Urobilinogen	1–3.5 mg/day
VMA	<8 mg/day

BLOOD

Acetoacetic acid	<0.3 mmol/liter
Acid phosphatase	1.0–5.0 King-Armstrong units
Alkaline phosphatase	20–90 IU/liter
Amino nitrogen	3.5–5.5 mg/dL
Amylase	60–180 somogyi units
Ascorbic acid	0.4–1.0 mg/dL
Bicarbonate	23–29 mmol/liter
Bilirubin	Total 0.3–1.0 mg/dL. Direct 0.1–0.3 mg/dL
	Indirect 0.2–0.7 mg/dL
Calcium	9–11 mg/dL
	Ionized—4.5–5.6 mg/dL
CO_2 in plasma	20–30 mmol/l (50–70 volume %)
CO_2 tension in artery	35–45 Hg
Ceruloplasmin	27–37 mg/dL
Chlorides	98–106 mmol/L
Cholesterol—total	150–250 mg%
Copper	115 + or –15 μg/dL
Cortisol	5-20 μg/dL
Creatine phosphokinase (CPK)	25–90 units/mL, in males. 10–70 units/mL in females
Creatinine	<1.5 mg/dL
Free fatty acids	0.7 mmol/liter
Gastrin	40–200 mg/dL
Glucose	70–110 mg/dL
17-OH corticosteroids	2–10 mg/day
IgG	800–1500 mg/dL
IgM	40–150 mg/dL
IgA	90–320 mg/dL
Insulin	6–26 uU/mL
17-ketosteroids	7–25 mg/day in males. 4 –15 mg/day in females
Lipase	1.5 units
Magnesium	0.8–1.3 mmol/liter

*It's not that I'm so smart, it's just that I stay with problems longer—**Albert Einstein***

5' nucleotidase	0.3–2.6 Bodansky units/dL
Osmolality	280–300 mOsm/kg of water
Oxygen	17–21 volume % in arterial blood
	10–16 volume % in venous blood
Oxygen saturation	97% in arterial blood. 60–85% in venous blood
pH of blood	7.36–7.44
Phosphorus, inorganic	1–1.4 mmol/liter
Potassium	3.5–5.0 mmol/liter
Protein—total	5.5–8.0 g/dL
Albumin	3.5–5.5 g/dL
Globulin	2.0–3.5 g/dL
Sodium	136–145 mmol/liter
Sulfate inorganic	0.8–1.2 mg/liter
Testosterone	<100 ng/dL in females. 300–1000 ng/dL in males
TSH	0–5 IU/mL plasma
Thyroxine (T_4)	5–12 µg/dL
Triiodothyronine (T_3)	80–200 ng/dL
SGOT/AST	6–18 units/liter
SGPT/ALT	3–26 units/liter
Uric acid	2.5–8.0 mg/dL—males
	1.5–6.9 mg/dL—females
Urea nitrogen (BUN)	10–20 mg/dL
RBC count	4.6–6.2 millions/mm³ in males
	4.2–5.4 millions/mm³ in females
	4.5–5.1 millions/mm³ in children
Reticulocyte count	25,000–75,000/mm³
WBC count	4,300–10,000/mm³
Platelet count	1,50,000–4,40,000/cu mm
Bleeding time	1–4 minutes
Hematocrit	40–54 mL/100 mL
Clotting time	2–15 minutes
Clot retraction time	Apparent in 60 minutes, complete in 24 hours
	Usually <6 hours
Plasma fibrinogen	160–400 mg/dL
Partial thromboplastin time	68–82 seconds
	Activated is 32–46 seconds
Prothrombin time	11–15 seconds
Hemoglobin	14–18 mg/dL—males
	12–16 mg/dL—females
	11–16 mg/dL—children
	16–19 mg/dL—newborn
Fetal hemoglobin	<2%
Hemoglobin A_2	1.5–3.5%

You can never get enough of what you don't really need—**Eric Hoffer**

Osmotic fragility	Begins in 0.45–0.39% NaCl and completes in 0.33–0.30%
Sedimentation rate (ESR)	<10 mm in one hour in males
	<20 mm in one hour in females

STOOL EXAMINATION

Bulk	100–200 g
Water	75%
Osmolarity	250 mOsm/L
Color	Brown
-pH	7.0–7.5
Fat	<7 g/day
Stercobilinogen	50–280 mg/day
Urobilinogen	30–200 mg/100 g
Nitrogen	<2.5 g/day
Calcium	0.6 g/24 hours
Trypsin	20–90 unit/gram

Index

0'-p DDD (Mitotane) 395
5-Fluorouracil 395

A

Abbe switch flap 378
Abbe-Estlander's rotation flap 378
Abbreviated injury scale (AIS) 167
Abdominal aneurysms 202
Abdominal aorta 185
Abdominal compartment syndrome 173
Abdominal trauma 170
Abrasion 29
Abscess, cold 62
Abscess, cold, sequelae 64
Abscess, cold, sites of origin 63
Abscess, cold, treatment 64
Abscess, complication 61
Abscess, external 60
Abscess, factors precipitating 60
Abscess, Hilton's method of draining 61
Abscess, internal 60
Abscess, metastatic 61
Abscess, parapharyngeal 292
Abscess, pyogenic 59
Abscess, retropharyngeal 293
Abscess, sites 60
Abscess, treatment 61
ABVD regime 243
Acceleration injuries 377
Achalasia cardia 367
Achalasia cardia, clinical features 367
Achalasia cardia, etiology
Achondroplasia 356
Acid-base balance 20
Acinic cell tumor 354
Acoustic neuroma.488
Acquired AVF 213

Acral lentiginous melanoma 281
Acriflavine 9
Acrocyanosis 182
Actinomyces Israelii 75
Actinomycosis 75
Actinomycosis, clinical features 75
Actinomycosis, clinical types 75
Actinomycosis, pathogenesis 75
Actinomycosis, treatment 75
Acute arterial occlusion 197
Acute compartment syndrome 198
Acute pyomyositis 82
Acute retropharyngeal abscess 293
Acute suppurative tenosynovitis 159
Adamantinoma 314
Adelaide Coma Scale 379, 380
Adenoid cystic carcinoma 352
Adenolymphoma 351
Adiposis dolorosa 97
Adrenal gland left 337
Adrenal gland, arterial supply 337
Adrenal gland, embryology 337
Adrenal gland, right 336
Adrenal gland, structure 337
Adrenal gland, venous drainage 337
Adrenal glands, surgical anatomy 336
Adrenocortical carcinoma 338
Adrenocortical tumors 337
Adrenocortical tumors, benign 337
Adriamycin 395
Adson's test 179, 187, 349
Advanced ultrasound techniques 317
AGES scoring, thyroid 321, 323
Aggressive fibromatosis 107
Agranulocytosis 318

Ainhum 209
Air embolism 200
Alexander Fleming 2
Alexis Carrel 2
Alfred Blalock 2
Allen's test 188, 349
Allograft 142
Alveolar abscess 317
Ambroise Pare 1
Ambulatory venous pressure 224
Amelanotic melanoma 281
Ameloblastoma 314
AMES scoring, thyroid, papillary carcinoma 321, 323
Aminoglutethimide 396
Amputation, below knee 207
Amputation, Burgess 207
Amputation, Gritti Stokes 207
Amputation, Ray 207
Amputations 207
Amyloid stroma 325
Anaesthesia, postoperative care 324
Anaesthesia, premedication 322
Anaesthesia, preoperative assessment 322
Anaplasia, features of 258
Anaplastic carcinoma of thyroid 325
Anatomy of lymphatics of head and neck 285
Anesthesia, caudal 327
Anesthesia, epidural 327
Anesthesia, general 322
Anesthesia, instruments 323
Anesthesia, intravenous regional 326
Anesthesia, regional 325
Anesthesia, spinal 326
Anesthesia, topical 326
Anesthetics, gaseous 322
Anesthetics, intravenous 322
Anesthetics, volatile 322

Aneurysm needle 309
Aneurysm, carotid artery 205
Aneurysm, cirsoid 212
Aneurysm, dissecting 204
Aneurysm, false 201
Aneurysm, popliteal 204
Aneurysm, true 201
Aneurysms 201
Aneurysms, abdominal 202
Aneurysms, Berrys 202
Aneurysms, clinical features 202
Aneurysms, peripheral 203
Aneurysms, types 201
Angelchik prosthesis 369
Angina, Ludwig's 291
Angiogram, direct aortic 190
Angiogram, transbrachial 193
Angiography 189
Angiography, digital substraction 190
Angiography, Seldinger 189
Anion gap 19
Ankle-brachial pressure index 189
Ankylosing spondylitis 359
Ann Arbor staging 241
Anterior tibial artery 350
Anterior transpositioning of the ulnar nerve 254
Anthrax 79
Anthrax, types 79
Anticoagulants 230
Anticoagulants, oral 231
Anti-HIV antibody 87
Antimalignancy drugs 395
Antirabies vaccination, indications 78
Antisepsis 3
Antithyroid drugs 317
Antituberculous drugs 246
Aortoiliac block 187
Ape or Simian thumb deformity 252
Aphthous ulcer 381
Aphthous ulcer, herpetiform 381
Aphthous ulcers, major 381
Aphthous ulcers, minor 381
Apple-gelly nodule 55
Apudomas 335
Arm-foot venous pressure 224
Arterial disease, examination in 346

Arterial diseases 174, 185
Arterial diseases, investigation 189
Arterial diseases, treatment 193
Arterial emboli 198
Arterial embolism, effects of 198
Arterial embolism, investigations of 199
Arterial grafts 194
Arteries of upper limb 175
Arteries, lower limb 185
Arteries, superficial femoral and deep femoral 185
Arteriovenous fistula 212
Arteritis temporal 184
Arteritis, Thakayasu's 183
Artery, anterior tibial 185, 188
Artery, axillary 175, 188
Artery, brachial 175, 188
Artery, common carotid 188, 185
Artery, deep femoral 185
Artery, dorsalis pedis 188
Artery, external iliac 185
Artery, facial 188
Artery, femoral 188
Artery, peroneal 185, 188
Artery, popliteal 188
Artery, posterior tibial 185, 188
Artery, radial 175, 188
Artery, right subclavian 175
Artery, subclavian 188
Artery, superficial 185
Artery, superficial temporal 189
Artery, ulnar 175
Artery, ulnar 188
Arthritis 357
Arthritis, acute pyogenic 357
Arthritis, chronic pyogenic 357
Arthritis, rheumatoid 357
Arthritis, rheumatoid, treatment 358
Arthritis, types 358
Arthrodesis 351
Arthroplasty 351
Arthroplasty, excision 351
Arthroplasty, total replacement 352
Artificial blood 130
Arytenoids cartilages 395
Ascending venography 224
Asepsis 3
Astrocytomas 387

Atherectomy 193
Atherosclerosis 190
Atherosclerosis, features and evaluation 191
Atherosclerosis, management 191
Atherosclerosis, pathogenesis 191
Atracurium 323
Atraumatic needle 302
Attitude 330
Autoclave 4
Autograft 142
Axillary artery 351
Axillary nerve injuries 255
Axillary vein thrombosis 218
Axonotmesis 248
Azathioprine 396

B

Bacillus anthracis 79
Bacteremia 67
Bamboo spine 359
Barium swallow X-ray 366
Barium swallow, achalasia cardia, 368
Barrett's ulcer 371
Bartonella henselae 240
Basal cell carcinoma 277
Base ball finger 163
Basedow's disease 313
Basophil adenomas 390
BCC 277
BCC, basisquamous 278
BCC, clinical features of 278
BCC, geographic 277
BCC, morphia type 278
BCC, pigmented 277
BCC, treatment of 278
Bed sore 48
Behcet's syndrome 381
Belsey Mark-4 operation 369
Bence Jones proteins 363
Bends disease 201
Benzopyrones 236
Bernard von Langenbeck 2
Berry picking 323
Berry's aneurysms 386
Berry's ligament 304
Berry's sign 324
Berrys aneurysms 202
Beta-propiolactone 9
Bier's block 326

Biobrane 137
Biopsy 262
Biopsy, excision 262
Biopsy, incision 262
Biopsy, trucut 263
Biopsy, wedge 46
Bisgaard method 229
Blair's incision 345
Blast injuries 170
Blast injuries, management 170
Blended current 313
Bleomycin 395
Block dissection neck 301
Block dissection, complications 302
Blood clotting factors 123
Blood coagulation, mechanism 122
Blood fractions 128
Blood loss, measurement 125
Blood substitutes 129
Blood transfusion 127
Blood transfusion, complications 129
Blood transfusion, indication 127
Blood transfusion, massive 129
Blowout fracture 327
Blue leg 219
Boil 64
Bone disease of hyperparathyroidism 355
Bone tumors 360
Bone tumors, benign 360
Bone tumors, malignant 362
Bone tumors, secondaries 363
Bone, infections 353
Bone, anatomy 345
Bone, Paget's disease of 354
Bowen's disease 274
Boyd's classification of claudication 185
Boyle's apparatus 323
BPL inactivated vaccine 78
Brachial artery 351
Brachial plexus injuries 250
Brachytherapy 393
Brachytherapy, advantages 394
Brachytherapy, disadvantages 394
Brachytherapy, types 394
Brain tumors, primary 387
Brain tumors, special features 389
Brain tumors, treatment 389

Branchial cyst 287
Branchial fistula 287
Branhan's sign 214
Breslow's classification 281
Broder's grading of squamous cell carcinoma 262, 276
Brodie's abscess 354
Brodie-Trendelenburg test 222, 354
Brown-Séquard syndrome 169
Brunner's grading of lymphedema 235
Bubonocele 389
Buerger's angle of vascular insufficiency 187
Buerger's postural test 187, 348
Buerger's vascular angle of insufficiency 348
Buffalo hump 235
Buffers 20
Bullet injuries 169
Bullet injuries, management 169
Bunion 109
Burkitt's lymphoma 244
Burns 132
Burns contracture 137
Burns contracture, prevention 137
Burns contracture, problems 137
Burns contracture, treatment 137
Burns injury, effects 135
Burns, biological dressings 137
Burns, classification 132
Burns, fluid resuscitation 136
Burns, full thickness 134
Burns, local management 136
Burns, management 135
Burns, partial thickness 134
Burns, pathophysiology 134
Burns, rule of nine 133
Burns, sepsis 135
Burns, synthetic dressings 137
Burns, types 132
Bursa anserine 109
Bursa, anatomical 108
Bursa, psoas 108
Bursa, semimembranosus 109
Bursa, subacromial 108
Bursa, subhyoid 108
Bursa, tailor's 109
Bursae 108
Bursitis 108
Bursitis, bicipitoradial 108

Bursitis, infrapatellar 109
Bursitis, olecranon 108
Bursitis, prepatellar 109
Bursitis, retro-Achilis 109
Bursitis, retrocalcaneum 109
Bursitis, semimembranosus 109
Busulfan 395

C

Cadaver donor 151
Café au lait spots 106
Caison's disease 201
Calcinosis cutis 110
Calcitonin 325
Caldwell-Luc operation 392
Calf musculovenous pump 217
Callosity 163
Canal, Guyon's 253
Cancrum oris 366
Capillary filling time 348, 349
Capillary hemangioma 210
Capillary vascular malformations 210
Carbimazole 317
Carbogen 322
Carbuncle 65
Carcinoma 259
Carcinoma , gingivobuccal complex 370
Carcinoma alveolus 388
Carcinoma cheek 370
Carcinoma cheek, biological behavior 371
Carcinoma esophagus, 373
Carcinoma esophagus, barium swallow 374
Carcinoma esophagus, clinical features 374
Carcinoma esophagus, intubation 376
Carcinoma esophagus, lower third growth 375
Carcinoma esophagus, middle third growth 375
Carcinoma esophagus, palliative treatment 376
Carcinoma esophagus, terminal events 376
Carcinoma esophagus, types 374
Carcinoma esophagus, upper third growth 375

Carcinoma floor of the mouth 388
Carcinoma hard palate 392
Carcinoma posterior one third tongue 387
Carcinoma tongue 384
Carcinoma tongue, clinical features 384
Carcinoma tongue, prognostic factors 387
Carcinoma tongue, spread 385
Carcinoma tongue, treatment 386
Carcinoma, Merkel cell 272
Card test 253
Cardiac arrest 120
Carotid artery aneurysm 205
Carotid artery, ligation 303
Carotid blowout 303
Carotid body tumor 294
Carotid body tumor, Shamblin classification of 295
Carotid subclavian bypass 177
Carpal tunnel 252
Carpal tunnel syndrome 252
Carpopedal spasm 335
Cartilage 345
Cartilage, elastic 346
Cartilage, hyaline 345
Cartilage, types 345
Cartilage, white 346
Cat scratch fever 240
Catgut, chromic 310
Catgut, plain 310
Catheter based interventions 177
Catheter, Foley's 306
Catheter, Malecot 306
Caudal anesthesia 327
Caudal anesthesia, complications 327
Caudal anesthesia, indication 327
Caudal anesthesia, procedure 327
Causalgia 251
Causes of secondary lymphedema 234
Cautery, coagulation 313
Cautery, cutting 313
Cavernous hemangioma 211
Cavernous lymphangioma 289
CEAP classification of lower limb varicose veins 221
Cell culture vaccines 79
Cellulitis 56
Cellulitis, clinical features 57

Cellulitis, management 57
Cellulitis, orbital 57
Cellulitis, sequelae 57
Cellulitis, special sites 57
Celsus 1
Central cord syndrome 168
Central venous pressure 117
Central venous pressure, complications 118
Cerebellar vermis tumors 389
Cerebral concussion 377
Cerebral contusion 377
Cerebral laceration 377
Cervical rib 179
Cervical rib, investigations 180
Cervical rib, pathology 179
Cervical rib, treatment 179
Cervical sinus 287
Cervical sympathectomy 181
Cervicothoracic canal 174
Cetrimide 8
Charle's operation 237, 238
Charles B Huggins 2
Chassaignac tubercle 189
Cheek 361
Cheilitis 377
Chemical burns 140
Chemical sympathectomy 196
Chemotherapy 394
Cherubism 318
Chimney sweep cancer 275, 381
Chlorhexidine 8
Chloroxylenol 9
Cholesterol crystals 287
Chondroma 361
Chondroma, types 361
Chondromas, multiple 361
Chondrosarcoma 270
Chordoma 111
Christiaan Neethling Barnard 2
Christmas disease 123
Chromophobe adenomas 390
Chronic retropharyngeal abscess 293
Chronic subdural empyema 383
Chylocele 392
Cidex 7
Cilastozol 177
Cimino fistula 152, 214
Cinthol 8
Circumvallate papillae 362
Cirsoid aneurysm 212

Cisplatin 396
Clamp, Moynihan's occlusion 303
Clamp, Payr's crushing 303
Clark's classification 281
Clark's concept 281
Classic radical neck dissection 301
Classification, Breslow's 281
Classification, CEAP, of lower limb varicose veins 221
Classification, Clark's 281
Classification, Dunhill, thyroid neoplasm 321
Classification, Rye's 241
Classification, Seddon's 248
Classification, Sunderland's 249
Claudication, classification 185
Claudication, intermittent 185
Claudication, upper limb 176
Claudio 185
Claw hand 253
Claw hand deformity 253
Cleft disorders, LAHS classification 308
Cleft disorders, problems 308
Cleft lip 308
Cleft lip and palate 307
Cleft lip repair, principles of 309
Cleft lip, treatment 309
Cleft palate 310
Cleft palate, treatment 310
Clergyman's knee 109
Clostridium tetani 68
Clostridium Welchii 71
Clostridium Welchii, exotoxins 71
Clubbing 331
Coagulation cascade system 122
Cock's peculiar tumor 104
Cockett and Dodd, subfacial ligation 227
Cold and warm water test 350
Coleman's sign 334
Collagen vascular diseases 181
Collar stud abscess 157
Collis' vertical gastroplasty 369
Colloid cyst 389
Colloid goiter 310
Colonic injury 172
Commando operation (combined mandibular dissection and neck dissection) 302
Common carotid artery 352

Common peroneal nerve 255
Compartment injuries 161
Compartment resection 267
Compartment syndrome 197, 36
Complex decongestive therapy 237
Complications of multinodular goiter 311
Complications of venous ulcers 229
Compound palmar ganglion 156, 161
Compressibility 345
Condylar fracture 332
Congenital AVF 212
Coning 378, 382
Conservative functional block dissection 301
Consistency 343
Corn 163
Corn, types 163
Costoclavicular compression maneuver 188, 349
Costoclavicular space 174, 178
Cresol 5
Crest syndrome 181
Cretinism 331
Cricoid cartilage 395
Cricopharyngeal myotomy 289
Cricothyroid 395
Crile's grading 316, 558
Criles' operation 301
Critical limb ischemia 186
Cross fluctuation 344, 386
Crossed leg test 350
Crush injury 29
Crush syndrome 36
Crutch palsy 255
Cryoprecipitate 128
Cryosurgery 314
Cryosurgery, advantages 315
Cryosurgery, indications 315
Cryptorchidism 382
CSF rhinorrhea 381
CT scan 318
CT scan, advantages 318
CT scan, contrast agents 318
Curling's ulcer 135
Cyanosis 331
Cyclophosphamide 395
Cyclosporine 396
Cyclosporine A 153

Cyst 100
Cyst, acquired 100
Cyst, apoplectic 100
Cyst, branchial 287
Cyst, congenital 100
Cyst, dermoids 100
Cyst, distention 100
Cyst, effects 101
Cyst, epidermal 103
Cyst, false 100
Cyst, Morrant Baker 110
Cyst, retention 100
Cyst, sebaceous 103
Cyst, thyroglossal 307
Cyst, traumatic 101
Cyst, true 100
Cyst, tubulodermoid 100, 102
Cystic hygroma 289
Cytosine arabinoside 395

 D

Dalrymple's sign 314
Damage control surgery 168
Dangerous area of face 59
Day care surgery 315
Day care surgery, precaution 315
De Quervain's subacute granulomatous thyroiditis 327
DeBakey's classification 204, 205
Deceleration injuries 377
Decompression disease 201
Deep palmar arch 154
Deep palmar space infection 159
Deep ring occlusion test 385
Deep vein thrombosis 218
Deep veins 216
Defibrillation technique 121
Degloving injuries 161
Delayed capillary filling 187
Delayed primary suturing 35
Delayed venous filling 187
Delphian node 306
Demarcation, line of 186
Demodex folliculorum 103
Dental abscess 317
Dental cyst 316
Dental ulcer 381
Dentigerous cyst 315
Dentoalveolar fracture 332

Depressed skull fracture 384
Depressed skull fracture, problems 384
deQuervain's autoimmune thyroiditis 310, 327
Dercum's disease 97
Dermal flares 220
Dermatofibroma 272
Dermatofibrosacroma protuberans 272
Dermoid, angular 101
Dermoid, external angular 101
Dermoid, implantation 102
Dermoid, internal angular 101
Dermoid, sequestration 101
Dermoid, teratomatous 103
Dermoids 101
Descending venogram 224
Desmoid tumor 107
Detegents 8
Dettol 9
Dexon 310
Dextran 40 129
Diabetic foot 49, 207
Diabetic foot, pathogenesis 208
Diabetic gangrene 207
Diagnostic indices of Wayne's, thyrotoxicosis 315
Diagnostic peritoneal lavage 171
Diaphyseal achalasia 356
Diathermy 313
Diathermy, types 313
Differential diagnosis of TOS 178
Differentiated thyroid carcinoma 321
Diffuse hyperplastic goiter 310
Digital substraction angiography 190
Dilator, Bake's 303
Dilator, Lister's urethral 307
Direct aortic angiogram 190
Disappearing pulse syndrome 187, 350
Disease, Basedow's 313
Disease, Bowen's 274
Disease, Meige's 233
Disease, Milroy's 233
Disease, Plummer's 310, 313
Diseases of the arteries 190
Disinfection 4
Disinfection, different methods 4

Dissecting aneurysm 204
Distal run off 189
Dominant nodule 312
Donor criteria 127
Doppler 317
Doppler, advantages 317
Doppler, types 317
Doppler, uses 317
Doppler, venous 223
Dorsalis pedis artery 188, 350
Double barrelled aorta 204, 205
Drain systems, classification of 305
Drain, closed suction 305
Drain, corrugated rubber 304
Drain, Jackson-Pratt 305
Drain, Redivac 305
Drain, sump suction 305
Drain, under water seal 306
Drains 304
Drains, closed siphon 305
Drains, indications 306
Drains, open (static) 305
Drains, problems in 306
Drains, types 304
DSA 190
DTC 321
DTC, TNM staging 321
DTIC 284
Duck embryo vaccine 79
Dumb bell tumor 294, 350
Dunhill classification 321
Duodenal injury 171
Duodenal injury, complications 172
Duoderm 137
Duplex scan 224
Duplex scanning 317
Dupuytren's contracture 162
DVT, prevention 219
Dyes 8
Dyschondroplasia 361
Dyshormonogenesis 309
Dysphagia 366
Dysplasia 259

E

EAST 179, 187
Ecchondroma 361
ECF excess 12
ECF loss 12

Ectopic thyroid 306
Eddie's current 179
Edwin Smith Papyrus 1
Effects and sequelae of DVT 220
Effects of arterial embolism 198
Electrical burns 137
Electrocautery 313
Elephantiasis 234
Elevated arm stress test 179, 187, 349
Embolectomy 177, 199
Embolectomy, brachial 177
Emboli, arterial 198
Emboli, venous 198
Embolism 175, 198
Embolism, air 200
Embolism, fat 200
Embolism, upper limb ischemia 175
Embolization spread 260
Embolization, therapeutic 200
Embolus, saddle 199
Embolus, treatment of 177
Emil Theodor Kocher 2, 330
Enchondroma 361
Enchondromatosis 357
Encysted hydrocele of the cord 391
Endarterectomy 193
Endotracheal tube 323
Endovenous laser ablation 228
Endrophonium 323
Enflurane 322
Enroth sign 315
Enteral nutrition 24
Enterocele 388
Eosinophil (acidophil) adenomas 390
Ependymomas 388
Epididymo-orchitis, acute 386
Epidural anesthesia 327
Epidural anesthesia, advantages 327
Epiglottic cartilage 395
Epignathus 110
Epineurorrhaphy 249
Epiperineurorrhaphy 249
Epiplocele 388
Epithelial pearls 275
Epithelioid cells 246
Epithelioma 52, 274

Epulis 313
Epulis 368, 371
Epulis fissuratum 314
Epulis, carcinomatous 314
Epulis, congenital 313
Epulis, fibrosarcomatous 314
Epulis, fibrous 314
Epulis, Giant cell 314
Epulis, granulomatous 314
Epulis, myelomatous 314
Epulis, pregnancy 314
Erb-Duchenne paralysis 251
Erysipelas 59
Erythralgia 184
Erythrocyanosis frigida 44
Erythromelalgia 184
Erythroplakia 367
Eschar 133, 137
Eschar, circumferential 137
Escharotomy 137
Eschmann blade 143
Esophageal endosonography 367
Esophagectomy, thoracoscopic-laparoscopic 375
Esophagectomy, transhiatal blind total 375
Esophagitis, reflux 371
Esophagocardiomyotomy 368
Esophagoscopy 366
Esophagoscopy, fiberoptic flexible 467
Esophagoscopy, rigid 367
Esophagoscopy, types 367
Esophagus 364
Esophagus, Auerbach's plexus 365
Esophagus, abdominal 365
Esophagus, anatomic narrowing 365
Esophagus, anatomy 364
Esophagus, arterial supply 365
Esophagus, Barrett's 370
Esophagus, cervical 364
Esophagus, corrosive stricture 371
Esophagus, lymphatic drainage 365
Esophagus, Meissner's plexus 365
Esophagus, nerve supply 365
Esophagus, parts 364
Esophagus, thoracic 365
Esophagus, venous drainage 365
Ethambutol 246
Ether 322

Ethylene oxide sterilization 9
Etoposide 496
Eusol bath 6
Eve's disease 314
EVLA 228
Ewing's sarcoma 363
Exophthalmos 315, 362
Exophthalmos severe 316
Exophthalmos, malignant 316
Expansile impulse 343
External cardiac compression (massage) 120
Extradural abscess 385
Extradural hematoma 381
Extradural hematoma, lucid interval 382
Extradural hematoma, pathology 382
Extradural hematoma, treatment 382
Extradural hematomas 378
Extrinsic healing method 256
Eye signs in toxic goiter 314

F

Face, development 307
Facial artery 351
Facial nerve 341
Facial nerve palsy 360
Facial nerve palsy, features of 379
Facial nerve palsy, surgeries 360
Facial nerve sacrifice 356
Facial nerve, branches 342
Faciovenous plane of Patey 342
Fasciotomies 36
Fat embolism 200, 348
Features of secondaries in neck 297
Fegan's technique 225
Fegan's test 223, 355
Felon 155, 157
Femoral artery 351
Fibrin cuff theory 221
Fibrinogen 128
Fibroma 107
Fibroma, classification 107
Fibroma, hard 107
Fibroma, soft 107
Fibrosarcoma 269
Fibrous dysplasia of bone 318
Fibrous dysplasia of jaw 319

Fibrous dysplasia, complications 320
Fibrous dysplasia, treatment 320
Field block 326
Filarial lymphedema 234
Filiform papillae 362
Fine needle aspiration cytology 262
Finger invagination test 385
Fistula 39
Fistula, acquired 40
Fistula, arteriovenous 212
Fistula, branchial 287
Fistula, Cimino 214
Fistula, congenital 40
Fistula, external 40
Fistula, internal 40
Fistula, thyroglossal 308
Fixed thrombus 219
Fixity to deeper structures 345
Fixity to the skin 345
Flap, axial pattern 146
Flap, cross leg 149
Flap, cutaneous 146
Flap, faciocutaneous 146
Flap, forehead 147
Flap, groin 148
Flap, muscle 146
Flap, myocutaneous 146
Flap, osteomyocutaneous 146
Flap, pectoralis major myocutaneous 148
Flap, radial forearm 150
Flap, random pattern 146
Flap, salutatory 146
Flaps 142, 145
Flaps, free 146, 150
Flaps, types 146
Flexor retinaculum 154
Fluctuation 344
Fluctuation 385
Fluid therapy 22
Fluid therapy, principles 23
Fluid therapy, problems 23
FNAC 262
FNAC of thyroid 309
Foam sclerotherapy by Tessari 226
Foliate papillae 362
Follicular carcinoma thyroid 323
Follicular odontome 315
Foot 163
Foot drop 255

Foramen cecum 362
Forceps, Allis tissue holding 399
Forceps, artery 399
Forceps, artery, types 399
Forceps, artery, uses 399
Forceps, Babcock's 300
Forceps, Cheatle's 398
Forceps, Desjardin's choledocholithotomy 303
Forceps, dissecting 301
Forceps, Kocher's 399
Forceps, Lane's tissue holding 300
Forceps, plain nontoothed dissecting 302
Forceps, right angle 399
Forceps, sinus (Lister's) 304
Forceps, sponge holding (Rampley's) 398
Forceps, toothed dissecting 302
Formaldehyde 6, 10
Fournier's gangrene 384
Fovea palatine 363
Fowler's operation 164
Fracture 346
Fracture healing, factors affecting 348
Fracture healing, stages 347
Fracture mandible 330
Fracture mandible 331
Fracture mandible, complications 335
Fracture mandible, management 333, 335
Fracture mandible, of Symphysis 335
Fracture mandible, ramus or angle 334
Fracture middle third area 323
Fracture middle third area, classification 324
Fracture middle third area, Le Fort classification 324
Fracture, avulsion 347
Fracture, causes 346
Fracture, clinical features 347
Fracture, closed 346
Fracture, comminuted 347
Fracture, complicated 347
Fracture, complications 348
Fracture, compound'446
Fracture, depressed 347
Fracture, Greenstick 346

Fracture, nasoethmoid complex 324
Fracture, open 346
Fracture, stellate 347
Fracture, transverse 346
Fracture, types 346
Fracture, zygomatic arch 327
Fracture, zygomatic complex 325
Fractures middle third area, management 328
Francis D Moore 2
Freckle, Hutchinson's 279
Free thrombus 219
French disease 74
Frenulum linguae 362
Fresh frozen plasma 128
Fries' modified Bernard facial flap 378
Frog hand 155, 159
Froment's sign 253, 254
Frontal lobe tumors 389
Fuchsig's test 350
Fungiform papillae 362
Funicular 389
Furuncle 64
Fusobacterium fusiformis 54

 G

Gadolinium 319
Gaiter's zone 54
Gallamine 323
Ganglion 107
Ganglioneuroma 105
Gangrene 186, 206
Gangrene, dry 186, 206
Gangrene, moist 206
Gangrene, wet 186, 206
Gas gangrene 71
Gas gangrene, clinical features 72
Gas gangrene, clinical types 72
Gas gangrene, treatment 72
Gaseous sterilization 9
Gaspare Tagliacozzi 2
Gastroesophageal reflux disease (GERD) 366, 368
Gastroesophageal reflux disease, complications 369
Gastroesophageal reflux disease, surgical treatment 369
Gastroesophageal reflux disease, treatment 369

Gastroesophageal reflux disease, types 369
Gastrostomy 25
Gastrostomy, Janeway's mucus lined permanent 25
Gastrostomy, Kader-Senn temporary 25
Gastrostomy, percutaneous, endoscopic 25
Gastrostomy, Stamm's temporary 25
Gene therapy 397
General anesthesia, complications 324
General anesthesia, components 324
General anesthesia, steps 324
General physical examination 330
Generalized neurofibromatosis 106
Geographic tongue 383
Giant cell reparative granuloma 315
Gieger Muller's gamma ray counter 320
Gigli's wire/saw 308
Gingivae 362
Gingivitis, ulcerative 365
Glioma, distal 248
Gliomas 387
Glomangioma 104
Glomus tumor 104
Glossitis 382
Glossitis migrans 383
Glossitis, chronic superficial 383
Glossitis, Hunter's 383
Glossitis, median rhomboid 383
Glossitis, pellagra 383
Glove drain 304
Gluck-Sorenson's laryngectomy 301
Glutaraldehyde 7
Goiter, classification of 310
Goiter, colloid 310
Goiter, nodular 311
Goiter, plunging 313
Goldner method 257
Gonorrhea 91
Gonorrhea, treatment 92
Grading of tumor 261

Grading, Crile's 316
Graft 142
Graft rejection 152
Graft, contracture 144
Graft, full thickness 145
Graft, partial thickness 142
Graft, split skin 142
Graft, Thiersch 142
Graft, Wolfe 145
Grafts, arterial 194
Graftversushost disease 152
Granular cell myoblastoma 382
Granulation tissue 45
Granulation tissue, exuberant 46
Granulation tissue, healthy 45
Granulation tissue, unhealthy 45
Grave's disease 310, 313
Great pox 74
Great saphenous vein 216
Guerin's fracture 324
Gustatory sweating 359
Guyon's canal 253

 H

Haimovici triad 198
Halogens 5
Halsted test 349
Hamartomata 210
Hand infections 155
Hand infections, complications 156
Hand infections, general principles of managing 156
Hand injuries 160
Hand injuries, classification 160
Hand injuries, treatment 161
Hand, surgical anatomy 151
Handley's wide local excision 283
Hard palate 363
Harvey's sign 187
Harvey's venous refilling test 349
Hashimoto's autoimmune thyroiditis 310, 326
Hashimoto's thyroiditis c326
Head injuries, clinical approach 379
Head injuries, complications 381
Head injuries, mechanism 377
Head injuries, treatment 380
Heberden's nodes 163
Helicobacter pylori 259

Hemangioma 209
Hemangioma, capillary 210
Hemangioma, cavernous 210
Hemangioma, strawberry 210
Hemangiosarcoma 260
Hemiarthroplasty 351
Hemithyroidectomy 319, 327
Hemophilia, classic 123
Hemorrhage 123
Hemorrhage, acute 124
Hemorrhage, acute on chronic 124
Hemorrhage, arterial 123
Hemorrhage, capillary 123
Hemorrhage, chronic 124
Hemorrhage, clinical features 125
Hemorrhage, pathophysiology 125
Hemorrhage, primary 124
Hemorrhage, reactionary 124
Hemorrhage, secondary 124
Hemorrhage, treatment 126
Hemorrhage, venous 123
Hemostat 399
Henderson equation 21
Henderson-Hasselbalch equation 21
Heparin 230
Heparin antagonists 231
Hepatitis 83
Hepatitis A virus 83
Hepatitis A virus, treatment 84
Hepatitis B and pregnancy 85
Hepatitis B virus 84
Hepatitis B virus, post-exposure prophylaxis 86
Hepatitis B virus, pre-exposure prophylaxis 85
Hepatitis B virus, serology 84
Hepatitis B virus, standard precautions 85
Hepatitis B virus, treatment 85
Hepatitis C virus 86
Hepatitis C virus, features 86
Hepatitis D virus 83
Hepatitis E virus 83
Hepatitis G virus flavirus 83
Hepatitis viruses 83
Hepatitis, infectious 83
Hernia 387
Hernia, classification 388
Hernia, direct 389

Hernia, hiatus 370
Hernia, indirect 389
Hernia, inflamed 388
Hernia, inguinal 387
Hernia, irreducible 388
Hernia, Littre's 388
Hernia, obstructed 388
Hernia, paraesophageal 371
Hernia, reducible 388
Hernia, Richter's 388
Hernia, rolling 371
Hernia, sac 388
Hernia, strangulated 388
Hernioplasty 390
Herpes labialis 377
Herpetic lingual ulcer 382
Hexachlorophone 8
Hibernoma 97
Hibitane 8
High molecular weight dextran 130
High resolution CT 319
High ulnar palsy 254
Hippocrates 1
History taking 329
Hitch stitches 381, 383
HIV infection and AIDS 87
HIV infection, gastrointestinal problems 88
HIV infection, hospital and surgeon 89
HIV infection, neurological problems 89
HIV infection, pathogenesis 88
HIV infection, prevention 89
HIV infection, pulmonary problems 88
HIV infection, treatment 89
HIV infection, tumors in 88
HIV infection, universal precaution 90
HIV, tests for 87
Hockey stick incision 302
Hodgkin's lymphoma 240
Homan's operation 237
Homan's sign 219
Homan's test 356
Home parenteral nutrition 27
Hood sign 308
Hormone antagonists 396

Hormone therapy 396
Horner's syndrome 298, 299, 303
Horse antirabies serum 79
Hospital-acquired infection 80
Hot-air oven 4
Hounsfield number 318
Housemaid's knee 109
Hudson brace with perforator and burr 309
Human albumin 4.5% 128, 129
Human immunodeficiency virus 87
Human rabies immunoglobulin 79
Humby's knife 143
Hunter's ligation 215
Hunterian chancre 74
Hurthle cell carcinoma of thyroid 325
Hutchinson's triad 75
Hutchinson' teeth 367
Hutchinson's freckle 279
Hybridoma 397
Hydrocele en bisac 391
Hydrocele, complications of 392
Hydrocele, congenital 391
Hydrocele, examination of 391
Hydrocele, filarial 392
Hydrocele, secondary 391
Hydrocele, treatment 392
Hydrocele, vaginal 391
Hydrocephalus 386
Hydrocephalus, acquired 387
Hydrocephalus, classification 386, 387
Hydrocephalus, congenital 387
Hydrocephalus, treatment 387
Hydrogen peroxide 8
Hypaque 343
Hyperabduction maneuver 188, 349
Hyperbaric oxygen 120
Hyperdynamic (warm) shock 114
Hyperkalemia 18
Hypernatremia 15
Hypernatremia, acute 15
Hypernatremia, causes 15
Hypernatremia, treatment 15
Hyperparathyroidism 333
Hyperparathyroidism, acute 333
Hyperparathyroidism, primary 333
Hyperparathyroidism, secondary 333

Hyperparathyroidism, tertiary 333
Hyperthyroidism 313
Hyperthyroidism, signs 314
Hyperthyroidism, symptoms 314
Hypertrophic scar 38
Hypodynamic hypovolemic septic shock 114
Hypoglossal nerve palsy 380
Hypokalemia 16
Hypokalemia, causes 16
Hypokalemia, treatment 17
Hypokalemic alkalosis 21
Hypokalemic periodic paralysis 17
Hyponatremia 12
Hyponatremia, acute 14
Hyponatremia, chronic 14
Hyponatremia, classification 12
Hyponatremia, euvolemic 13
Hyponatremia, hypervolemic 13
Hyponatremia, hypotonic 13
Hyponatremia, hypovolemic 13
Hyponatremia, treatment 14
Hypoparathyroidism 329
Hypothenar muscles 155
Hypothyroidism 330
Hypovolemia, covert compensated 115
Hypovolemia, types 115
Hypovolemia. decompensated 115

I

Ian-Aird test 355
Icterus 331
Ileal mucosal patch 237
Immunohistochemistry 263
Immunosuppression 396
Immunosuppressive agents 153
Immunotherapy 396
Immunotherapy agents 396
Impulse on coughing 385
In situ saphenous vein graft 194
In transit nodules 260
Incision, Blair's 345
Induration 46
Infectious mononucleosis 239
Inferior thyroid artery 332
Infiltration block 326
Inflammation 31
Inflammation, acute 32

Inflammation, chemical mediators 32
Inflammation, management 33
Inflammation, phases 32
Ingrowing toe nail 164
Inguinal canal, 389
Inguinal canal, boundaries 390
Inguinal canal, surgical anatomy of 389
Inguinal ring, deep
Inguinal ring, superficial 389
Inguinoscrotal swellings, examination of 381
Inhalation burns 140
Inhalation burns, clinical features 140
Inhalation burns, management 140
Injection sclerotherapy 225
Injuries, brachial plexus 250
Injuries, radial nerve 254
Injuries, ulnar nerve 253
Injury severity score (ISS) 167
Injury, reperfusion 197
Inner lymphatic ring 285
Instruments 398
Integra 137
Intermittent claudication 185
Internal open cardiac massage 121
Intervertebral disc prolapse 359
Intra-arterial thrombolysis using fibrinolysins 199
Intracerebral abscess 385
Intracerebral hematoma 378
Intracranial abscess 385
Intracranial abscess, treatment 386
Intracranial aneurysm 386
Intracranial aneurysm, subclinoid type 386
Intracranial aneurysm, supraclinoid type 386
Intracranial aneurysm, types 486
Intracranial tumors 387
Intrinsic healing method 256
Intrinsic minus deformity 253
Intrinsic plus deformity 253
Involucrum 354
Iodophors 5
IOHEXOL (Omnipaque), 318
Iopamiro 318

Ischemia, chronic, treatment 177
Ischemia, critical limb 186
Ischemia, features of 187
Ischemia, upper limb 175
Ischemia, upper limb chronic type 176
Ischemia, upper limb investigations 176
Ischemia, upper limb, acute type 175
Ischemia, upper limb, types 175
Isoflurane 322
Isograft 142
Isolated limb perfusion 283
Isotope lymphoscintigraphy 233
Ivor Lewis operation 375

J

Jaw and temporomandibular joint, examination of 371
Jaw tumors 312
Jaw tumors, classification 312
Jejunostomy 25
Jejunostomy, needle 25
Jejunostomy, Witzel 25
Jellinek's sign 315
Jod Basedow thyrotoxicosis 314
Joffroy's sign 315
John H Gibbon 2
John Hunter 1
Jonathan Rhoads 2
Joseph Lister 1, 3
Jugular lymph trunk 286
Juvenile melanoma, 279

K

Kang cancer 275
Kangri cancer 275
Kaposi's sarcoma 270
Kasabach-Merritt syndrome 211
Keloid 37
Keratin pearls 275
Keratoacanthoma 273
Kernohan's notch effect 378, 382
Kessler method 257
Ketamine 322
Killian's dehiscence 288, 364
Kinmoth classification 233
Kiss cancer 260

Klippel-Trenauny-Weber syndrome 211
Klumpke's paralysis 251
Knie's sign 315
Knots, types 311
Kocher, Emil, Theodor 330
Kocher's sign 315
Kocher's test 361
Kondolean's operation 237, 238
Kuntz nerve 182
Kyphosis 359

L

Lahey's test 312
Langhan's cells 246
Laparoscopic fundoplication 369
Laryngeal cartilages 394
Laryngeal intrinsic muscles 395
Laryngeal joints 396
Laryngeal ligaments 396
Laryngeal papilloma 397
Laryngocele 289
Larynx, actions of 396
Larynx, benign lesions 397
Larynx, cavity of 396
Larynx, lymphatic drainage 396
Larynx, malignant tumor 398
Larynx, malignant tumor, anatomical types 398
Larynx, malignant tumor, conservative surgery 300
Larynx, malignant tumor, etiology 398
Larynx, malignant tumor, staging 399
Larynx, malignant tumor, treatment 300
Larynx, spaces of 396
Larynx, surgical anatomy 394
Lasers in surgery 314
Lateral aberrant thyroid 308
Lateral neck dissection 302
Leiomyosarcoma 269
Lentigo maligna melanoma 281
Leprosy 73
Leprosy, surgical complications 74
Leprosy, types 73
Leriche's syndrome 185
Lethal triad 126
Leukoplakia 366
Leukoplakia, causes 366

Leukoplakia, histological grading 367
Leukoplakia, types 366
Levels in neck nodes 297
Lid Lag's sign 314
Lid retraction 314
Ligneus thyroiditis 327
Limb saving procedures 207
Line of demarcation 186
Line of Sebileau 390
Lingual thyroid 307
Lip 376
Lip, carcinoma 377
Lip, carcinoma, clinical features 378
Lip, neoplasm 377
Lipedema 236
Lipoma 97
Lipoma, complications 98
Lipoma, treatment 98
Liposarcoma 98, 264, 269
Lips 361
Livedo reticularis 184
Liver injury 172
Liver injury, complications 173
Loewi's sign 315
Long thoracic nerve 256
Lord's plication 392
Louis Pasteur 1
Low molecular weight dextran 129
Low molecular weight heparin 230
Low temperature steam formaldehyde sterilizer 10
Low ulnar palsy 254
Lower esophageal sphincter 365
Lower plexus injury 251
Lucid interval 382
Ludwig's angina 58, 291
Lugol's iodine 318
Lumbar sympathectomy 193, 194
Lumbricals 155
Lupus vulgaris 55
Lymph scrotum 384
Lymphadenitis, acute suppurative 239
Lymphadenitis, chronic nonspecific 239
Lymphadenitis, tuberculous 239, 245
Lymphadenopathy, cervical 238

Lymphangiographic classification of lymphedema 232
Lymphangiography 232
Lymphangiosarcoma 270
Lymphangitis 58, 233
Lymphangitis, management 59
Lymphatic mapping and sentinel node biopsy 283
Lymphatic ring 285
Lymphatics 232
Lymphedema 58, 233
Lymphedema classification 233
Lymphedema, clinical features 235
Lymphedema, filarial 234
Lymphedema, grading of Brunner's 235
Lymphedema, lymphangiographic classification 232
Lymphedema, secondary causes 234
Lymphedema, pathology 234
Lymphoma, Burkitt's 244
Lymphoma, Hodgkin's 240
Lymphoma, Hodgkin's Ann Arbor staging 241
Lymphoma, Hodgkin's, treatment of 242
Lymphoma, non-Hodgkin's 243
Lymphoma, non-Hodgkin's, treatment 244
Lymphoma, Rapport classification 243
Lymphoma, REAL classification 240
Lymphoma, Reed-Sternberg cell 240, 241
Lymphoma, Rye's classification 241
Lymphomas 240
Lymphovenous shunt 237
Lyre sign 295
Lysol 5

M

Macrocheilia 366, 377
Macroglossia 366, 383
Madura foot 39, 76

Madura foot, pathogenesis 77
Madura hand 77
Mafenide acetate 136, 140
Maffucci syndrome 211
Magnetic resonance
  cholangiopancreatography
  (MRCP) 320
Magnetic resonance imaging 319
Magnetic resonance imaging,
  advantages 320
Magnetic resonance imaging,
  contraindication 320
Magnetic resonance imaging,
  disadvantages 320
Magnetic resonance imaging,
  uses 319
Malignant edema 71
Malignant exophthalmos 316
Malignant hyperthermia 324
Malignant lymphoma 326
Malignant mixed tumor 353
Malignant mixed tumor, types 353
Malignant neurilemmoma 270
Malignant pustule 80
Malignant salivary tumors,
  complications of surgery
  356
Malignant salivary tumors,
  general features 354
Malignant salivary tumors,
  indications for radiotherapy
  357
Malignant salivary tumors,
  indications for surgery 356
Malignant salivary tumors,
  management 355
Malignant salivary tumors, TNM
  staging 355
Malignant salivary tumors,
  treatment 356
Mallet finger 163
Management of fracture,
  principles of 348
Mandible, dislocation of the 336
Mandible, examination of 372
Mandible, surgical anatomy 330
Maneuver, costoclavicular
  compression 188
Maneuver, hyperabduction 188
Manual lymphatic drainage 237
Marjolin's ulcer 138

Marjolin's ulcer 275, 276
Marker stitches 249
Marsupialization 364
Maxilla, anatomy of 371
Maxillary antrum 372
Maxillary tumors 389
Maxillary tumors, behavior and
  presentation 390
Maxillary tumors, Lederman's
  classification 390
Maxillary tumors, Ohngren's
  classification 390
Maxillary tumors, TNM staging
  391
Maxillofacial injuries,
  complications 337
Maxillofacial injuries,
  hemorrhage 322
Maxillofacial injuries, primary
  care 321
Maxon 310
Mayo's towel clip 398
McCune Albright's syndrome 319
McFee incision 302
MCR chappals 255
MCR chappals 50
Median claw hand 254
Median nerve injuries 251
Median nerve palsy, clinical
  features of 252
Medullary carcinoma of thyroid
  325
Medulloblastoma 388
Meglumine iothalamate, 318
Meige's disease 233
Melanoma 280
Melanoma, ABCDE 282
Melanoma, classifications 281
Melanoma, clinical features of 281
Melanoma, immunotherapy 284
Melanoma, juvenile 279
Melanoma, TNM staging 282
Melanoma, treatment of 283
Melanotic skin cancers (MSC) 271
Melanuria 282
Melphalan 283, 284, 395
Memorial Sloan-Kettering
  Cancer Center leveling of
  neck nodes 297
MEN II syndrome 326
MEN syndrome 97

Meningiomas 388
Meningocele 391
Mercaptopurine 395
Merkel cell carcinoma 272
Mesher 144
Mesna 268
Metabolic acidosis 21, 22
Methimazole 318
Michael E DeBakey 2
Microchelia 366
Microsclerotherapy 225
Middle third area, surgical
  anatomy 323
Mikulicz disease 348
Millard cleft lip repair 309
Milroy's disease 233
Miner's elbow 108
Modified Heller's operation 368
Modified Perthe's test 223
Modified radical neck dissection
  301
Moebius sign 315
Molluscum sebaceum 273
Monks localizing zones 172
Monoclonal antibodies 397
Monocryl (polyglecaprone) 310
MOPP regime 243
Morrissey's cough impulse test 223
Mose's sign 219, 356
Mousseau-Barbin tube 376
Mouth-to-mouth breathing 120
MR spectroscopy 320
MRND 301
MRND types 301
Mucoepidermoid tumor 352
Muir and Burclay regime 136
Mule spinner's disease 381
Multilocular cystic disease of the
  jaw 314
Multiorgan dysfunction
  syndrome (MODS) 68
Multiple chondromatosis 361
Multiple exostoses 356
Multiple myeloma 363
Muscle relaxants 322
Muscle relaxants, depolarizing
  322
Mycetoma pedis 76
Mycobacterium leprae 73
Mycobacterium tuberculosis 72
Mycotic aneurysms 386

Index

Myelomeningocele 391
Myer's stripper 226
Myopathy 316
Myositis ossificans 348
Myxedema madness 331
Myxedema, features of 357
Myxoedema, pretibial 316

N

Naevi 279
Naffziger's sign 315
Nasal bone fracture, mode of injury 324
Nasal bone fracture, treatment 324
Nasolabial flap 378
Nasopharyngeal carcinoma 388
Near total thyroidectomy 327
Neck dissection, classic radical 301
Neck dissection, lateral 302
Neck dissection, modified radical 301
Neck dissection, types 301
Neck injuries 169
Neck injuries, treatment 169
Necrosis 186
Necrotizing fasciitis 81
Necrotizing fasciitis, management 82
Needle holder 302
Needle stick injury in surgical practice 90
Needle stick injury in surgical practice, management 91
Needle stick injury in surgical practice, prevention 91
Negri bodies 78
Negus hydrostatic dilatation 368
Neonatal thyrotoxicosis 314
Neoplasia, classification 258
Neoplasm 258
Neoplasm, definition 258
Neoplasm, investigations for 262
Neostigmine 323
Nerve block 326
Nerve injuries, prognostic factors 250
Nerve of Bell 256
Nerve repair, primary 249
Nerve repair, secondary 250

Nerve suturing, types 249
Neumann's tumor 313
Neurilemmoma 107
Neurilemmoma, malignant 270
Neuroblastoma 338
Neuroblastoma, Hutchinson's type 338
Neuroblastoma, pepper type 338
Neurofibroma 105
Neurofibroma, complications 106
Neurofibroma, elephantiatic 106
Neurofibroma, nodular 105
Neurofibroma, plexiform 106
Neurolipoma 97
Neuroma 105
Neuroma, end 105
Neuroma, false 105
Neuroma, lateral 105
Neuroma, proximal 248
Neuropraxia 248
Neurotmesis 248
Nevi 279
Nevus compound 279
Nevus, blue 279
Nevus, junctional 279
Nicoladoni's sign 214
Nissen's fundoplication 368, 369
Nitrous oxide 322
No reflow phenomenon 198
Nodal staging in secondaries 300
Nodovenous shunt 237
Nodular goiter 311
Nodule, dominant 312
Nodule, retrosternal 312
Noma 366
Non chromaffin paraganglioma 294
Nondepolarizing muscle relaxants 323
Nonmelanotic skin cancers (NMSC) 271
Non-odontogenic tumors 313
Nosocomial infection 80
Nosocomial infection, prevention 80
Nosocomial infection, sources 80
Nourishment 330
Nutrition 23

O

Obesity 27
Obesity, causes 27
Obesity, complications 27
Obesity, surgery 27

Obesity, treatment 27
Oblique arytenoids 395
Occipital lobe tumors 389
Ochsner's clasping test 252
Odontogenic tumors 312
Ollier's disease 357, 361
Omentocele 388
Omentoplasty 193, 196, 237
Oncocytoma 352
Onychocryptosis 164
Operation, Charle's 237, 238
Operation, Criles 301
Operation, Homan's 237
Operation, Kondolean's 237
Operation, Paul Braund's 254
Operation, Sistrunk 237
Operation, Sistrunk, thyroid 308
Operation, StyeBunnell's 254
Operation, Thompson's 237, 238
Ophthalmometer 315
Opportunistic infections 81
Opsite 137
Oral and upper aerodigestive cancers 368
Oral anticoagulants 231
Oral carcinomas, problems with 393
Oral carcinomas, prognostic factors 393
Oral cavity cancer, Broder's histological grading 373
Oral cavity cancer, reconstruction after surgery 375
Oral cavity cancer, TNM staging 372
Oral cavity malignancies 370
Oral cavity, examination of 364, 370
Oral cavity, premalignant conditions 368
Oral cavity, verrucous carcinoma 371
Oral malignancies, treatment strategy 393
Oral submucosal fibrosis 367
Oral submucosal fibrosis, treatment 367
Organ of Zuckerkand 339
Orphan Annie eye 322
Orrhinger and Orrhinger approach 375

Orthopantomogram 311
Oschner's Mahoner's test 355
Osmotic demyelination
    syndrome 14
Ossification, cartilaginous 346
Ossification, membranous 346
Osteitis deformans 354
Osteitis fibrosa cystica 355
Osteoarthrosis 358
Osteoarthrosis, primary 358
Osteoarthrosis, secondary 358
Osteoblastic secondaries 260
Osteochondroma 361
Osteoclastoma 361
Osteogenesis imperfect 356
Osteoma 360
Osteoma, cancellous 361
Osteoma, ivory 360
Osteoma, types 360
Osteomalacia 355
Osteomyelitis of jaw 317
Osteomyelitis, acute 353
Osteomyelitis, chronic 353
Osteomyelitis, chronic,
    treatment 354
Osteoporosis 355
Osteosarcoma 264, 362
Osteotomy 352
Outer lymphatic ring 285
Owen H Wangensteen 2
Oxygen 322
Oxygen therapy 119

 P

Pachydermatocele 106
Pack years index 192
Packed cells 128
Paget's disease of nipple 274
Paget's test 102, 108, 344
Painful arc syndrome 356
Palate 362
Palate, diseases of the 311
Palatoplasty, treatment 311
Palmar aponeurosis 154
Palpation of blood vessels 188
Panarteritis 192
Pancoast tumor 303
Pancreatic injury 172
Pancreatic injury, complications
    172

Pancuronium bromide
    (Pavulon) 323
Panda sign 327
Pannus 357
Papillary carcinoma of thyroid
    322
Papillary carcinoma of thyroid,
    treatment of 323
Papillary cystadeno-
    lymphomatosum 351
Papilloma 99
Papilloma, complications 100
Papilloma, infective 99
Papilloma, skin 99
Papilloma, treatment 100
Papilloma, true 99
Parafollicular 'C' cells 325
Paraneoplastic syndromes 261
Parapharyngeal abscess 292
Parathyroid hormone 332
Parathyroid, anatomy 332
Parathyroidectomy, indications
    for 334
Parathyroidectomy, problems 335
Parathyroidectomy, surgical
    aspects 335
Parietal lobe tumors 389
Parkland regime 136
Parona's space 160
Paronychia, acute 156
Paronychia, chronic 157
Parotid abscess 345
Parotid abscess, complications 346
Parotid duct (Stensen's) 341
parotid enlargement, differential
    diagnosis 380
Parotid fistula 346
Parotid fistula, duct 347
Parotid fistula, gland 347
Parotid fistula, treatment 347
Parotid gland, anatomy 341
Parotid gland, parts 341
Parotid swelling, features of 378
Parotid tumor, clinical features 349
Parotid, accessory 341
Parotid, acute suppurative
    sialadenitis 345
Parotid, bidigital palpation 379
Parotidectomy 357
Parotidectomy, complications 359
Parotidectomy, extended total 359

Parotidectomy, patial
    (functional) 358
Parotidectomy, radical 358
Parotidectomy, superficial/
    lateral 358
Parotidectomy, suprafacial
    extracapsular 359
Parotidectomy, total
    conservative 358
Parotidectomy, types 358
Partial thyroidectomy 327
Patey, faciovenous plane 342
Patterson operation 374
Paul Braund's operation 254
PDS 310
Pedal edema 332
Pembertones'sign 313
Pen test 252
Penetrating injury 170
Percussion 333
Percutaneous transluminal
    angioplasty 192
Perfluorocarbon 130
Periapical cyst 316
Periostitis 229
Peripheral aneurysms 203
Peripheral heart 216
Peripheral nerve injuries 248
Peritonsillar abscess 304
Peritonsillar abscess, clinical
    features 304
Peritonsillar abscess, treatment
    304
Permeation spread 260
Perniosis 55
Perthe's test 223
Perthe's test, modified 223, 356
Perthes test 356
Phagedena 54
Pharyngeal pouch 288
Pharyngitis, acute 306
Phenol 5
Pheochromocytoma 339
Philtrum 361
Phlegmasia alba dolens 219
Phlegmasia cerulea dolens 219
Physiology of venous blood flow
    in lower limb 217
Pindborg's tumor 313
Pituitary tumors 390
Pituitary tumors, classification 390
Pituitary tumors, treatment 390

pKa 20
Plantar fasciitis 164
Plasma 128
Plasma osmolality 15
Plaster of Paris 350
Platelet concentrate 128
Platelet-rich plasma 128
Pleomorphic adenomas 350
Plethysmography 224
Plummer's disease 310, 313
Plunging goiter 313
Pointing index 252
Policeman's heel 164
Poly-dioxanone suture material 310
Polyarteritis nodosa 182
Polyethylene (ethylene) 311
Polyglactic acid 310
Polyglecaprone 310
Polyglycolic acid 310
Polyostotic fibrous dysplasia 319
Polypropylene (prolene) 310
Popliteal aneurysm 204
Popliteal artery 351
Position of trachea 362
Postcricoid tumor 375
Posterior cricoarytenoid 395
Posterior tibial artery 350
Postoperative thrombosis 218
Postphlebitic limb 54, 229
Post-thrombotic ulcer 54
Potato tumor 294
Pott's puffy tumor 66, 385
Pott's puffy tumor, complication 66
Pott's puffy tumor, treatment 66
Povidone iodine 6
Pratt's test 223, 355
Preauricular sinus 312
Precancerous condition 368
Precancerous lesion 368
Pregangrene 186
Premalignant conditions of skin 274
Pressure sore 48
Pretibial myxedema 316
PriceHill regimen 387
Primary nerve suturing 249
Primary suturing 35
Primary suturing after wound excision 35
Primary thyrotoxicosis 317
Pringle maneuver 173

Procarbazin 395
Proctoscope 309
Proflavine 9
Profundaplasty 193, 194
Prolactin secreting adenomas 390
Propanidid 322
Propofol 322
Propranolol 318
Propylthiouracil 318
Proud flesh 46
Psammoma bodies 322, 323
Pseudohyperkalemia 19
Pseudohypokalemia 17
Pseudosynapsis 359
PTA 192
Pulmonary capillary wedge pressure 118
Pulsatility 345
Pyemia 68
Pyogenic granuloma 46, 66
Pyorrhea alveolaris 367, 368
Pyrazinamide 246
Pyrosis 369

 Q

Quadruple ligation 214
Quaternary ammonium compounds (quats) 8
Quinsy 304

 R

Rabies 77
Rabies, active immunization 78
Rabies, clinical features 78
Rabies, passive immunization 79
Rabies, pathogenesis 77
Rabies, post-exposure prophylaxis 78
Rabies, vaccines for 78
Radial artery 351
Radial bursa 159
Radial nerve injuries 254
Radiation absorbed dose (RAD) 393
Radicular cyst 316
Radio sensitive tumors 392
Radioactive iodine 320
Radiofrequency ablation (RFA) method 227
Radioiodine therapy 319
Radio-resistant tumors 392
Radiotherapy 392

Radiotherapy, care of patients on 394
Radiotherapy, problems in 394
Radiotherapy, sources 393
Ranula 364
Ranula, treatment 364
Rapport classification 243
Raynaud's disease 181
Raynaud's phenomenon 180
Raynaud's phenomenon, causes 181
Raynaud's phenomenon, pathology 181
Raynaud's phenomenon, treatment 178, 181
Raynaud's phenomenon, types 181
Raynaud's syndrome 180
REAL classification 240
Recurrent fibroid of Paget's 107
Recurrent laryngeal nerve 306
Recurrent laryngeal nerve palsy 329
Recycled blood 130
Reducibility 343, 345
Reed-Sternberg cell 240, 241
Reinke's edema 397
Renal injury 173
Reperfusion injury 197
Respiratory acidosis 22
Rest pain 186
Reticular varices 220
Retractor, Czerney's 300
Retractor, Deaver's 301
Retractor, Doyen's 301
Retractor, hernia 300
Retractor, Joll's thyroid 303
Retractor, Morris' 301
Retractor, self-retaining 301
Retractor, single hook 300
Retractor, Volkmann's 300
Retrograde lymphatic spread 260
Retrograde transfemoral Seldinger angiography 189, 193
Retromolar trigone 362
Retropharyngeal abscess 293
Retrosternal nodule 312
Reversal agents 323
Rhabdomyosarcoma 269
Rheomacrodex 129
Rhinophyma 273
Ricketic rosary 355
Rickets 355
Rickets, renal 355

Riedel's thyroiditis 327
Rifampicin 246
Ripple bed 49
Risus sardonicus 69
Rocuronium 323
Rodent ulcer 277
Roentgen unit 393
Roos test 179, 349
Rosenbach's sign 315
Rubidomycin 395
Rudolph Matas 2
Rule of 7 in the neck 287
Rye's classification 240

S

Saddle embolus 199
SAG-M blood 128
Saliva 340
Salivary calculi 345
Salivary calculus 343
Salivary fistula 377
Salivary gland tumors, minor 357
Salivary gland, ectopic 340
Salivary gland, examination 375
Salivary glands, adenocarcinoma of 354
Salivary glands, squamous cell carcinoma of 354
Salivary neoplasms 348
Salivary neoplasms, classification 348
Salivary tumors, pain in 351
Saphena varix 226
Sarcoma 259
Sarcoma, Kaposi's 270
Sarcoma, synovial 269
Sarcomas 263
Saturday night palsy 255
Savlon 8
Scabbard trachea 331
Scalene triangle 174, 178
Scalpel with blades 309
Schobinger incision 302
Schwannoma 107, 388
Schwartz test 223, 355
Scissors 308
Scleroderma 183
Sclerosants 225
Sclerosing angioma 272
Scoliosis 359
Scurvy 356

Secondaries in neck lymph nodes 240, 297
Secondaries in neck, treatment of 301
Secondaries in neck, types of 299
Secondaries in the neck with an occult primary 299, 300
Secondary nerve suturing 249
Secondary suturing 35
Secondary thyrotoxicosis 317
Seddon's classification 248
Seedling 260
Seldinger technique 189
SEPS 228
Septicemia 67
Septicemia, Gram-negative 67
Septicemia, Gram-positive 67
Sequestrum 186
Sequestrum 354
Shamblin classification of carotid body tumor 295
Shamida 338
Shock 112
Shock, anaphylactic 113, 115
Shock, cardiogenic 112, 116
Shock, cardiogenic, management 117
Shock, causes 112
Shock, effects 114
Shock, hypovolemic 112
Shock, neurogenic 113
Shock, pathophysiology of 113
Shock, septic 113, 114
Shock, septic, stages 114
Shock, stages 114
Shock, treatment 115
Shouldering sign 374
Sialadenitis 343, 345
Sialadenitis, acute bacterial suppurative 345
Sialadenitis, chronic 345
Sialectasis 345
Sialography 343
Sialosis 345
Sick cell syndrome 125
Sign Berry's 324
Sign, 'sun-setting' 387
Sign, 'V' 158
Sign, Berry's 362
Sign, Branham's/Nicoladoni's 349
Sign, Branhan's 214
Sign, Chvostek's 335

Sign, Coleman's 334
Sign, curtain 350, 377
Sign, Dalrymple's 314, 362
Sign, Enroth 315
Sign, Froment's 253
Sign, Harvey's 187
Sign, Homan's 219
Sign, Hood 308
Sign, Hook 159
Sign, Jellink's 315
Sign, Joffroy's 315, 362
Sign, Kanavel 159
Sign, Knie's 315
Sign, Kocher's 315
Sign, Lid Lag's 314, 362
Sign, Loewi's 315
Sign, Lyre 295
Sign, Milian's ear 59
Sign, Moebius 315, 563
Sign, Moses 219
Sign, Naffziger's 315, 362
Sign, Nicoladoni's 214
Sign, Panda 327
Sign, Pemberton's 361
Sign, Pembertones' 313
Sign, Racoon's eye 338
Sign, Rosenbach's 315
Sign, Rust's 63
Sign, slip 98, 343
Sign, Stellwag's 314, 362
Sign, Stemmer's 235
Sign, Tinel's 250
Sign, trail 362
Sign, Trousseau's 230, 335
Sign, von Graefe's 314, 362
Signaloc 4
Signs 329
Silk 310
Singer's/screamer's nodule 397
Sinus 39
Sinus or fistula, clinical examination of 335
Sinus, cervical 287
Sinus, median mental 39, 41
Sinus, pilonidal 39
Sinus, tuberculous 39
Sipple's disease 336
Sir Astley Cooper 1
Sistrunk operation 237
Sistrunk operation, thyroid 308
Sjögren's syndrome 347
Sjögren's syndrome, primary 347

Sjögren's syndrome, secondary 347
Skin adnexal tumors 271
Skin cancers, melanotic 271
Skin cancers, non-melanotic 271
Skin grafting 142
Skin tumors 271
Skin tumors, classification of 271
Skip lesions 348
Sleeping pulse rate 316, 358
Slip sign 98
Sloan Kettering scoring, thyroid DTC 321
Slough 186
Small bowel injury 172
Small saphenous vein 217
Smoker's ulcer 382
Smoking index 192
Sodium deficit formula 14
Sodium diatrizoate, 318
Soft palate 363
Soft tissue sarcoma, clinical features of 264
Soft tissue sarcoma, treatment of 267
Soft tissue tumors 263, 265
Solitary thyroid nodule 312
Space of Gillette 293
Spina bifida 390
Spina bifida aperta 391
Spina bifida occulta 390
Spina bifida, treatment 391
Spina bifida, types 390
Spina ventosa 163
Spinal anesthesia, advantages 327
Spinal anesthesia, complications 327
Spinal anesthesia, contraindications 327
Spinal anesthesia, disadvantages 327
Spinal anesthesia, drugs used 327
Spinal anesthesia, technique 326
Spinal anesthesia, types 327
Spinal injury 168
Spiral CT scan 318
Spiral CT scan, advantages 319
Splenectomy, complications 173
Splenic injury 173
Splenic injury, management 173
Spondylolisthesis 359
Spongioblastoma polare 388

Spontaneous thrombosis 218
Spread of malignant tumors 260
Squamous cell carcinoma 52, 274
Stafne bone cyst 340
Stages of tuberculous lymphadenitis 245
Staging laparotomy 242
Staging of the tumor 261
Staging, Ann Arbor 241
Stanford classification 204
Starch iodine test 359
Starry night pattern 244
Starry sky pattern 244
Stellwag's sign 314
Stemmer's sign 235
Stenson's duct 341
Stenson's duct examination 376
Sterilization 4
Sternomastoid tumor 296
Stomatitis 365
Stomatitis, angular 366
Stomatitis, aphthous 365
Stomatitis, candida 365
Stomatitis, nutritional 365
Stomatitis, traumatic 365
Stomatitis, Vincent's ulcerative 365
Strawberry hemangioma 210
Stridor 313
Stripper, Myer's 226
Stripper, Myer's vein 308
Stripping of vein 226
Student's elbow 108
Sturge-Weber syndrome 211
Stye-Bunnell's operation 254
Subarachnoid hemorrhage 384
Subclavian artery 351
Subclavian artery, right 175
Subclavian steal syndrome 184
Subdelphian node 306
Subdural abscess 385
Subdural hematoma 378
Subdural hematoma, acute 383
Subdural hematoma, chronic 383
Subdural hygroma 383
Subepithelial benign nodular fibrosis 272
Subfascial endoscopic perforator ligation surgery 227
Subfascial ligation of Cockett and Dodd 227
Subhyoid bursa 296
Subhyoid bursitis 296

Sublingual dermoid 365
Submandibular calculus 376
Submandibular duct (Wharton's) 343
Submandibular salivary gland 342
Submandibular salivary gland enlargement, differential diagnosis 381
Submandibular salivary gland excision 344
Submandibular salivary gland swelling 378
Submandibular salivary gland tumors 354
Submandibular salivary gland tumors, benign 354
Submandibular salivary gland tumors, malignant 354
Submandibular salivary gland, parts 342
Subtotal thyroidectomy 327
Sunderland's classification 249
Superficial palmar arch 154
Superficial temporal artery 352
Superior laryngeal nerve 306
Superior sulcus tumor 303
Supraomohyoid block 301
Surgical anatomy of thoracic outlet 174
Surgical needles 302
Surgical needles, types 302
Surgical site infection 92
Surgical site infection, classification 94
Surgical site infection, management 96
Surgical site infection, prevention 95
Surgical wounds, classification 93
Surgical wounds, physical status classification 93
Sushruta 1
Suture materials 310
Suture materials, absorbable 310
Suture materials, absorbable, uses 310
Suture materials, braided 311
Suture materials, classification 310
Suture materials, coated 311
Suture materials, monofilament 311

Suture materials, multifilament 311
Suture materials, natural 311
Suture materials, non-absorbable 310
Suture materials, non-absorbable, uses 311
Suture materials, numbering 311
Suture materials, synthetic 311
Suture materials, twisted 511
Suture materials, uncoated 511
Suturing, types 311
Suxamethonium chloride (scoline) 322
Swelling/lump, examination of 340
Sympathectomy, cervical 181
Sympathectomy, chemical 196
Sympathectomy, lumbar 193, 194
Symptoms 329
Syndactyly 162
Syndrome, acute compartment 198
Syndrome, auriculotemporal 359
Syndrome, Boerhaave's 372
Syndrome, Brown-Séquard 169
Syndrome, central cord 168
Syndrome, compartment 36, 197
Syndrome, Conn's 338
Syndrome, crest 181
Syndrome, crush 36
Syndrome, Cushing's 338
Syndrome, DiGeorge's 333
Syndrome, disappearing pulse 187
Syndrome, Frey's 359
Syndrome, Frey's, treatment 360
Syndrome, Horner's 298, 299, 303
Syndrome, Kasabacch Merritt 211
Syndrome, Klippel-Trenauny-Weber 211
Syndrome, Leriche's 185
Syndrome, Maffucci 211
Syndrome, Mallory-Weiss 372
Syndrome, MEA 335
Syndrome, MEN 97, 335
Syndrome, MEN, types 336
Syndrome, Mendelson's 324
Syndrome, Mikulicz 375
Syndrome, Patterson-Kelly 372
Syndrome, Plummer-Vinson 372
Syndrome, Raynaud's 180
Syndrome, Sjogren 375
Syndrome, Sturge Weber 211
Syndrome, subclavian steal 184
Syndrome, thoracic outlet 174, 178
Syndrome, Treacher-Collins 312
Syndrome, Wermer's 336
Syndromes, paraneoplastic 261
Synovial sarcoma 269
Syphilis 74
Syphilis, congenital 75
Syphilis, early 74
Syphilis, late 74
Syphilis, latent 74
Syphilis, primary 74
Syphilis, secondary 74
Systemic inflammatory response syndrome (SIRS) 119
Systemic sclerosis 183

T

T1 relaxation time 319
T2 relaxation time 319
Talipes equinovarus 229
TAO 192
Tear cancer 277
Technetium-99 pertechnetate scan 352
Technetium-99m labeled Sestamibi isotope scan 334
Temporal arteritis 184
Temporal lobe tumors 389
Temporomandibular joint, examination of 374
Temporomandibular joint, movements of 374
Tendinitis 356
Tendon 256
Tendon graft 257
Tendon healing, stages 257
Tendon repair 257
Tendon transfer 257
Tendon, types of suturing 257
Tenoma 257
Terminal pulp space infection 157
Tessari, foam sclerotherapy 226
Test, Adson's 179, 187
Test, Allen's 188
Test, Brodie-Trendelenburg 222
Test, Buerger's postural 187
Test, card 253
Test, elevated arm stress 179, 187
Test, Fegan's 223
Test, Lahey's 312
Test, modified Perthe's 223
Test, Morrissey's cough impulse 223
Test, Ochsner's clasping 252
Test, pen 252
Test, Perthe's 223
Test, Pratt's 223
Test, Roos 179
Test, Schwartz 223
Test, three-tourniquet 223
Testicular sensation 386
Tests, thyroid function 309
Tetanus 68
Tetanus toxoid 71
Tetanus, clinical features 69
Tetanus, different postures in 70
Tetanus, staging of 70
Tetanus, treatment 70
Tetanus, types of 70
Tetany 21
Tetany 335
Thakayasu's arteritis 183
Thenar muscles 155
Theodor Billroth 2
Therapeutic emblization 200
Thermoablation of varicose veins 227
Thiersch graft 229
Thiopentone 322
Thompson's operation 237, 238
Thoracic outlet syndrome 174, 178
Thread veins 220
Three/multiple tourniquet test 355
Three-tourniquet test 223
Thrombectomy 193
Thromboangiitis obliterans 192
Thrombophlebitis 230
Thrombophlebitis migrans 230
Thrombosis, deep vein 218
Thrombus, blue 219
Thrombus, fixed 219
Thyroarytenoid 395
Thyrocardiac 320
Thyroglobulin estimation 324
Thyroglossal cyst 307
Thyroglossal fistula 308
Thyroid 304
Thyroid acropachy 316
Thyroid cartilage 394
Thyroid crisis 330

Thyroid disease, investigations 364
Thyroid FNAC of thyroid 309
Thyroid function tests 309
Thyroid gland, examination of 356
Thyroid malignancy, etiology 322
Thyroid neoplasm 321
Thyroid neoplasm, Dunhill classification 321
Thyroid nodule, solitary 312
Thyroid steal 328
Thyroid storm 330
Thyroid toxicity, features of 357
Thyroid, Pizzillo's method of palpation
Thyroid, agenesis 308
Thyroid, AGES scoring 321, 323
Thyroid, AMES scoring 321, 323
Thyroid, anaplastic carcinoma 325
Thyroid, anatomy 304
Thyroid, blood supply 305
Thyroid, congenital anomalies 306
Thyroid, development of 304
Thyroid, DTC, TNM staging 321
Thyroid, ectopic 306
Thyroid, follicular carcinoma 323
Thyroid, Hurthle cell carcinoma 325
Thyroid, Lahey's method of examination 360
Thyroid, lateral aberrant 308
Thyroid, lateral aberrant 363
Thyroid, lingual 307
Thyroid, lymphatic drainage 306
Thyroid, medullary carcinoma of 325
Thyroid, papillary carcinoma 322
Thyroid, pyramidal lobe 304
Thyroid, thrill 360
Thyroid, toxic, in children 320
Thyroid, toxic, in pregnancy 320
Thyroidea ima artery 305
Thyroidectomy 327
Thyroidectomy, complications of 328, 329
Thyroidectomy, hemi 319, 327
Thyroidectomy, near total 327
Thyroidectomy, partial 327
Thyroidectomy, subtotal 318, 327
Thyroidectomy, total 327
Thyroiditis 310
Thyroiditis ligneous 327

Thyroiditis, Hashimoto's 326
Thyroiditis, Riedel's 327
Thyroiditis, woody 327
Thyrotoxic crisis 330
Thyrotoxicosis 313
Thyrotoxicosis factitia 313
Thyrotoxicosis, diagnostic indices, Wayne's 314
Thyrotoxicosis, investigations 317
Thyrotoxicosis, Jod Basedow 314
Thyrotoxicosis, neonatal 314
Thyrotoxicosis, treatment 317
Time motion mode 316
Tinel's sign 250
TNM staging 261
TNM staging for DTCs 321
TNM staging of melanoma 282
TNM staging of, soft tissue sarcoma 266
Tongue 362
Tongue fissure 382
Tongue tie 366, 383
Tongue ulcers, differential diagnosis 381
Tongue, benign tumors 382
Tongue, development and nerve supply 380
Tongue, hairy 383
Tongue, lymphatic drainage 379
Tongue, syphilitic ulcer 381
Tongue, tuberculous ulcer 382
Tonsillar bed 302
Tonsillar position 305
Tonsillectomy 305
Tonsillectomy, complications 306
Tonsillectomy, nursing care 305
Tonsillitis, acute 303
Tonsillitis, acute catarrhal 303
Tonsillitis, acute follicular 303
Tonsillitis, acute membranous 303
Tonsillitis, acute parenchymatous 303
Tonsillitis, chronic 303
Tonsillitis, chronic fibroid 304
Tonsillitis, chronic follicular 304
Tonsillitis, chronic parenchymatous 304
Tonsillitis, chronic, complications 304
Tonsillitis, chronic, treatment 304
Tonsillitis, clinical features 303
Tonsillolith 304

Tonsils, anatomy 302
Torticollis 295
Total laryngectomy 301
Total laryngectomy, after care 301
Total parenteral nutrition 26
Total thyroidectomy 327
Touhy needle 327
Tourniquet palsy 255
Tourniquet, complications 131
Tourniquet, elastic bandage 130
Tourniquet, pneumatic 130
Tourniquet, rubber 130
Tourniquets 130
Toxic shock syndrome 135
Toxic thyroid in children 320
Toxic thyroid in pregnancy 320
Toxoplasmosis 239
Tracheoesophageal fistula 373
Tracheoesophageal fistula, treatment 373
Tracheostomy 339
Tracheostomy care 343
Tracheostomy complications 343
Tracheostomy functions 343
Tracheostomy nursing care 343
Tracheostomy tube 304
Tracheostomy tube, Fuller's bivalved 304, 339
Tracheostomy tube, Jackson's 304, 339
Tracheostomy tube, polyvinyl chloride (PVC) 304
Tracheostomy tube, Shiley's fenestrated 339
Tracheostomy tubes 339
Tracheostomy, approaches 342
Tracheostomy, high 339
Tracheostomy, indication 341
Tracheostomy, indications for 304
Tracheostomy, low 339
Tracheostomy, mid 339
Tracheostomy, technique 341
Tracheostomy, types 339, 342
Traction test 386
Transcoelomic spread 261
Transcyte 137
Transillumination 386
Transillumination test 344, 372
Transluminal balloon angioplasty 193
Transplantation 151

Transplantation, bone-marrow 152
Transplantation, donor criteria 151
Transplantation, heterotopic 151
Transplantation, liver 152
Transplantation, renal 151
Transplantation, renal, complications 151
Trans-tubular potassium gradient (TTKG) 17
Transverse arytenoid 395
Traumatic arterial occlusion 197
Traumatic needle 302
Treatment of chronic ischemia 177
Trendelenburg operation 226
Trendelenburg test II, 355
Triad, Haimovici 198
Triad, Virchow's 218
Triage 165
Triage algorithm 165
Triangle, scalene 174, 178
Triclosan 5
Trigeminal neuralgia 256
Trismus 69, 374, 393
Trismus, grading 393
Trismus, problems 393
Trotter's triad 389
Trousseau's sign 230
Trucut biopsy 263
Ttransplantation, orthotopic 151
Tube drains 304
Tube drains, advantages 305
Tube, infant feeding 307
Tube, Kehr's 'T' 308
Tube, red rubber 306
Tube, Ryle's
Tube, Ryle's, indication 307
Tubercle, Chassaignac 189
Tuberculosis 72
Tuberculosis, pathogenesis 72
Tuberculous dactylitis 163
Tuberculous epididymitis 384
Tuberculous lymphadenitis, stages 245
Tubocurarine 323
Tugging sensation 308
Tumor markers 263
Tumor, carotid body 294
Tumor, dumb bell 294, 350
Tumor, grading 261
Tumor, pancoast 303
Tumor, potato 294

Tumor, staging of 261
Tumor, sternomastoid 296
Tumor, Warthin's 351
Type of neck dissection 301

 U

Ulcer 42
Ulcer, arterial 51
Ulcer, base 339
Ulcer, base 43
Ulcer, Bazin's 44
Ulcer, callous 44
Ulcer, carcinomatous 52
Ulcer, chilblains 55
Ulcer, classification 43
Ulcer, cortisol 45
Ulcer, debridement 47
Ulcer, definition 42
Ulcer, diabetic 48, 49
Ulcer, dressing 47
Ulcer, edge 42, 338
Ulcer, examination 336
Ulcer, floor 43, 338, 339
Ulcer, frost bite 55
Ulcer, gravitational 54
Ulcer, healing 43
Ulcer, ischemic 51
Ulcer, management 47
Ulcer, margin 42, 338
Ulcer, Marjolin's 52, 55, 229, 275, 276
Ulcer, Martorell's 44
Ulcer, melanotic 53
Ulcer, Meleney's 51
Ulcer, mobility 339
Ulcer, neurogenic 48
Ulcer, neuropathic 48
Ulcer, nonhealing 43
Ulcer, parts 42
Ulcer, penetrating 48
Ulcer, perforating 48
Ulcer, rodent 277
Ulcer, rodent 53
Ulcer, spreading 43
Ulcer, syphilitic 44
Ulcer, traumatic 51
Ulcer, treatment 47
Ulcer, trophic 48, 53
Ulcer, tuberculous 55
Ulcer, venous 228
Ulcer, venous 54

Ulnar artery 351
Ulnar bursa 159
Ulnar nerve injuries 253
Ulnar paradox 253
Ultrasound 316
Ultrasound, advantages 316
Ultrasound, A-mode 316
Ultrasound, B-mode 316
Ultrasound, disadvantages 317
Ultrasound, M-mode 316
Ultrasound, therapeutic use 317
Ultrasound, uses 316
Upper limb claudication 176
Upper limb ischemia 175
Upper limb ischemia, bypass surgeries 177
Upper limb ischemia, investigations 176
Upper limb ischemia, management 177
Upper plexus injury 251
Upprt limb edema 332
Urinary bladder injury 173

 V

VACTER anomalies 373
Vaptans 14
Varicose vein surgery, complications of 228
Varicose veins 220
Varicose veins, clinical features 222
Varicose veins, complications of 228
Varicose veins, EVLA 228
Varicose veins, examination of 353
Varicose veins, thermoablation 227
Varicose veins, treatment 225
Varicosities, primary 221
Varicosities, secondary 221
Vascular anomalies 209
Vascular malformations 210
Vascular malformations, capillary 210
Vecuronium bromide 323
Vein, great saphenous 216
Vein, small saphenous 217
Vein, stripping 226
Veins of conduit 216
Veins, pumping 216
Veins, thread 220

Veins, varicose 220
Venography 224
Venography, ascending 224
Venography, descending 224
Venous Doppler 223
Venous emboli 198
Venous refilling time 348
Venous return, factors affecting 217, 218
Venous ulcer 228
Venous ulcers, complications of 229
Venturi phenomenon 179
Verrucous carcinoma , 52, 275
Vicryl 310
Vinca alkaloids 395
Vincent's angina 365
Virchow's triad 218
VNUS closure 227
Vocal nodule 3987
Vocal polyp 397
Volkmann's scoop 309
von Graefe's sign 314
von Recklinghausen's disease 106, 333
von Willebrand's disease 123
von Willebrand's factor 123

W

Waldeyer's ring inner 285
Waldeyer's ring outer 285

Wallace's rule of '9 133
Warfarin sodium 231
Warthin Starry' 240
Warthin's tumor 351
Water excess 11
Water loss 11
Watering can perineum 382
Wayne's diagnostic indices (clinical) of thyrotoxicosis 315
Webspaces, infection 158
Webspaces, surgical anatomy 158
Wen 103
Wharthin's duct 343
Wharton's duct examination 376
White cell trapping theory 221
White leg 219
Wick drain 304
Wilhelm K Rontgen 2
William S Halsted 2
William TG Morton 1
Willis definition of neoplasm 258
Winging of the scapula 256
Woody thyroiditis 327
Woolsorter's disease 80
Wound 28
Wound debridement 34
Wound dehiscence 36
Wound healing 33

Wound healing, phases 34
Wound healing, types 33
Wound infection 36
Wound, classification 28
Wound, clean 30
Wound, clean contaminated 31
Wound, clean incised 29
Wound, contaminated 31
Wound, definition 28
Wound, dirty 31
Wound, lacerated 29
Wound, surgical 30
Wound, tidy 28
Wound, untidy 28
Wounds, clean 93
Wounds, clean-contaminated 93
Wounds, contaminated 93
Wounds, dirty 93
Wounds, management 34
Wrist drop 255
Wry neck 295
Wuchereria Bancrofti 58

X

Xenograft 142
Xeroderma pigmentosa 274

Z

Zadik's operation 164
Zieman's test 385